Microwave
Engineering

Microwave Engineering

V Krishnamurthi BE, MSc (Engg), PhD

Former Professor and Head
Department of Electronics and Communication Engineering
College of Engineering, Anna University
Chennai, India

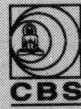

CBS

CBS Publishers & Distributors Pvt Ltd

New Delhi • Bengaluru • Chennai • Kochi • Kolkata • Mumbai
Bhopal • Bhubaneswar • Hyderabad • Jharkhand • Nagpur • Patna • Pune • Uttarakhand • Dhaka (Bangladesh)

Microwave Engineering

ISBN: 978-93-88178-72-3

First Edition: 2019

Published by Satish Kumar Jain and produced by Varun Jain for

CBS Publishers & Distributors Pvt Ltd

4819/XI Prahlad Street, 24 Ansari Road, Daryaganj, New Delhi 110 002, India.
Ph: 23289259, 23266861, 23266867   Fax: 011-23243014   Website: www.cbspd.com
e-mail: delhi@cbspd.com; cbspubs@airtelmail.in

Corporate Office: 204 FIE, Industrial Area, Patparganj, Delhi 110 092
Ph: 4934 4934   Fax: 4934 4935   e-mail: publishing@cbspd.com;   publicity@cbspd.com

Branches

- **Bengaluru:** Seema House, 2975, 17th Cross, K.R. Road,
  Banasankari 2nd Stage, Bengaluru 560 070, Karnataka
  Ph: +91-80-26771678/79   Fax: +91-80-26771680   e-mail: bangalore@cbspd.com
- **Chennai:** 7, Subbaraya Street, Shenoy Nagar, Chennai 600 030, Tamil Nadu
  Ph: +91-44-26680620, 26681266   Fax: +91-44-42032115   e-mail: chennai@cbspd.com
- **Kochi:** 42/1325, 1326, Power House Road, Opposite KSEB Power House,
  Ernakulam 682 018, Kochi, Kerala
  Ph: +91-484-4059061-65   Fax: +91-484-4059065   e-mail: kochi@cbspd.com
- **Kolkata:** 6/B, Ground Floor, Rameswar Shaw Road, Kolkata-700 014, West Bengal
  Ph: +91-33-22891126, 22891127, 22891128   e-mail: kolkata@cbspd.com
- **Mumbai:** 83-C, Dr E Moses Road, Worli, Mumbai-400018, Maharashtra
  Ph: +91-22-24902340/41   Fax: +91-22-24902342   e-mail: mumbai@cbspd.com

Representatives

• Bhopal	0-8319310552	• Bhubaneswar	0-9911037372	• Hyderabad	0-9885175004	• Jharkhand	0-9811541605
• Nagpur	0-9021734563	• Patna	0-9334159340	• Pune	0-9623451994	• Uttarakhand	0-9716462459
• Dhaka (Bangladesh)	01912-003485						

Printed at: Glorious Printers, Daryaganj, New Delhi

Preface

This book on *Microwave Engineering* is the outcome of many years of teaching this course to undergraduate engineering students. The rich experience gained is fully utilized in the preparation of this book. All available books in the market on this course encompass a large spectrum that they are not suitable for the one semester course.

This book is mainly intended for a semester course on BE, BTech, AMIE, AMIETE, HNC and City & Guilds students specializing in ECE/telecommunication engineering and BSc, MTech and MSc (electronics) students. As the syllabi of most of the Indian universities are covered in this book, it is useful as a textbook for students as well as a reference to practising engineers and for self-study.

The fundamental concepts and principles of microwave engineering are explained in a simple, lucid and easy-to-understand language so that the reader is able to follow them without any difficulty. Each chapter deals with a specific topic and includes a large number of illustrations and numerical examples. Chapter-end key points, review and descriptive questions and exercise problems with answers facilitate students to reinforce the concepts and principles easily and will enhance their problem-solving skills.

Chapter 1 introduces the propagation of electromagnetic waves followed by properties and generation of radio waves, modulation and sidebands, transmission, reception, detection and reproduction of radio waves. Further, it presents the classification of microwave frequencies characteristics of microwaves and microwave measurements. It also deals with the important milestones in the development of microwave engineering and applications.

Chapter 2 deals with the characteristics of various transmission line coefficients and their relationships. It then discusses the concept of standing wave and standing wave ratio. Further, it explains the construction, characteristics and utilization of Smith chart.

Chapter 3 encompasses the classification of microwave transmission lines and their characteristics. The planar microwave transmission line structures such as microstrip lines, dielectric strip waveguides, slot lines, shielded strip lines and coplanar strip lines are discussed. Finally, the merits and demerits of planar transmission lines are presented.

Chapter 4 describes various types of waveguides such as rectangular and circular waveguides and special configuration of waveguides such as capacitively loaded rectangular waveguides, ridge waveguides, dielectric loaded waveguides, surface waveguides and dielectric rod waveguides and their characteristics, modes of operation and power handling capacity. Finally, it discusses the advantages of waveguides over coaxial lines and comparison between them.

In **Chapter 5**, the electric two-port network theory is reviewed and the Z, Y, h and $ABCD$ lumped parameters are defined. It has been brought out clearly why these parameters cannot be used to describe the microwave (MW) networks and the concept of scattering matrix is introduced. The scattering parameters or S-parameters of two-port and multi-port MW networks are derived. Properties of S-parameters are discussed in detail and the relationships between S-parameters and Z, Y, and $ABCD$ parameters are derived.

Chapter 6 describes the MW passive components commonly employed in MW communication systems such as waveguide flanges, matched terminations, short-circuit plungers, waveguide corners and windows, tuning screws, adopters, coupling loops, apertures, attenuators and phase shifters. The E-plane and H-plane tees and magic tee are discussed and their S-matrix are derived. The applications of magic tee are explained in detail.

In **Chapter 7**, MW passive devices such as isolators, circulators and directional couplers are described, their S-matrices are derived and the step-by-step design procedure of binomial and Tchebyshev couplers are discussed and illustrated.

In **Chapter 8**, MW resonator parameters and their types such as coaxial cavity resonators, waveguide cavity resonators, Q of cavities and shunt impedance of cavity resonators are detailed.

Chapter 9 deals with classification of MW filters, filter parameters, insertion loss, series and shunt filters elements. Design of prototype filter and transformation of prototype filter design to high-pass, band-pass and band-rejection and MW filter designs are discussed.

Chapter 10 brings out the limitations of conventional vacuum tubes at MW frequencies and describes the constructional details and operating principle of klystron amplifiers. Its characteristic, advantages and applications are numerated.

In **Chapter 11**, the constructional details and operating principle of klystron oscillators are described. The various modes of operation, their characteristics, advantages and applications are explained.

Chapter 12 deals with the constructional details and operating principle of traveling wave tube amplifiers. Their characteristics, advantages and applications are explained and compared with those of klystron amplifiers.

In **Chapter 13**, the construction and mechanism of operation of magnetron oscillators are described. Mode separation, phase focusing and tuning are explained. Hull cut-off magnetic field and voltage are also derived.

Chapter 14 describes the construction and operating principle of crystal and Schottky diodes followed by their applications. PIN devices and their applications as switches, phase shifters, attenuators, modulators and limiters are also explained.

In **Chapter 15**, the Gunn diode, a transferred electron device (TED) is described. Its operating principle, various modes of operation and applications are illustrated in detail.

Chapter 16 describes avalanche transit-time devices (ATTD) and discusses the construction and mechanism of operation and applications.

In **Chapter 17**, the fabrication and operating principle of tunnel diode are described. Its application as amplifier and oscillator is explained in detail. The characteristics of tunnel diodes are compared with those of pn junction diode.

Chapter 18 describes the structure of a varactor diode and its operating principle. Its applications as frequency multiplier and tuner are discussed.

In **Chapter 19**, the operating principle of parametric amplifier is explained and Manley-Rowe power relation is derived. The types of parametric amplifiers and their merits and limitations are discussed.

Chapter 20 discusses the limitations of low frequency transistors at MW frequencies and describes the construction and operation of MW BJTs and FETs.

Chapter 21 discusses the MW communication system, terminal stations, frequency scheme, repeaters, radio horizon, contour maps, Fresnel zone, ground reflections and diversity systems. Finally, MW link design, system gain and advantages of MW communication system are described in detail.

In **Chapter 22**, communication satellites, advantages of geostationery satellite, satellite communication systems, ground station, transponder, link losses and link budget calculations are discussed.

In **Chapter 23**, the classification of radars, radar frequencies and basic radar system are discussed. Radar range equation and maximum range equation are derived. Duplexer, pulsed radar, frequency modulated continuous wave radar and FM Doppler radar are discussed in detail.

Chapter 24 deals with industrial applications of microwaves such as MW heating, domestic MW ovens, MW dryers, plasma generators, measurement of moisture, thickness and medical applications such as diagnostic, therapeutic and monitoring.

In **Chapter 25**, classification of integrated circuits is discussed followed by the scale of integration of circuits and components, advantages and disadvantages of integrated circuits. Further, the monolithic microwave integrated circuits (MMICs) fabrication materials, their properties and substrate material selection are discussed. The properties of conductors, dielectric and resistive materials are explained. Finally, the fabrication methods of MMICs and MOSFETs are discussed.

Chapter 26 deals with the MW measurement devices such as tunable detectors, and slotted line probes. Further, the voltage standing wave ratio (VSWR) meter is explained. The spectrum and network analyzers and their applications are discussed. The principle of operation of power sensors and their applications are described.

In **Chapter 27**, the measurement of low, medium and high MW power, insertion loss, VSWR, impedance, frequency, Q of a cavity, dielectric constant, antenna parameters and noise factors are discussed in detail.

Chapter 28 describes the features of MW radiation and its biological effects and safe levels and protection.

In **Chapter 29**, the characteristics such as efficiency, gain, directivity, effective area of aperture, radiation pattern, beam width and polarization are described. Then the classification of MW antennas and various types of MW antennas such as half-wave dipole antenna, horn antenna, reflector antenna, lens antenna, slot antenna, microstrip antenna and semiconductor antenna and their characteristics are explained.

V Krishnamurthi

Contents

1

Introduction to Microwaves

Objectives

- Understand the propagation, properties and classification of radio waves.
- Learn the method of generation, modulation, transmission and reception of radio waves.
- Understand the electromagnetic spectrum and microwave bands.
- Obtain an idea of the development and applications of microwaves.

1.1 INTRODUCTION

Every electrical circuit carrying alternating current radiates a certain amount of electrical energy in the form of electromagnetic waves. But the amount of energy thus radiated is extremely small since the dimensions of the circuit are much less when compared to its wavelength. Thus, for a power line, carrying 50 Hz current with 6 m spacing between the conductors, will radiate practically no energy because the wavelength at 50 Hz is 6 million meters and 6 m is negligible in comparison to this. On the other hand, a coil of 6 m diameter carrying a 3 MHz current will radiate a considerable amount of energy because 6 m is comparable with 100 m wavelength of the radiated wave. It is thus apparent that the size of the radiator required is *inversely proportional* to the frequency. Therefore, low frequency waves require a large antenna system for effective radiation whereas a small size radiator can radiate high frequency waves.

Every radiator has directional characteristics. Hence, it radiates stronger power in certain directions than others. Directional characteristics of antennas are utilized to concentrate the radiation towards the desired direction or to favour the reception of energy from a particular direction. This property is the basis for *microwave* (MW) *communication*.

1.2 PROPAGATION OF ELECTROMAGNETIC WAVES

The electrical energy that has been radiated into free space exists in the form of electromagnetic (EM) waves. These waves are known as *radio waves*. They travel with the velocity of light. They consist of magnetic and electric fields that are perpendicular to each other and also at right angles to the direction of travel or *propagation*. If these fields could actually be seen, the wave would appear as indicated in Fig. 1.1. One half of the electrical energy contained in the wave is in the form of *electric energy* and the other half is in the form of *magnetic energy*.

1.3 PROPERTIES OF RADIO WAVES

The important properties of radio waves are *frequency, intensity, direction of propagation* and *plane of polarization.* The radio waves will vary in intensity with the frequency of the current and will therefore be alternately *positive* and *negative* as shown in Fig. 1.1(b). The distance occupied by one complete cycle of the wave is called *wavelength* λ and is equal to the velocity of the wave or light divided by the frequency f. The relationship between the velocity c in meters/sec, wavelength λ in meters and the frequency f in Hz is given by

$$\lambda = c/f = 300 \times 10^6/f \qquad (1.1)$$

It can be seen from Eq. (1.1), that a low frequency wave has a long wavelength while a high frequency wave has a short wavelength.

The strength of a radio wave is measured in terms of the voltage stress produced in space by the electric field. It is usually expressed in $\mu V/m$. It is also exactly the same voltage induced in a conductor 1 m long by the magnetic field sweeping across the conductor with the velocity of light. The minimum field strength required for satisfactory reception of a radio wave depends upon a number of factors such as frequency, type of signal involved and the amount of interference present. Under certain conditions, radio waves with signal strength as low as $0.1\ \mu V/m$ are adequate. Occasionally, signal strengths exceeding $1000\ \mu V/m$ are required to ensure satisfactory reception at all times. In most cases, the useful signal strength lies between these two extremes.

A plane parallel to the mutually perpendicular lines of the electric and magnetic flux is called the *wave front*. The wave always travels in a direction perpendicular to the wave front. But whether it is forward or backward direction depends on the relative direction of the lines of electric and magnetic flux. If the direction of either the magnetic flux or the electric flux is reversed, the direction of travel is reversed. However, reversing both the sets of flux has no effect. The direction of electric lines of flux is called the direction of *polarization* of the wave. If the electric flux lines are vertical as shown in Fig. 1.1, the wave is vertically polarized. If the electric flux lines are horizontal and the electromagnetic flux lines are vertical, then it is horizontally polarized.

As radio waves travel away from their point of origin, they get attenuated due to (i) spreading of the waves, (ii) absorption by the ground or ionosphere, and (iii) reflection or refraction by ionosphere or lower atmosphere or ground. The resulting situation is quite complex and differs greatly depending on the frequency of radio waves. Table 1.1 summarizes the bahaviour of different classes of radio waves.

Example 1.1: Find the range of wavelength for very low frequency range 10 kHz to 30 kHz.

Solution: From Eq. (1.1), the wavelength is given by

$$\lambda = c/f = 300 \times 10^6/f\ m$$

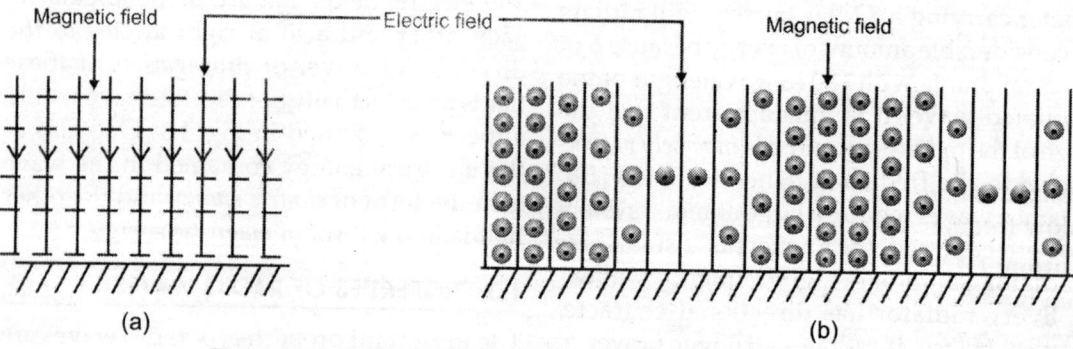

Fig. 1.1: Vertically polarized wave (a) Front view (b) Side view

Table 1.1: Classification of radio waves

Class	Frequency range	Wavelength range	Propagation characteristics	Typical uses
Very low frequency (VLF)	10 kHz–30 kHz	30,000 m – 10,000 m	Low attenuation; very reliable	Long distance point-to-point communication
Low frequency (LF)	30 kHz–300 kHz	10,000 m – 1,000 m	Night propagation same as VLF; day time absorption greater; less reliable	Long distance point-to-point comunication, marine communication navigational aids
Medium frequency (MF)	300 kHz–3 MHz	1,000 m – 100 m	Low night and high day attenuation	Broadcasting; marine navigational aids
High frequency (HF)	3 MHz–30 MHz	100 m – 10 m	Ionosphere propagation; varies with time of the day, season and frequency	All types of moderate to long distance communication
Very high frequency	30 MHz–300 MHz	10 m – 1 m	Line of sight propagation; not affected by ionosphere	Short distance communication, TV, FM, radar, aircraft navigation
Ultra-high frequency (UHF)	300 MHz–3 GHz	100 cm – 10 cm	Same as above	Short distance communication, TV, FM, radar, aircraft navigation, radio relay system
Super-high frequency (SHF)	3 GHz–30 GHz	10 cm – 1 cm	Same as above	Radar, navigation, radio relay systems
Extra-high frequency (EHF)	30 GHz–300 GHz	1 cm – 1 mm	Same as above	Radar, navigation, radio relay systems

For $\quad f_1 = 10,000$ Hz,
$\quad \lambda_1 = 300 \times 10^6/10,000 = \mathbf{30,000}$ **m**

For $\quad f_2 = 30,000$ Hz,
$\quad \lambda_2 = 300 \times 10^6/30,000 = \mathbf{10,000}$ **m**

Example 1.2: Find the range of wavelength for low frequency range 30 kHz to 300 kHz.

Solution: From Eq. (1.1), the wavelength is given by

$$\lambda = c/f = 300 \times 10^6/f \text{ m}$$

For $\quad f_1 = 30,000$ Hz

$\lambda_1 = 300 \times 10^6/30,000$
$\quad = \mathbf{10,000}$ **m**

For $\quad f_2 = 300,000$ Hz,
$\lambda_2 = 300 \times 10^6/300,000$
$\quad = \mathbf{1000}$ **m**

Example 1.3: Find the range of wavelength for medium frequency range 300 kHz to 3 MHz.

Solution: From Eq. (1.1), the wavelength is given by

$$\lambda = c/f = 300 \times 10^6/f \text{ m}$$

For $f_1 = 300,000$ Hz,
    $\lambda_1 = 300 \times 10^6/300,000$
    $= \mathbf{1000}$ **m**
For $f_2 = 3 \times 10^6$ Hz,
    $\lambda_2 = 300 \times 10^6/3 \times 10^6$
    $= \mathbf{100}$ **m**

Example 1.4: Find the range of wavelength for high frequency range 3 MHz to 30 MHz.

Solution: From Eq. (1.1), the wavelength is given by

$$\lambda = c/f = 300 \times 10^6/f \ \text{m}$$

For $f_1 = 3 \times 10^6$ Hz,
    $\lambda_1 = 300 \times 10^6/3 \times 10^6$
    $= \mathbf{100}$ **m**
For $f_2 = 30 \times 10^6$ Hz,
    $\lambda_2 = 300 \times 10^6/30 \times 10^6$
    $= \mathbf{10}$ **m**

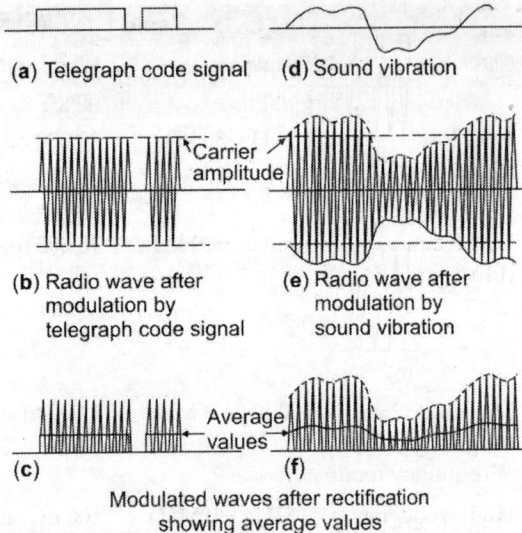

(a) Telegraph code signal   (d) Sound vibration

(b) Radio wave after modulation by telegraph code signal

(e) Radio wave after modulation by sound vibration

(c)   (f)

Modulated waves after rectification showing average values

Fig. 1.2: (a) Telegraph code signal (b) Modulated wave (c) Detected wave of (b) with average value (d) Acoustic wave (e) Modulated wave and (f) Detected wave of (e) with average value

1.4 GENERATION OF RADIO WAVES

The radio frequency power required by a transmitter is always obtained from vacuum tube or solid-state oscillators. These devices convert dc power into RF power. At frequencies over 1 GHz, the power generated is of the order of kilowatts.

1.5 MODULATION

If an RF wave is to convey a message, some features of the wave must be varied in accordance with the information or message to be transmitted. The process of performing this is called *modulation*. There are two important and common types of modulation: *amplitude modulation* and *frequency modulation*. In amplitude modulation, the amplitude of the high frequency carrier wave is varied in accordance with the instantaneous value of the message wave. For example, in radiotelegraphy, the RF transmitter is turned ON and OFF in accordance with the telegraph code as illustrated in Figs 1.2 (a) and (b). In radiotelephony, the RF signal amplitude is varied in accordance with the strength

of the sound wave being transmitted as shown in Figs. 1.2 (d) and (e). Figures 1.2 (c) and (f) show the waves after detection along with the average values that are similar to the telegraph and sound signals. Similarly, in picture transmission, the RF signal amplitude is varied in accordance with the light intensity of the part of the picture that is being transmitted at that instant. In the frequency modulation, the RF signal frequency is varied in accordance with the instantaneous value of the message signal. The frequency modulation is widely used in high frequency communication systems. Figure 1.3 shows the amplitude and frequency modulated waves by a single frequency sine wave for the purpose of comparison.

1.6 NATURE OF MODULATED WAVE

A modulated wave is a mixer of several waves of different frequencies superimposed upon each other. The actual nature of the modulated wave can be studied by analyzing its equation mathematically. Thus, with a sine wave amplitude modulation as in

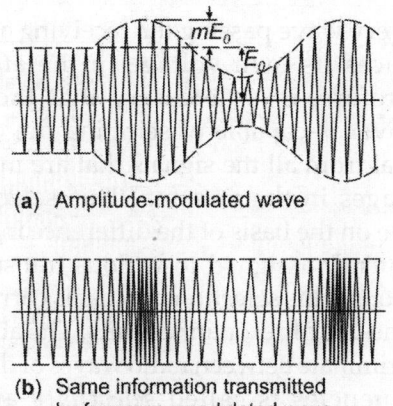

(a) Amplitude-modulated wave

(b) Same information transmitted
by frequency-modulated wave

Fig. 1.3: (a) Amplitude-modulated wave (b) Frequency-modulated wave

Fig. 1.3 (a), the amplitude of RF oscillation is given by $V = V_c + mV_c \sin 2\pi f_s t$. V_c represents the amplitude of the carrier wave, f_s is the signal or message frequency and m is the *degree of modulation* or *modulation index*. Hence, the amplitude-modulated wave can be mathematically represented by

$$v = V_c(1 + m \sin 2\pi f_s t) \sin 2\pi f_c t \qquad (1.2)$$

where f_c is the carrier frequency. Eq. (1.2) may be written as

$$v = V_c \sin 2\pi f_c t + m \sin 2\pi f_s t \sin 2\pi f_c t \qquad (1.3)$$

By expanding the last term in Eq. (1.2), we get

$$v = V_c \sin 2\pi f_c t + (mV_c/2) \cos 2\pi (f_c - f_s)t$$
$$- (mV_c/2) \cos 2\pi (f_c + f_s)t \qquad (1.4)$$

Thus, the amplitude-modulated (AM) wave consists of *three separate waves*. One of them is the carrier wave. Its amplitude is independent of the presence or absence of modulation. The magnitude of the other two components are the same but their frequencies differ, one of them is less than the carrier frequency by the signal or message or *modulating* frequency and the other one is more than the carrier frequency by the signal or message or *modulation* frequency. These two frequencies are called *sideband frequencies*. The lower frequency band is called *lower*

sideband and the higher frequency band is called *upper sideband* frequencies. Both the sidebands carry the message or intelligence that is being transmitted. The frequency of the sideband components relative to the carrier frequency is determined by the modulation frequency. The relative amplitudes of the sideband components is determined by the amplitude of the modulation signal, or in other words, on the modulation index.

When the modulation signal is more complex than a simple sine wave, it results in the occurrence of additional sideband frequencies. Thus, if the modulation signal has a frequency band of 300 Hz to 3,500 Hz and the carrier frequency is 1000 kHz, then the modulated wave will contain two sidebands, the lower sideband will be from 996.5 kHz to 999.7 kHz, and the upper sideband will be from 1000.3 kHz to 1003.5 kHz.

The analysis of the frequency-modulated (FM) wave is more complex. However, the result is analogous to amplitude modulation. The principal difference is that the frequency-modulated wave contains not only the same sideband frequencies as that of amplitude-modulated wave but also contains higher order sidebands. For example, if the modulation signal has a frequency of 1000 Hz and the carrier frequency is 1000 kHz, then the modulated wave will not only contain two sidebands of 999 kHz and 1001 kHz but also contain 998 kHz and 1002 kHz sidebands and possibly 997 kHz to 1003 kHz sidebands. The amplitudes of the various sidebands will depend on the extent and the rate of frequency variation.

1.7 SIGNIFICANCE OF SIDEBANDS

The carrier and sideband frequencies are present in the modulated wave and can be separated from each other by suitable filters. The sideband frequencies are generated as a result of modulation. Their magnitude and frequency are dependent upon the type of the modulation. Thus, it is seen that the transmission of message requires the use of a band of frequencies rather than a single frequency. The frequency components involved in standard broadcasting of speech and quality music are from 100 Hz to 5000 Hz. When modulated, the total bandwidth required is 10 kHz. Hence, each transmitting station would have been assigned a carrier frequency with a bandwidth of 5 kHz on either side of the carrier frequency. If this entire band of frequencies is not fully received due to attenuation in propagation paths, then the quality of reception will be poor.

1.8 TRANSMISSION OF RADIO SIGNALS

The modulated wave is further amplified and its power is boosted to the required level. Then, it is radiated into the space by means of transmitting antenna. In this way, a number of broadcasting stations will be transmitting the electromagnetic waves into the space. Each broadcasting station has been assigned a specific carrier frequency and a bandwidth of 10 kHz. Signals will be simultaneously available in the space from all these stations. The desired station program is selected at the receiver end by means of tuning.

1.9 RECEPTION OF RADIO SIGNALS

To receive radio signals, it is first necessary to abstract energy from the radio waves passing the receiving point. Any antenna capable of radiating electrical energy is also able to absorb energy from the passing radio waves. This is because the electromagnetic flux of the wave cuts across the antenna and induces in the antenna a voltage that varies in time in exactly the same way as the current flowing in the transmitting antenna. The induced voltage and the associated current produced represent the radio frequency energy absorbed from the passing wave.

Every wave passing the receiving antenna induces its own voltage in the antenna. Therefore, it is necessary that the radio receiver is capable of selecting the desired signal from all the signals that are inducing voltages in the antenna. This selection is made on the basis of the difference in carrier frequency assigned to various transmitting stations. This selection process is carried out by the use of resonant circuits. The ability to discriminate between radio waves of different frequencies is called *selectivity* and the process of adjusting circuits to resonance with the frequency of the desired signal is known as *tuning*.

Radio signals at the receiving antennae will be very weak as the broadcasting stations are thousands of kilometers away from the receiving point. For satisfactory reproduction, the received signal needs to be amplified further. If the amplification takes place before detection, it is radio-frequency amplification and if the amplification takes place after detection, it is audio-frequency amplification. The amplification of the signals is necessary for the satisfactory reception of signals from waves that are otherwise too weak to produce audible response. This amplification can be obtained by using vacuum tubes or transistors.

1.10 DETECTION OF RADIO SIGNALS

The process by which the transmitted message or intelligence is retrieved from the modulated wave is called *demodulation* or *detection* and the circuit is known as *detector* or *demodulator*. With amplitude-modulated waves, the detection is accomplished by rectifying the wave to produce a current that varies in accordance with the modulation of the received wave. Thus, when the modulated wave shown in Fig. 1.2(e) is rectified, the resulting current has an average value that varies in accordance with the instantaneous value of the original signal as shown in Fig. 1.2(f). In the case of telegraph codes, rectified current reproduces the dots and dashes of the telegraph code as shown in Fig. 1.2(c) and can be used to operate a telegraph sounder.

The detection of a frequency-modulated wave is accomplished by passing the wave through a circuit in which the relative response depends on the frequency. This circuit is known as a *frequency discriminator*. The average value of the output of the discriminator varies in accordance with the instantaneous value of the original signal.

Example 1.5: A carrier frequency of 1.5 MHz is amplitude modulated by a low frequency signal of 1 kHz. Find the sideband frequencies.

Solution: $f_c = 1500$ kHz; $f_m = 1$ kHz.

Lower sideband (LSB) frequency is given by

$$LSB = f_c - f_m = 1,500 - 1 = 1499 \text{ kHz}.$$

Upper sideband (USB) frequency is given by

$$USB = f_c + f_m = 1,500 + 1 = 1501 \text{ kHz}.$$

Example 1.6: A carrier frequency of 1.5 MHz is amplitude modulated by a low frequency signal of frequencies 500 Hz to 3 kHz. Find the sideband frequencies.

Solution: $f_c = 1500$ kHz;

$$f_{m_1} = 0.5 \text{ kHz and } f_{m_2} = 3 \text{ kHz}$$

Lower sideband (LSB) frequencies are given by

$$LSB_1 = f_c - f_{m_1}$$
$$= 1,500 - 0.5 = 1499.5 \text{ kHz}.$$
$$LSB_2 = f_c - f_{m_2}$$
$$= 1,500 - 3 = 1497 \text{ kHz}.$$

Thus, LSB = 1497 kHz to 1499.5 kHz.

Upper sideband (USB) frequencies are given by

$$USB_1 = f_c + f_{m_1}$$
$$= 1,500 + 0.5 = 1500.5 \text{ kHz}.$$
$$USB_1 = f_c + f_{m_1}$$
$$= 1,500 + 3 = 1503 \text{ kHz}$$

Thus, USB = **1500.5 kHz to 1503 kHz.**

Example 1.7: If the carrier power and modulation index of amplitude modulated wave are 10 kW and 0.6 kW respectively, find the power in each sideband.

Solution: The power in each sideband is given by

$$P_{sb} = (m^2/4)\, P_c$$
$$m = 0.6, P_c = 10 \text{ kW}$$
$$P_{sb} = (0.6^2/4) \times 10 \text{ kW} = \mathbf{0.9 \text{ kW}}$$

1.11 REPRODUCTION OF RADIO SIGNALS

The detected waves are audio frequency waves. They are still weak signals. Hence they are further amplified by a series of voltage amplifiers and finally by a power amplifier. The output of the power amplifier is fed to a loudspeaker. The loudspeaker converts the varying audio frequency current in its coil into acoustic waves or into an audible response that is almost same as the original message or information.

1.12 MICROWAVE FREQUENCIES

The term *microwave* is used to describe electromagnetic (EM) waves with wavelengths ranging from 30 cm to 3 mm. The microwave (MW) frequency range is from 1 GHz (10^9 Hz) to 100 GHz (10^{11} Hz). Electromagnetic waves with wavelengths ranging from 1 mm to 10 mm are known as millimeter waves. The free space is characterized by the following electrical medium parameters: (i) Permittivity $\varepsilon_0 = 8.854 \times 10^{-12}$ F/m, (ii) Conductivity $\sigma_0 = 10^{-14}$ mho/m and (iii) Permeability $\mu_0 = 4\pi \times 10^{-7}$ H/m. Figure 1.4 shows the electromagnetic frequency spectrum. Because of short wavelengths, microwaves are not reflected by the ionosphere. During World War II, there was tremendous development in the field of microwaves for defense purposes.

Different classification schemes are used to designate MW frequency bands. Table 1.2 shows the new and old US military MW bands and IEEE MW frequency bands and their designations.[1]

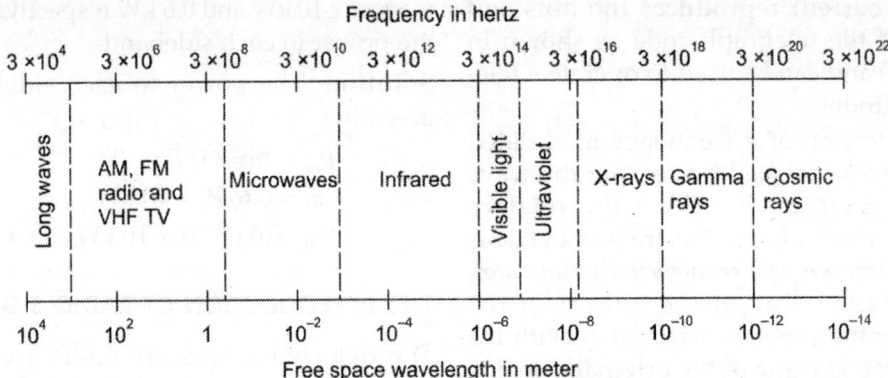

Fig. 1.4: The electromagnetic spectrum

1.13 CHARACTERISTICS OF MICROWAVES

There are three important characteristics that differentiate MW engineering from low and optical frequencies. They are:

(i) The size of most of the MW components is comparable with wavelengths at MW frequencies.

(ii) Currents at MW frequencies tend to flow along the surface of conductors. This increases dramatically the resistive effect. Therefore, special techniques are required to minimize the circuit losses at MW frequencies. Hence, silver-plating and polishing of metallic surfaces of certain MW components are essential.

(iii) At MW frequencies, voltages and currents are uniquely defined and hence cannot be measured directly as in the case of low-frequency circuits.

1.14 MICROWAVE DEVICES

Conventional lines will radiate considerable amount of power because of their comparable lengths with the wavelengths of the microwaves. This results in losses in micro-

Table 1.2: Classification of MW frequencies

US Military MW bands				IEEE MW band	
New bands	*Frequency range (GHz)*	*Old bands*	*Frequency range (GHZ)*	*Band*	*Frequency range (GHZ)*
A band	0.10–0.25	P band	0.225–0.390	HF band	0.003–0.030
B band	0.25–0.50	L band	0.390–1.550	VHF band	0.030–0.300
C band	0.50–1.00	S band	1.550–3.900	UHF band	0.300–1.000
D band	1.00–2.00	C band	3.900–6.200	L band	1.000–2.000
E band	2.00–3.00	X band	6.200–10.900	S band	2.000–4.000
F band	3.00–4.00	K band	10.900–36.00	C band	4.000–8.000
G band	4.00–6.00	Q band	36.00–46.00	X band	8.000–12.000
H band	6.00–8.00	V band	46.00–56.00	Ku band	12.000–18.000
I band	8.00–10.00	W band	56.00–100.00	K band	18.000–27.000
J band	10.00–20.00			Ka band	27.000–40.000
K band	20.00–40.00			Millimeter	40.000–300.000
L band	40.00–60.00			Submillimeter	> 300.000
M band	60.00–100.00				

wave energy. Therefore special active and passive devices are required for the generation and transmission of signals at microwave frequencies. The microwaves can be generated using vacuum tubes such as reflex klystron, magnetrons and backward wave oscillators or solid-state devices such as Gunn diodes, tunnel diodes and varactor diodes. They are amplified using multi-cavity klystron and traveling wave tube amplifiers or solid-state amplifiers such as parametric amplifiers and metal-semiconductor field effect transistors (MESFETs).

Microwaves are transmitted through coaxial lines, waveguides, strip lines, micro-strip lines and other devices such as attenuators, phase shifters, circulators, isolators and directional couplers. All these devices will be described in the text.

1.15 MICROWAVE SYSTEMS

A microwave system normally consists of a transmitting subsystem and a receiver subsystem. The transmitting system includes a microwave source or oscillator, wave-guides and a transmitting antenna. The receiver system includes a receiving antenna, transmission lines or waveguide, a microwave amplifier and a receiver. A typical microwave system is shown in Fig. 1.5.

1.16 MICROWAVE UNITS

Different units are used in microwave measurements. Of these, the meter-kilogram-

Table 1.3: MKS units		
Quantity	*Unit*	*Symbol*
Resistance	Ohm	Ω
Conductance	Mho	℧
Inductance	Henry	H
Capacitance	Farad	F
Voltage	Volt	V
Current	Ampere	A
Power	Watt	W
Charge	Coulomb	Q
Field	Volt/meter	E
Flux linkage	Weber	ψ
Frequency	Hertz	Hz
Length	Meter	m
Time	Second	s
Velocity	Meter/Second	v

second units (the International System of Units) are used internationally. We shall follow this system throughout. Table 1.3 shows the most commonly used MKS units.

1.17 HISTORICAL BACKGROUND

In this section, we shall deal with the important milestones in the development of MW engineering.[2,3,4]

1845: Michael Faraday studied the effect of magnetic field on the propagation of light through glass. He established the existence of relationship between electromagnetic waves and light. He speculated that light might have wave like characters.

1865: James Clerk Maxwell published a paper "A dynamical theory of the electromagnetic

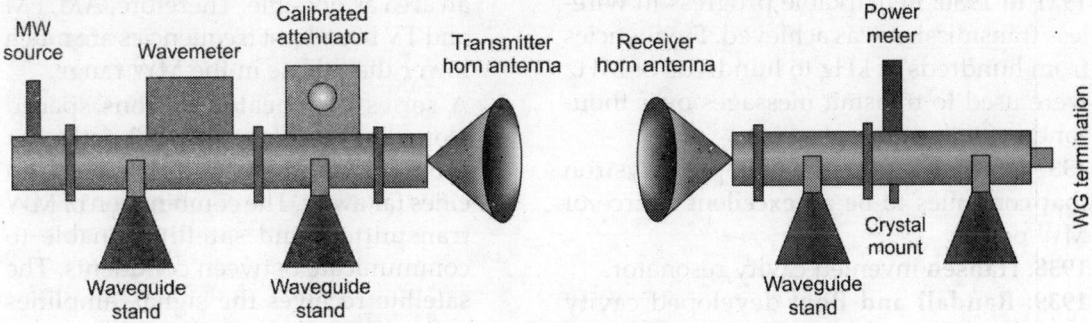

Fig. 1.5: A typical microwave system

field". He developed four basic equations known as Maxwell's equations and demonstrated that the electromagnetic fields travel at the speed of light.

1888: Heinrich Hertz generated 30 MHz signal and validated the Maxwell's theory. Established the relationship $f \lambda_0 = c$, where λ_0 is the free space wavelength and c is the velocity of light (3×10^8 m/s.).

1893: Heinrich Hertz demonstrated that parabolic reflectors concentrate the EM energy, thus improving the efficiency of transmission. Parabolic reflectors are used even today as efficient MW antennas.

1895: Guglielmo Marconi transmitted radio signals over 1 mile; thus demonstrating the first practical application of EM waves in the field of communication. The transmission distance was increased to 4 miles by using parabolic reflectors with an operating frequency of 1.2 GHz.

1897: Lord Rayleigh theoretically proved that EM waves could propagate through hollow metal tubes (waveguides).

1897: Oliver Lodge demonstrated EM wave propagation in waveguides at 1.5 and 4 GHz.

1901: Guglielmo Marconi transmitted successfully the first transatlantic wireless message from England to Newfoundland at a distance of 3,000 miles.

1919: Barkhausen and Kurz developed positive grid MW oscillators.

1921: Hull developed smooth bore Magnetron for MW signal generation.

1921 to 1930: Remarkable progress in wireless transmission was achieved. Frequencies from hundreds of kHz to hundreds of MHz were used to transmit messages over thousands of miles through space.

1937: Varian Brothers developed Klystron that continues to be an excellent source of MW power.

1938: Hansen invented cavity resonator.

1939: Randall and Boot developed cavity magnetrons to produce 400 W of power at 3 GHz.

1944: R Kompfner developed helix-type traveling wave tube.

1957: L Esaki developed tunnel diode.

1958: WT Reed developed IMPATT-type oscillators.

1963: JB Gunn developed Gunn-effect diodes.

1965: MW transistors were developed.

1966: Mead proposed **metal semiconductor FET**

1969: Middlebrook realized MESFET (metal-oxide semiconductor field effect transistor).

With the development of MW repeater stations and satellite communication, microwave technology has been recognized as a major field for commercial and military purposes.

1.18 MICROWAVE APPLICATIONS

Two of the earliest MW uses are for point-to-point communication and radars. Some of the most important uses of MW are discussed below:

(i) **Point-to-point communication:** For point-to-point communication, it is important that the transmitted signal is sharply focused and aimed at the receiving antenna. Since these abilities can easily be achieved at MW frequencies, they are ideally suited for point-to-point communication. The function of the radio and TV broadcasting is to *broadcast* the radio signals over as *broad* an area as possible. Therefore, AM, FM and TV broadcast frequencies are much lower than those in the MW range.

A series of repeater stations spaced along the line of sight (LOS) paths can provide a communication link between cities far away. The combination of MW transmitters and satellites enable to communicate between continents. The satellite receives the signal, amplifies and retransmits it to a large area. Since atmospheric noise is low in the frequency band 3 to 6 GHz, most satellite communication systems operate within this frequency band.

Communication theory states that the amount of information that can be transmitted is directly proportional to the available bandwidth. The MW spectrum contains a wide band of frequencies. This is advantageous for use in transmitting information. It can therefore accommodate many more communication channels than the conventional radio and TV frequencies.

(ii) **Radar systems:** Another major application of microwaves is radar systems. They are used to detect enemy aircrafts and guide missiles, to control flight traffic at airports and to observe and track weather patterns. Radars are also used in garage-door openers, burglar alarms and vehicle speed detectors. MW is extremely useful in radar systems because it can be sharply focused. For instance, an airport-radar must be able to detect separate planes in the traffic pattern. Hence, the radar beam must be sufficiently narrow so that the received signal is reflected from one aircraft only and not from any other in the vicinity of 15°. This necessitates the use of a very narrow beam and therefore MW frequencies are used. Sharply focused MW beams from an aircraft are also used to map the terrain of a large area.

(iii) **Commercial and industrial applications:** MW ovens are typical examples of commercial and industrial applications. In MW ovens, the entire volume of food is heated directly and uniformly. As a result, the cooking time is reduced. Heating property of microwaves is also used in drying potato chips, grains, paper, coffee beans etc. Microwaves are used to measure precisely the thickness of metal sheets in rolling mills and also to determine moisture content in substances. Because

MW penetrates the ionosphere, they are used in radio astronomy and for communication with space vehicles.

1.19 ADDITIONAL EXAMPLES

Example 1.8: Find the wavelength of the MW signal at 1 GHz.

Solution: From Eq. (1.1), the wavelength is given by
$$\lambda = c/f = 300 \times 10^6/f \text{ m}$$
$$f = 10^9 \text{ Hz}$$
$$\lambda = 300 \times 10^6/10^9 = 0.3 \text{ m} = \textbf{30 cm}.$$

Example 1.9: Find the range of wavelength of the X-band MW signal (8 to 12 GHz).

Solution: From Eq. (1.1), the wavelength is given by
$$\lambda = c/f = 300 \times 10^6/f \text{ m}$$
$$f_1 = 8 \times 10^9; \ f_2 = 12 \times 10^9$$
$$\lambda_1 = 300 \times 10^6/8 \times 10^9 = 0.0375 \text{ m}$$
$$= \textbf{3.75 cm}$$
$$\lambda_2 = 300 \times 10^6/12 \times 10^9 = 0.0275 \text{ m}$$
$$= \textbf{2.75 cm}$$

Range of wavelength is from 2.75 cm to 3.75 cm.

Example 1.10: Find the wavelength of the MW signal at 300 GHz.

Solution: From Eq. (1.1), the wavelength is given by
$$\lambda = c/f = 300 \times 10^6/f \text{ m}$$
$$f = 300 \times 10^9 \text{ Hz}$$
$$\lambda = 300 \times 10^6/300 \times 10^9 = 0.001 \text{ m}$$
$$= \textbf{1 mm}.$$

Example 1.11: The carrier frequency in amplitude modulation is 2 MHz and the modulation frequency is 1 kHz. Find the sideband frequencies.

Solution: Given: $f_c = 2000$ kHz; $f_m = 1$ KHz. The sideband frequencies are given by
$$f_{\text{sideband}} = f_c \pm f_m = 2000 \pm 1$$
$$= \textbf{1999} \text{ and } \textbf{2001} \text{ kHz}.$$

Example 1.12: If the 2 MHz carrier-frequency is modulated by a band of frequencies from 1 kHz to 4 kHz, find the sideband frequencies.

Solutions: Given:

$$f_c = 2000 \text{ kHz}; \ f_m = 1 \text{ to } 4 \text{ kHz}$$

$$f_{\text{sideband}} = f_c \pm f_m = 2000 \pm (1 \text{ to } 4)$$

The lower sideband is given by

$$\text{LSB} = 2000 - (1 \text{ to } 4)$$

$$= \mathbf{1996} \text{ to } \mathbf{1999} \text{ kHz}$$

The upper sideband is given by

$$\text{USB} = 2000 + (1 \text{ to } 4)$$

$$= \mathbf{2001} \text{ to } \mathbf{2004} \text{ kHz}$$

Example 1.13: The amplitude of the carrier is two times that of modulation signal, find the modulation index and amplitude of each sideband.

Solution: Given: $V_c / V_m = 2$

The modulation index is given by

$$m = V_m / \text{amplitude of each sideband}$$

$$= 1/2 = \mathbf{0.5}$$

The amplitude of each sideband is given by

$$V_{\text{sideband}} = (m/2)V_c = \mathbf{0.25} V_c$$

Example 1.14: If the modulation index $m = 0.4$, find the power in each sideband.

Solution: Given: $m = 0.4$

The power in each sideband is given by

$$P_{\text{sideband}} = (m^2/4) \, P_c = \mathbf{0.04} \, P_c$$

Example 1.15: The sideband frequencies of a transmitting station is 10.005 and 9.995 MHz. What is its carrier frequency?

Solution: The sideband frequencies are given by

$$\text{LSB} = f_c - f_m = \mathbf{9.995} \text{ MHz}$$

$$\text{USB} = f_c + f_m = \mathbf{10.005} \text{ MHz}$$

$$\text{LSB} + \text{USB} = 2f_c = 20 \text{ MHz}.$$

$$\therefore \qquad f_c = 10 \text{ MHz}.$$

KEY POINTS

- A small size radiator can radiate considerable energy at high frequencies. The wavelength of the radio waves (RF) is short and comparable with the dimensions of the RF components.

- Every radiator radiates stronger power in certain directions than others.

- RF waves are radiated into free space in the form of electromagnetic (EM) waves at the velocity of light.

- Important properties of radio waves: frequency, intensity, direction of propagation and plane of polarization.

- $\lambda = \lambda c / f$; λ is in meters, $c = 300 \times 10^6$ and f is in Hz.

- The strength of a radio wave is measured in mV/m.

- Wave front is a plane parallel to the mutually perpendicular lines of the electric and electromagnetic flux.

- The direction of wave polarization is the direction of electric lines of flux.

- The radio frequency power is generated using vacuum tube or solid-state oscillators.

- The process of varying a feature of a carrier wave is called modulation.

- In amplitude modulation, the amplitude of the high frequency carrier wave is varied in accordance with the instantaneous value of the message wave and its frequency remains constant.

- The amplitude-modulated wave consists of the carrier wave and two sidebands. The magnitudes of the two sidebands are the same but the frequencies differ. Both the sidebands carry the message or intelligence. The process by which the transmitted message or intelligence is retrieved from the modulated wave is called demodulation or detection.

- In the frequency modulation, the RF signal frequency is varied in accordance with the instantaneous value of the message signal and its amplitude remains constant.

- The detection of a frequency-modulated wave is accomplished by passing the wave through a circuit in which the relative response depends on the frequency. This circuit is known as frequency discriminator.

- Loudspeakers convert the varying audio frequency current in its coil into acoustic waves.

- Microwaves are electromagnetic (EM) waves with wavelengths ranging from 30 cm to 3 mm. The microwave (MW) frequency range is from 1 GHz (10^9 Hz) to 100 GHz (10^{11} Hz).
- An antenna radiates electrical energy and also absorbs energy from the passing radio waves.

FURTHER READINGS

1. Altman JL (1962). *Microwave Circuits*, New Jersey, Van Nostrand.
2. Atwater HA (1962). *Introduction to Microwave Theory*, New York: McGraw Hill.
3. Collin, RE (1966). *Foundations of Microwave Engineering*, New York: McGraw Hill.
4. Historical Perspectives of Microwave Engineering – Special centennial issue, *IEEE Trans*. Vol. MTT – 32, Sept., 1984.
5. Gandhi OP (1981). *Microwave Engineering*, New York: McGraw Hill.
6. Pozar DM (1990), *Microwave Engineering*, Addison-Wesley, Mass.

REVIEW QUESTIONS

1.1 Why does an electrical transmission line not radiate considerable amount of energy?

1.2 At higher frequencies, considerable energy is radiated. Explain.

1.3 What is meant by directional characteristic?

1.4 What are the components of radio waves? What is their velocity of propagation?

1.5 Mention the important properties of a radio wave.

1.6 Write down the relationship between wave length and the frequency.

1.7 In what units the strength of a radio wave is measured.

1.8 What is a wave front?

1.9 What is meant by polarization?

1.10 Define modulation.

1.11 Mention the two common types of modulation.

1.12 Define amplitude modulation.

1.13 Define modulation index.

1.14 Define frequency modulation.

1.15 How many sidebands are present in amplitude modulation?

1.16 How many sidebands are present in frequency modulation?

1.17 Name the circuits used for detection.

1.18 What are microwaves?

1.19 Mention the MW bands with their frequency range.

1.20 Mention the different classification of frequency spectrum.

1.21 What is the important property of MW used in communication?

1.22 What is the important property of MW used in radar systems?

1.23 What is the important property of MW used in MW oven?

1.24 Mention four uses of MW in domestic and industrial applications.

DESCRIPTIVE QUESTIONS

1.1 Explain briefly the propagation of radio waves.

1.2 Describe the process of modulation.

1.3 Describe the process of detection.

1.4 Explain the nature of the modulated wave and the significance of sidebands.

1.5 Draw the electromagnetic frequency spectrum and indicate the relevant details.

1.6 Explain the classification of radio waves with their frequency range, wavelength range, characteristics and uses.

1.7 Give the classification of microwaves and their most important properties.

1.8 Explain the applications of microwaves in (i) point-to-point communication, (ii) radar systems and (iii) commercial applications.

PRACTICE PROBLEMS

1.1 Find the range of wavelength for very high frequency range 30 MHz to 300 MHz. (**Ans:** 1 m to 10 m)

1.2 Find the range of wavelength for ultra-high frequency range 300 MHz to 3 GHz. (**Ans:** 10 cm to 1 m)

1.3 Find the range of wavelength for super-high frequency range 3 GHz to 30 GHz. (**Ans:** 1 cm to 10 cm)

1.4 Find the range of wavelength for extra-high frequency range 30 GHz to 300 GHz. (**Ans:** 1 cm to 1 mm)

1.5 The carrier frequency in amplitude modulation is 1 MHz and the modulation frequency is 1 kHz. Find the sideband frequencies. (**Ans:** 999 and 1001 kHz)

1.6 If the 1 MHz carrier frequency is modulated by a band of frequencies from 500 Hz to 4 kHz, find the sideband frequencies.
(**Ans:** 996 to 999.5 kHz and 1000.5 to 1004 kHz)

1.7 The amplitude of the carrier is four times that of modulating signal, find the modulation index and amplitude of each sideband.
(**Ans:** 0.25 , 0.125 V_c)

1.8 If the modulation index $m = 0.6$, find the power in each sideband.
(**Ans:** 0.09 P_c)

1.9 A transmission line having a solid dielectric reduces the phase velocity to 2×10^8 m/s from its free space value. Find the wavelength of a 500 MHz sine wave on the line.
(**Ans:** 40 cm)

1.10 A 500 MHz sine wave is propagated over a matched transmission line that has air dielectric. The phase velocity in the air is 3×10^8 m/s. Find the wavelength of the signal on the line.
(**Ans:** 60 cm)

REFERENCES

1. Terman FE (1955). *Electronic and Radio Engineering*, New York, McGraw Hill Intl. Ed.

2. Liao SY (2003). *Microwave Devices and Circuits*, Pearson, India.

3. Das A and Das SK (2004). *Microwave Engineering*, TMH, New Delhi.

4. Historical Perspectives of Microwave Engineering – Special centennial issue, IEEE Trans. Vol. MTT – 32, Sept. 1984.

Transmission Line Theory and Impedance Matching

Objectives

- Understand the transmission line characteristics and derive the relevant equations.
- Define the transmission line coefficients and derive the relationship.
- Develop the concept of standing waves and define standing wave ratio.
- Construct the Smith chart and use it for solving transmission line problems.
- Know the conditions of impedance matching.
- Understand the design of single and double stub-matching
- Study the broadband matching techniques.
- Describe various methods of matching device.

2.1 INTRODUCTION

In conventional circuit theory, all circuit elements such as resistance, conductance, inductance and capacitance are lumped constants. This is not true at high frequencies. At high frequencies, these circuit elements are distributed along the length of the line. Thus, the microwave transmission lines are analyzed in terms of voltage, current and impedance by distributed circuit theory.

Transmission lines find several uses in radio works. They are employed

(i) to transmit electromagnetic energy,
(ii) as resonant circuits at very high frequencies,
(iii) as measuring devices at high frequencies,
(iv) as aids to obtain impedance matching.

The transmission line theory forms the basis for the study of microwave transmission lines.

2.2 TRANSMISSION LINE EQUATIONS WITH SINUSOIDAL EXCITATION

In this section, we will analyze the microwave transmission lines with sinusoidal excitation by distributed-circuit theory in terms of voltage, current and impedance. A transmission line with distributed circuit elements having a resistance R, a conductance G, an inductance L and a capacitance C per unit length is shown in Fig. 2.1. All these parameters are per unit length of the line.

Consider a very short length dz of the transmission line. In this short distance, the series line resistance is $R\,dz$ and the inductance is $L\,dz$, shunt conductance is $G\,dz$ and capacitance is $C\,dz$, as shown in Fig. 2.1. The voltage across the wires decreases an amount dV due to the voltage drop produced by the line current I flowing through $R\,dz$ and $L\,dz$. Similarly, the current decreases a small

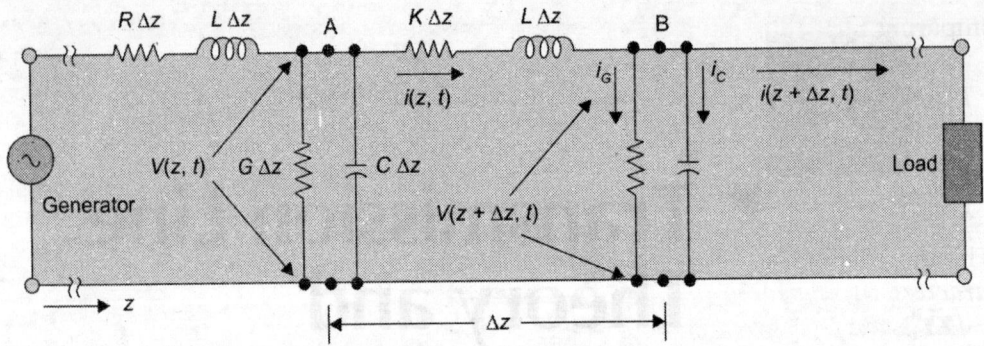

Fig. 2.1: Short section of a transmission line

amount dI in the short length of the line as a result of current flow through $G\,dz$ and $C\,dz$. Therefore, the transmission line equations may be written as

$$dV/dz = -I \times \text{impedance of length } dz$$
$$= -I\,(R + j\omega L)\,dz = -ZI \qquad (2.1a)$$

$$dI/dz = -V \times \text{admittance of length } dz$$
$$= -V\,(G + j\omega C)\,dz = -YV \qquad (2.1b)$$

where

V = voltage across line at distance z from the sending end

I = current in the line at distance z from the sending end

z = distance from the sending end

R = resistance per unit length in ohm

L = inductance per unit length in henry

C = capacitance per unit length in farad

G = conductance per unit length in mho

$Z = (R + j\omega L)$ = series line impedance per unit length in ohm

$Y = (G + j\omega C)$ = shunt admittance per unit length in mho

$\omega = 2\pi f$ = frequency in radian.

Differentiating Eqs (2.1a) and (2.1b) with respect to dz, we get

$$\frac{d^2V}{dz^2} = \frac{-Z\,dI}{dz} = ZYV = \gamma^2 V \qquad (2.2a)$$

$$\frac{d^2I}{dz^2} = \frac{-Y\,dV}{dz} = ZYI = \gamma^2 I \qquad (2.2b)$$

Equations (2.2a) and (2.2b) are the standard differential equations of wave propagation. One possible solution is

$$V = V_s\,e^{-\sqrt{ZY}\cdot Z} + V_r\,e^{\sqrt{ZY}\cdot Z}$$
$$= V_s\,e^{-\gamma z} + V_r\,e^{\gamma z} \qquad (2.3a)$$

$$I = I_s\,e^{-\sqrt{ZY}\cdot Z} + I_r\,e^{\sqrt{ZY}\cdot Z}$$
$$= I_s\,e^{-\gamma z} + I_r\,e^{\gamma z} \qquad (2.3b)$$

Here,

V_s = sending-end voltage amplitude

V_r = receiving-end voltage amplitude

I_s = sending-end current amplitude

I_r = receiving-end current amplitude

$\gamma = \sqrt{ZY}$ = propagation constant.

The first term in the right-hand side of Eq. (2.3a) and (2.3b) represents the incident wave and the other term the reflected wave.

2.3 TRANSMISSION LINE CONSTANTS

The electrical properties of a transmission line are determined by resistance, conductance, inductance and capacitance per unit length of the line, i.e. R, G, L and C. Differentiating Eq. (2.3a), we get

$$\frac{dV}{dz} = -\sqrt{ZY}\,V_s e^{-\sqrt{ZY}\cdot Z} + \sqrt{ZY}\,V_r e^{-\sqrt{ZY}\cdot Z}$$

$$= -ZI \qquad (2.4)$$

$$\text{or, } I = \frac{-\sqrt{ZY}\,V_s\,e^{-\sqrt{ZY}\cdot Z} + \sqrt{ZY}\,V_r\,e^{\sqrt{ZY}\cdot Z}}{(-Z)}$$

$$= \left(\frac{V_s}{\sqrt{Z/Y}}\right)e^{-\sqrt{ZY}\cdot Z} - \left(\frac{V_r}{\sqrt{Z/Y}}\right)e^{\sqrt{ZY}\cdot Z}$$

$$(2.5)$$

Comparing Eq. (2.3b) and (2.5), we obtain

$$I_s = \left(\frac{V_s}{\sqrt{Z/Y}} \right) = \left(\frac{V_s}{Z_0} \right) \quad (2.6a)$$

$$I_r = \left(\frac{V_r}{\sqrt{Z/Y}} \right) = -\frac{V_r}{Z_0} \quad (2.6b)$$

The impedance $Z_0 = \sqrt{Z/Y}$ is called the *characteristic impedance* of the line and $\gamma = \sqrt{ZY}$ is the *propagation constant*. Thus, the electrical properties of the transmission line enter into the line equations through the impedance Z_0 and the propagation constant γ.

2.3.1 Lossy Line

The transmission line with comparable R and G is called *lossy line* as these parameters contribute for losses that occur in the line.

$$Z_0 = \sqrt{\frac{Z}{Y}} = \sqrt{(R + j\omega L)/(G + j\omega C)} \quad (2.7)$$

$$\gamma = \sqrt{ZY} = \sqrt{(R + j\omega L)(G + j\omega C)} \quad (2.8a)$$

$$= \alpha + j\beta \quad (2.8b)$$

where α is the *attenuation constant* and β is the *phase constant*.

The *characteristic impedance* Z_0 is the ratio of the voltage to the current in an individual wave. It is also the impedance of a finite length of line when $Z_L = Z_0$.

The *attenuation constant* α increases with frequency. At high frequencies, the series resistance R and the shunt conductance G are proportional to the square root and the first power of frequency respectively. At low frequencies, in lines with solid dielectric, the line loss is mostly caused by the resistance while at high frequencies, line loss occurs due to shunt conductance.

The *phase constant* β of a high-frequency line is proportional to the frequency and to the square root of the product LC of the line inductance and capacitance but is independent of both resistance and conductance. The use of dielectric insulation in lines, as in the case of coaxial lines, increases the capacitance of the line, and thereby, the phase constant β is increased in proportion to $\sqrt{k}$, where k is the dielectric constant of the insulation. The length of the line βz is called *electrical length* of the line.

The *wavelength* λ of a transmission line is defined as the distance that a wave has to travel along the line in order that the total phase shift to be 2π radians. Hence,

$$\beta\lambda = 2\pi \quad \text{and} \quad \lambda = 2\pi/\beta \quad (2.9)$$

In case of radio frequency lines with air dielectric, λ is approximately equal to the free space wavelength of the wave of the same frequency. In the case of coaxial cables with solid dielectric with a dielectric constant k, the wavelength is very closely equal to the free-space wavelength divided by $\sqrt{k}$.

The *phase velocity* v_p of a transmission line is defined as the product of the wavelength λ and the corresponding frequency f. Thus,

$$\text{phase velocity } v_p = f\lambda = \frac{2\pi f}{\beta} \quad (2.10)$$

The phase velocity approximates very closely the velocity of light in high-frequency lines having air dielectric. In lines with solid dielectric, the phase velocity is equal to the velocity of light divided by $\sqrt{k}$, where k is the dielectric constant of the insulation.

2.3.2 Low-Loss Line

The transmission line with low values of R and G is called *low-loss line* as these parameters contribute negligible losses in the line.[2] The characteristic impedance is given by

$$Z_0 = \sqrt{\frac{(R + j\omega L)}{(G + j\omega C)}}$$

$$= \sqrt{\left(\frac{L}{C}\right)\left[\left(\frac{1 + R}{j\omega L}\right) \Big/ \left(\frac{1 + G}{j\omega C}\right)^{\frac{1}{2}}\right]}$$

$$= \sqrt{\left(\frac{L}{C}\right)\left[\left(\frac{1 + R}{j\omega L}\right)^{\frac{1}{2}}\left(\frac{1 + G}{j\omega C}\right)^{-\frac{1}{2}}\right]}$$

For low-loss lines, $R \ll \omega L$ and $G \ll \omega C$, Z_0 becomes

$$= \sqrt{\left(\frac{L}{C}\right)\left[\left(1 + \frac{\frac{1}{2}R}{j\omega L}\right)\left(1 - \frac{1}{2}\frac{G}{j\omega C}\right)\right]}$$

$$= \sqrt{\left(\frac{L}{C}\right)}\left[\left(1+\frac{1}{2}\frac{R}{j\omega L}-\frac{1}{2}\frac{G}{j\omega C}-\frac{1}{4}\frac{RG}{(j\omega)^2 LC}\right)\right]$$

$$= \sqrt{\left(\frac{L}{C}\right)}\left[\left(1+\frac{1}{2}\frac{R}{j\omega L}-\frac{1}{2}\frac{G}{j\omega C}\right)\right]$$

since RG is very small

$$= \sqrt{\left(\frac{L}{C}\right)}\left[1+\frac{1}{2}\left(\frac{R}{j\omega L}-\frac{G}{j\omega C}\right)\right] \quad (2.11)$$

The propagation constant is given by

$$\gamma = \sqrt{(R+j\omega L)(G+j\omega C)}$$

$$= j\omega\sqrt{LC}\left[\left(1+\frac{R}{j\omega L}\right)\left(1+\frac{G}{j\omega C}\right)\right]^{\frac{1}{2}}$$

Since $R \ll \omega L$ and $G \ll \omega C$, the propagation constant γ reduces to

$$= j\omega\sqrt{LC}\left[\left(1+\frac{\frac{1}{2}R}{j\omega L}\right)\left(1+\frac{\frac{1}{2}G}{j\omega C}\right)\right]$$

$$= j\omega\sqrt{LC}\left[1+\frac{1}{2}\left(\frac{R}{j\omega L}+\frac{G}{j\omega C}\right)\right]$$

$$= \frac{1}{2}\left(R\sqrt{\frac{C}{L}}+G\sqrt{\frac{L}{C}}\right)+j\omega\sqrt{LC}$$

$$= \alpha + j\beta \quad (2.12)$$

Therefore, the attenuation constant α and the phase constant β are given by

$$\alpha = \frac{1}{2}\left(R\sqrt{\frac{C}{L}}+G\sqrt{\frac{L}{C}}\right) \quad (2.13a)$$

$$\beta = \omega\sqrt{LC} \quad (2.13b)$$

The phase velocity is given by

$$v_p = \frac{2\pi f}{\beta} = \frac{1}{\sqrt{LC}} \quad (2.14)$$

The product $LC = 1/\mu\varepsilon$ is independent of the size and separation of the conductors. It depends only on the permeability μ and permittivity ε of the insulating medium.

2.3.3 Lossless Lines

A transmission line is said to be lossless if its resistance R and conductance G are zero. In the case of high frequency lines, $R \ll j\omega L$ and $G \ll j\omega C$. Therefore, the transmission line equations are

$$\frac{dV}{dz} = -j\omega LI \quad (2.15a)$$

$$\frac{dI}{dz} = -j\omega CV \quad (2.15b)$$

$$\frac{d^2V}{dz^2} = -\omega^2 LCV = (j\beta)^2 V \quad (2.16a)$$

$$\frac{d^2I}{dz^2} = -\omega^2 LCI = (j\beta)^2 I \quad (2.16b)$$

The solution of the above equations is:

$$V = V_s\, e^{-j\beta z} + V_r\, e^{j\beta z} \quad (2.17a)$$

$$I = I_s\, e^{-j\beta z} + I_r\, e^{j\beta z} \quad (2.17b)$$

The characteristic impedance is given by

$$Z_0 = \sqrt{\frac{(R+j\omega L)}{(G+j\omega C)}} = \sqrt{\frac{(j\omega L)}{(j\omega C)}}$$

$$= \sqrt{\frac{L}{C}} \quad (2.18)$$

The propagation constant is given by

$$\gamma = \sqrt{(R+j\omega L)(G+j\omega C)}$$

$$= j\omega\sqrt{LC} = \alpha + j\beta \quad (2.19)$$

Therefore, the attenuation and phase constants are given by

$$\alpha = 0 \quad (2.20a)$$

$$\beta = \omega\sqrt{LC} \quad (2.20b)$$

The phase velocity is given by

$$v_p = \frac{\omega}{\beta} = \frac{1}{\sqrt{LC}} \quad (2.21)$$

[Above 2.4]

Example 2.1: The primary constants of a coaxial cable at 50 MHz are $L = 234$ nH/m, $C = 93.5$ pF/m, $R = 0.6$ ohm/m and $G = 0$. Find (a) the attenuation constant, (b) the phase constant and (c) the phase velocity.

Solution: Given: $f = 50$ MHz, $L = 234$ nH/m, $C = 93.5$ pF/m, $R = 0.6$ ohm/m and $G = 0$

$\omega L = 2\pi \times 50 \times 10^6 \times 234 \times 10^{-9} = 73.5$ ohms

Since $\omega L \gg R$ and $G = 0$, from Eq. (2.18),

$$Z_0 = \sqrt{\frac{L}{C}} = \sqrt{234 \times 10^{-9}/93.5 \times 10^{-12}}$$

$$= 50 \text{ ohms}$$

(a) From Eq. (2.13a),

$$\alpha = R \frac{\sqrt{(C/L)}}{2} = \frac{R}{2\sqrt{L/C}}$$

$$= \frac{0.6}{2 \times 50} = 0.006 \; \text{Np/m}.$$

(b) From Eq. (2.13b),

$$\beta = \omega\sqrt{LC}$$
$$= 2\pi \times 50 \times 10^6 \times$$
$$\quad (234 \times 10^{-9} \times 93.5 \times 10^{-12})^{1/2}$$
$$= 100 \, \pi \times 10^6 \times 46.8 \times 10^{-10}$$
$$= 0.468 \, \pi \; \text{rad/m}.$$

(c) From Eq. (2.14),

$$v_p = \frac{1}{\sqrt{LC}} = \frac{1}{(46.8 \times 10^{-10})}$$
$$= 2.14 \times 10^8 \; \text{m/s}.$$

2.4 IMPEDANCE AND ADMITTANCE EQUATIONS

Figure 2.2 shows a short length of a transmission line. Along the transmission line, two waves are present: (i) incident wave and (ii) reflected wave. The incident wave travels from the source or generator end towards the load or receiving end whereas the reflected wave travels from the load or receiving end towards source or generator end. Thus, the voltage or current along the transmission line is the sum of the incident and reflected voltages or currents. Thus,

$$V = V_{\text{inc}} + V_{\text{ref}}$$
$$= V_s \, e^{-\gamma z} + V_r \, e^{\gamma z} \qquad (2.22a)$$
$$I = I_{\text{inc}} + I_{\text{ref}}$$
$$= I_s \, e^{-\gamma z} - I_r \, e^{\gamma z}$$
$$= (V_s \, e^{-\gamma z} - V_r \, e^{\gamma z})/Z_0 \qquad (2.22b)$$

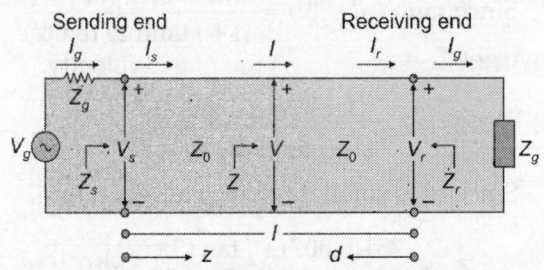

Fig. 2.2: A transmission line of length *l*

2.4.1 Line Impedance

The line impedance of a transmission line is defined as the ratio of the voltage at any point to the current at that point. Thus,

$$Z = \frac{V}{I} \qquad (2.23)$$

As z = 0 at the sending end, from Eqs (2.22a) and (2.22b), we obtain

$$I_s Z_s = V_s + V_r \qquad (2.24a)$$
$$I_s Z_0 = V_s - V_r \qquad (2.24b)$$

Adding Eqs (2.24a) and (2.24b) and re-arranging, we get

$$V_s = I_s \frac{(Z_s - Z_0)}{2} \qquad (2.25a)$$

Subtracting Eq. (2.24b) from Eq. (2.24a) and rearranging, we have

$$V_r = I_s \frac{(Z_s - Z_0)}{2} \qquad (2.25b)$$

Substituting these values in Eqs (2.22a) and (2.22b), we obtain

$$V = \left(\frac{I_s}{2}\right)\left[(Z_s + Z_0)e^{-\gamma z} + (Z_s - Z_0)e^{\gamma z}\right] \qquad (2.26a)$$

$$I = \left(\frac{I_s}{2Z_0}\right)\left[(Z_s + Z_0)e^{-\gamma z} - (Z_s - Z_0)e^{\gamma z}\right] \qquad (2.26b)$$

2.4.2 Z from Sourced End

At any point z from the sending or generator end, the line impedance Z may be expressed in terms of Z_s and Z_0. From, Eq. (2.26a) and (2.26b), it is given as

$$Z = \frac{V}{I}$$

$$= Z_0 \frac{(Z_s + Z_0)e^{-\gamma z} + (Z_s - Z_0)e^{\gamma z}}{(Z_s + Z_0)e^{-\gamma z} - (Z_s - Z_0)e^{\gamma z}} \qquad (2.27)$$

Using the relation $e^{\pm \gamma z} = \cosh(\gamma z) \pm \sinh(\gamma z)$, the line impedance Z may be expressed in hyperbolic functions. Thus,

$$Z = Z_0 \frac{Z_s \cosh \gamma z - Z_0 \sinh \gamma z}{Z_0 \cosh \gamma z - Z_s \sinh \gamma z} \qquad (2.28)$$

2.4.3 Z from Load End

At the receiving or load end, $z = l$ and the line impedance at the receiving end in terms of Z_s and Z_0 is given by

$$Z = Z_0 \frac{(Z_s + Z_0)e^{-\gamma l} + (Z_s - Z_0)e^{\gamma l}}{(Z_s + Z_0)e^{-\gamma l} - (Z_s + Z_0)e^{\gamma l}} \quad (2.29)$$

This equation in hyperbolic function is given by

$$Z = Z_0 \frac{Z_s \cosh \gamma l - Z_0 \sinh \gamma l}{Z_0 \cosh \gamma l - Z_s \sinh \gamma l} \quad (2.30)$$

2.4.4 Z in terms of Z_l and Z_0

Sometimes, it is necessary to express the line impedance in terms of Z_l and Z_0. At the load end, $z = l$. Hence, the voltage at the load end is $V_l = I_l Z_l$. Then,

$$I_l Z_l = V_s e^{-\gamma l} + V_r e^{\gamma l} \quad (2.31a)$$
$$I_l Z_0 = V_s e^{-\gamma l} - V_r e^{\gamma l} \quad (2.31b)$$

From these equations we get

$$V_s = \left(\frac{I_l}{2}\right)(Z_l + Z_0)e^{\gamma l} \quad (2.32a)$$

$$V_r = \left(\frac{I_l}{2}\right)(Z_l - Z_0)e^{-\gamma l} \quad (2.32b)$$

Substituting Eqs (2.32a) and (2.32b) in Eqs (2.22a) and (2.22b) and letting $z = l - d$, we get

$$V = \left(\frac{I_l}{2}\right)\left[(Z_l + Z_0)e^{\gamma d} + (Z_l - Z_0)e^{-\gamma d}\right] \quad (2.33a)$$

$$I = \left(\frac{I_l}{2Z_0}\right)\left[(Z_l + Z_0)e^{\gamma d} - (Z_l - Z_0)e^{-\gamma d}\right] \quad (2.33b)$$

At any point from the receiving or load end, the impedance Z in terms of Z_l and Z_0 is given by

$$Z = Z_0 \frac{(Z_l + Z_0)e^{\gamma d} + (Z_l - Z_0)e^{-\gamma d}}{(Z_l + Z_0)e^{\gamma d} - (Z_l - Z_0)e^{-\gamma d}} \quad (2.34)$$

Using the relation $e^{\pm\gamma d} = \cosh(\gamma d) \pm \sinh(\gamma d)$, the Eq. (2.34) can be expressed as

$$Z = Z_0 \frac{Z_l \cosh \gamma d + Z_0 \sinh \gamma d}{Z_0 \cosh \gamma d + Z_l \sinh \gamma d} \quad (2.35)$$

From Eq. (2.35), the line impedance at the sending or generator end can be found by substituting $d = l$. Thus

$$Z_s = Z_0 \frac{(Z_l + Z_0)e^{\gamma l} + (Z_l + Z_0)e^{-\gamma l}}{(Z_l + Z_0)e^{\gamma l} - (Z_l + Z_0)e^{-\gamma l}} \quad (2.36)$$

Equation (2.36) in hyperbolic functions is given by

$$Z = Z_0 \frac{Z_l \cosh \gamma l + Z_0 \sinh \gamma l}{Z_0 \cosh \gamma l + Z_l \sinh \gamma l} \quad (2.37)$$

Example 2.2: An air-insulated coaxial cable of length 15 cm, $Z_0 = 75$ ohms and $\alpha = 0.4$ dB/m is terminated with a short circuit. Compute the input impedance at 1.5 GHz and 2 GHz.

Solution: Given: $l = 15$ cm, $Z_0 = 75$ ohms. $\alpha = 0.4$ dB/m and $f = 1.5$ and 2 GHz.

For an air-insulated coaxial cable $\lambda = \lambda_0$.

(a) At 1.5 GHz:

$$\lambda_o = 300 \times \frac{10^8}{1.5 \times 10^9} = 20 \text{ cm}$$

$$\beta l = \left(\frac{2\pi}{\lambda}\right) l = \left(\frac{2\pi}{20}\right) \times 15 = \frac{3\pi}{2} \text{ rad}$$

$$\alpha l = 0.4 \times 15 = 0.06 \text{ dB or } \frac{0.06}{0.8686}$$
$$= 0.007 \text{ Np/m}$$

Since $Z_l = 0$, Eq.(2.37) reduces to

$$Z_{in} = Z_0 \left(\frac{Z_0 \sinh \gamma l}{Z_0 \cosh \gamma l}\right)$$
$$= Z_0 \tanh \gamma l$$
$$= Z_0 \tanh (\alpha l + j\beta l)$$

Since $\tanh (\alpha l + j\beta l) = \dfrac{(\tanh \alpha l + j \tan \beta l)}{(1 + j \tanh \alpha l \tan \beta l)}$, we get

$$Z_{in} = Z_0 \frac{(\tanh \alpha l + j \tan \beta l)}{(1 + j \tanh \alpha l \tan \beta l)}$$

Since αl is small, $\tanh \alpha l = \alpha l$. Therefore,

$$Z_{in} = \frac{75\left[(0.007) + j \tan (3\pi/2)\right]}{\left[1 + j \, 00.7 \tan (3\pi/2)\right]}$$

$$= \frac{75\left[\dfrac{0.007}{\tan(3\pi/2)} + j1\right]}{\dfrac{1}{\tan(3\pi/2)} + j\,0.007}$$

As $\tan\left(\dfrac{3\pi}{2}\right) = -\infty$, the input impedance is given by

$$Z_{in} = \frac{j\,75}{j\,0.007} = \mathbf{10{,}714 \text{ ohms.}}$$

(b) At 2 GHz:

$$\lambda_o = 300 \times \frac{10^8}{2} \times 10^9 = 15 \text{ cm}$$

$$\beta l = \left(\frac{2\pi}{\lambda}\right) l = \left(\frac{2\pi}{15}\right) \times 15 = 2\pi \text{ rad.}$$

$$\alpha l = 0.4 \times 15 = 0.06 \text{ dB or } \frac{0.06}{0.8686}$$

$$= 0.007 \text{ Np/m}$$

$$Z_{in} = \frac{75\,[(0.007) + j\tan(2\pi)]}{1 + j\,0.007\tan(2\pi)}$$

$$= 75 \times 0.007 \text{ since } \tan 2\pi = 0$$

$$= \mathbf{0.525 \text{ ohms}}$$

2.4.5 Impedance of a Lossless Line

For a lossless transmission line, $\alpha = 0$, and hence, $\gamma = j\beta$. The characteristic impedance of a lossless line is pure resistance R_o. Therefore, the line impedance from the sending end is given by

$$Z = R_0 \frac{Z_s \cos\beta z - jR_o \sin\beta z}{R_o \cos\beta z - jZ_s \sin\beta z} \qquad (2.38)$$

Equation (2.38) is obtained by using the trigonometric relations,

$\sin h\,(j\beta z) = j\sin\beta z$ and $\cosh(j\beta z) = \cos\beta z$

The line impedance from the receiving or load end is given by,

$$Z = R_o \frac{Z_l \cos\beta d + jR_o \sin\beta d}{R_o \cos\beta d + jZ_l \sin\beta d} \qquad (2.39)$$

2.4.6 Determination of Z_0

The characteristic impedance Z_0 and the propagation constant γ of a transmission line

can be obtained by taking measurements with the *receiving* or load end short-circuited and open-circuited. Thus, when the load end is shorted, $Z_l = 0$ and hence $V_l = 0$. The short-circuited impedance Z_{sc} measured at the sending or generator end is given by substituting $Z_l = 0$ in Eq. (2.37). We then obtain

$$Z_{sc} = Z_0 \frac{Z_0 \sinh\gamma l}{Z_0 \cosh\gamma l} = Z_0\tanh\gamma l \qquad (2.40)$$

Similarly, when the receiving or load end is open-circuited, $Z_l = \infty$ and hence $I_l = 0$. The open-circuited impedance Z_{oc} measured at the sending or generator end is given by substituting $Z_l = \infty$ in Eq. (2.37). We then obtain

$$Z_{oc} = Z_0 \frac{Z_0 \cosh\gamma l}{Z_0 \sinh\gamma l} = Z_0\coth\gamma l \qquad (2.41)$$

Therefore, the characteristic impedance Z_0 can be obtained from Eq. (2.40) and (2.41). Thus,

$$Z_{sc}\cdot Z_{oc} = Z_0\coth\gamma l\cdot Z_0\tanh\gamma l = Z_0^2$$

$$\therefore \qquad Z_0 = \sqrt{Z_{oc}\,Z_{sc}} \qquad (2.42)$$

The propagation constant γ of the line can be obtained from Z_{oc} and Z_{sc}. Thus,

$$\frac{Z_{sc}}{Z_{oc}} = Z_0\tanh\lambda l Z_0\coth\gamma l = \tanh^2\gamma l$$

$$\therefore \qquad \gamma = \left(\frac{1}{l}\right)\tanh^{-1}\sqrt{\frac{Z_{sc}}{Z_{oc}}}$$

$$= \alpha + j\beta \qquad (2.43)$$

2.4.7 Normalized Impedance

The ratio of the line impedance to its characteristic impedance is known as the normalized impedance z of a transmission line. Thus,

$$z = \frac{\text{line impedance}}{\text{characteristic impedance}}$$

$$= \left(\frac{Z}{Z_0}\right) = r \pm jx \qquad (2.44)$$

It is a common practice to use the lower case letters to represent normalized quantities in describing distributed transmission-line circuits.

2.4.8 Line Admittance

The transmission-line equations for the line voltage, current and transmitted power may be solved in terms of the line admittance.

The line admittance Y is the reciprocal of the line impedance Z. Thus,

$$Y = \left(\frac{1}{Z}\right)$$

$$= \frac{(Z_s + Z_0)e^{-\gamma z} - (Z_s - Z_0)e^{\gamma z}}{Z_0(Z_s + Z_0)e^{-\gamma z} + (Z_s - Z_0)e^{\gamma z}} \quad (2.45a)$$

after substituting for Z from Eq. (2.27). Using the relationship $Y_s = 1/Z_s$ and $Y_0 = 1/Z_0$, we get

$$Y = Y_0 \frac{(Y_0 + Y_s)e^{-\gamma z} - (Y_0 - Y_s)e^{\gamma z}}{(Y_0 + Y_s)e^{-\gamma z} + (Y_0 - Y_s)e^{\gamma z}} \quad (2.45b)$$

$$= G \pm jB$$

where the characteristic admittance Y_0 is the reciprocal of the characteristic impedance Z_0. Thus,

$$Y_0 = \left(\frac{1}{Z_0}\right) = G_o \pm jB_o \quad (2.46)$$

The normalized admittance y of a transmission line is defined as the ratio of the line admittance to its characteristic admittance. Thus,

$$y = \frac{Y}{Y_0} = g \pm jb \quad (2.47a)$$

The normalized admittance y of a transmission line is the reciprocal of the normalized impedance z. Thus,

$$y = \frac{1}{z} = \frac{Z_0}{Z} = g \pm jb \quad (2.47b)$$

2.5 REFLECTION COEFFICIENT

The travelling wave along the transmission line consists of the following two components:

i. Incident wave travelling in the positive z-direction from the source towards the receiving or load end.

ii. Reflected wave travelling in the negative z-direction from the load end towards the sending or generator end.

A transmission line terminated in a load impedance Z_l is shown in Fig. 2.3. The incident voltage and current waves are

$$V = V_s e^{-\gamma z} + V_r e^{\gamma z} \quad (2.48a)$$

$$I = I_s e^{-\gamma z} + I_r e^{\gamma z} \quad (2.48b)$$

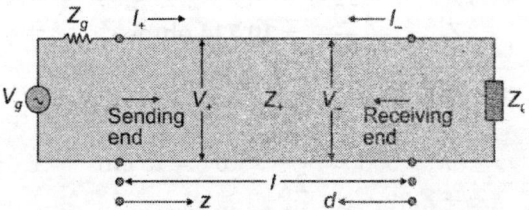

Fig. 2.3: Transmission line with load impedance

Since $I_s = V_s/Z_0$ and $I_r = -V_r/Z_0$, the current wave can be expressed in terms of the voltage as

$$I = (V_s/Z_0)\, e^{-\gamma z} - (V_r/Z_0)\, e^{\gamma z} \quad (2.49)$$

Assuming the length of the line is l, the voltage and current at the receiving or load end is obtained by letting $z = l$ in Eqs (2.48a) and (2.48b). Thus,

$$V_l = V_s e^{-\gamma l} + V_r e^{\gamma l} \quad (2.50a)$$

$$I_l = (V_s e^{-\gamma l} - V_r e^{\gamma l})/Z_0 \quad (2.50b)$$

Z_l, the load impedance, is the ratio of the load voltage to the load current at the receiving end. It is given by

$$Z_l = \frac{V_l}{I_l} = Z_0 \frac{V_s e^{-\gamma l} + V_r e^{\gamma l}}{V_s e^{-\gamma l} - V_r e^{\gamma l}} \quad (2.51)$$

The *reflection coefficient* Γ is defined as the ratio of the reflected voltage or current to the incident voltage or current. Thus,

$$\Gamma = V_{ref}/V_{inc} = -I_{ref}/I_{inc} \quad (2.52)$$

From Eq. (2.51), it can be seen that the reflected voltage at the receiving or load end is $V_r e^{\gamma l}$ and the incident voltage is $V_s e^{-\gamma l}$. Therefore, the load reflection coefficient Γ_l at the *receiving or load end* is given by

$$\Gamma_l = \frac{V_{ref} \text{ at the receiving or load end}}{V_{inc} \text{ at the receiving or load end}}$$

$$= V_r e^{\gamma l}/V_s e^{-\gamma l} \quad (2.53a)$$

From Eq. (2.51), we get

$$Z_l/Z_0 = \frac{V_s e^{-\gamma l} + V_r e^{\gamma l}}{V_s e^{-\gamma l} - V_r e^{\gamma l}} \qquad (2.53b)$$

Subtracting unity from both side and rearranging, we get

$$\left(\frac{Z_l}{Z_0}\right) - 1 = \frac{(V_s e^{-\gamma l} + V_r e^{\gamma l}) - (V_s e^{-\gamma l} - V_r e^{\gamma l})}{V_s e^{-\gamma l} - V_r e^{\gamma l}}$$

$$\frac{(Z_l - Z_0)}{Z_0} = \frac{2 V_r e^{\gamma l}}{(V_s e^{-\gamma l} - V_r e^{\gamma l})} \qquad (2.53c)$$

Similarly, it can be shown that

$$\frac{(Z_l + Z_0)}{Z_0} = \frac{2 V_s e^{-\gamma l}}{V_s e^{-\gamma l} - V_r e^{\gamma l})} \qquad (2.53d)$$

From Eqs (2.53c) and (2.53d), we obtain

$$\Gamma_l = \frac{V_r e^{\gamma l}}{V_s e^{-\gamma l}}$$

$$= \frac{(Z_l - Z_0)}{(Z_l + Z_0)} \qquad (2.53e)$$

Since the load and characteristic impedances are usually complex quantities, the load reflection coefficient is also complex quantity. Thus,

$$\Gamma_l = |\Gamma_l| e^{j\theta_l} = |\Gamma_l| \angle\theta_l \qquad (2.54)$$

From Eq. (2.53e) it can be seen that $|\Gamma_l|$ is always less than or equal to 1. θ_l, the phase angle of the load-reflection coefficient is the phase angle between the incident and reflected voltages at the receiving end. The reflection coefficient at any point z along the transmission line from the generator or sending end is given by

$$\Gamma = \frac{V_r e^{\gamma z}}{V_s e^{-\gamma z}} \qquad (2.55)$$

Then, the reflection coefficient at any point along the transmission line from the receiving or load end is obtained by substituting $z = l - d$ in Eq. (2.55). Thus, the reflection coefficient at any point along the trans-

mission line from the receiving or load end is given by

$$\Gamma_d = \frac{V_r e^{\gamma(l-d)}}{V_s e^{-\gamma(l-d)}}$$

$$= \left(\frac{V_r e^{\gamma l}}{V_s e^{-\gamma l}}\right) e^{-2\gamma d}$$

$$= \Gamma_l e^{-2\gamma d}$$

$$= |\Gamma_l| e^{-2\alpha d} e^{j(\theta_l - 2\beta d)} \qquad (2.56)$$

since $\gamma = \alpha + j\beta$.

The reflection coefficient at any point along the line from the receiving or load end can be determined from Eq. (2.56). Figure 2.4 shows the variation in the magnitude and phase of the reflection coefficient for a lossy line. Both quantities change in an inward-spiral way. Since for a lossless line, the attenuation $\alpha = 0$, the magnitude of the reflection coefficient remains constant. However, the phase angle of the reflection coefficient varies circularly towards the generator or sending end by an angle of $-2\beta d$ and is shown in Fig. 2.5.

From Eq. (2.53), it is evident that

(i) If the load impedance Z_l equals the characteristic impedance Z_0 of the line, then there is no reflection since the total power is delivered to the load. Hence, the reflected wave does not exist. Hence,

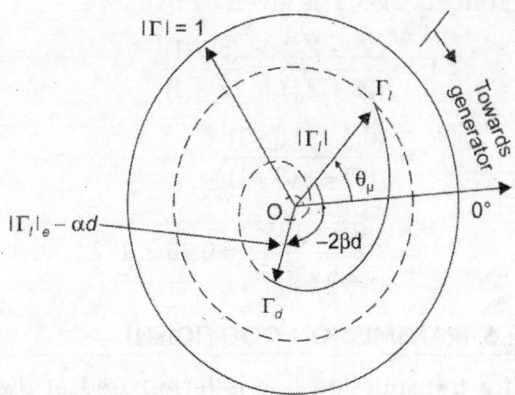

Fig. 2.4: Locus of reflection coefficient of a lossy line

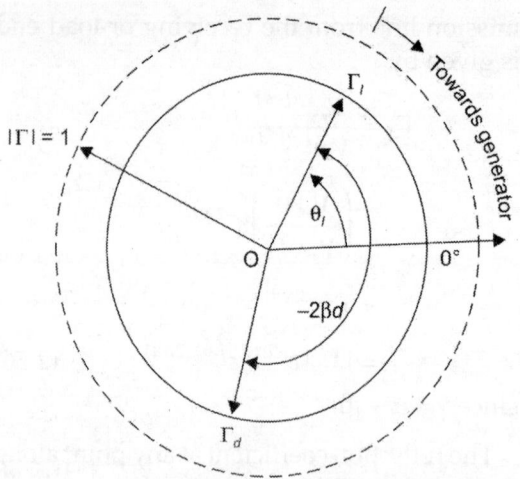

Fig. 2.5: Locus of reflection coefficient of a lossless line

the reflection coefficient is zero and there is no reflection from the load end.

(ii) If the terminating impedance differs from the characteristic impedance, then a reflected wave exists and travels towards the sending or generator end. If the generator impedance is different from the characteristic impedance, it will be reflected back at the generator.

Example 2.3: The normalized impedance of a transmission line is $z_l = 0.5 + j0.5$. Show that the reflection coefficient is given by $0.45 \angle 117°$.

Solution: Given $z_l = 0.5 + j0.5$

From Eq. 2.53, Γ is given by

$$\Gamma = \frac{(Z_l - Z_0)}{(Z_l + Z_0)} = \frac{(z_l - 1)}{(z_l + 1)}$$

$$= \frac{(0.5 + j0.5 - 1)}{(0.5 + j0.5 + 1)}$$

$$= \frac{\sqrt{0.5} \angle 135°}{\sqrt{2.5} \angle 18°} = 0.45 \angle 117°$$

2.6 TRANSMISSION COEFFICIENT

If a transmission line is terminated at the receiving or load end in its characteristic impedance Z_0, the total power is absorbed by the load and it does not reflect any wave from the load end. Such a line is said to be a *matched or properly terminated line*. If the line is not terminated in its characteristic impedance, there exists a reflected wave that travels towards the source. Such a line is said to be a *mismatched or improperly terminated line*. The reflection coefficient Γ is present at all points along the mismatched transmission line.[3]

The *transmission coefficient T* is defined as the ratio of the transmitted voltage or current to the incident voltage or current. Thus,

$$T = \frac{\text{Transmitted voltage or current}}{\text{Incident voltage or current}}$$

$$= \frac{V_{tr}}{V_{inc}} = \frac{I_{tr}}{I_{inc}} \tag{2.57}$$

The incident voltage is V_{inc}, the transmitted voltage is V_{tr}, the incident current is I_{inc} and the transmitted current is I_{tr}.

The transmitted voltage at the receiving or load end is assumed to be

$$V_{tr}e^{-\gamma l} = V_s e^{-\gamma l} + V_r e^{\gamma l} \tag{2.58}$$

$$= V_s e^{-\gamma l} \left(1 + \frac{V_r e^{\gamma l}}{V_s e^{-\gamma l}}\right)$$

or $\quad \dfrac{V_{tr}}{V_s} = \left(1 + \dfrac{V_r e^{\gamma l}}{V_s e^{-\gamma l}}\right)$

From Eq. (2.57), the transmission coefficient T is given by

$$T = \frac{V_{tr}}{V_s} = \left(1 + \frac{V_r e^{\gamma l}}{V_s e^{-\gamma l}}\right) = (1 + |\Gamma_l|) \tag{2.59}$$

Substituting for $|\Gamma_l|$ from Eq. (2.53e), we obtain

$$T = 1 + |\Gamma_l|$$

$$= 1 + \frac{(Z_l - Z_0)}{(Z_l + Z_0)}$$

$$= \frac{2Z_l}{(Z_l + Z_0)} \tag{2.60}$$

2.6.1 Transmitted Power

Let the incident power be P_{inc}, the reflected power be P_{ref} and the transmitted power be P_{tr}. The transmission of power along a transmission line is shown in Fig. 2.6.

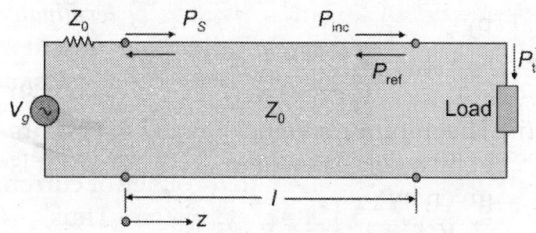

Fig. 2.6: Power transmission along a line

The power transmitted to the load is given by

$$P_{tr} = \text{incident power} - \text{reflected power}$$
$$= P_{inc} - P_{ref} \tag{2.61}$$

or $\quad P_{tr} = (P_{inc} - P_{ref}) = P_{inc}(1 - P_{ref}/P_{inc})$

$$P_{ref} = |V_r|^2/2Z_0, \ P_{inc} = |V_s|^2/2Z_0$$

$$P_{tr}/P_{inc} = 1 - |V_r|^2/|V_s|^2 = 1 - |\Gamma_l|^2 \tag{2.62}$$

Substituting for $|\Gamma_l| = [(Z_l - Z_0)/(Z_l + Z_0)]$ in Eq. (2.62), we get

$$1 - |\Gamma_l|^2 = 1 - [(Z_l - Z_0)/(Z_l + Z_0)]^2$$
$$= [(Z_l + Z_0)^2 - (Z_l - Z_0)^2]/(Z_l + Z_0)]^2$$
$$= 4Z_l Z_0/(Z_l + Z_0)^2$$
$$= (Z_0/Z_l)\,[2Z_l/(Z_l + Z_0)]^2$$
$$= (Z_0/Z_l)\,T^2 \tag{2.63}$$

Therefore, the transmitted power is given by

$$P_{tr} = (1 - |\Gamma_l|^2)\,P_{inc}$$
$$= (Z_0/Z_l)T^2\,P_{inc} \tag{2.64}$$

Example 2.4: An antenna having an impedance of 75 + j50 ohms is fed by a 50 ohms lossless line. Find the reflection coefficient.

Solution: The reflection coefficient is given by
$$\Gamma_l = (Z_l - Z_0)/(Z_l + Z_0)$$
$$= (75 + j50 - 50)/(75 + j50 + 50)$$
$$= (25 + j50)/(125 + j50)$$
$$= (1 + j2)/(5 + j2)$$

$$= 2.236 \angle 63.4°/5.385 \angle 21.8°$$
$$= \mathbf{0.415 \angle 41.6°}$$

Example 2.5: A transmission line with a characteristic impedance of 50 + j1 feeds a load of 50 + j50. Find (i) the reflection coefficient, (ii) the transmission coefficient.

Solution: (i) The reflection coefficient is given by
$$\Gamma_l = (Z_l - Z_0)/(Z_l + Z_0)$$
$$= (50 + j50 - 50 - j1)/(50 + j50 + 50 + j1)$$
$$= j49/(100 + j51)$$
$$= 49 \angle 90°/112.5 \angle 27°$$
$$= \mathbf{0.436 \angle 63°}$$

(ii) The transmission coefficient is given by
$$T = 2Z_l/(Z_l + Z_0)$$
$$= 2(50 + j50)/(50 + j50 + 50 + j1)$$
$$= (1 + j1)/(1 + j0.51)$$
$$= 0.707 \angle 45°/1.1 \angle 27°$$
$$= \mathbf{0.645 \angle 18°}$$

Example 2.6: A transmission line with a characteristic impedance of 50 + j50 feeds a load of 50 − j50. Find (i) the reflection coefficient, (ii) the transmission coefficient. Verify that (iii) $T = 1 + \Gamma_l$ and (iv) $T^2 = (1 - \Gamma_l)^2\,Z_l/Z_0$.

Solution: (i) The reflection coefficient is given by
$$\Gamma_l = (Z_l - Z_0)/(Z_l + Z_0)$$
$$= (50 - j50 - 50 - j50)/(50 - j50 + 50 + j50)$$
$$= -j100/100 = \mathbf{1 \angle -90°}$$

(ii) The transmission coefficient is given by
$$T = 2Z_l/(Z_l + Z_0)$$
$$= 2(50 - j50)/(50 - j50 + 50 + j50)$$
$$= (1 - j1) = \mathbf{\sqrt{2} \angle -45°}$$

(iii) $T = (1 - j1)$
$$= 1 + 1 \angle -90°$$
$$= 1 + \Gamma_l$$

(iv) $T^2 = (\sqrt{2} \angle -45°)^2 = \mathbf{2 \angle -90°}$

$$(1 - \Gamma_l^2)Z_l Z_0 = \frac{\left[1 - (1 \angle -90°)^2\right](50 - j50)}{(50 + j50)}$$

$$= \frac{(1+1)(1-j1)}{(1+j1)}$$

$$= \frac{2 \times \sqrt{2} \angle -45°}{\sqrt{2} < 45°}$$

$$= 2 \angle -45° - 45°$$

$$= 2 \angle -90° = T^2$$

2.7 STANDING WAVE

The two waves propagating along a transmission line are (i) the incident wave travelling from the source towards the load end and reflected waves from the load end towards the source. They, thus, travel in opposite directions with unequal amplitudes. These are given in Eqs (2.2a) and (2.3b).

2.7.1 Voltage Standing Wave Equation

Substitution of $\gamma = \alpha + j\beta$ in Eq. (2.3a), we obtain

$$V = V_s e^{-\alpha z} e^{-j\beta z} + V_r e^{+\alpha z} e^{+j\beta z} \quad (2.65)$$

Using the relationship $e^{\pm j\beta z} = \cos \beta z \pm j \sin \beta z$, we get

$$V = V_s e^{-\alpha z} [\cos \beta z - j \sin \beta z]$$
$$+ V_r e^{\alpha z} [\cos \beta z + j \sin \beta z]$$

Rearranging this equation, we have

$$= [V_s e^{-\alpha z} + V_r e^{\alpha z}] \cos \beta z - j [V_s e^{-\alpha z} - V_r e^{\alpha z}] \sin bz$$

$$= V_0 e^{-j\phi} \quad (2.66)$$

This is known as the *voltage standing wave equation.*

2.7.2 Standing Wave Pattern

The voltage V_0 is given by

$$V_0 = [(V_s e^{-\alpha z} + V_r e^{\alpha z})^2 \cos^2 \beta z$$
$$+ (V_s e^{-\alpha z} - V_r e^{\alpha z})^2 \sin^2 \beta z]^{1/2} \quad (2.67)$$

Equation (2.67) is known as *standing wave pattern* of the voltage wave or *amplitude of the standing wave.*

2.7.3 Standing Wave Phase Pattern

The phase angle ϕ is given by

$$\phi = \tan^{-1} \left(\frac{V_s e^{-\alpha z} - V_r e^{\alpha z}}{V_s e^{-\alpha z} + V_r e^{\alpha z}} \tan \beta z \right) \quad (2.68)$$

This equation is known as *phase pattern of the standing wave.*

The following results can be obtained from Eq. (2.67).

(i) The maximum value of Eq. (2.67) occurs at $\beta z = n\pi$ where $n = 0, \pm 1, \pm 2$. It is given by

$$V_{max} = V_s e^{-\alpha z} + V_r e^{\alpha z}$$
$$= V_s e^{-\alpha z} (1 + |\Gamma_l|) \quad (2.69)$$

(ii) The minimum value of Eq. (2.67) occurs at $\beta z = (2n-1)\pi$ where $n = 0, \pm 1, \pm 2,$. It is given by

$$V_{min} = V_s e^{-\alpha z} - V_r e^{\alpha z}$$
$$= V_s e^{-\alpha z} (1 - |\Gamma_l|) \quad (2.70)$$

(iii) The maxima occur at $\beta z = n\pi$, i.e. $z = n\pi/\beta$ and $\beta = 2\pi/\lambda$. Hence, $z = n\lambda/2$, $n = 0, \pm 1, \pm 2,...$ i.e. at $0, \pm \lambda/2, \pm \lambda,...,$

(iv) The minima occur at $\beta z = (2n-1)\pi/2$, i.e., $z = (2n-1)\pi/2\beta$ and $\beta = 2\pi/\lambda$. Hence, $z = (2n-1)\lambda/4$, $n = 0, \pm 1, \pm 2,...$ i.e. at $\pm \lambda/4$, $\pm 3\lambda/4,...$

Thus, the successive *maxima* or *minima* occur at an interval of $\lambda/2$.

It is evident that the minimum value is not zero.

In a similar way, the maximum and minimum values of current are given by

$$I_{max} = I_s e^{-\alpha z} + I_r e^{\alpha z}$$
$$= I e^{-\alpha z} (1 + |\Gamma_l|) \quad (2.71)$$

$$I_{min} = I_s e^{-\alpha z} - I_r e^{\alpha z}$$
$$= I_s e^{-\alpha z} (1 - |\Gamma_l|) \quad (2.72)$$

Figure 2.7 shows the standing wave pattern of two oppositely travelling waves with unequal amplitude in a lossy line.[4]

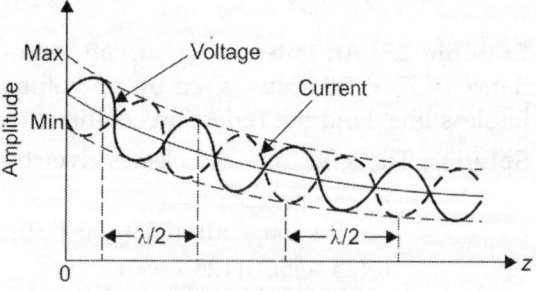

Fig. 2.7: Standing wave pattern in a lossy line

Along the transmission line, the current and voltage waves are 90° out of phase. Hence, the current distribution has minima where the voltage has maxima and *vice versa*. This is because of the fact that the current of the reflected wave has the opposite phase from the reflected voltage. As a result, the currents in the two waves add whenever the voltages subtract and *vice versa*.

The variations in both the voltage and current distributions repeat their general character every half wavelength. This is characteristic of all distributions on transmission lines.

2.7.4 Special Cases

The nature of voltage and current distribution along a transmission line can be understood by considering a number of special cases in detail.[5,6] It is assumed that the attenuation constant α is very small.

2.7.4.1 Open-Circuited Line

When the line is open-circuited, $Z_l = \infty$; hence, $\Gamma_l = 1 \angle 0°$. Therefore, the incident and reflected waves are equal in magnitude and phase. The line voltage is, therefore, their sum and is the maximum at the load. The currents due to these voltages are equal in magnitude but opposite in phase; hence, they cancel and the line current is zero as must be the case for an open-circuited line.

As the waves advance towards the sending end, the phase of the incident wave increases and that of the reflected wave decreases by β radians per unit length of the line. However, the magnitudes do not change as α is very small. At a distance $d = \lambda/8$ from the load, $\beta d = \pi/4$. Hence, the line voltage is the vector sum of the two voltages that are 90° apart and is less than that at the load.

As the waves travel further, the phases change. At $d = \lambda/4$ from the load, $\beta d = \pi/2$ and the two voltages differ by 180°. Hence, the line voltage is their difference and quite small as α is very small. The line voltage will

not be zero since some attenuation is always present. This causes the reflected wave to be smaller than the incident wave.

As d further increases, the phase angles also increases. At $d = \lambda/2$ from the load, $\beta d = \pi$ and the two voltages are in phase and the line voltage is their sum once again. The current distribution has minima where the voltage has maxima and *vice versa*. This cycle repeats itself for every half wavelength. This is illustrated in Fig. 2.8(a).

2.7.4.2 Short-Circuited Line

When the line is short-circuited, $Z_l = 0$; hence $\Gamma_l = 1 \angle 180°$. Therefore, the incident and reflected waves are equal in magnitude but out of phase. The line voltage is their sum and is zero at the load. The currents due to these voltages are equal in magnitude and are in phase; hence, they add up and the line current is the maximum, as must be the case, for a short-circuited line.

At $d = \lambda/4$ from the load, $\beta d = \pi/2$ and the two voltages are in phase. Hence, the line voltage is their sum and is the maximum. However, the currents are out of phase, and hence, minimum but not zero because the reflected current is smaller than the incident current.

As d further increases, the phase angles also increase. At $d = \lambda/2$ from the load, $\beta d = \pi$ and the two voltages are out of phase and the line voltage is minimum once again. However, the currents are in phase, and hence, they add up. The current distribution has minima where the voltage has maxima and *vice versa*. This cycle repeats itself for every half wavelength. This is illustrated in Fig. 2.8(b).

2.7.4.3 Matched Line

When the line is matched, $Z_l = Z_0$; hence $\Gamma_l = 0$. Hence, there is no reflection. The voltage and current distributions are flat or constant as shown in Fig. 2.8(c).

2.7.4.4 *Resistance Terminated Line*

Case 1: *The load impedance is greater than the characteristic impedance* $(Z_l > Z_0)$.

When the line is terminated with a resistance $R_l > Z_0$, the amplitude of the reflected wave at the load is less than that of the incident wave but is in phase as in the open-circuited case. As a result, the voltage and current distributions are similar to those in an open-circuit and the maxima and minima occur at exactly the same places as in the case of an open-circuited load. However, the reflected-wave amplitude is less in this case, and hence, the minima is higher than in an open-circuit as shown in Fig. 2.8(d).

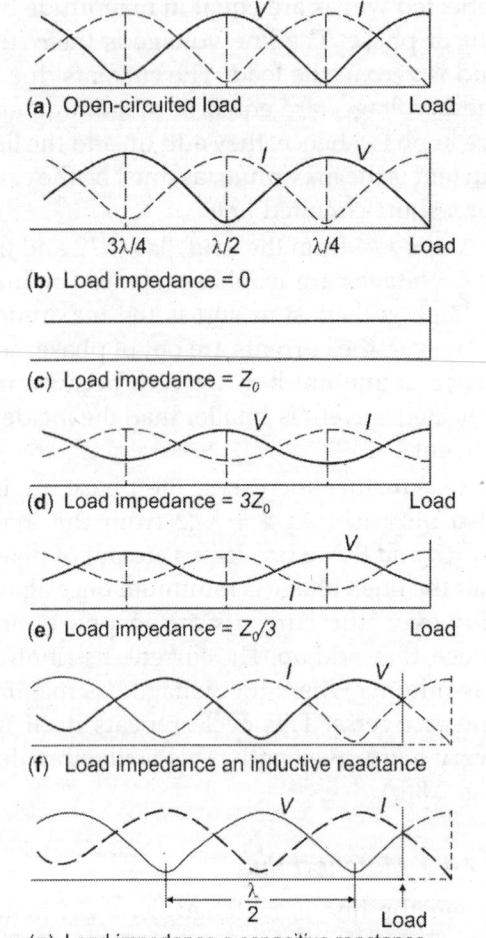

(a) Open-circuited load   Load

$3\lambda/4$ $\lambda/2$ $\lambda/4$ Load

(b) Load impedance = 0

(c) Load impedance = Z_0

(d) Load impedance = $3Z_0$ Load

(e) Load impedance = $Z_0/3$ Load

(f) Load impedance an inductive reactance

$\dfrac{\lambda}{2}$ Load

(g) Load impedance a capacitive reactance

Fig. 2.8: Voltage and current distribution for different loads

Case 2: *The load impedance is less than the characteristic impedance* $(Z_l < Z_0)$

When the line is terminated with a resistance $R_l < Z_0$, the amplitude of the reflected wave at the load is less than that of the incident wave and has the same-phase relation with respect to the incident wave as in the short-circuited case. As a result, the voltage and current distributions are similar to that in the short-circuited case and the maxima and minima occur at exactly the same places as in short-circuited load. However, the reflected-wave amplitude is less in this case, and hence, the maxima is not as large and the minima not as small as in the short-circuited case as shown in Fig. 2.8(e).

2.7.4.5 *Reactance Terminated Line*

Case 1: *Inductive reactance load impedance* $(Z_l = jX_l)$

When the line is terminated with an inductive reactance jX_l and $Z_0 = R_0$, then $G_l = 1 \angle \tan^{-1} X_l / R_0$. As a result, the voltage and current distributions vary in the same way and to the same extent as in an open-circuited or a short-circuited case. However, the reactive impedance causes the minima to be displaced with respect to the minima for open-circuited load as shown in Fig. 2.8(f).

Case 2: *Capacitive reactance load impedance* $(Z_l < -jX_l)$

When the line is terminated with a capacitive reactance $-jX_l$ and $Z_0 = R_0$, then $\Gamma_l = 1 \angle \tan^{-1} (-X_l/R_0)$. As a result, the first minimum in the voltage distribution occurs closer to the load than a quarter wavelength as shown in Fig. 2.8(g). This is because for capacitive loads, the phase angle of the reflection coefficient is negative and the reflected wave lags behind the incident wave at the load. Thus, with a capacitive load, the distance from the load at which the reflected wave lags $180°$ behind the incident wave is less than a quarter wavelength.

2.7.4.6 Lossless Line

The behaviour of an ideal transmission line with zero losses is important because, under practical conditions, it is permissible to neglect the losses at high frequencies. In this case, $\alpha = 0$ and the amplitudes of incident and reflected waves do not change as they travel along the transmission line. The voltage and current distribution are shown in Fig. 2.9(a). As the reflection coefficient is unity, the distributions are half sine waves that become zero at the minima. Figure 2.9(b) shows the voltage and current distributions that indicate the magnitude and phase simultaneously.

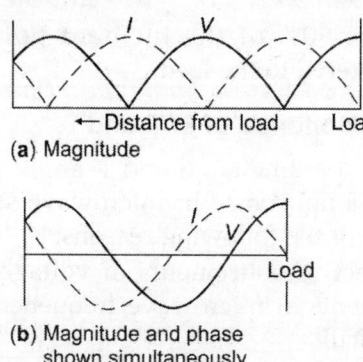

(a) Magnitude

(b) Magnitude and phase shown simultaneously

Fig. 2.9: Voltage and current relations on an open-circuited transmission line

Example 2.7: To design a MW amplifier, an inductance is required to series resonate with a capacitive reactance of 15,000 ohms. If the inductor consists of a short-circuited line with $Z_0 = 75$ ohms, $\alpha = 0.002$ dB/m and $\lambda = 10$ cm, find the length of the line and Z_{in}.

Solution: Given: $X_c = 15{,}000$ ohms, $Z_0 = 75$ ohms, $\alpha = 0.002$ dB/m and $\lambda = 10$ cm.

To series resonate with $-j15{,}000$ ohms, the input impedance of the short-circuited line should be $+j15{,}000$ ohms. Therefore,

$$Z_{in} = j15{,}000 = j75 \tan \beta l$$

Hence, $\quad \beta l = \tan^{-1} 15{,}000/75 = \tan^{-1} 200$

$$= \pi/2 - 1/200$$

$$\therefore \quad l = (\lambda/2\pi)(\pi/2 - 1/200)$$

$$= \lambda/4 \,(1 - 1/100\pi)$$

$$= \lambda/4 \,(1 - 0.003)$$

$$= \mathbf{0.997} \,(\lambda/4)$$

Thus, a short-circuited line of length about 0.3% less than $\lambda/4$ would provide the desired inductive reactance without adding any resistance.

$$\alpha l = 0.002 \times \lambda/4 = 0.002 \times 2.5$$

$$= 0.005 \text{ dB/m} = 5.76 \times 10^{-4} \text{ Np/m}.$$

Since αl is small, $\tanh \alpha l = \alpha l$ and $\tan \beta l = 200$, we have

$$Z_{in} = \frac{Z_0(\tanh \alpha l + j \tan \beta l)}{(1 + j \tanh \alpha l \tan \beta l)}$$

$$= \frac{75(5.76 \times 10^{-4} + j200)}{(1 + j5.76 \times 10^{-4} \times j200)}$$

$$= \mathbf{1700 + j15{,}800 \text{ ohms}}$$

2.8 STANDING WAVE RATIO (SWR)

Along a transmission line, the presence of the standing wave is due to the simultaneous propagation of the incident and reflected waves travelling in opposite directions with unequal amplitude. The standing wave ratio (SWR) S is defined as the ratio of the maximum voltage or current to the minimum voltage or current on the standing wave pattern,[1] as shown in Fig. 2.10. Thus, the standing wave ratio S is given by

$$S = \frac{\text{Maximum voltage or current}}{\text{Minimum voltage or current}}$$

$$= \frac{|V_{max}|}{|V_{min}|} = \frac{|I_{max}|}{|I_{min}|} \qquad (2.73)$$

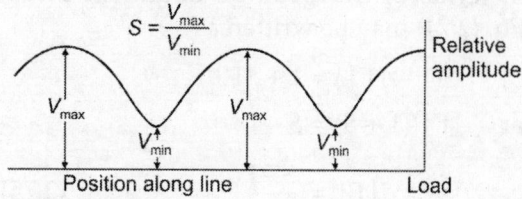

Fig. 2.10: Parameters defining the standing-wave ratio

The standing-wave ratio is also a measure of the amplitude ratio of the reflected to incident waves. The distance between two successive maxima or minima is $\lambda/2$. The standing wave ratio of *unity* denotes the absence of the reflected wave and the transmission line is known as *flat line*. A very high standing-wave ratio indicates that the reflected wave is almost as large as the incident wave. Theoretically, with zero attenuation, the standing wave ratio is *infinity* when the line is either open-circuited or short-circuited or terminated with a lossless reactance. On a lossless line, the standing-wave ratio is constant throughout the transmission line. For a lossy-line, SWR cannot be defined because the standing-wave pattern markedly changes along the transmission line.

2.8.1 SWR and Reflection Coefficient Γ

The standing-wave ratio S is related to the reflection coefficient Γ. The exact relation between the two is derived below.

$$S = V_{max}/V_{min}$$

Substitution of V_{max} and V_{min} from Eqs (2.69) and (2.70) yields

$$S = \frac{V_s e^{-\alpha z}(1+|\Gamma_l|)}{V_s e^{-\alpha z}(1-|\Gamma_l|)}$$

$$= \frac{1+|\Gamma|}{1-|\Gamma|} \qquad (2.74)$$

From Eq. (2.74), the reflection coefficient in terms of SWR can be obtained. Thus, Eq. (2.74) may be written as

$$S(1 - |\Gamma|) = 1 + |\Gamma|$$

or $\quad |\Gamma| (1 + S) = S - 1$

$\therefore \qquad |\Gamma| = \dfrac{S-1}{S+1} \qquad (2.75)$

Example 2.8: A 1.25 GHz propagating along a transmission line has an SWR = 1.94. Find (a) the reflection coefficient (b) the reflected power and (c) the power delivered to the load.

Solution: Given: SWR = 1.94, f = 1.25 GHz.

(a) From Eq. (2.75),

$$|\Gamma| = \frac{(S-1)}{(S+1)} = \frac{(1.94-1)}{(1.94+1)}$$

$$= \frac{0.94}{2.94} = 0.316$$

(b) The reflected power is given by

$$|\Gamma|^2 \, P_{in} = (0.316)^2 \, P_{in} = 0.10 \, P_{in}$$

Thus 10% of the incident power is reflected back.

(c) The power delivered to the load is given by

$$(1 - |\Gamma|^2) \, P_{in} = (1 - 0.1) \, P_{in} = 0.9 P_{in}$$

Thus 90% of the incident power is delivered to the load.

2.8.2 Importance of SWR and Γ

The two parameters S and Γ are of considerable importance in microwave studies because of the following reasons:

(i) Direct measurements of voltages and currents at microwave frequencies are difficult.

(ii) Indirect methods of measuring the above two quantities are easier. The voltages at microwave frequencies can be measured by using a probe connected to a crystal detector. The probe output current is proportional to the voltages at the probe point.

(iii) The probe can easily be moved along the transmission line and the maxima and minima of the voltage or current can be directly measured. Hence, the SWR can be computed from these measurements.

(iv) Since SWR is known, Γ_l can be obtained.

(v) The phase angle of Γ_l can be evaluated from the voltage-minimum location.

(vi) Since Γ_l has been obtained, the normalized impedance z can be calculated from Eq. (2.59) and is given by

$$z = Z_l /Z_0 = (1 + \Gamma_l)/(1 - \Gamma_l),$$

Figure 2.11 shows the relationship between the SWR and Γ_l. Table 2.1 shows the values of standing-wave ratio S and the reflection coefficient Γ for various loads.

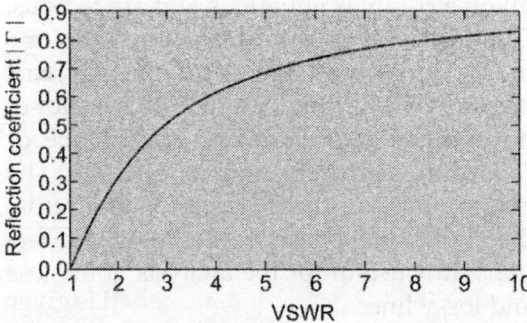

Fig. 2.11: Relationship between the SWR and the reflection coefficient

Table 2.1: Reflection coefficient and SWR		
Load Z_l	*Reflection coefficient Γ*	*SWR*
Z_0	0	1
∞ (open)	$1\angle 0°$	∞
0 (short)	$1\angle 180°$	∞
$+jX$ (inductive)	$\exp[j2\tan^{-1}(X/Z_0)]$	∞
$-jX$ (capacitive)	$\exp[-j2\tan^{-1}(X/Z_0)]$	∞

The importance of the standing-wave ratio arises from the fact that it can be very easily measured experimentally. Further, the standing-wave ratio indicates directly the extent to which reflected waves exist on the line. In addition, standing-wave ratio measurements provide an important means of measuring impedance.

2.8.3 Z_{max}, Z_{min} and Z in Terms of SWR and Γ

When a lossless transmission line is terminated with real characteristic impedance $Z_0 = R_0$, its line impedances at the voltage maximum and minimum points are purely real. The maximum line impedance Z_{max} at voltage maximum or current minimum is given by

$$Z_{max} = V_{max}/I_{min}$$
$$= V_{max}/(V_{min}/Z_0)$$
$$= Z_0(V_{max}/V_{min})$$

$$= Z_0 S = Z_0 \frac{1+|\Gamma|}{1-|\Gamma|} \qquad (2.76a)$$

The maximum normalized impedance z_{max} is given by

$$z_{max} = Z_{max}/Z_0 = S$$
$$= (1+|\Gamma|)/(1-|\Gamma|) \qquad (2.76b)$$

The minimum line impedance Z_{min} at voltage minimum or current maximum is given by

$$Z_{min} = V_{min}/I_{max}$$
$$= V_{min}/(V_{max}/Z_0)$$
$$= Z_0(V_{min}/V_{max})$$

$$= Z_0/S = Z_0 \frac{1-|\Gamma|}{1+|\Gamma|} \qquad (2.77a)$$

The minimum normalized impedance z_{min} is given by

$$z_{min} = Z_{min}/Z_0 = 1/S$$
$$= (1-|\Gamma|)/(1+|\Gamma|) \qquad (2.77b)$$

Example 2.9: The reflection coefficient of a transmission line is $0.4\angle-45°$. Find the SWR.

Solution: The SWR S is given by
$$S = (1+|\Gamma|)/(1-|\Gamma|)$$
$$= (1+0.4)/(1-0.4)$$
$$= 1.4/0.6 = \textbf{2.33}$$

Example 2.10: The SWR of a transmission line is 1.5. Find the reflection coefficient.

Solution: The reflection coefficient is given by
$$|\Gamma| = (S-1)/(S+1)$$
$$= (1.5-1)/(1.5+1)$$
$$= 0.5/2.5 = \textbf{0.2}$$

Example 2.11: Find the impedances at voltage maximum and minimum points if $S = 1.2$ and $Z_0 = 50$ ohms.

Solution: The impedance at voltage maximum is given by
$$Z_{max} = S Z_0$$
$$= 1.2 \times 50 = \textbf{60 ohms}$$

The impedance at voltage minimum is given by

$$Z_{min} = S/Z_0$$
$$= 1.2/50 = \mathbf{0.024} \text{ ohms}$$

Example 2.12: A 600 MHz generator with $V_g = 10$ V and $Z_g = 0$ is connected to a load of $150 + j90$ ohms by means of an air-insulated coaxial cable with $Z_0 = 75$ ohms and $l = 15$ cm. (i) Assuming $\alpha = 0$, find Γ_l, Γ_{in} and SWR. (ii) Calculate V_{max} on the line. (iii) If $\alpha = 2.0$ dB/m, and $l = \lambda$, determine $|\Gamma_{in}|$.

Solution: Given: $f = 600$ MHz, $V_g = 10$ V, $Z_g = 0$, $Z_l = 150 + j90$ ohms, $Z_0 = 75$ ohms and $l = 15$ cm

(i) $\Gamma_l = (Z_l - Z_0)/(Z_l + Z_0)$
$$= (150 + j90 - 75)/(150 + j90 + 75)$$
$$= (75 + j90)/(225 + j90)$$
$$= (1 + j1.2)/(3 + j1.2)$$
$$= 1.56 \angle 50.2/3.23 \angle 21.8$$
$$= \mathbf{0.48} \angle \mathbf{28.4^\circ}$$

At 600 MHz, $\lambda_0 = 50$ cm $= \lambda$ since it is an air-insulated line.

$\beta l = (2\pi/\lambda)l = (2\pi/50)15 = 0.6\pi$ rad. or 108°

Since $\alpha = 0$,

$\Gamma_{in} = \Gamma_l \angle -2\beta l = 0.48 \angle (28.4^\circ - 2 \times 108^\circ)$
$$= \mathbf{0.48} \angle \mathbf{-187.6^\circ}$$

SWR $= (1 + |\Gamma_l|)/(1 - |\Gamma_l|)$
$$= 1.48/0.52 = \mathbf{2.85}$$

(ii) $V_s = V_q/(1 + \Gamma_{in})$
$$= 10/(1 - 0.476 + j0.06)$$
$$= 10/(0.524 + j0.06)$$
$$= 19 \angle 6.5^\circ$$

$V_{max} = (1 + |\Gamma|)V_s$

For a lossless line, $|\Gamma| = |\Gamma_{in}|$. Therefore, from Eq. (2.69),

$V_{max} = (1 + |\Gamma_{in}|) V_s$
$$= 1.48 \times 19$$
$$= \mathbf{28.12} \text{ V}$$

(iii) $\alpha = 2.0$ dB/m $= 0.23$ Np/m, and $l = \lambda = 0.5$ m

$al = 0.23 \times 0.5 = 0.115$ Np

$\Gamma_{in} = \Gamma_l e^{-\alpha l}$
$$= 0.48 \, e^{-0.115} = \mathbf{0.429}$$

2.9 SMITH CHART

Solutions of transmission line problems involve complex equations and are tedious. Out of many graphical methods, the one most commonly used is the Smith chart, devised by Philip H. Smith.[6,7] It is a plot of normalized impedance or admittance or reflection coefficient in a unity circle. The magnitudes are directly read in the radial directions and phase in the angular directions. It is useful for the analysis of lossless and lossy lines.

2.9.1 Construction of Smith Chart

The construction of the Smith chart is based on two sets of orthogonal circles.[8] One set of circles represents the ratio $r = R/Z_0$ and the other set of circles represents the ratio $x = X/Z_o$ where R and X are the resistance and reactance component of the line impedance respectively. Z_0 is the characteristic impedance and is a pure resistance for a lossless line.

The normalized impedance along a transmission line is given by

$$z = Z/Z_0$$
$$= (1 + \Gamma_l e^{-2\gamma d})/(1 - \Gamma_l e^{-2\gamma d}) \quad (2.78)$$

At the load end, $d = 0$, and hence

$$z = (1 + \Gamma_l)/(1 - \Gamma_l)$$
$$= Z_l/Z_0$$
$$= (R_l + jX_l)/Z_0 = r + jx \quad (2.79)$$

From the above equation, we may express the reflection coefficient Γ_l in terms of z. It is given by

$$\Gamma_l = (z - 1)/(z + 1) = \Gamma_r + j\Gamma_i \quad (2.80)$$

Substituting Eq. (2.80) in Eq. (2.79), we obtain

$$z = (1 + \Gamma_l)/(1 - \Gamma_l)$$
$$- (1 + \Gamma_r + j\Gamma_i)/(1 - \Gamma_r - j\Gamma_i)$$

Γ_r is the real part and Γ_j is the imaginary part of Γ_l.

Multiplying the numerator and denominator by the conjugate of the denominator, we obtain

$$z = \frac{(1-\Gamma_r^2-\Gamma_i^2)+2j\Gamma_i}{(1-\Gamma_r)^2+\Gamma_i^2}$$

$$\therefore \quad r = \frac{(1-\Gamma_r^2-\Gamma_i^2)}{[(1-\Gamma_r)^2+\Gamma_i^2]} \tag{2.81}$$

$$x = \frac{2\Gamma_i}{[(1-\Gamma_r)^2+\Gamma_i^2]} \tag{2.82}$$

These two equations can be rearranged as equations of circles as detailed below.

2.9.2 Resistance Circles

Equation (2.81) may be written as

$$r[(1-\Gamma_r)^2-\Gamma_i{}^2] = 1-\Gamma_r^2-\Gamma_i{}^2$$

Expanding and rearranging, we get

$$r - 2r\Gamma_r + r\Gamma_r^2 + r\Gamma_i{}^2 + \Gamma_r^2 + \Gamma_i{}^2 = 1$$

$$\Gamma_r^2(r+1) + \Gamma_i{}^2(r+1) - 2r\Gamma_r = 1-r$$

or, $\quad \Gamma_r^2 + \dfrac{-2r\Gamma_r}{r+1} + \Gamma_i{}^2 = \dfrac{1}{r+1} - \dfrac{r}{r+1}$

By adding $[r/(r+1)]^2$ on either side, we obtain

$$\Gamma_r^2 - 2r\Gamma_r/(r+1) + [r/(r+1)]^2 + \Gamma_i{}^2$$
$$= 1/(r+1) - r/(r+1) + [r/(r+1)]^2$$

i.e., $\quad [\Gamma_r - r/(r+1)]^2 + \Gamma_i{}^2 = [1/(r+1)]^2 \tag{2.83}$

Equation (2.83) represents a family of resistance circles having a constant resistance r with centre at $r/(r+1)$ and radius of $1/(r+1)$. All constant resistance circles are plotted in Fig. 2.12.

2.9.3 Reactance Circles

Equation (2.82) may be written as

$$(1-\Gamma_r)^2 + \Gamma_i^2 - \frac{2\Gamma_i}{x} = 0$$

Expanding and rearranging, we get

$$1 - 2\Gamma_r + \Gamma_r^2 + \Gamma_i^2 - \frac{2\Gamma_i}{x} = 0$$

$$(\Gamma_r - 1)^2 + \Gamma_i^2 - \frac{2\Gamma_i}{x} = 0$$

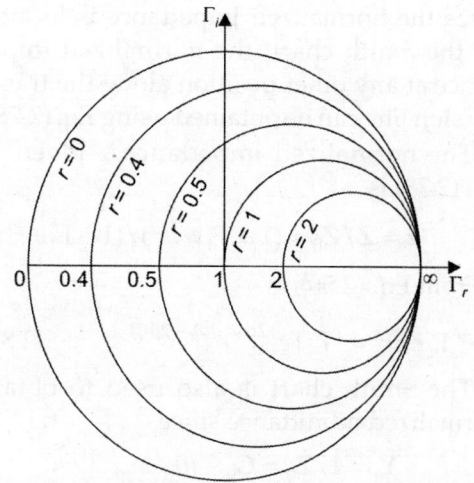

Fig. 2.12: Constant resistance circles

By adding $(1/x)^2$ on either side and rearranging, we obtain

$$(\Gamma_r - 1)^2 + [\Gamma_i - (1/x)]^2 = (1/x)^2 \tag{2.84}$$

Equation (2.84) represents a family of reactance circles having a constant reactance x with centre at $(1, 1/x)$ and radius of $1/x$. All constant reactance circles are plotted in Fig. 2.13.

Along the circumference of the Smith chart are shown the relative distance scales in wavelength and a phase angle scale specifying the angle of reflection coefficient.

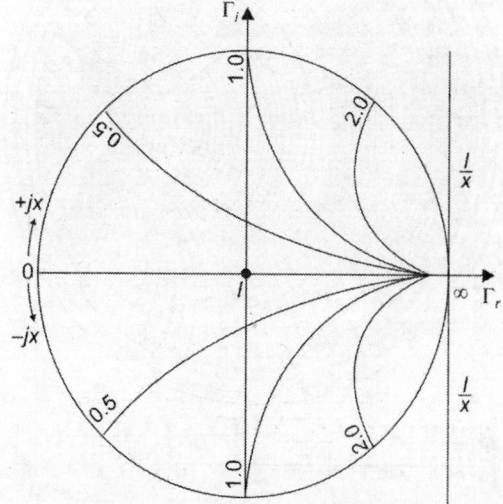

Fig. 2.13: Constant reactance circles

Once the normalized impedance is located on the Smith chart, the normalized impedance at any other position along the transmission line can be obtained using Eq. (2.78).

The normalized impedance z given in Eq. (2.78) is

$$z = Z/Z_0 = (1 + \Gamma_1 e^{-2\gamma d})/(1 - \Gamma_1 e^{-2\gamma d})$$

From Eq. (2.56),

$$\Gamma_l e^{-2\gamma d} = |\Gamma_l| e^{-2\alpha d} e^{j(\theta_l - 2\beta d)} \qquad (2.85)$$

The Smith chart is also used to obtain normalized admittance since

$$Y_o = 1/Z_0 = G_0 - jB_0$$

and $\qquad Y = G + jB \qquad (2.86)$

The normalized admittance is then

$$y = Y/Y_0 = Z_0/Z$$
$$= 1/z = g + jb \qquad (2.87)$$

The Smith chart is obtained by superposing constant r and x circles. Thus, Figs (2.12) and (2.13) superimposed one over the other result in the Smith chart. This is shown in Fig. 2.14.

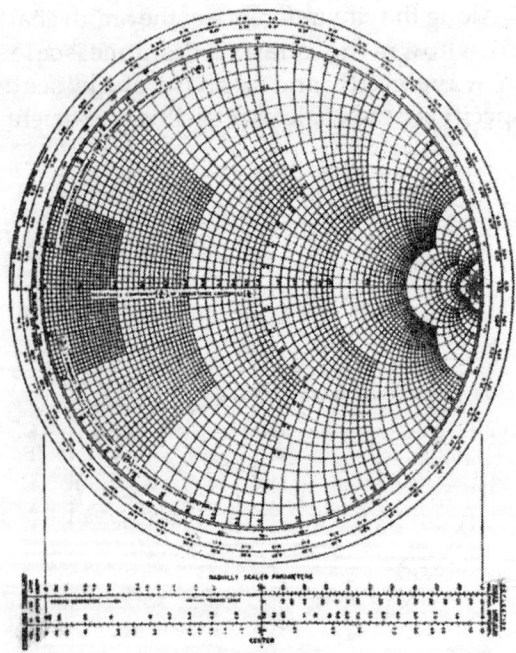

Fig. 2.14: Smith chart

2.9.4 Characteristics of Smith Chart

The important characteristics of a Smith chart are:

1. A Smith chart consists of two families of orthogonal circles: (i) constant r loci, and (ii) constant x loci.

2. The radius of the constant r circles is $1/(r + 1)$ and the coordinates of the centre are $[r/(r + 1), 0]$.

3. The radius of the constant x circles is $1/x$ and the coordinates of the centre are $(1, 1/x)$.

4. All the constant r circles pass through the points $\Gamma_r = \infty$ and $\Gamma_i = 0$.

5. All the constant x circles pass through the point $(\infty, 0)$.

6. The inductive reactance $(+jx)$ is represented in the upper half of the Smith chart and the capacitive reactance $(-jx)$ is represented in the lower half of the Smith chart.

7. A Smith chart can also be used for normalized admittance. In this case, the constant r and constant x circles become constant g (conductance) and constant b (susceptance) circles respectively.

8. The distance around the Smith chart is $\lambda/2$ (half-wavelength).

9. At the V_{max} point, $z_{max} = S$.

10. At the V_{min} point, $z_{min} = 1/S$.

11. The horizontal radius to the right of the center $(1, 0)$ of the Smith chart corresponds to $V_{max}, I_{min}, z_{max}$ and S.

12. The horizontal radius to the left of the center $(1,0)$ of the Smith chart corresponds to $V_{min}, I_{max}, z_{min}$ and $1/S$.

13. The normalized admittance y is the reciprocal of normalized impedance z. Hence, the corresponding quantities in the admittance chart are 180° out of phase with those in the impedance chart.

14. The normalized z or y is repeated for every half wavelength of distance.

15. The distances are in wavelengths towards the generator and also towards the load.

The standing-wave pattern can be measured using Smith chart or a slotted line directly. Then, the magnitude of reflection coefficient, reflected power, transmitted power and load impedance can be calculated from the chart.

2.9.5 Applications of Smith Chart

The various applications of the Smith chart are listed below:[9]

1. For a specified load impedance Z_l, the corresponding SWR can be directly obtained from the Smith chart.
2. For a specified SWR and the line impedance at any one point on the transmission line, the impedance at any other point can be found.
3. Once the SWR is known, the magnitude and the phase angle of the reflection coefficient can be obtained.
4. For a specified SWR and the location of the voltage minima, the input and output impedances can be found.

5. Smith chart is also useful for stub matching of the transmission lines.

(i) Determination of z of a lossless line of length l terminated with Z_l.

The steps to obtain normalized impedance of a lossless line terminated with load impedance Z_l from the Smith chart are listed below:

1. On the Smith chart, locate the normalized load impedance $z = Z_l/Z_0$. Let it be point P as shown in Fig. 2.15.
2. Draw a line joining the centre point O and P, extend it to intersect the circumference at Q.
3. From P, move towards generator by a distance l/λ to reach the point R on the unit circle. R corresponds to the input point of the line. While moving, Γ and S do not change.
4. Draw a circular arc with O as centre and OP as radius to intersect the line OR at T.
5. The impedance at T gives the normalized input impedance z. The input impedance is then $Z = z \times Z_0$.

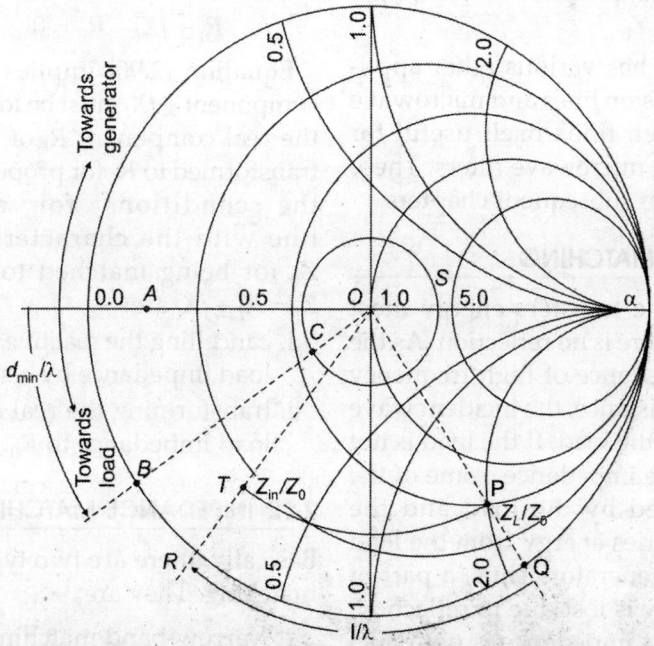

Fig. 2.15: Determination of impedance using Smith chart

(ii) Determination of Z_l for a given SWR and position of voltage minimum.

The Smith chart simplifies the solution of load impedance provided the SWR and the position of the first voltage minimum are available from measurements in the laboratory. The steps are as follows:

1. Draw the S-circle for the given SWR with center O as shown in Fig. 2.15.

2. With the transmission line shorted, the first voltage minimum occurs at the load. When the line is loaded, it shifts towards the generator by an amount d_{min}/λ. The impedance at voltage minimum is the normalized resistance of magnitude $1/S$. It corresponds to the point A on the left half of the real axis of the Smith chart.

3. From the point A, move along the circumference towards the load a distance d_{min}/λ. Let this point be B.

4. Draw a line joining the points O and B. Let the point of intersection between the line OB and the S-circle be the point C.

5. Point G corresponds to the normalized load impedance z_l. Then, the load impedance $Z_l = z_l \times Z_0$.

The Smith chart has various other applications in transmission lines and microwave engineering. It even finds itself useful for stub matching and microwave filters. These will be discussed in subsequent chapters.

2.10 IMPEDANCE MATCHING

A transmission line transfers energy most efficiently when there is no reflection. As the characteristic impedance of high frequency line is always a resistance, the incident wave delivers energy to the load. If the load is not matched to the line impedance, some of the energy is reflected by the load and the reflected wave carries energy from the load end towards the generator. Thus, a part of the incident energy is lost due to reflection. Generally, the load impedance is not equal to the characteristic impedance. In such cases,

to transfer maximum energy to the load, it is necessary to match the load impedance to the characteristic impedance of the transmission line. It is also desirable that the line impedance is independent of the length of the line. Similarly, in many measurement systems involving transmission lines, it is necessary that there is no reflection.

2.11 CONDITION FOR IMPEDANCE MATCHING

If the transmission line is not matched with the load, there will be reflection at the load end. The load reflection coefficient Γ_l is given by

$$\Gamma_l = (Z_l - Z_0)/(Z_l - Z_0) \qquad (2.88)$$

At high frequencies, the characteristic impedance Z_0 of a lossless line is purely resistive and is equal to R_0. Z_l is the load impedance. Assuming the load impedance is a complex load, we have $Z_l = R_l \pm jX_l$. Substituting this in Eq. (2.88), we obtain

$$\Gamma_l = (R_l \pm jX_l - R_0)/(R_l \pm jX_l + R_0) \qquad (2.89)$$

If the line is matched with the load, $\Gamma_l = 0$. Hence

$$R_l \pm jX_l - R_0 = 0 \qquad (2.90)$$

Equation (2.90) implies that the reactive component $\pm jX_l$ must be identically zero and the real component R_l of the load must be transformed to R_0 for proper matching. Thus, the conditions for a transmission line with the characteristic impedance Z_0 for being matched to a complex load $Z_l = R_l \pm jX_l$ are:

i. cancelling the reactive component of the load impedance by a suitable element

ii. transforming the real component of the load impedance to R_0.

2.12 IMPEDANCE MATCHING METHODS

Basically, there are two types of impedance matching. They are:

i. Narrow-band matching

ii. Broad-band matching

In narrow-band matching, the impedance is matched over a narrow band of frequencies. This method uses reactive elements such as shunt and series stubs, reactive irises and tuning screws for matching. In broad-band matching, the impedance is matched for a wide or broad-band of frequencies. This is accomplished using quarter-wave transformers, tapered lines and matched terminations.

2.12.1 Narrow-Band Matching

In narrow-band matching, the methods used are:

  i. Single stub matching
  ii. Double stub matching
  iii. Waveguide windows or reactive irises
  iv. Tuning screws
  v. Inductive and capacitive hosts
  vi. Waveguide stub matching
  vii. Coaxial line stub matching

These matching methods are discussed in the following subsections.

2.12.1.1 Single Stub Matching

In this method, a short section of the short-circuited transmission line called *stub*, is used in shunt with the transmission line as shown in Fig. 2.16. Short-circuited sections are preferred to open-circuited ones because a good short-circuit is easier to obtain than a good open-circuit. The distance d from the load and the the length l of the stub are so choosen that the reflected wave generated by the shunting impedance of the stub is *equal in magnitude and opposite in phase* to the reflected wave of the transmission line at this point due to mismatch. Although a reflected wave is present along the distance d because of the reflection from the load, there is no reflected wave on the generator side of the stub line due to cancellation of the two reflected waves.

Since the matching involves parallel or shunt connection of transmission line and the stub, the design of single stub matching is carried out with *admittances*. The Smith chart, as explained earlier, can be used as the admittance chart as well.

  i. *Design concept for single stub matching*: In a lossless transmission line, as we move away from the complex load towards the generator, a voltage minimum occurs at which the input admittance is solely conductance and hence, $Y_{11} = g = S$. Likewise, at a voltage maximum, the

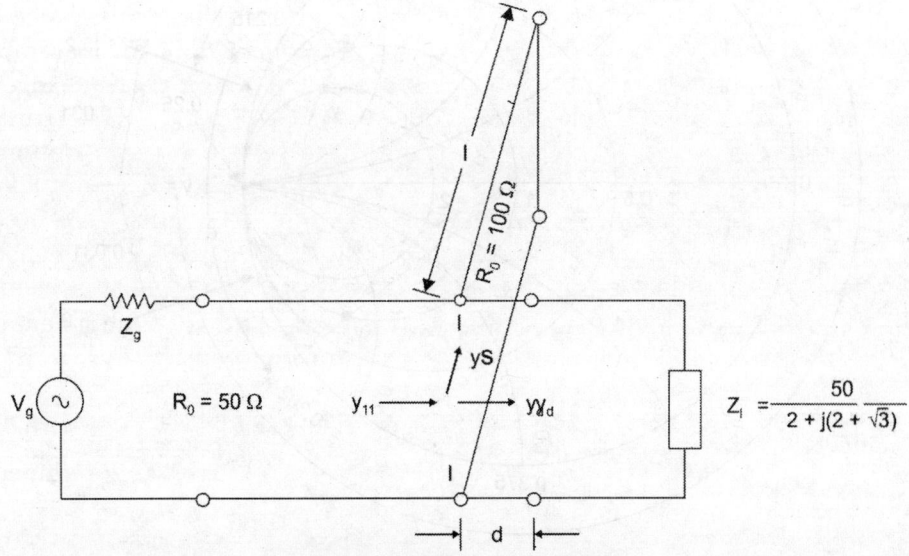

Fig. 2.16: Single stub matching

input admittance is pure conductance and $Y_{11} = g = 1/S$, where $S = $ SWR. Hence, between the voltage minimum and maximum points there must exist a point, at a certain distance from the first voltage minimum at which the real part of the normalized admittance is unity, i.e. $y = 1 + jb$. The reactive component $\pm jb$ of the admittance can be cancelled by an equal and opposite susceptance $\mp jb$ of a parallel stub line of length l located at that point and having characteristic admittance equal to that of the transmission line Y_0.

Then, the total normalized admittance y_{11} of the transmission line and the stub looking towards the load side is given by

$$y_{11} = 1 \pm jb \mp jb = 1 \qquad (2.91)$$

for proper matching. The distance d from the load is given by

$$d = (\lambda/4\pi)\cos^{-1}[(S-1)/(S+1)] \qquad (2.92)$$

The length l of the stub is given by

$$l = \left(\frac{\lambda}{2\pi}\right)\tan^{-1}\left(\frac{\sqrt{S}}{S-1}\right) \qquad (2.93)$$

ii. *Design steps for single step matching*: **The** steps involved in the design of **a single** shunt stub using the Smith **chart** are listed below:

a. Locate the normalized load admittance y_l point on the Smith chart as shown in Fig. 2.17.

b. Draw a S-circle through y_l as shown in Fig. 2.17, so that it intersects the unity circle at y_d. Choose the y_d which is nearest to the load.

c. The characteristic admittance of the stub is usually different from that of the transmission line. Therefore, the condition for matching at the junction is

$$Y_{11} = Y_d + Y_s \qquad (2.94)$$

where Y_s is the susceptance that the stub provides. The stub and the

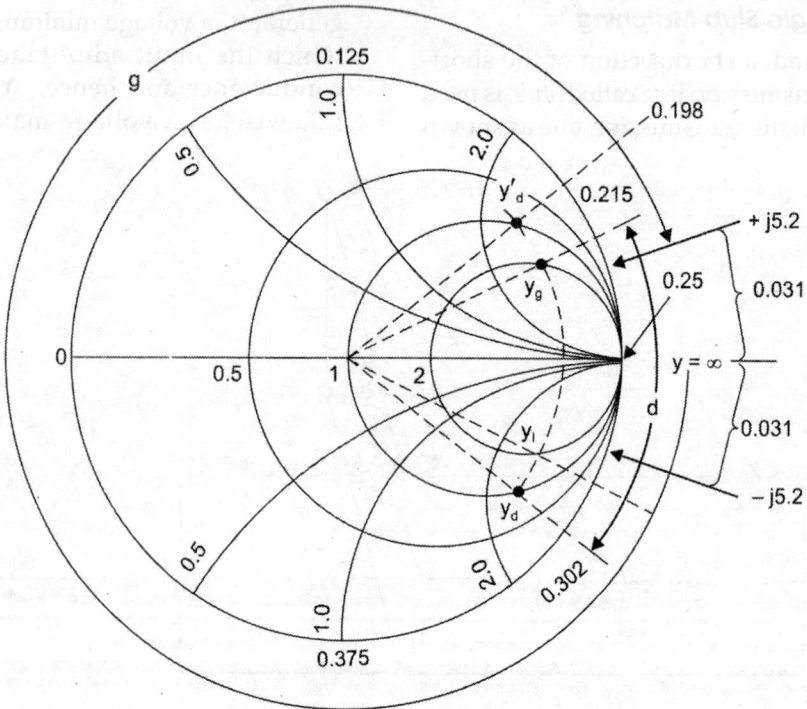

Fig. 2.17: Illustration of single stub match design technique

section of the transmission line from the load to the junction are in parallel. For matching the admittances, they must be converted to normalized values using the Smith chart. Thus,

$$y_{11}Y_0 = y_d Y_0 + y_s Y_{os}$$
$$y_s = (y_{11} - y_d)(Y_0/Y_{os}) \quad (2.95)$$

d. The distance between the load and the stub position is obtained from the distance scale.

e. The stub provides a susceptance of $+jb$. Locate this on the Smith chart.

f. The required distance l from the short-circuited end where $z = 0$ and $y = \infty$, by traversing the chart towards the generator until $+jb$ is reached. This distance is the stub length.

As the line is matched at the junction, there will not be any standing wave in the transmission line from the stub to the generator.

The practical design of single stub matching can be carried out with the aid of Fig. 2.18. It gives the length l of the stub and its position d with respect to the standing wave ratio. Such a stub will enable any load impedance to be matched to the characteristic impedance of the transmission line, provided that the load is *not an open-circuit, short-circuit* or *pure reactance*.

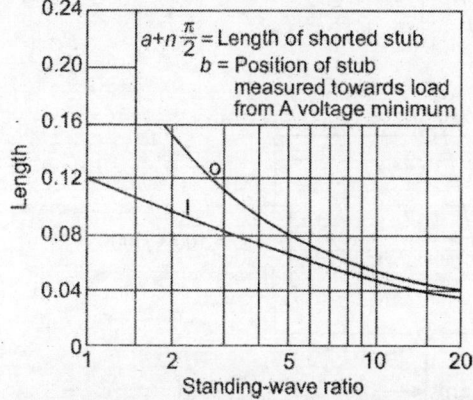

Fig. 2.18: Graph for single stub match design

Example 2.13: A lossless transmission line has a characteristic impedance $R_0 = 50\Omega$. It is to be matched with a load impedance of $50/[2 + j(2 + \sqrt{3})]\Omega$ using a lossless short-circuited stub. The stub has a characteristic impedance of $100\ \Omega$. Find the step position nearest to the load and its length for impedance matching.

Solution: Given $R_0 = 50\Omega$, $Z_l = \dfrac{50}{2 + j(2 + \sqrt{3})}\Omega$, $Z_s = 100$ W.

a. Locate the normalized load admittance y_l point on the Smith chart shown in Fig. 2.17

$$y_l = \frac{R_0}{Z_l} = \frac{50}{50[2 + j(2 + \sqrt{3}]}$$
$$= 2 + j3.732$$

b. Draw S-circle through y_l as shown in Fig. 2.17 so that it intersects the unit resistance circle at y_d.
$$y_d = 1 - j2.6$$

c. Since $Z_s = 100\ \Omega$ and $R_0 = 50\ \Omega$, the condition for matching is given by
$$Y_{11} = Y_d + Y_s$$
Y_s is the susceptance that the stub will provide. These admittances are to be converted to normalized values for matching using Smith chart. Thus
$$y_{11}Y_0 = y_d Y_0 + y_s Y_{os}$$
or $\quad y_s = (y_{11} - y_d)(Y_0/Y_{os})$
$$= [1 - (1 - j2.6)](100/50)$$
$$= +j5.20$$

d. The distance between the load and the stub position is obtained from the distance scale. Thus
$$d = (0.302 - 0.215)\lambda$$
$$= 0.087\lambda$$

e. The stub provides a susceptance of $+j5.20$. Locate $+j5.20$ point on the Smith chart. Let this distance be l_1.

f. The requied distance l from the short-circuited end where $z = 0$ and $y = \infty$ by traversing the chart towards the generator until the point $+j5.20$ is reached.

This gives the stub length l/λ. Thus

$$l = (0.50 - l_1)\,\lambda$$
$$= (0.50 - 0.031)\,\lambda$$
$$= 0.469\,\lambda$$

As the transmission line is matched at the junction, there is no standing wave on the transmission line from the stub junction to the generator.

2.12.1.2 Double Stub Matching

The problem with single stub matching is that it is sometimes impractical because the stub cannot be placed physically at the ideal location. In such cases, double stub matching is used. It consists of two or double short-circuited stubs connected in parallel with a fixed length $3\lambda/8$ between them as shown in Fig. 2.19. The stub nearest to the load is used to adjust the susceptance. It is located at a specified wavelength from the constant conductance unity circle on an appropriate constant S-circle. Assuming that the stubs and the transmission line have the same characteristic impedance, the admittance of the line at the second stub is given by

$$y_{22} = y_{d2} \pm y_{s2} \tag{2.96}$$

The position and lengths of the stubs are so choosen that there is no standing wave on the transmission line to the left of the second stub.

i. *Design steps for double stub matching*: The steps involved in the design of a double shunt stub using the Smith chart are listed under:

a. Locate the normalized load impedance z_l point on the Smiuth chart as shown in Fig. 2.20.

b. Draw a S-circle through z_l as shown in Fig. 2.20 and read the normalized admittance y_l 180° out of phase with z_l on the SWR circle.

c. Draw the spacing circle of $3\lambda/8$ by rotating the constant conductance unity circle ($g = 1$). Through a phase angle $\phi = [2\beta d = 2 \cdot (2\pi/\lambda)(3\lambda/8)] = 3\pi/2$ towards the load. Since y_{d2} is on the $g = 1$ circle and y_{11} and y_{d2} are $3\lambda/8$ apart, y_{11} lies on the spacing circle.

d. Read y_{d1} on the Smith chart by moving y_l for a distance of d along the S-circle towards the generator.

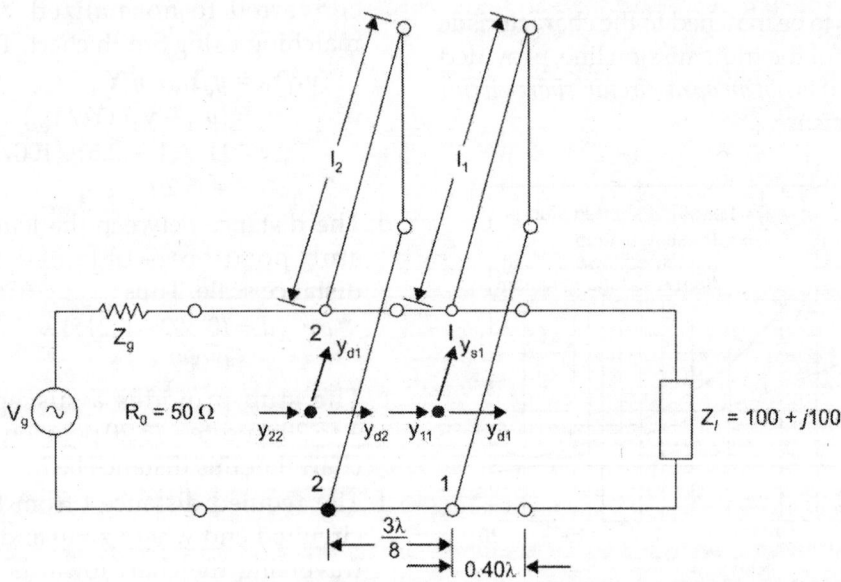

Fig. 2.19: Double stub matching

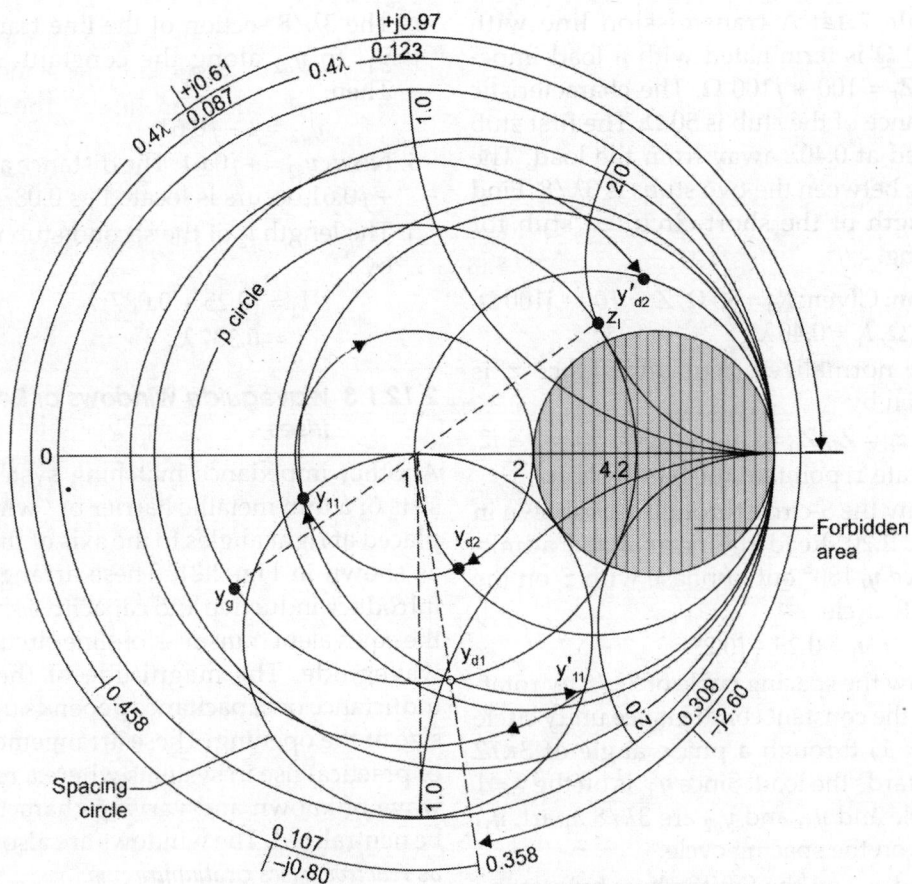

Fig. 2.20: Illustration of double stub match design

e. The intersection of the spacing circle and the constant g circle on which y_{d1} is located is y_{11}.

f. At the junction 1-1 of Fig. 2.19, $y_{11} = y_{d1} + y_{s1}$ where y_{s1} is the normalized admittance of the first stub.

$$\therefore \quad y_{s1} = y_{11} - y_{d1} = +jb_{s1} \qquad (2.97)$$

g. The length l_1 of the first stub is the distance traversed from the short-circuited end towards the generator until the point $+jb_{s1}$ is reached.

h. The $(3\lambda/8)$ section of the line transforms $y_{11} = y_{d2}$ along the constant S-circle. Then

$$y_{d2} = 1 - jb_{s2} \qquad (2.98)$$

i. Now, $y_{s2} = +jb_{s2}$. Locate the distance l_{s2} at which $+jb_{s2}$ occurs.

j. The length l_2 of the second stub is the distance traversed from the short-circuited end towards the generator until the point $+jb_{s2}$ is reached.

As the transmission line is matched, there is no standing wave on the transmission line to the left of stub 2.

ii. *Limitation of double stub matching*: The double stub method cannot be used to match all impedances. For example, if the normalized conductance exceeds $\csc^2\beta$, it cannot be used since matching conditions are not satisfied. Further, if g_l is greater than 2, the spacing circle and $g = 2$ circle do not intersect. The area of $g = 2$ circle is known as *forbidden region* of the normalized load admittance for possible matching.

Example 2.14: A transmission line with $R_0 = 50\ \Omega$ is terminated with a load impedance $Z_l = 100 + j100\ \Omega$. The characteristic impedance of the stub is $50\ \Omega$. The first stub is placed at 0.40λ away from the load. The spacing between the two stubs is $3\lambda/8$. Find the length of the short-circuited stub for matching.

Solution: Given: $R_0 = 50\ \Omega$, $Z_l = 100 + j100\ \Omega$, $Z_s = 50\ \Omega$, $l_1 = 0.40\ \lambda$.

a. The normalized load impedance z_l is given by
$$z_l = Z_l/Z_0 = (100 + j100)/50 = 2 + j2$$
Locate z_l point on the Smith chart.

b. Draw the S-circle through z_l as shown in Fig. 2.20. Read the normalized admittance y_l 180° out of phase with z_l on the SWR circle.
$$y_l = 0.25 - j0.25$$

c. Draw the spacing circle of $3\lambda/8$ by rotating the constant conductance unity circle ($g = 1$) through a phase angle of $3\pi/2$ towards the load. Since y_{d2} is on the $g = 1$ circle and y_{11} and y_{d2} are $3\lambda/8$ apart, y_{11} lies on the spacing cycle.

d. Read y_{d1} on the Smith chart by moving y_l for a distance of 0.4λ from 0.458 to 0.358 along the S-circle towards the generator. Thus,
$$y_{d1} = 0.55 - j1.08$$

e. y_{11} is found by carrying y_{d1} along the constant g-circle that intersects the spacing circle at y_{11}. It is given by
$$y_{11} = 0.55 - j0.11$$

f. Now, $y_{11} = y_{d1} + y_{s1}$, where y_{s1} is the normalized admittance of the first stub. y_{s1} is given by
$$\begin{aligned} y_{s1} &= y_{11} - y_{d1} \\ &= (0.55 - j0.11) - (0.55 - j1.08) \\ &= +j0.97 \end{aligned}$$

g. The distance at which $+j0.97$ occurs is located as 0.123λ. Therefore, the length of the first stub is
$$\begin{aligned} l_1 &= (0.25 - 0.123)\lambda \\ &= \mathbf{0.373\lambda} \end{aligned}$$

h. The $3\lambda/8$ section of the line transforms y_{11} to y_{d2} along the constant S-circle. Then,
$$y_{d2} = 1 - j0.61$$

i. Now, $y_{s2} = +j0.61$. The distance at which $+j0.61$ occurs is located as 0.087λ.

j. The length l_2 of the second stub is given by
$$\begin{aligned} l_2 &= (0.25 + 0.087)\lambda \\ &= \mathbf{0.337\lambda} \end{aligned}$$

2.12.1.3 Waveguide Windows or Reactive Irises

Another impedance matching system consists of a thin metallic barrier or "windows" placed at right angles to the axis of the guide as shown in Fig. 2.21. These arrangements introduce inductive and capacitive shunts in the equivalent transmission-line circuit of the waveguide. The magnitude of the shunt inductance or capacitance depends upon the size of the opening. These arrangements are of practical use in systems where a reflected wave of known and varying character is to be neutralized. The windows are also known as *reactive irises* or *diaphragms*.

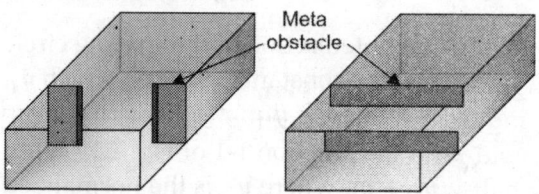

Fig. 2.21: Waveguide windows (a) Inductive (b) Capacitive

2.12.1.4 Turning Screws

Tuning screws are used as tuning devices for impedance matching because of the reactive nature of the screws. Figure 2.22(a) shows an adjustable or tuning screw. The screw projects into the waveguide in a direction parallel to the electric field. Such an arrangement has same effect as shunting a capacitive load across the equivalent transmission-line circuit of the waveguide.

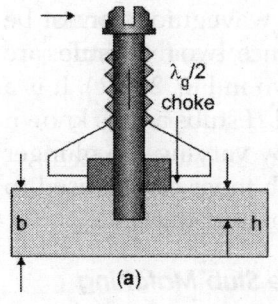 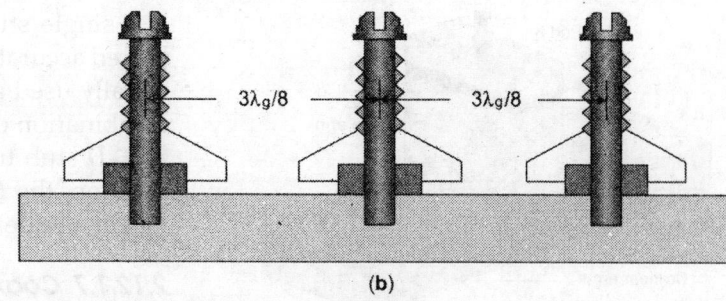

Fig. 2.22: (a) Tuning screw (b) Three-screw tuner

The susceptance of this capacitive load increases with the penetration into the guide up to the point where the equivalent penetration is $\lambda_g/4$. Then, the probe becomes resonant. The system acts as though a series resonant circuit of low resistance is connected in shunt with the waveguide. Thus, the extent to which the screw projects into the waveguide determines the magnitude of the compensating reflections. The position of the screw with respect to the standing wave pattern that is to be eliminated determines the phasing of the reflected wave. To adjust the axial position of the screw, a longitudinal slot is provided in the middle of the broad side of the guide.

A thin screw of diameter very much less than $\lambda_g/4$ offers capacitive susceptance when $h < \lambda_g/4$, infinite susceptance when $h = \lambda_g/4$ and inductive susceptance when $h > \lambda_g/4$. To avoid power leakage through the screw gap, half-wavelength choke is used at the screw insertion junction as shown.

The above tuning screw shown in Fig. 2.22(a) can be slided along the waveguide axis through a longitudinal slot which is centered in the broad wall. With this provision, both the penetration and the position of the tuning screw can be varied along a longitudinal distance of half guide wavelength $\lambda_g/2$ for better matching with ease. These devices are known as *slide screw tuners*. With a three-screw tuner shown in Fig. 2.22(b), a greater range of impedance matching can be achieved.

2.12.1.5 *Inductive and Capacitive Posts*

Inductive and capacitive posts are also used as matching devices. A thin conductive cylindrical post extending fully across the narrow width of the waveguide at the centre of the broad wall provides an inductive susceptance across the waveguide operated in TE_{10} mode. If the post is located across the waveguide at right angles to the electric field of the TE_{10} mode, it offers capacitive susceptance across the waveguide. As the diameter of the post increases, the susceptance also increases. Thsese posts are shown in Fig. 2.23.

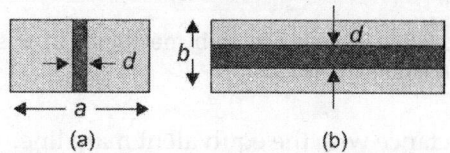

Fig. 2.23: Posts (a) Inductive (b) Capacitive

2.12.1.6 *Waveguide Stub Matching*

Stub matching can be used to match the waveguides. The three types of stub matching in rectangular waveguides are (i) *E* stub, (ii) *H* stub and (iii) *E-H* stub tuners. In a rectangular waveguide, the stub is connected in the *E* or *H* plane by placing the waveguide short plunger across the wide or narrow dimensions respectively as shown in Fig. 2.24(a) and (b). For an *E* stub, the dielectric field lines penetrate from the waveguide into the stub whereas in *H* stub, the magnetic field lines penetrate from the waveguide into the stub. Thus, the *E* stub offers a series

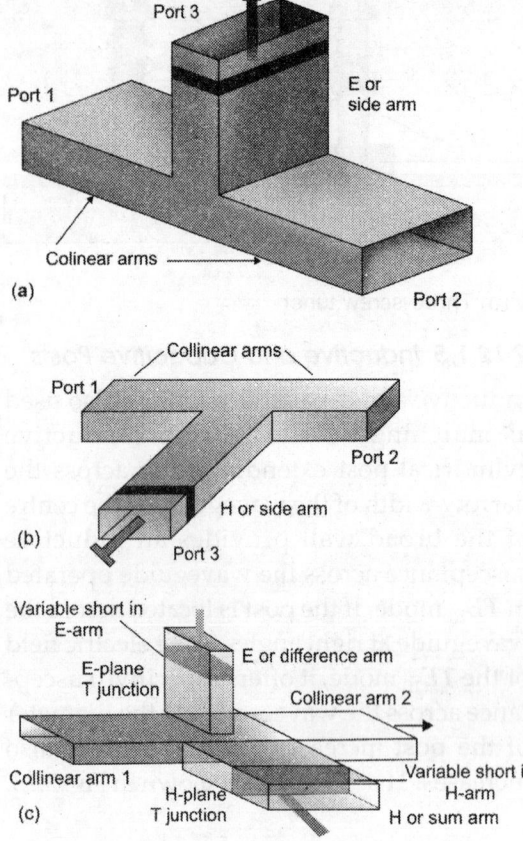

(a)

(b)

(c)

Fig. 2.24: Waveguide stub matching (a) *E* stub (b) *H* stub (c) *E-H* tuner

reactance with the equivalent main line. The *H* stub offers a shunt susceptance across the waveguide.

A single stub in a waveguide cannot be placed accurately. Hence, two fixed stubs are usually used as shown in Fig. 2.24(c). It is a combination of *E* and *H* stubs and is known as *E-H* stub tuner . By varying the plunger position, the *E-H* stub tuner can be used to match a wide range of impedances.

2.12.1.7 Coaxial Line Stub Matching

For matching a two-conductor coaxial lines, the stub is realized by a *T*-junction placed at the stub position as shown in Fig. 2.25. The step length is adjusted by a movable plunger. The stub position is adjusted by a sliding arrangement. A longitudinal slot on the outer conductor of the coaxial line allows the movement of the centre conductor of the stub. This is a complicated process. Therefore, two fixed double stub of variable length is used for the coaxial line matching. The double shunt stubs are easy to construct for coaxial lines.

2.12.2 Broadband Matching

In broadband matching, the methods used are:

  i. Quarter-wave transformer matching
 ii. Multisection quarter-wave transformer matching
iii. Tapered transmission lines
 iv. Matched terminations

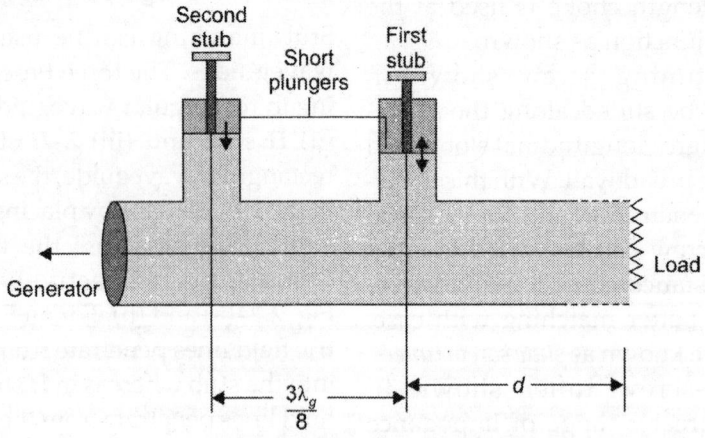

Fig. 2.25: Coaxial line stub matching

2.12.2.1 Quarter-wave Transformer Matching

Sections of transmission lines that are exactly a quarter-wave length long have the unique impedance transforming property. This property is frequently made use of for matching purposes. Consider a transmission line with characteristic impedance Z_2 and an electrical length $\beta l = \pi/2$. If it is terminated with an impedance Z_3, the input impedance of the line is given by

$$Z_{in} = Z_2 \frac{Z_3 + jZ_2 \tan \beta l}{Z_2 + jZ_3 \tan \beta l}$$

$$= Z_2 \frac{(Z_3/\tan \beta l) + jZ_2}{(Z_2/\tan \beta l) + jZ_3} \quad (2.99)$$

Since $\beta l = \pi/2$, $\tan \beta l = \infty$. Therefore Z_{in} reduces to

$$Z_{in} = Z_2^2 / Z_3 \quad (2.100)$$

If Z_{in} is to be matched to the generator of impedance $Z_1 = Z_{in}$, then at $\beta l = \pi/2$, Z_2 is

$$Z_2 = \sqrt{Z_1 Z_3} \quad (2.101)$$

Thus, a load Z_3 can be matched to the generator impedance Z_1 by inserting a line of length $l = \lambda_g/4$ and a characteristic impedance of $\sqrt{Z_1 Z_3}$. This matching section of the line is known as its *quarter-wave transformer*. It is shown in Fig. 2.26. When the generator impedance Z_1 and the load impedance Z_3 are widely different, a multisection quarter-wave transformer is used to obtain better matching.

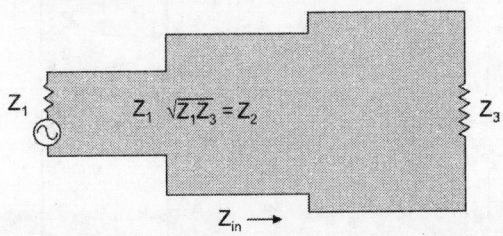

Fig. 2.26: Single section quarter-wave transformer

i. Bandwidth of a Quarter-wave Transformer

A perfect impedance matching is provided by a single section quarter-wave at frequencies for which $\lambda_{g0}/4$ where λ_{g0} is the guide wavelength. Thus, a perfect matching is obtained with a single section quarter-wave transformer at a designated frequency f_0 and at its odd harmonics. The bandwidth of this line is determined by considering an electrical length $\beta l = \theta$ at any frequency f_1 other than f_0 and the input reflection coefficient Γ.

Assume that a quarter-wave transformer is to match a load $Z_3 = Z_l$ to a transmission line of impedance Z_1, then, the input reflection coefficient is given by

$$\Gamma = (Z_{in} - Z_1)/(Z_{in} + Z_1) \quad (2.102)$$

The input impedance Z_{in} is given by

$$Z_{in} = Z_2 \frac{Z_l + jZ_2 \tan \theta}{Z_2 + jZ_l \tan \theta} \quad (2.103)$$

Since $\theta = \beta l = \pi/2$, Z_{in} becomes

$$Z_{in} = Z_2^2 / Z_l \quad (2.104)$$

If Z_2 is choosen to be equal to $\sqrt{Z_1 Z_l}$ then $Z_{in} = Z_1$ and the load is matched to the main transmission line. Thus the intermediate section of the transmission line of quarter-wavelength transforms the load impedance Z_l into an impedance Z_1. Hence, it acts as an ideal transformer with a turn ratio of $\sqrt{Z_l/Z_1}$.

A perfect match is obtained only at that frequency for which the transformer is a quarter-wave ($\lambda/4 + n\lambda/2$) long.

Let $\theta = \beta l$ be electrical length of the quarter-wave transformer at a frequency f. For a **TEM** wave in an air-filled line, $\beta l = (2\pi/\lambda) l = 2\pi f l / c$. The input impedance presented to the main transmission line at any frequency is given by

$$Z_{in} = Z_2 \frac{Z_l + jZ_2 \tan \theta}{Z_2 + jZ_l \tan \theta} \quad (2.105)$$

Therefore, the reflection coefficient is

$$\Gamma = (Z_{in} - Z_1)/(Z_{in} + Z_1) \quad (2.106)$$

Substitution of Eq. (2.105) in Eq. (2.106) yields

$$\Gamma = \frac{Z_2(Z_l - Z_1) + j(Z_2^2 - Z_1 Z_l)\tan\theta}{Z_2(Z_l + Z_1) + j(Z_2^2 + Z_1 Z_l)\tan\theta} \quad (2.107)$$

Substituting $Z_2^2 = Z_1 Z_l$ in Eq. (2.107), we get

$$\Gamma = \frac{Z_l - Z_1}{(Z_l + Z_1 + j2\sqrt{Z_1 Z_2}\tan\theta)} \quad (2.108)$$

It can be seen that the input reflection coefficient is a periodic function that varies with frequency. The bandwidth Δf of the quarter-wave transformer is defined for the range of $|\Gamma|$ having the maximum allowable limit $|\Gamma_m|$ around the mid frequency f_0 where $|\Gamma| = 0$ and $\theta = \pi/2$. For **TEM** wave, $\theta = \beta l = (\pi/2)(f/f_0)$. At θ_m, $f_m = 2f_0\theta_m/\pi$. Therefore, the bandwidth is given by

$$\Delta f = 2(f_0 - f_m) = 2(f_0 - 2f_0\theta_m\pi)$$
$$= 2f_0(1 - 2\theta_m\pi) \quad (2.109)$$

and the fractional bandwidth $\Delta f/f_0$ is given by

$$\Delta f/f_0 = 2(1 - 2\theta_m\pi) \quad (2.110)$$

where $\theta_m = \cos^{-1}\dfrac{2|\Gamma_m|\sqrt{Z_1 Z_l}}{(Z_l - Z_1)\sqrt{1 - |\Gamma_m|}}$ (2.110a)

At the lower edge of the band, $\theta_1 = \pi f_1/2f_0$ and $\lambda_g = \lambda_{g1}$. At the upper edge of the band, $\theta_2 = \pi f_2/2f_0$ and $\lambda_g = \lambda_{g2}$. Thus, the length of the quarter-wave transformer and the fractional bandwidths are given by

$$l = \frac{\lambda_{g0}}{4} = \frac{\lambda_{g1}\lambda_{g2}}{2(\lambda_{g1} + \lambda_{g2})} \quad (2.111)$$

$$\Delta f/f_0 = \frac{2(\lambda_{g1} - \lambda_{g2})}{(\lambda_{g1} + \lambda_{g2})}$$
$$= \frac{2(f_2 - f_1)}{(f_2 + f_1)} \quad (2.112)$$

Thus, the bandwidth of a single section quarter-wave transformer is small. Therefore, for wide bandwidth, multi-section quarter-wave transformers are used.

ii. Multi Reflections at the Junctions

The overall input reflection coefficient of a single section quarter-wave transformer can be evaluated by considering all reflections at the junctions and neglecting all higher order reflections. Two discontinuties of a single section quarter-wave transformer at which the reflection coefficient Γ and transmission coefficient T are shown in Fig. 2.27. For each junction, the reflection and transmission coefficients are

$$\Gamma_1 = \frac{Z_2 - Z_1}{Z_2 + Z_1}; \Gamma_2 = -\Gamma_1; \Gamma_3 = \frac{Z_3 - Z_2}{Z_3 + Z_2}$$

$$T_{12} = 1 + \Gamma_2 = \frac{2Z_1}{Z_1 + Z_2}$$

$$T_{21} = 1 + \Gamma_1 = \frac{2Z_2}{Z_1 + Z_2} \quad (2.113)$$

For simplicity, let a unit amplitude wave be incident at the input. The overall input reflection coefficient Γ due to infinite number of multiple reflections is given by

$$\Gamma = \Gamma_1 + T_{12}T_{21}\Gamma_3 e^{-2j\theta} + T_{12}T_{21}\Gamma_3^2\Gamma_2 e^{-4j\theta} + \dots$$

$$= \Gamma_1 + T_{12}T_{21}\Gamma_3 e^{-2j\theta}\sum_{n=0}^{\infty}\Gamma_2^n\Gamma_3^n e^{-j2n\theta} \quad (2.114)$$

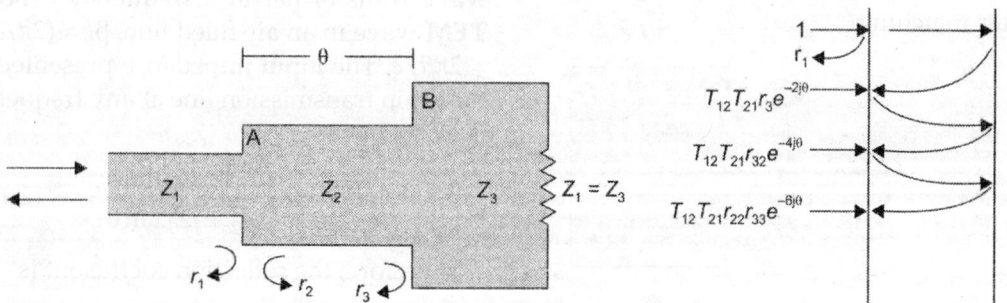

Fig. 2.27: Multiple reflections

Using the relationship $\sum\limits_{n=0}^{\infty} x^n = \dfrac{1}{1-x}$, Eq. (2.114) reduces to

$$\Gamma = \Gamma_1 + \frac{T_{12}T_{21}\Gamma_3 e^{-2j\theta}}{1 - \Gamma_2\Gamma_3 e^{-2j\theta}} \qquad (2.115)$$

Replacing $T_{12} = 1 + \Gamma_2 = 1 - \Gamma_1$ and $T_{21} = 1 + \Gamma_2$ gives

$$\Gamma = \frac{\Gamma_1\Gamma_3 e^{-2j\theta}}{1 + \Gamma_1\Gamma_3 e^{-2j\theta}} \qquad (2.116)$$

If $|\Gamma_1| \ll 1$ and $|\Gamma_3| \ll 1$, Γ becomes

$$\Gamma = \Gamma_1\Gamma_3 e^{-2j\theta} \qquad (2.117)$$

The maximum error in this approximate evaluation is about 4% for $|\Gamma_1|$ and $|\Gamma_3| \leq 0.2$.

2.12.2.2 Multisection Quarter-wave Transformers

Multisection quarter-wave transformers have gradually varying step size. They are used for impedance matching whenever wide bandwidth is required. It is shown in Fig. 2.28 with n section. The two impedances Z_1 and Z_{n+1} are to be matched by $(n-1)$ sections of the quarter-wave transformer. Z_1 is the impedance of the first section and Z_{n+1} is the load impedance. The impedance at each step or junction is given by

$$Z_2 = \sqrt{Z_1 Z_3}\,;\, Z_3 = \sqrt{Z_2 Z_4}\,;\, Z_4 = \sqrt{Z_3 Z_5}\,;\,...$$

$$Z_{n-1} = \sqrt{Z_{n-2} Z_n}\,;\, Z_n = \sqrt{Z_{n-1} Z_{n+1}} \qquad (2.118)$$

Thus, the impedance at the junction is given by

$$Z_i = \sqrt{Z_{i-1} Z_{i+1}} \qquad (2.119)$$

The discontinuity at each junction or step generates a reflection coefficient. Because of discontinuities at the junctions or steps, each component wave undergoes multiple reflections back and forth between any two successive functions. Hence, at any frequency f, the total reflection coefficient Γ_t is given by

$$\Gamma_t = \Gamma_1 + \Gamma_2 e^{-j2\theta} + \Gamma_3 e^{-j4\theta} + ... + \Gamma_n e^{-j2n\theta}$$

$$(2.120)$$

For small reflections, the reflection coefficient Γ_i at the junction of ith and $(i+1)^{th}$ section is given by

$$\Gamma_i = (Z_{i+1} - Z_i)/(Z_{i+1} + Z_i) \qquad (2.121)$$

The last reflection coefficient Γ_n is

$$\Gamma_n = (Z_l - Z_n)/(Z_l + Z_n) \qquad (2.122)$$

2.12.2.3 Tapered Transmission Lines

A length of transmission line whose characteristic impedance varies gradually and continuously is known as *tapered transmission line*. A travelling wave passing such a section will have its voltage to current ratio transformed in accordance with the ratio of the characteristic impedances involved. The requirement for a satisfactory taper is that the change in the characteristic impedance per wavelength should not be too large. Otherwise, tapered section will cause reflections. Figure 2.29 shows a coaxial tapered and a two-wire tapered sections.

The impedance of the tapered line is a function of z in the longitudinal direction. For analysis purpose, the tapered line is assumed to consist of a large number of elementary sections of length dz with incre-

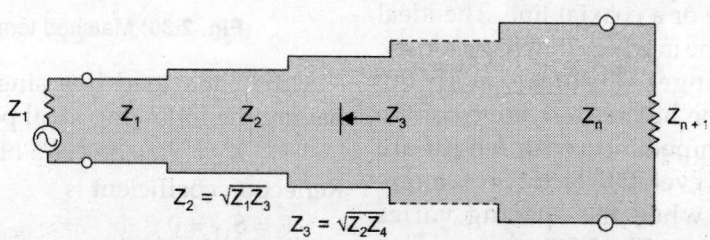

Fig. 2.28: Multisection quarter-wave transformer

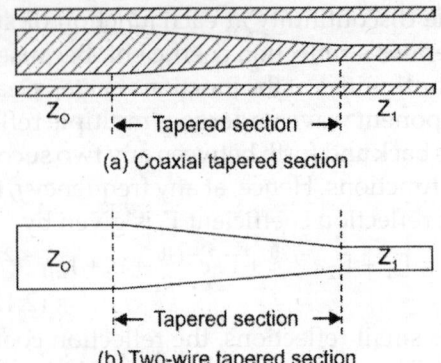

(a) Coaxial tapered section

(b) Two-wire tapered section

Fig. 2.29: Tapered lines (a) Coaxial line and (b) Two-wire line

mental impedance dZ and a differential reflection coefficient $d\Gamma$. The differential reflection coefficient is given by

$$d\Gamma = [(Z + dZ) - Z]/(Z + dZ) + Z]$$
$$= dZ/(2Z + dZ) \qquad (2.123)$$

Since $dZ \ll Z$,

$$d\Gamma = \frac{dZ}{2Z} = \frac{1}{2}d\ln Z \qquad (2.124)$$

Hence, the reflection coefficient at the input of a tapered line of length l is

$$\Gamma_i = \frac{1}{2}\int_0^l d(\ln Z)e^{-j2\beta z} \qquad (2.125)$$

Γ_i can be obtained from the known values of $Z(z)$ or from the frequency response characteristic of Γ_i. A tapered section of a transmission line acts as a perfect impedance matching transformer at high frequencies.

A transmission line can be tapered by varying the spacing between the two conductors in the two-wire lines or by varying the diameter of the inner (or outer) conductor of a concentric line or a coaxial line. The ideal type of taper is one in which the characteristic impedance changes uniformly with the length so that the higher derivatives of the characteristic impedance with length are minimized. However, satisfactory results are obtained even when the spacing varies linearly as shown in Fig. 2.29.

2.12.2.4 Matched Terminations

Matched terminations are extensively used in the laboratory when measuring impedance or scattering parameters. The matched load provides a termination that absorbs all the incident power and hence it is equivalent to termination of the line in its characteristic impedance. They are used in coaxial lines and waveguides to absorb the incident power without any reflection and radiation.

The matched load for a waveguide is a tapered wedge or slab of lossy dielectric placed at the end of a shorted line as shown in Fig. 2.30. Since the dielectric is lossy, the incident power is absorbed. Reflections are avoided by tapering the lossy dielectric into a wedge. Thus the termination may be viewed as a lossy tapered transmission line. An overall length of one or more wavelengths at the lowest frequency of operation is sufficient enough to provide a matched load with an input standing wave ratio of 1.01 or less.

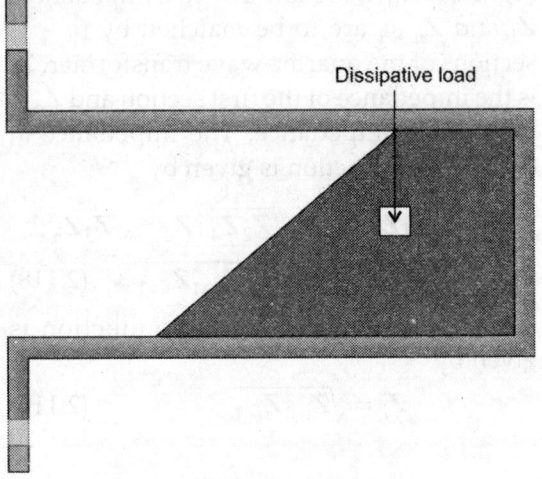

Dissipative load

Fig. 2.30: Matched termination

A matched load is a single port device having the following ideal parameters.

$$Z_{in} = Z_0 = 50 \text{ or } 75 \text{ ohms}$$

Reflection coefficient is

$$\Gamma = S_{11} = 0$$
$$VSWR = 1.0$$

Example 2.15: Determine the length and impedance of a quarter-wave transformer to match a load of 100 Ω to a line with characteristic impedance of 50 Ω at a frequency of 10 GHz for (a) rectangular waveguide with $a = 2.286$ cm and (b) coaxial cable. Find the frequency band over which the reflection coefficient remains less than 0.1.

Solution: Given: $Z_l = 100$ Ω, $Z_1 = 50$ Ω, $f_0 = 10$ GHz, $a = 2.286$ cm, $\Gamma_m = 0.1$.

a. *Rectangular waveguide:*

$$\lambda_0 = \frac{c}{f_0} = \frac{3 \times 10^{10}}{10^{10}} = 3 \text{ cm}$$

$$\lambda_g = \lambda_0 / \sqrt{1 - (\lambda_0 / 2a)^2}$$

$$= 3 / \sqrt{1 - (3/2 \times 2.286)^2}$$

$$= 3 / \sqrt{1 - 0.43}$$

$$= 4 \text{ cm}$$

Hence the length of the quarter-wave transformer is

$$l = \lambda_g / 4 = \textbf{1 cm}$$

b. *Coaxial line:* For air-filled coaxial line, $\lambda_g = \lambda_0 = 3$ cm.
Hence, the length of the quarter-wave transformer is

$$l = \lambda_g / 4 = \textbf{0.75 cm}$$

The characteristic impedance of the matching section is given by

$$Z_2 = \sqrt{Z_1 Z_l} = \sqrt{50 \times 100} = \textbf{70.71 Ω}$$

c. The bandwidth Δf is given by

$$\Delta f = 2f_0(1 - 2\theta_m / \pi)$$

$$\theta_m = \cos^{-1} \left| \frac{2/\Gamma/\sqrt{Z_1 Z_l}}{(Z_l - Z_1)\sqrt{1 - |\Gamma_m|}} \right|$$

$$= \cos^{-1} \left| \frac{2 \times 0.1 \times 70.71}{100 - 50} \sqrt{1 - (0.1)^2} \right|$$

$$= \cos^{-1} \left| \frac{0.2 \times 7071}{50 \times 0.99} \right|$$

$$= \cos^{-1} \left| \frac{0.289}{0.99} \right| = 73.5°$$

$$\Delta f = 2f_0(1 - 2\theta_m / \pi)$$
$$= 2 \times 10(1 - 2 \times 73.5 / 180)$$
$$= \textbf{3.67 GHz}$$

2.13 ADDITIONAL EXAMPLES

Example 2.16: A transmission line with solid dielectric reduces the phase velocity to 2×10^8 m/sec. from its air value. Find the wavelength of a 500 MHz sine wave on this line.

Solution: Given: $v_p = 2 \times 10^8$; $f = 500$ MHz. From Eq. (2.10), the wavelength is given by

$$\lambda = v_p / f$$
$$= 2 \times 10^8 / 500 \times 10^6 = 0.4 \text{ m or } \textbf{40 cm}$$

Example 2.17: A 50 ohms lossless line feeds an antenna of impedance of $(50 + j50)$ ohms at a frequency of 2 GHz. Calculate the voltage reflection coefficient at the load end and determine the VSWR produced.

Solution: Given: $Z_0 = 50$; $Z_l = 50 + j50$
From Eq. (2.53),

$$\Gamma_l = (Z_l - Z_0)/(Z_l + Z_0)$$
$$= (50 + j50 - 50)/(50 + j50 + 50)$$
$$= j50/(100 + j50) = \textbf{0.4472} \angle\textbf{63.4°}$$

The VSWR at the load end is given by Eq. (2.74).

$$S = (1 + |\Gamma_l|)/(1 - |\Gamma_l|)$$
$$= (1 + 0.4472)/(1 - 0.4472)$$
$$= 2.4472/0.5528 = \textbf{2.618}$$

Example 2.18: A transmission line has $Z_o = 75 + j0.01$ ohm and $Z_l = 70 + j50$ ohm. Calculate (a) Γ_l, and (b) T, (c) Verify that $T = 1 + \Gamma_L$ and (d) $T^2 = (1 - \Gamma_L^2) Z_l / Z_0$.

Solution: Given:

$$Z_0 = 75 + j0.01 \text{ ohm,}$$
$$Z_l = 70 + j50 \text{ ohm}$$

(a) From Eq. (2.53),

$$\Gamma_l = (Z_l - Z_0)/(Z_l + Z_0)$$

$$= \frac{[70 + j50 - (75 + j0.01)]}{[70 + j50 + 75 + j0.01]}$$

$$= 50.24 \angle 95.7° / 153.48 \angle 19.0°$$
$$= 0.33 \angle 76.7° = \textbf{0.08 + j0.32}$$

(b) From Eq. (2.60),
$$T = 2Z_l/(Z_l + Z_0)$$

$$= \frac{[2(70 + j50)]}{[70 + j50 + 75 + j0.01]}$$

$$= 172.05 \angle 35.5°/153.48 \angle 19.0°$$

$$= 1.12 \angle 16.5° = \mathbf{1.08 + j0.32}$$

(c) $T = 1.08 + j0.32 = 1 + 0.08 + j0.32 = 1 + \Gamma_l$

(d) $T^2 = [1.12 \angle 16.5°]^2 = \mathbf{1.25 \angle 33°}$

$(1 - \Gamma^2) Z_l / Z_0 = [1 - (0.33 \angle 76.7°)^2] \times$
$$[(70 + j50)/(75 + j0.01)]$$

$$= (86 \angle 35.5°/75 \angle 0°) \times 1.1 \angle -2.5°$$

$$= \mathbf{1.25 \angle 33°}$$

Example 2.19: A transmission line has $Z_0 = 50 + j0.01$ ohm and $Z_l = 73 - j42.5$ ohm. Find: (a) Γ_l and (b) S.

Solution: Given:
$$Z_0 = 50 + j0.01 \text{ ohm,}$$
$$Z_l = 73 - j42.5 \text{ ohm}$$

(a) From Eq. (2.53),
$$\Gamma_1 = (Z_l - Z_0)/(Z_l + Z_0)$$

$$= \frac{[(73 - j42.5) - (50 + j0.01)]}{[70 - j42.5 + 50 + j0.01]}$$

$$= 0.337 \angle -42.7°$$

(c) From Eq. (2.74).
$$S = (1 + |\Gamma_1|)/(1 - |\Gamma_1|)$$
$$= (1 + 0.337)/(1 - 0.337) = \mathbf{2.21}$$

Example 2.20: A lossless transmission line has $Z_0 = 50$ ohm and $Z_l = 75$ ohm. The line is connected to a generator of 50 ohm and a voltage of 30 V (rms). The line is a quarter wavelength. Find (a) the input impedance, (b) the magnitude of instantaneous load voltage, and (c) the instantaneous power delivered to the load.

Solution: Given:
$$Z_0 = 50 \text{ ohm, } Z_l = 75 \text{ ohm, } d = \lambda/4$$
(a) $\beta d = (2\pi/\lambda) \times (\lambda/4) = \pi/2$.

From Eq. (2.39),
$$Z_{in} = R_0^2/R_l = (50)^2/75 = \mathbf{33.3 \text{ ohm.}}$$

(b) The magnitude of the instantaneous voltage at the load is $|V_l| = V_s (1 + \Gamma_l)$. From Eq. (2.53),
$$\Gamma_l = (R_l - R_0)/(R_l + R_0)$$
$$= [75 - 50)/(75 + 50) = \mathbf{0.20}$$
$$\therefore |V_l| = V_s (1 + \Gamma_l) = 30 (1 + 0.20) = \mathbf{36 \text{ V}}$$

(c) The instantaneous power delivered to the load is
$$P_l = (|V_l|)^2/Z_l = 36^2/75 = \mathbf{17.28 \text{ W}}$$

Example 2.21: A lossless transmission line of 80 cm long is operated at 600 MHz. The line parameters are: $L = 0.25$ μH/m, $C = 100$ pF/m. Find: (a) Z_0, (b) β, (c) v_p and (d) Z_{in}.

Solution: Given:
$$L = 0.25 \text{ μH/m, } C = 100 \text{ pF/m}$$
$$f = 600 \text{ MHz, } d = 80 \text{ cm}$$

(a) Since the line is lossless, $R = G = 0$.
From Eq. (2.11),
$$Z_0 = \sqrt{\frac{L}{C}} = \sqrt{\frac{0.25 \times 10^{-6}}{100 \times 10^{-12}}} = \mathbf{50 \text{ ohms}}$$

(b) From Eq. (2.13b),
$$\beta = \omega\sqrt{LC}$$
$$= 2 \times 3.14 \times 600 \times 10^6$$
$$(0.25 \times 10^{-6} \times 100 \times 10^{-12})^{1/2}$$
$$= \mathbf{18.85 \text{ rad} = 1080°}$$

(c) From Eq. (2.14),
$$v_p = \frac{\omega}{\beta} = 1/\sqrt{LC}$$

$$= \left(\frac{1}{0.25 \times 10^{-6} \times 100 \times 10^{-12}}\right)^{1/2}$$

$$= \mathbf{2 \times 10^8 \text{ m/s.}}$$

(d) From Eq. (2.39),
$$Z_{in} = R_0 \frac{Z_l \cos\beta d + jR_0 \sin\beta d}{R_0 \cos\beta d + jZ_l \sin\beta d}$$

$$= 50 [(100 \times \cos(18.85 \times 0.8) + j50 \sin(18.85 \times 0.8)]$$
$$\div [(50 \times \cos(18.85 \times 0.8) + j100 \sin(18.85 \times 0.8)]$$

$= 50 \times (100 \times \cos 864.4° + j50 \sin 864.4°)/$
$\qquad (50 \times \cos 864.4° + j\,100 \sin 864.4°)$
$= 50 \times [-80.9) + j29.5]/(-40.45 + j58.7)$
$= 50 \times 86.1 \angle -19.9°/71.3 \angle -55.4$
$= \mathbf{60.3 \angle 35.5° = 49.1 + j35}$

Example 2.22: A generator of 60 V and 300 ohms delivers power at 100 MHz by means of transmission line of 300 ohms impedance to two 300 ohms load that are in parallel with a capacitive impedance of $-j300$ ohms. Calculate (a) Z_{in} and (b) power dlivered to each load. Assume $\beta l = 288°$

Solution: Given:

$$V_g = 60 \text{ V}, Z_g = 300 \text{ ohms},$$
$$f = 100 \text{ MHz}, Z_0 = 300 \text{ ohms}$$

The effective load impedance is

$$\frac{300 \times 300}{600} = j300.$$

Hence, $Z_{el} = \dfrac{150(-j300)}{(150 - j300)}$

$$= \frac{-j300}{(1 - j2)} = 120 - j60$$

From Eq. (2.39),

$Z_{in} = 300\,[(120 - j60)\cos 288° + j300 \sin 288°]$
$\qquad /[300 \cos 288° + j[(120 - j60) \sin 288°]$

$\qquad = \mathbf{755 - j138.5 \text{ ohms}}$

$$I_g = \frac{V_g}{(Z_g + Z_{in})} = \frac{60}{(300 + 755 - j138.5)}$$

$$= 0.0564 \angle 7.47° \text{ A}$$

The average power delivered to the input of the line is $P_{in} = \frac{1}{2}I_g^2 \times 755 = \mathbf{1.2 \text{ W}}$

Since the line is lossless, the load power is also equal to 1.2 W. Hence, each load receives **0.6 W.**

Example 2.23: A transmission line with $Z_0 = 300$ ohms is terminated with a capacitive impedance of $-j300$ ohms. Calculate (a) Reflection coefficient, (b) SWR and (c) power delivered to the load. Assume $\beta l = 288°$.

Solution: Given: $Z_0 = 300$, $Z_l = -j300$

From Eq. (2.53),

$$\Gamma = \frac{(Z_l - Z_0)}{(Z_l + Z_0)} = \frac{(-j300 - 300)}{(-j300 + 300)}$$

$$= \frac{(-j1 - 1)}{(-j1 + 1)} = -\frac{(1 + j1)}{(1 - j1)}$$

$$= \mathbf{1 \angle 90°}$$

From Eq. (2.74),

$$S = \frac{(1 + |\Gamma|)}{(1 - |\Gamma|)} = \frac{(1 + 1)}{(1 - 1)} = \infty$$

From Eq. (2.39)

$Z_{in} = 300\,[-j300 \cos(288°) + j300 \sin(288°)]/$
$\qquad [-j300 \cos(288°) + j300 \sin(288°)]$
$\qquad = -j300\,(0.95 + 0.309)/(0.309 - 0.95)$
$\qquad = \mathbf{j589 \text{ ohms}}$

Since, Z_{in} is purely inductive impedance, no power can be transferred by the source to the load and hence, no power is delivered to the load.

Example 2.24: A 50 Ω lossless line has a length of 0.4 λ. The operating frequency is 300 MHz. A load of $40 + j30$ is connected at $z = 0$. The source at $z = -l$ is 12 $\angle 0°$ V in series with 50 ohms. Find (a) reflection coefficient, (b) SWR and (c) Z_{in}. Assume $\beta l = 288°$.

Solution: Given:

$$Z_l = 40 + j30, Z_0 = 50,$$
$$f = 300 \text{ MHz}, V_g = 12 \angle 0° \text{ V}$$

(a) From Eq. (2.53),

$$\Gamma = \frac{(Z_l - Z_0)}{(Z_l + Z_0)} = \frac{(40 + j30 - 50)}{(40 + j30 + 50)}$$

$$= \frac{(-1 + j3)}{(9 + j3)} = 0.333 \angle 90°$$

(b) From Eq. (2.74),

$$S = \frac{(1 + |\Gamma|)}{(1 - |\Gamma|)} = \frac{1.333}{0.667} = 2.0$$

(c) From Eq. (2.39),

$Z_{in} = 50\,[(40 + j30) \cos 288° + j50 \sin 288°]/$
$\qquad [50 \cos 288° + j(40 + j30) \sin 288°]$
$\qquad = \mathbf{25.5 + j5.90}$

Example 2.25: The normalized load impedance of a transmission line is $1 + j1$ and the operating wavelength is 5 cm. Using a Smith chart, find the first V_{max}, first V_{min} from the load end and S.

Solution: Given: $z = 1 + j1$, $\lambda = 5$ cm

1. Locate $z_l = 1 + j1$ on the chart as shown in Fig. 2.31.
2. Draw a dashed straight line from the center of the chart through $(1+ j1)$ intersecting the distance scale and read the distance as 0.162 λ.
3. Move from the 0.162 λ point towards the generator and first stop at voltage maximum point on the right hand side of the real axis at 0.25 λ.

$$d_1(V_{max}) = (0.25 - 0.162)\lambda$$
$$= 0.088 \times 5 = \textbf{0.44 cm}$$

4. Similarly, move from this point towards the generator by 0.162 λ and stop at voltage maximum point on the right hand side of the real axis at 0.5 λ. Then

$$d_2(V_{max}) = (0.5 - 0.162)\lambda$$
$$= 0.338 \times 5 = \textbf{1.69 cm}$$

5. Draw the S-circle with center at $(1, 0)$ and passing through the point $(1 + j1)$.
6. The intersection of the circle on the right side of the real axis gives the SWR. Thus, $S = \textbf{2.6}$.

Example 2.26: A transmission line has $Z_0 = 50$ ohm and $S = 2$ when the line is loaded. When the line is shorted, the voltage minimum shifts by 0.15 λ towards the load. Determine the load impedance using a Smith chart.

Solution: Given: $Z_0 = 50$ ohm, $S = 2$

1. When the line is shorted, the first voltage minimum occurs at the load point itself as shown in Fig. 2.32.
2. When the line is loaded, the first voltage minimum shifts 0.15λ from the load. The distance between two successive minima is $\lambda/2$.
3. Draw the S-circle for $S = 2$.
4. Move along the distance scale towards the load a distance 0.15 λ from the minimum point and stop at 0.15 λ.
5. Draw a straight line from this point to the center of the Smith chart.
6. The intersection point between the line and the S-circle is

$$z_l = 1 - j0.65$$

7. The load impedance is

$$Z_l = (1 - j0.65) \times 50 = \textbf{(50 - j32.5) ohm}.$$

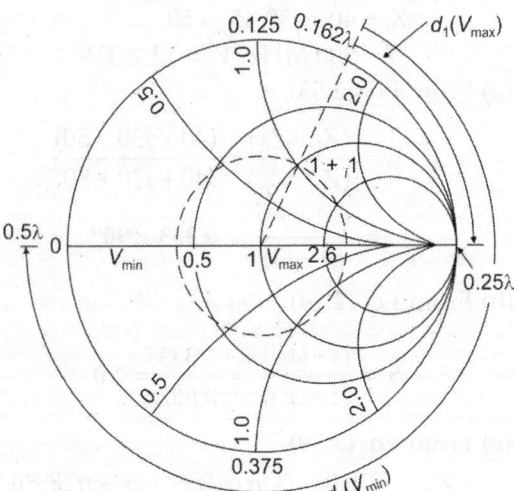

Fig. 2.31: Solution for example 2.25 using Smith chart

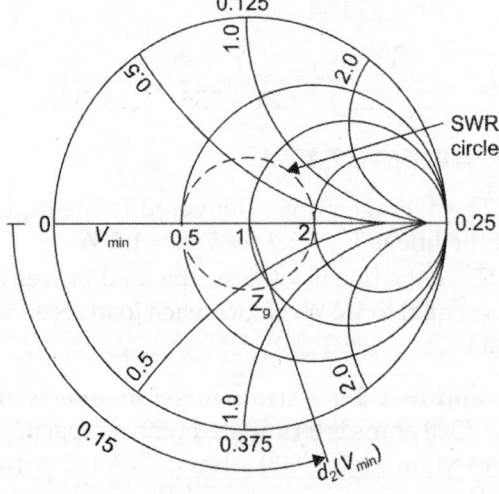

Fig. 2.32: Solution for example 2.26 using a Smith chart

KEY POINTS

- Microwave transmission lines are analyzed in terms of voltage, current and impedance by distributed-circuit theory.

- Transmission lines are employed (i) to transmit electromagnetic energy, (ii) as resonant circuits at very high frequencies, (iii) as measuring devices at high frequencies and (iv) to obtain impedance matching.

- The characteristic impedance Z_0 is the ratio of the voltage and current in an individual wave. It is also the impedance of a finite length of line when $Z_L = Z_0$.

- The propagation constant $\gamma = \alpha + j\beta$ where α is the attenuation constant and β is the phase constant.

- The phase velocity v_p of a transmission line is defined as the product of the wavelength λ and the corresponding frequency f. Thus, phase velocity $v_p = f\lambda = 2\pi f/\beta$

- The normalized impedance z of a transmission line is defined as the ratio of the line impedance to its characteristic impedance. Thus,

$$z = (Z/Z_0) = r \pm jx.$$

The normalized admittance **y** is given by

$$y = Y/Y_0 = Z_0/Z = 1/z = g \pm jb.$$

- The general solution of transmission line equation consists of two waves, incident and reflected waves, travelling in opposite directions with varying amplitudes. This results in the standing waves on the line.

- The reflection coefficient Γ is defined as the ratio of the reflected voltage or current to the incident voltage or current. It is given by

$$\Gamma = V_{ref}/V_{inc} = -I_{ref}/I_{inc}.$$

- Similarly, the reflection coefficient at the load end or the load reflection coefficient is defined as

$$\Gamma_l = V_r e^{\gamma l}/V_s e^{-\gamma l} = (Z_l - Z_0)/(Z_l + Z_0)$$

- The transmission coefficient T is defined as the ratio of the transmitted voltage or current to the incident voltage or current. Thus, transmission coefficient

$$T = V_{tr}/V_{inc} = I_{tr}/I_{inc}.$$

- The standing wave ratio (SWR) S is defined as the ratio of the maximum voltage or current to the minimum voltage or current on the standing wave pattern. Thus, standing wave ratio

$$S = V_{max}/V_{min} = I_{max}/I_{min}.$$

- The standing wave ratio S is related to the reflection coefficient Γ. The exact relations between the two are

$$S = (1 + |\Gamma|)/(1 - |\Gamma|) \text{ and } |\Gamma| = (S - 1)/(S + 1)$$

- The line impedance at voltage maximum or current minimum is given by $Z_{max} = Z_0 S$ and the line impedance at voltage minimum or current maximum is given by $Z_{min} = Z_0/S$.

- The most commonly used graphical tool to solve transmission line problems is the Smith chart. The Smith chart is based on two sets of orthogonal circles. One set of circles represents the ratio $r = R/Z_0$ and other set of circles represents the ratio $x = X/Z_0$ where R and X are the resistance and reactance component of the line impedance and the characteristic impedance Z_0 is a pure resistance for a lossless-line.

- The distance when travelled once around the smith chart is $\lambda/2$ The normalized z or y is repeated for every half wavelength of distance. SWR and impedance at any point on the line can easily be found from the Smith chart.

- Maximum energy is transferred to the load when the load impedance is matched with the characteristic impedance of line.

- A transmission line with characteristic impedance R_0 is matched to a complex load impedance $Z_l = R_l \pm jX_l$ by cancelling the reactive component of the load by a suitable element and transforming the real component to R_0.

- The two methods of impedance matching are narrow band and broadband matching.

- In narrow band matching, single stub, double stub, reactive irises and tuning screws are used.

- In single stub matching, a short section of a short-circuited transmission line, called stub, is used in shunt with the transmission line.

- In double stub matching, two short-circuited stubs with a fixed distance $3\lambda/8$ between them are used in shunt with the transmission line.

- Tuning screws provide the inductance or capacitive reactance required for matching.

- Waveguide windows or irises or diaphragms are used to match the waveguides. They are placed at right angles to the axis of the waveguide.

- In broadband matching, single and multisection quarter-wave transformers, tapered transmission lines and matched terminations are used.

- A quarter-wave transformer is a section of a transmission line that is exactly quarter wavelength.

- A multisection quarter-wave transformer consists of *n*-sections of quarter-wave transformers with gradually varying steps.
- A tapered transmission line is one whose characteristic impedance varies gradually and continuously along the length of the transmission line.
- Matched termination or matched load for a waveguide is a tapered slab or a wedge of loosy dielectric placed at the end of a shorted waveguide.

FURTHER READING

1. Hayt Jr WH and Buck JA (2001). *Engineering Electromagnetics*, New Delhi, TMH.
2. Jordan EC and Balmain KG (1999). *Electromagnetic Waves and Radiating Systems*, New Delhi, PHI.
3. Kuo FF (1965). *Network Analysis and Synthesis*, Singapore, John Wiely.
4. Ryder JD (1997). *Networks, Lines and Fields*, New Delhi, PHI.

REVIEW QUESTIONS

2.1. How does standing wave occur?
2.2. Define standing wave ratio.
2.3. Express S in terms of reflection coefficient $|\Gamma|$.
2.4. Express $|\Gamma|$ in terms of SWR S.
2.5. What is the value of SWR when the load end is shorted?
2.6. What is the value of SWR when the load end is open?
2.7. What is the value of SWR when the load end is terminated with Z_0?
2.8. What is the value of SWR when the load end is terminated with reactance?
2.9. Describe the Smith chart.
2.10. What is a reactance circle?
2.11. What is a resistance circle?
2.12. Mention the applications of the Smith chart.
2.13. What is meant by impedance matching?
2.14. Mention the two steps involved in matching.
2.15. What are the two types of matching methods?
2.16. What is narrow band matching?
2.17. What is single stub matching?
2.18. What is double stub matching?
2.19. Mention the devices used for matching waveguides.
2.20. What is broadband matching?

2.21. What is a quarter-wave transformer?
2.22. What is a tapered line?
2.23. What is a matched termination?

DESCRIPTIVE QUESTIONS

2.1 Derive the transmission line equations.
2.2 Derive from the transmission line equations, Z_0, λ, α, β and v_p for a lossless line.
2.3 Define reflection coefficient and derive the expression for the same.
2.4 Define transmission coefficient and derive the expression for the same.
2.5 Define standing wave ratio and derive the expression for the same.
2.6 Describe the construction of the Smith chart.
2.7 Explain the use of the Smith chart to determine Z of a lossless line of length l terminated with Z_l.
2.8 Explain the use of the Smith chart to determine Z_l from given SWR and position of voltage minima.
2.9 What is impedance matching? Why is it necessary? What are the conditions to be satisfied for proper impedance matching? What are the two methods of impedance matching?
2.10 What is a single stub matching? Explain its design procedure.
2.11 What is a double stub matching? Explain its design procedure.
2.12 Describe the tuning screws, waveguide windows and inductive and capacitive posts.
2.13 Explain how a single section quarter-wave transformer can be used for impedance matching. Derive its bandwidth and reflection coefficient.
2.14 Describe a multisection quarter-wave transformer. Derive an expression for the reflection coefficient.
2.15 Write brief notes on tapered lines and matched terminations.

PRACTICE PROBLEMS

2.1 A 60-ohm lossless transmission line feeds an antenna with $Z_0 = 75 + j75$ ohms at 2 GHz. Calculate Γ_L and VSWR.
[**Ans:** 0.495 $\angle 42.52°$, 2.946]
2.2 In a transmission line of $Z_0 = 50$ ohms, calculate the reflection coefficient for a

load impedance of 0, 50, 100, 160 and 250 ohms.

[**Ans:** −1, 0, 0.33, 0.5 and 0.67]

2.3 In a transmission line of Z_0 = 50 ohms, calculate the reflection coefficient for a load impedance of $-j100, -j50, 0, +j50$ and $+j100$ ohms.

[**Ans:** $1 \angle -53.1°, 1 \angle -90°, 1 \angle -180°, 1 \angle 90°$ and $1 \angle 53°$]

2.4 An impedance of 35 + $j75$ ohms is connected across the load end of a transmission line with Z_0 = 50 ohms. Calculate the reflection coefficient and SWR.

[**Ans:** $\Gamma_L = 0.653 \angle 70.11°$ and S = 4.76]

2.5 A load impedance of $70 \angle 30°$ is connected across the load end of a transmission line with Z_0 = 50 ohms. Calculate the reflection coefficient and SWR.

[**Ans:** $\Gamma_L = 0.315 \angle 55.59°$ and S = 2.92]

2.6 A 50 ohm lossless line connects a signal of 10 GHz to a load of 100 ohms. Calculate the reflection coefficient and VSWR.

[**Ans:** 0.3333, 2]

2.7 A transmission line of length 100 m and Z_0 = 100 ohm operating at 10 MHz is terminated by a load impedance Z_l = 100 − $j200$ ohm. Using smith chart, determine the line impedance and admittance at 25 m from the load.

[**Ans:** $(45 + j120)$ ohm, $(0.0027 - j0.0073)$ mho]

2.8 A lossless transmission line with Z_0 = 50 ohm is terminated with Z_l. The maximum and minimum standing wave voltage is 2.5 V and 1 V respectively and the distance between the successive minima is 5 cm. The line is first terminated by short, and then by the unknown load. The shift in the voltage minimum is 1.25 cm towards the generator. Using a Smith chart, determine the load impedance.

[**Ans:** 34.5 − $j36$ ohm]

2.9 Find the normalized admittance corresponding to a normalized impedance of $z = 0.5 + j0.5$ using Smith chart.

(**Ans:** $1 - j1$)

2.10 Measurements on a 50 ohm line yielded a VSWR of 2, I min_1 at 6 cm and I min_2 at 21 cm. Determine (a) the components of the equivalent series load impedance, and (b) the components of the equivalent parallel load impedance using a Smith chart.

(**Ans:** $77.5 - j34, 92.6 - j208$)

2.11 A load impedance of $(73 - j80)$ Ω is to be matched to a 50 Ω coaxial line, having a lossless dielectric constant of 4, using a short-circuited single stub at 500 MHz. The guide wavelength is 30 cm. Find the position and the length of the stub.

(**Ans:** d = 3.6 cm, l = 3.0 cm)

2.12 A 100 Ω line with air dielectric is terminated by a load of $(75 + j40)$ Ω. It is excited at 1 GHz by a matched generator. Determine the position and length of a single matching stub of 100 Ω impedance.

(**Ans:** d = 9.0 cm, l = 5.1 cm)

2.13 A lossless 50 Ω air dielectric line has V_{max} = 2.5 V and V_{min} = 1.0 V when terminated with an unknown load. The distance between the sucessive minima is 5 cm and the first minimum at the load end is at 1.25 cm. Design a single stub for impedance matching.

(**Ans:** d = 0.35 cm, l = 1.3 cm)

REFERENCES

1. Johnson WL (1980). *Transmission Lines and Networks*, New York, McGraw Hill.

2. Pramanik A (2003). *Electromagnetism, Theory and Applications*, New Delhi, PHI.

3. Rizzi PA (2001). *Microwave Engineering: Passive Circuits*, New Jersey, PH.

4. Collin RE (1992), *Foundations of Microwave Engineering*, McGraw Hill, New York.

5. Terman FE (1955). *Electronics and Radio Engineering*, McGraw Hill, New York

6. Smith PH (1939). *Transmisson Line Calculator, Electronics*, vol. 12 p. 29.

7. Smith PH (1944). *An Improved Transmisson Line Calculator*, Electronics, vol. 13, p 130.

8. Kraus HL (1949). *Transmission Line Charts*, Electrical, Engineering, vol. 68, p 767.

9. Smith PH (1969). *Electronic Applications of Smith Chart*, New York, McGraw Hill.

10. Seely S and Poularikas AD (1979). *Electromagnetics, Classical and Modern Theory and Applications*, Marcel Dekker, New York.

11. Skilling HH (1951). *Electrical Transmission Lines*, New York: McGraw Hill.

12. Liboff RL and Dalman GC (1985). *Transmission Lines, Wave Guides andSmith Charts*, Macmillan, New York.

13. Das A and Das SK (2000). *Microwave Engineering*, TMH, New Delhi.

3 ■ Multiconductor Microwave Transmission Lines

Objectives

- Understand the construction of coaxial cables.
- Discuss the power handling capacity of coaxial cables.
- Know the excitation modes of strip lines.
- Understand the losses that occur in the strip lines.
- Classify the MW strip lines.
- Learn the methods of excitation.
- Define Q of the strip lines.
- Discuss the advantages and disadvantages of coplanar transmission lines.

3.1 INTRODUCTION

Conventional open-wire lines are not suitable at microwave frequencies as transmission lines because of high radiation losses since the wavelength of the signal is smaller than the physical length of the lines at microwave frequencies. The microwave devices and circuits constitute a section or sections of microwave coaxial lines or waveguides. Microwave signals are therefore transmitted through these lines as electromagnetic waves. They are scattered at the junctions of these lines and travel in a well defined ports or directions.

3.2 CLASSIFICATION OF MW TRANSMISSION LINES

The microwave transmission lines are classified as: (i) Multiconductor lines, (ii) Single conductor lines, (iii) Open-boundary structures.

(i) *Multiconductor lines:* These lines have two or more conductors. They are coaxial, strip, slot, microstrip and coplanar lines. The mode of transmission in multiconductor lines is a **TEM** or **quasi-TEM** wave.

(ii) *Single conductor lines:* These are lines that have only one conductor. They are rectangular, circular and ridge waveguides. In single conductor lines, the modes of transmission are either **TE** or **TM** wave or both.

(iii) *Open-boundary structures:* These are dielectric rods. In an open-boundary structure, the mode of transmission is generally a combination of **TE** and **TM** waves known as hybrid **HE** modes.

In this chapter, we shall discuss the multiconductor lines and their characteristics.

3.3 COAXIAL CABLES

Transmission lines consist of two conductors used for carrying electromagnetic waves from one point to another point. They are available in various configurations. The most common forms are coaxial lines or cables. Because of its shielded nature, they are preferred for use at microwave frequencies.

There are three basic types of coaxial cables. They are:
(i) Flexible type
(ii) Semi-rigid type
(iii) Rigid type

These are shown in Fig. 3.1.

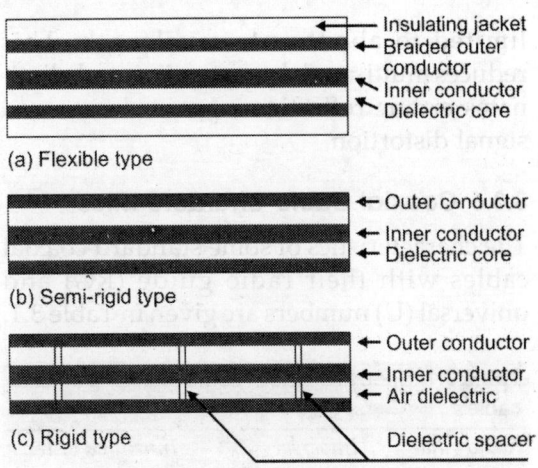

(a) Flexible type

(b) Semi-rigid type

(c) Rigid type

Fig. 3.1: Types of coaxial cables

3.3.1 Flexible Coaxial Cables

Flexible coaxial cable is shown in Fig. 3.1(a). Low loss solid or polyethylene dielectric is used in this type. The outer conductor of the flexible cable is single or double braided. It is constructed with knitted metal wire mesh so as to shield electromagnetic waves effectively.

3.3.2 Semi-Rigid Coaxial Cables

The semi-rigid coaxial cable is shown in Fig. 3.1(b). It has solid dielectric. Its outer conductor is made of thin copper. Hence it can be bent for convenient routing.

3.3.3 Rigid Coaxial Cables

The rigid coaxial cable is shown in Fig. 3.1(c). It uses air dielectric. Short dielectric spacers support the conductors so that no discontinuity is present for the flow of the microwave signal.

3.3.4 Characteristic Impedance of Coaxial Cables

These coaxial cables have a characteristic impedance of 50 ohms or 75 ohms. These cables are used up to microwave frequencies. The upper frequencies of operation of these cables are limited by its attenuation characteristic.

3.3.5 Shielding Effectiveness

The outer conductor shields the leakage of signal from outside to inside. The effectiveness of shielding of the outer conductor is expressed in terms of its transfer impedance Z_T. It is defined as the ratio of the longitudinal voltage V_i induced per unit length on the outside of the shield to the leakage current I_s flowing on the inside of the shield. Thus,

$$Z_T = V_i / I_s \qquad (3.1)$$

Shielding effectiveness of flexible type is low and that of rigid type is high.

Figure 3.2 shows a short section of the cable terminated with matched loads at both ends. The load voltage V_0 is

$$V_0 = V_i / 2 = I_s Z_T / 2 \qquad (3.2)$$

Hence, the transfer impedance Z_T is given by

$$Z_T = 2V_0 / I_s \qquad (3.3)$$

Generally, the average circumference of a coaxial cable for high frequency operation is

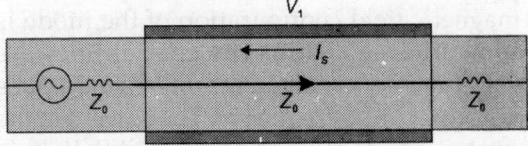

Fig. 3.2: Transfer impedance of a coaxial cable with matched terminations

limited to about one wavelength. This reduces multi-modal propagation and eliminates erratic reflections, power losses and signal distortion.

3.3.6 Coaxial Cable Characteristics

The characteristics of some standard coaxial cables with their radio guide (RG) and universal (U) numbers are given in Table 3.1.

Table 3.1: Specifications of some standard coaxial cables

Radio guide (RG) no.	Universal (U) no.	Z_0 Ω	Inner and outer conductors
RG 9	9/U	50	Silver-plated copper
RG 11	11/U	75	Tinned copper
RG 58A	58A/U	50	Tinned copper
RG 59	59/U	75	Copper
RG141A	141A/U	50	Silver-plated copper
RG179B	179B/U	75	Silver-plated copper
RG 214	214/U	50	Silver-plated copper

3.4 LOSSLESS OR IDEAL COAXIAL LINES

The most common form of microwave transmission lines is coaxial lines or cables. Because of its shielded nature, they are preferred for use at microwave frequencies. Loss-less or perfect coaxial lines consist of an inner perfect conductor and an outer perfect conductor with negligible resistance as shown in Fig. 3.3(a). The two conductors are at different potentials and the space between the two conductors is filled with a uniform loss-less homogeneous dielectric having a dielectric constant ε_r. In symmetrical coaxial lines, the dominant mode of propagation is *TEM* wave. The electric and magnetic field configuration of the mode is shown in Fig. 3.3(b). The coaxial lines are *broadband devices* since the *TEM* mode does not have cut-off frequency. The current in the center conductor of the coaxial line is assumed as

$$I_z = I_0 e^{-\beta g z} \qquad (3.4)$$

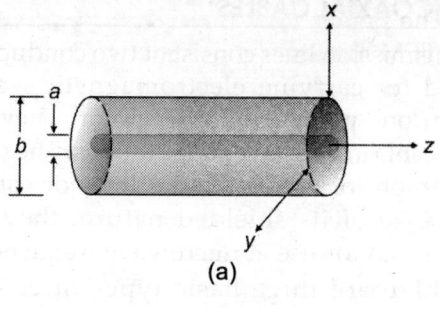

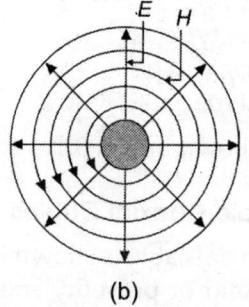

Fig. 3.3: (a) Coaxial line (b) Field configuration

Then, the magnetic intensity is induced by the current around the center conductor and is given by Ampere's law.

$$H_\phi = (I_0/2\pi r) e^{-\beta g z} \qquad (3.5)$$

The potential rise from the outer conductor to the center conductor is

$$V_r = (I_0 h/2\pi r) \ln (b/a) e^{-\beta g z} \qquad (3.6)$$

The characteristic impedance Z_0 of the symmetrical coaxial line with nonmagnetic dielectric is

$$Z_0 = \left(\frac{\eta}{2\pi}\right) \ln\left(\frac{b}{a}\right)$$

$$= \left(\frac{60}{\sqrt{\varepsilon_r}}\right) \ln\left(\frac{b}{a}\right) \text{ohm} \qquad (3.7)$$

Here $\eta = (\sqrt{\mu/\varepsilon})$ is the intrinsic impedance in an unbounded line, $\varepsilon_r = \varepsilon_0$, ε_0 is the dielectric constant of the dielectric medium between the conductors and a is the outer radius of the inner conductor and b is the inner radius of the outer conductor.

The power flow through the coaxial line in TEM modes is given by

$$P_{tr} = \pi V_0^2 /[\eta \ln(b/a)]$$

$$= (\eta I_0^2 /4\pi)(\ln(b/a) = \frac{1}{2} V_0 I_0 \quad (3.8)$$

after substituting for V_0 [from Eq. (3.7)]

3.4.1 Low-Loss Coaxial Lines

The power loss in a coaxial cable is due to the finite conductivity σ of the conductors and the dielectric loss in the medium between the two conductors. In a lossy dielectric, $\varepsilon = \varepsilon' - j\varepsilon'' << 1$ and $\sigma_d/\omega\varepsilon << 1$ where σ_d is the conductivity of the dielectric. Under these conditions, the propagation constant is given by

$$\gamma = \alpha + j\beta = j\omega\sqrt{\mu\varepsilon}\,(1 - j\sigma_d/2\omega\varepsilon)$$

$$= (\sigma_d/2)\left(\sqrt{\mu/\varepsilon}\right) + j\omega/\sqrt{\mu\varepsilon} \quad (3.9)$$

$$\alpha_d = (\sigma_d/2)\left(\sqrt{\mu/\varepsilon}\right) \quad (3.10)$$

$$\beta = \omega\sqrt{\mu\varepsilon} \quad (3.11)$$

Here α_d and β are the *attenuation constant* in the dielectric and the *phase constant* respectively.

The attenuation constant α_c due to power loss in the conductors is given by

$$\alpha_c = R_s \int_s |H|^2 \, dl / \sqrt{\mu/\varepsilon} \int_s |H|^2 \, ds \quad (3.12)$$

The integration is around the periphery of the two conductors $s = s_1 + s_2$. R_s is the surface resistance.

The *total attenuation constant* of the line is the sum of the two attenuation constants. Thus,

$$\alpha = \alpha_d + \alpha_c \quad (3.13)$$

The distributed parameters of the coaxial line are given by

$$R = (R_s/2\pi)\,(1/a + 1/b) \quad (3.14)$$

$$L = \sqrt{\mu_0 \varepsilon'} Z_0 = (\mu_0/2\pi)\ln b/a \quad (3.15)$$

$$G = \omega\varepsilon'' C/\varepsilon' \quad (3.16)$$

$$C = \sqrt{\mu_0\varepsilon'}/Z_0 = 2\pi\varepsilon'/\ln(b/a) \quad (3.17)$$

For low loss coaxial lines:

$$a_d = GZ_0/2, \quad a_c = R/2Z_0 \quad (3.18)$$

$$\alpha = \frac{1}{2}\left[R\sqrt{(C/L)} + G\sqrt{(L/C)}\right] \quad (3.19)$$

$$Z_0 = \sqrt{L/C} \quad (3.20)$$

The characteristic impedance of a coaxial line with $b/a = 3.6$ is equal to 76.86 ohm for air dielectric and it is 50.67 for solid polyethylene dielectric with minimum attenuation. The coaxial lines with 50 ohm are commonly used for minimum attenuation, as the attenuation coefficient does not vary considerably with b/a ratio.

3.4.2 Higher-Order Modes

Higher order modes are generated in a coaxial line at sufficiently high frequencies. The lower cut-off frequency of higher order modes is very high. Hence, higher order modes do not interfere at the normal lower operating frequencies. The lowest order higher order modes in coaxial lines are TE_{11} and TM_{01} modes. The cut-off wavelengths of these modes are:

(i) *For TE_{11} mode:*

$$\lambda_c = \pi(a + b) \quad (3.21)$$

(ii) *For TM_{01} mode:*

$$\lambda_c = 2(b - a) \quad (3.22)$$

The field configuration of the higher order modes are shown in Fig. 3.4. In order to prevent the higher order mode interference, the average circumference of the inner and outer conductors should be less than the wavelength at the operating frequency.

The two conductors of a coaxial line are *not* at equal and opposite potentials with respect to ground. Hence it is said to be an unbalanced line. The outer conductor is generally grounded and is ideally at ground potential whereas the inner conductor is at different potential with respect to ground. Any equipment connected between the lines introduces unequal impedances in both the lines. Hence, when coaxial cables are used

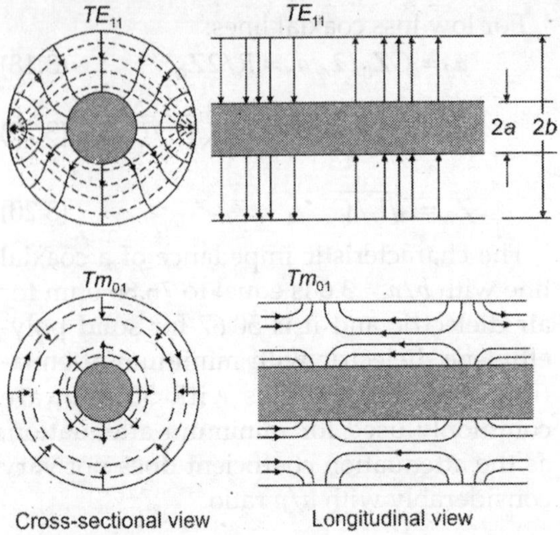

TE_{11} TE_{11}

$2a$ $2b$

Tm_{01} Tm_{01}

Cross-sectional view   Longitudinal view

Fig. 3.4: Higher order modes in coaxial lines (**E**-field), ... (**H**-field), ...

to feed balanced circuits such as parallel-wire lines or dipole antenna, impedance matching devices must be used for proper transfer of energy.

3.5 COAXIAL CABLE CONNECTORS AND ADAPTORS

Standard shielded connectors are used to terminate the coaxial cables or to connect to other components. To maintain low reflection or low VSWR, it is mandatory to standardize the coaxial connectors. These connectors are of various types depending on the frequency range and cable diameter. Several types of commonly used microwave coaxial connectors are described below.

3.5.1 Navy Type Connector

This type of connector is also known as N-type connector. It was mainly designed for defense applications during World War II. Its electrical and mechanical characteristics have been improved over the years. An improved version is shown in Fig. 3.5.

The right hand portion of the connected-pair is the *female* connector and the left portion is the *male* connector. It is the most commonly used connector in the frequency range of 1 to 18 GHz. Its characteristic impedance is 50 or 75 ohms with extremely low VSWR (<1.02). It is suitable for flexible or rigid cables.

The connectors are mated by threading them together until surface A of the male portion contacts firmly against surface A' of the female connector. When the connectors mate, the surfaces B and B' are separated by a few miles. Because of this discontinuity, a low reflection occurs. However, the gap is necessary to protect the center pin of the female conductor from getting mechanically damaged.

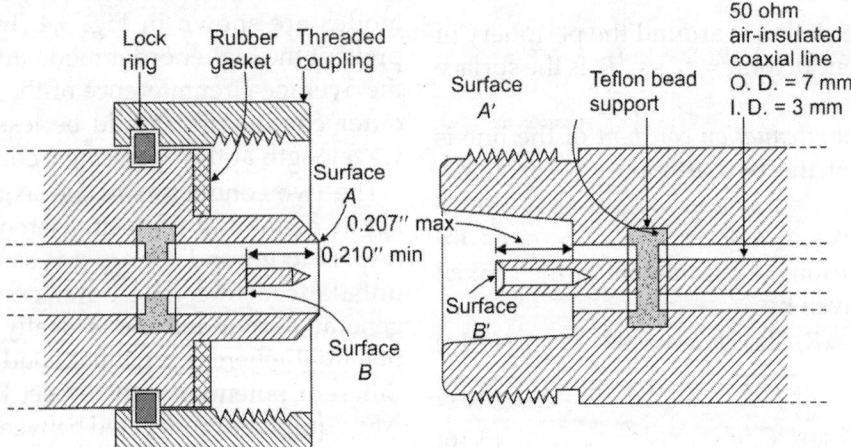

Fig. 3.5: N-type connector-pair for 50 ohm–7 mm lines

3.5.2 Bayonet Navy Type Connector

This type of connector is also known as **BNC** connector. It was originally designed for military applications during World War II. It is the most commonly used connector for frequencies up to 1 GHz. Its characteristic impedance is 50 or 75 ohms. It is suitable for flexible cables with diameters of up to 0.25 inch (6.35 mm).

3.5.3 Threaded Navy Type Connector

This type of connector is also known as **TNC** connector. The TNC is a threaded connector. The purpose of the thread is to make firm contact in the mating surface so as to prevent radiation at high frequencies. It can be used up to 12 GHz.

3.5.4 Subminiature Type-A Connector

This type of connector is also known as the SMA connector. It is used for thin flexible or semi-rigid cables. It is commonly used in low-power applications at higher MW frequencies, usually C, X and Ku bands. Figure 3.6 shows such a connector. They are designed for use with a Teflon-filled 50 ohms coaxial cable. Mating of the connectors is obtained by threading them together until surface A of the male portion contacts firmly against surface A' of the female connector. Since Teflon is compressible, threading the connector-pair together results in a firm contact between the corresponding Teflon surfaces.

The maximum frequency of operation is given by

$$f_{max} = 0.95c / \left[\pi(a+b)\sqrt{\mu_r \varepsilon_r} \right] \quad (3.23)$$

The frequency of operation is limited to 24 GHz because it generates higher-order modes beyond this frequency. The maximum SWR of the mated connector-pair is given by

$$SWR_{max} = 1.05 + 0.005f \quad (3.24)$$

where f is in GHz.

3.5.5 Subminiature Type-C Connector

This type of connector is also known as the SMC connector. It is smaller than SMA connector. It is a 50 Ω connector. It is suitable for flexible cables up to 0.125 inch or 3.17 mm. It can be used up to 7 GHZ.

3.5.6 Amphenol Precision Type Connector-7 mm

This type of connector is also known as **APC-7** connector. For precise measurements in coaxial systems, the two requirements are:

1. Reflection due to connector-pair is low, i.e. low SWR.
2. Connections are electrically repeatable even after many operations.

The APC-7 connectors satisfy these requirements fully. The APC-7 connector provides a unique coupling mechanism suitable for male or female connector. Since both male and female connectors are identical, they are known as *sexless* connectors.

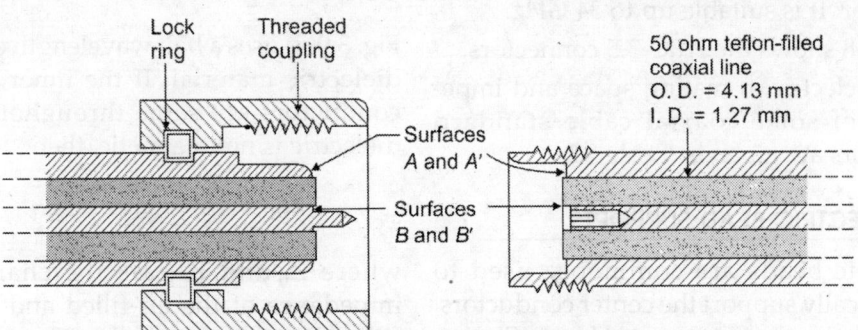

Fig. 3.6: SMA type connector-pair for teflon-filled 50 ohm lines

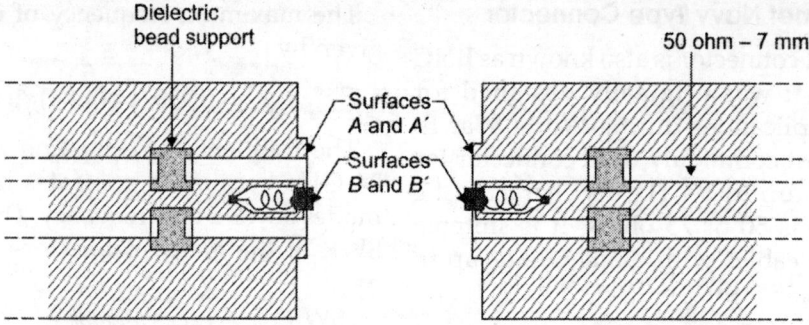

Dielectric bead support

Surfaces A and A'

Surfaces B and B'

50 ohm – 7 mm

Fig. 3.7: APC–7 connector-pair for use with 50 ohm–7 mm lines

Figure 3.7 shows such a connector. They are mated together by a threading arrangement. In this case, the surfaces *B* and *B'* touch first. The spring mechanism behind the surfaces *B* and *B'* cause them to retract until a firm contact is established between *A* and *A'*. Thus, both inner and outer conductors are in firm contact simultaneously. There is no center conductor discontinuity. Hence, this is the most repeatable 50-ohm connector with extremely low VSWR of 1.02. SWR value of this mated pair is repeatable within ±0.002 even after hundreds of operations. It is suitable up to 18 GHZ. Thus, this is an excellent connector for precise measurement.

3.5.7 Amphenol Precision Type Connector-3.5 mm

This type of connector is also known as **APC–3.5** connector. The APC-3.5 is used for repeatable connections. It is a 50-ohm connector with low VSWR. Its male or female end can mate with the opposite type SMA connector. It is suitable up to 34 GHz.

Fig. 3.8 shows the APC-3.5 connectors.

The dielectric in mating space and impedances of some coaxial cable standard connectors are given in Table 3.2.

3.6 DIELECTRIC BEAD SUPPORTS

Dielectric beads are commonly used to mechanically support the center conductors. Fig. 3.9 shows the four types of low-reflection bead supports. The first type shown in

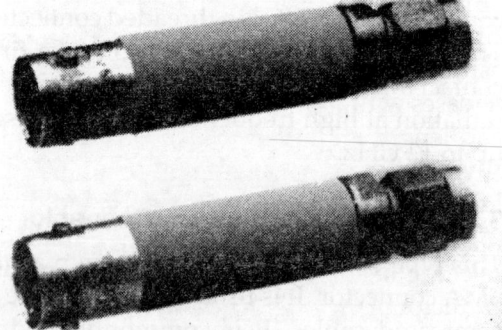

Fig. 3.8: APC-3.5

Table 3.2: Standard coaxial cable mating connectors

Type	Sex	Dielectric	Impedance
N	M/F	air	50/75
BNC	M/F	solid	50/75
TNC	M/F	solid	50/75
SMA	M/F	solid	50
APC-7	sexless	air	50
APC-3.5	sexed	air	50

Fig. 3.9(a) uses a half wavelength of low-loss dielectric material. If the inner and outer conductors are same throughout and the dielectric is nonmagnetic, then

$$Z_{01} = \frac{Z_0}{\sqrt{\varepsilon_r}} \tag{3.25}$$

where Z_0 and Z_{01} are the characteristic impedance of the air-filled and dielectric-filled lines respectively. The impedance repeats itself for every half wavelength.

Therefore, a matched load ($Z_{in} = Z_0$) connected to the air-filled line on the right side results in $Z_{in} = Z_0$ at the left edge of the dielectric. Thus, unity SWR is achieved along the Z_0 line. Hence, no reflection takes place. The disadvantage of this type of supports is that the SWR is dependent on the frequency since the bead can be one half of a wavelength only at the designated frequency.

The second type of bead support is shown in Fig. 3.9(b). It has a length of 0.02λ or less at the highest frequency of interest. The bead represents a very short length of low-impedance line. Hence, it is equivalent to a shunt capacitance. Therefore its SWR increases with the operating frequency. Since bead length is limited to 0.02λ, a mechanically rigid support is difficult to achieve at higher frequencies.

Figure 3.9(c) shows the third type of dielectric bead support. In this, the center conductor of the dielectric section is reduced such that the same characteristic impedance is maintained throughout the structure. Hence, we have

$$138 \log (b/a) = \left(\frac{138}{\sqrt{\varepsilon_r}}\right) \log \left(\frac{b}{a_1}\right) \quad (3.26)$$

Since the characteristic impedance is same in both air-filled and dielectric-filled lines, the SWR is practically unity at all frequencies. The radius b is so chosen as to avoid TE_{11} mode propagation. The dielectric bead is of $\lambda/4$ long at the highest frequency of interest so that the overall reflection is minimum.

The fourth type of dielectric bead support is shown in Fig. 3.9(d). This is used in both N-type and APC-7 type connectors. The dielectric material commonly used is Teflon or rexolite. The diameters of the conductors in the dielectric region are adjusted such that $Z_{01} = Z_0$. The capacitance effects due to the step discontinuities are compensated by under-cutting the dielectric on both ends as shown in Fig. 3.9(d). These behave like series inductances. For the Type-N connector, the Teflon bead is undercut by about 0.30 cm.

Adapters are passive devices having different connectors at the two ends. They

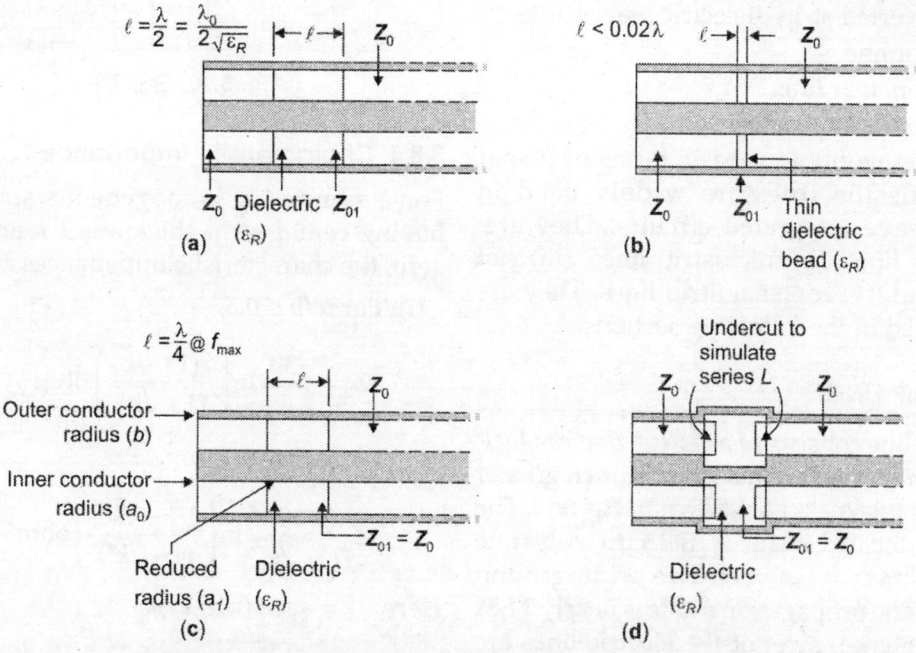

Fig 3.9: Four types of dielectric bead supports for coaxial lines

are used for interconnection between two different microwave ports.

3.7 PLANAR TRANSMISSION LINES

Planar transmission lines are *flat* transmission lines with low profile and light in weight. The development of planar transmission lines has led to miniaturization of microwave circuits. They may have two or more conductors. Because of the planar geometry, the line dimensions can be defined in a single plane to control their characteristic impedances. They are therefore suitable for microwave integrated circuits. The complete transmission line circuits can be fabricated in a single step using thin film technology and photolithography techniques.

Planar transmission lines are formed on different substrates and in various configurations. These structures are:

1. Microstrip line.
2. Inverted microstrip line.
3. Suspended microstrip line.
4. Microstrip with overlay.
5. Strip dielectric waveguide.
6. Inverted strip dielectric waveguide.
7. Slot line.
8. Coplanar line.
9. Coplanar strip line.

Of these, only four basic forms of planar transmission lines are widely used in microwave integrated circuits. They are: (i) strip lines, (ii) microstrip lines, (iii) slot lines and (iv) coplanar strip lines. They are discussed in the following sections.

3.8 STRIP LINES

A strip line consists of a central *thin conducting strip* of width w that is very much greater than its thickness t as shown in Fig. 3.10. The strip is located inside a dielectric substrate of thickness b between two wide ground plates. The propagation mode is nearly **TEM** mode. Hence, most of the electric lines are perpendicular to the center strip and the

ground plates and are concentrated over the width of the center conductor with fringe field lines at the edges of the center conductor. The fringe field lines extend up to certain distance from the edges of the center strip beyond which the field is practically zero. When the thickness $b < \lambda/2$, the field cannot propagate in the transverse direction and decreases exponentially. The energy is confined inside the strip line cross-section if the width of the ground plates $a > 5b$. Hence, vertical sidewalls are not necessary at the transverse ends. The commonly used dielectrics are teflon, polystyrene etc. The lines are suitable for use in the frequency range of 100 MHz to 30 GHz.

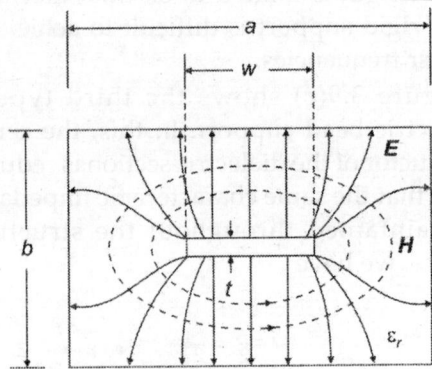

Fig. 3.10: Strip line

3.8.1 Characteristic Impedance

For a symmetric homogeneous strip line having center strip thickness t tending to zero, the characteristic impedances are:

(i) **For $w/b \leq 0.5$,**

$$Z_0 = \frac{30}{\sqrt{\varepsilon_r}} \ln\left(\frac{2(1+\sqrt{k})}{(1+\sqrt{k})}\right) \text{ohm} \qquad (3.27)$$

(ii) **For $w/b > 0.5$,**

$$Z_0 = \frac{30\pi^2}{\sqrt{\varepsilon_r}} \ln\left(\frac{2(1+\sqrt{k'})}{(1-\sqrt{k'})}\right) \text{ohm} \qquad (3.28)$$

Here $k = \text{sech}\,(\pi w/2b)$ $\qquad (3.29)$

$k' = \sqrt{(1-k^2)} = \tanh\,(\pi w/2b)$ $\qquad (3.30)$

When the center conductor of a symmetrical strip line $t \neq 0$, then an accurate value of the characteristic impedance can be found by method of moments.

For $w/b \geq 0.35$, the characteristic impedance of the symmetrical strip line is given by

$$Z_0 = \frac{94.15}{\sqrt{\varepsilon_r}} \left(\frac{wK}{b} + \frac{C_f}{8.854\varepsilon} \right)^{-1} \text{ ohm} \quad (3.31)$$

Here C_f is the fringe capacitance in pF/m due to fringe electric field at the edges of the strip and is given by

$$C_f = 8.854 \, \varepsilon_r \, [2K \ln (K + 1) - (K - 1)$$
$$\ln (K^2 - 1)] \text{ pF/m} \quad (3.32)$$
$$K = 1/(1 - t/b) \quad (3.33)$$

The variation of the characteristic impedance Z_0 of a partially shielded strip line with w/b for various values of t/b is shown in Fig. 3.11. The value of the characteristic impedance Z_0 decreases with increase in w/b and also with t/b. Practical microwave integrated circuits employ a thickness t of the order of 1.5 to 3 mils. Hence error introduced for zero thickness assumption is negligible.

When w/b is large, the strip line is completely shielded to avoid radiation. A shielded strip line consists of a *very thin* strip center conductor ($t/w \ll 1$) embedded in a low loss or loss-less dielectric medium enclosed in a rectangular metallic box. In the case of completely shielded strip line with large w, a more uniform **TEM** field region exists between the center strip and the horizontal plates. However, because of proximity between the edges and the sidewalls, fringe fields increase at the strip edges and some field lines terminate at the sidewalls. Hence fringe capacitance increases and the characteristic impedance Z_0 decreases considerably. Because w is large, the thickness of the strip is not negligible since it must have adequate mechanical strength to support the central strip when the dielectric is air. The variations of the characteristic impedance Z_0 are shown in Fig. 3.12 for a wide strip shielded in a rectangular box.

The electric field distribution in the cross-section of a typical shielded strip line where the fields are uniform within the range of the center conductor is shown in Fig. 3.13. As the propagation mode in strip lines is nearly **TEM** mode, the guide wavelength is given by $\frac{\lambda}{\sqrt{\varepsilon_r}}$.

3.8.2 Higher Modes in Strip Lines

The strip lines with **TEM** mode of propagation has considerably large operating bandwidth. The upper frequency limit is set by the presence of the nearest higher order **TE**$_{10}$ and **TM**$_{11}$ modes. Approximate expressions for the cut-off wavelength for these modes are:

$$\lambda_o(\textbf{TE}_{10}) = (2w + \pi b/2) \sqrt{\varepsilon_r} \quad (3.34)$$
$$\lambda_o(\textbf{TM}_{11}) = 2b \sqrt{\varepsilon_r} \quad (3.35)$$

When the strip is considerably wide, the cut-off conditions can be estimated by analyzing the cross-section by finite element method (FEM). Figure 3.14 shows the cut-off wavelengths for higher order modes for typical shielded strip lines.

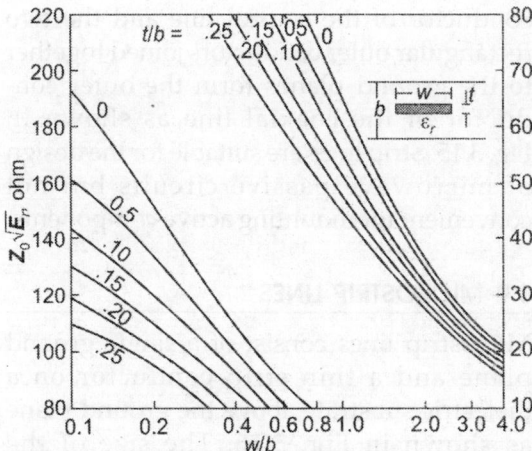

Fig. 3.11: Characteristic impedance Z_0 versus w/b plot

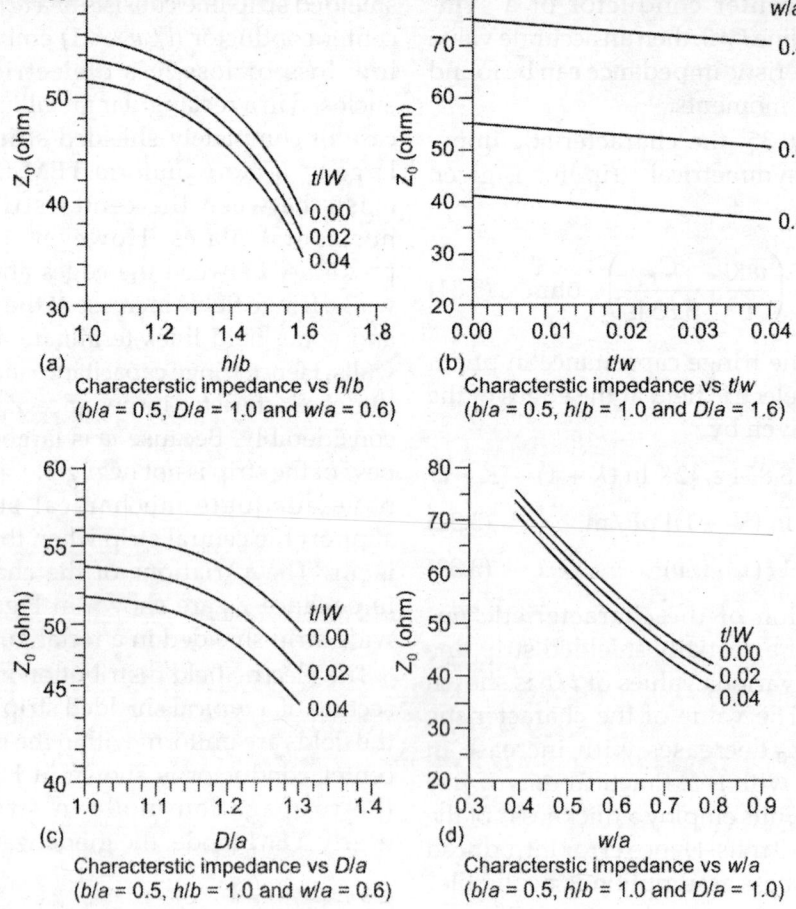

Fig. 3.12: Variation of characteristic impedance Z_0

3.8.3 Losses in Strip Lines

When the dielectric substrate is of low loss material, the attenuation factor in the strip line is due to the losses in the conductor. The attenuation factor is given by

For $w \geq 2b$ and $t \leq b/10$,

$$\alpha_c = \frac{(R_s/Z_0 b)[(\pi w/b) + \ln(4b/\pi t)]}{(\ln 2 + \pi w/2b)}$$
neper/unit length (3.36)

Here $R_s = \sqrt{\pi f \mu / \sigma}$

3.8.4 Excitation of Strip Lines

Coaxial lines with special connector or launcher are used as interface to excite the strip lines. The launcher consists of a *thin flat* *small center conductor*. This forms the center conductor of the coaxial line and the two rectangular outer conductors joined together to the ground planes form the outer conductor of the coaxial line as shown in Fig. 3.15. Strip lines are suitable for the design of microwave passive circuits but not convenient for mounting active components.

3.9 MICROSTRIP LINES

Microstrip lines consist of a single ground plane and a thin strip conductor on a dielectric substrate above the ground plane as shown in Fig. 3.16. The size of the microwave solid-state devices is very small, of the order of 0.008 to 0.08 mm^3. These

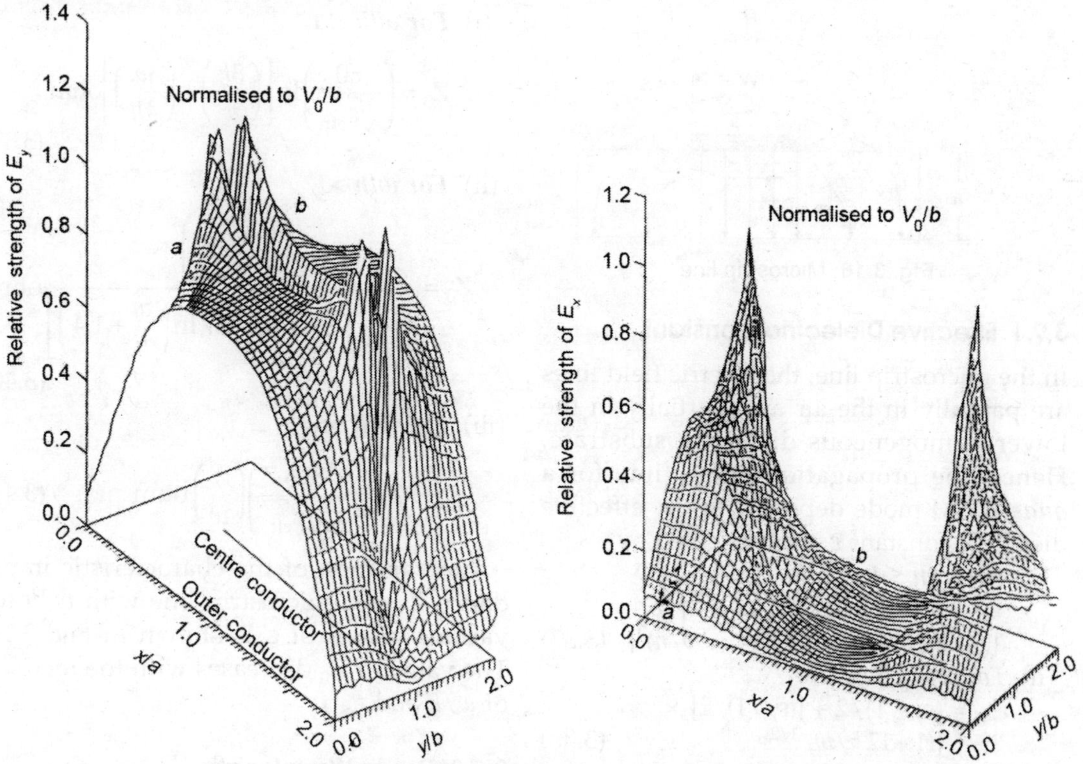

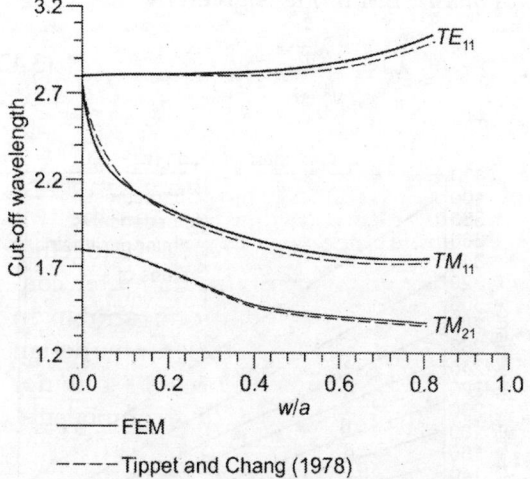

Fig. 3.13: Electric field distribution in a shielded strip line

Fig. 3.14: Cut-off wavelength versus *w/a*

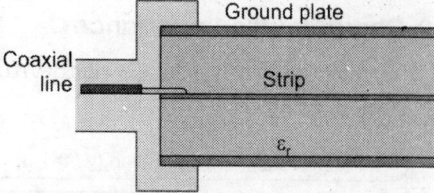

Fig. 3.15: Strip line launcher connector

devices are mounted on the microstrip lines for inputting the signal and extracting output power from them. Hence, the microstrip lines should be such that the devices are easily mounted on them. Since there is no ground plate and dielectric substrate is above the microstrip line, the electric field lines remain partially in the air and partially in the lower dielectric substrate. Because of this, the propagation mode is called *quasi*-**TEM** mode. The microstrip line radiates electro-magnetic energy due to open structure and possible discontinuity. The radiation loss is proportional to the square of the frequency. Thin and high dielectric materials are used to reduce the radiation loss of the open structure where the electric fields are mostly confined inside the dielectric.

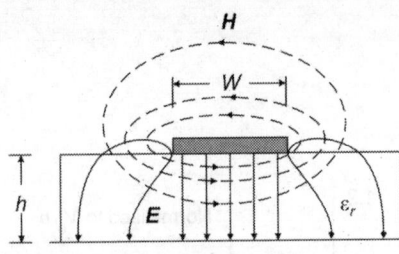

Fig. 3.16: Microstrip line

3.9.1 Effective Dielectric Constant

In the microstrip line, the electric field lines are partially in the air and partially in the lower homogeneous dielectric substrate. Hence, the propagation delay time for a *quasi*-TEM mode depends on the effective dielectric constant ε_{eff} and is given by

(i) *For w/h* ≤ 1:

$$\varepsilon_{eff} = (\varepsilon_r + 1)/2 + [(\varepsilon_r - 1)/2] \times$$
$$[(1 + 12\,h/w)^{-1/2} + 0.04\,(1 - w/h)^2] \quad (3.37)$$

(ii) *For w/h* $\gg 1$:

$$\varepsilon_{eff} = (\varepsilon_r + 1)/2 + [(\varepsilon_r - 1)/2] \times$$
$$[(1 + 12\,h/w)^{-1/2}] \quad (3.38)$$

Here ε_r is the relative dielectric constant of the substrate.

3.9.2 Characteristic Impedance

The characteristic impedance of the microstrip lines is given by:

(i) *For w/h* ≤ 1,

$$Z_0 = \left(\frac{60}{\sqrt{\varepsilon_{eff}}}\right) \ln\left[\left(\frac{8h}{w}\right) + \left(\frac{w}{4h}\right)\right] \text{ohm} \quad (3.39)$$

(ii) *For w/h* > 1,

$$Z_0 = \frac{\left(\dfrac{376.7}{\sqrt{\varepsilon_{eff}}}\right)}{\left[\left(\dfrac{w}{h}\right) + 1.4 + 0.667 \ln\left(\dfrac{w}{h} + 1.4\right)\right]} \text{ohm} \quad (3.40)$$

(iii) *For w/h* $\gg 1$,

$$Z_0 = \left(\frac{376.7}{\sqrt{\varepsilon_{eff}}}\right)\left(\frac{h}{w}\right) \text{ohm} \quad (3.41)$$

The variation of the characteristic impedance Z_0 of a microstrip line with w/h for various values of ε_r is shown in Fig. 3.17. The value of Z_0 decreases with the increase of w/h and ε_r.

3.9.3 Guide Wavelength

The guide wavelength for the propagation of *quasi*-TEM mode is given by

$$\lambda_g = \frac{\lambda_0}{\sqrt{\varepsilon_{eff}}} \quad (3.42)$$

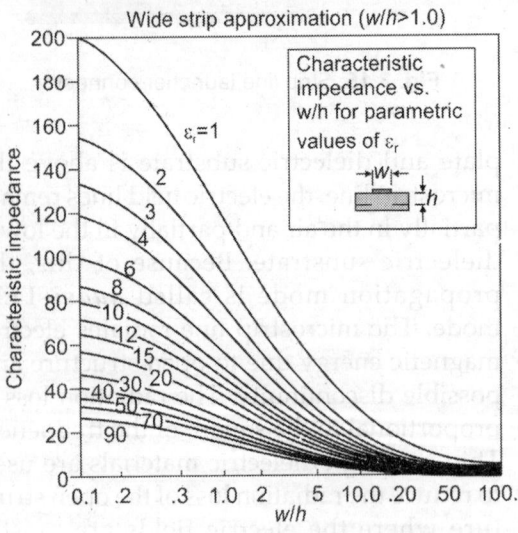

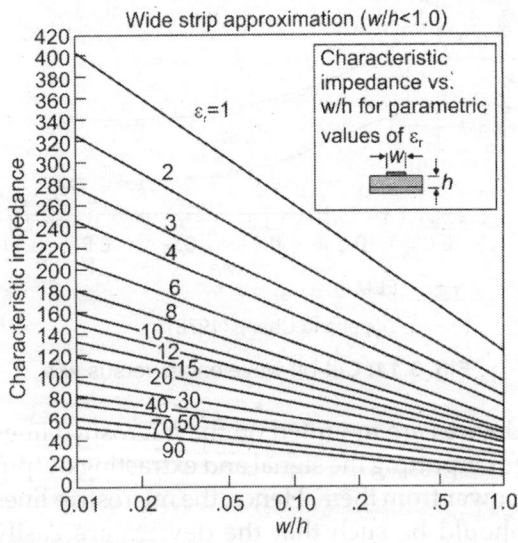

Fig. 3.17: Characteristic impedance Z_0 versus w/h

3.9.4 Losses in Microstrip Lines

Two types of losses occur in a microstrip line with nonmagnetic substrate for the signal attenuation. They are:

 (i) Dielectric loss in the substrate
 (ii) Ohmic loss in the strip conductor and the ground plane due to finite conductivity
 (iii) Radiation loss due to the thin open structure and possible discontinuity in the strip conductor.

The *total attenuation constant* of the line is the sum of the two attenuation constants; the dielectric attenuation constant α_d and ohmic attenuation constant α_c. Thus,

$$\alpha = \alpha_d + \alpha_c \qquad (3.43)$$

$$\alpha_d = (\sigma_d/2)\left(\sqrt{\mu/\varepsilon}\right) \qquad (3.44a)$$

$$= 27.3\,[(\varepsilon_{\text{eff}} - 1)/(\varepsilon_r - 1)]\,(\varepsilon_r/\varepsilon_{\text{eff}}) \times$$
$$(\tan\delta/\lambda_g)\ \text{dB/m} \qquad (4.44b)$$

Here σ_d is the conductivity of the dielectric substrate and $\tan\delta = \sigma_d/w\varepsilon$ *is the dielectric loss tangent.*

For a low loss dielectric substrate, the attenuation at microwave frequencies is mainly due to finite conductivity of strip conductor. This gives rise to ohmic losses due to current on the strip conductor. The distribution of current in the transverse plane is fairly uniform, with minimum value at the central axis and peaks to a maximum at the edges of the strip. Assuming uniform current distribution in the region $-w/2$ to $+w/2$, the attenuation constant due to ohmic loss of a wide line, $w/h > 1$, is given by

$$\alpha_c = \left(\frac{8.686}{Z_0 w}\right)\sqrt{\frac{\pi f\mu}{\sigma}}\ \text{dB/m} \qquad (3.45)$$

The variation of attenuation constant due to ohmic loss a_c for a wide range of w/h is shown in Fig. 3.18. Enclosing the microstrip with a metallic box with first resonance frequency much above the signal frequency eliminates the radiation loss of microstrip lines.

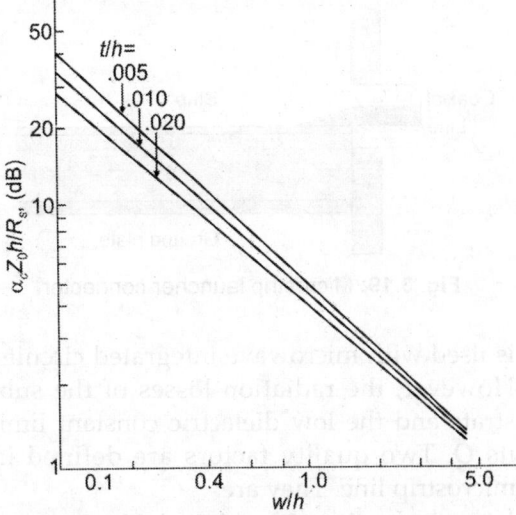

Fig. 3.18: Attenuation constant versus *w/h*

3.9.5 Substrate Materials

The widely used substrate materials for strip and microstrip lines and their electrical properties are given in Table 3.1.

Table 3.1: Substrate materials and their properties

Material	Dielectric constant ε	$\tan\delta$
Air	1	0
Alumina	9.6 to 10	0.0005 to 0.002
Polystyrene	2.53	4.7×10^{-4}
PTFE	2.2	0.0002 to 0.0005
Quartz	3.8	0.0001
RT/Duroid 5880	2.26	0.001
Sapphire	9.4	0.0002

3.9.6 Excitation of Microstrip Lines

Microstrip lines are excited by coaxial line through a launcher connector as shown in Fig. 3.19. Microstrip lines are highly suitable for the design of microwave passive circuits and series mounting of active devices across a gap in the strip.

3.9.7 Q of Microstrip Lines

Microwave integrated circuits require very high-Q resonant circuits. The quality factor Q of a microstrip line is very high. Hence, it

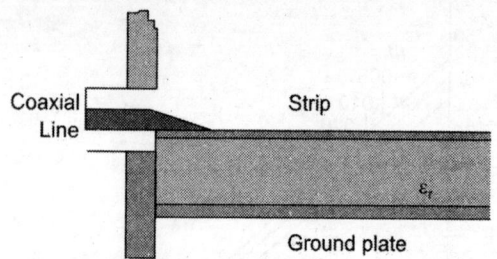

Fig. 3.19: Microstrip launcher connector

is used with microwave integrated circuits. However, the radiation losses of the substrate and the low dielectric constant limit its Q. Two quality factors are defined in microstrip line. They are:

(i) the quality factor Q_c related to the conductor attenuation constant and

(ii) the quality factor Q_d related to the dielectric attenuation constant.

(i) Quality factor Q_c

The ohmic attenuation constant in a wide microstrip line with uniform current distribution is given by

$$\alpha_c = \frac{8.686 R_s}{Z_0 w} \qquad (3.46)$$

Its characteristic impedance is given by

$$Z_0 = \left(\frac{h}{w}\right)\sqrt{\left(\frac{\mu}{\varepsilon}\right)} = \left(\frac{377}{\sqrt{\varepsilon_r}}\right)\left(\frac{h}{w}\right) \quad (3.47)$$

The wavelength in the microstrip line is given by

$$\lambda_g = \frac{30}{\left(f\sqrt{\varepsilon_r}\right)} \qquad (3.48)$$

In the above equation, f is in GHz.

Q_c is related to the conduction attenuation constant and is given by

$$Q_c = 27.3/a_c \qquad (3.49)$$

where α_c is in dB/λ_g. Substituting for α_c we obtain

$$Q_c = 39.5\,(h/R_s)\,f_{GHz} \qquad (3.50)$$

In the above equation, h is in cm and R_s is given by

$$R_s = \sqrt{\pi f \mu / \sigma}$$
$$= 2\pi\sqrt{f_{GHz}/\sigma} \text{ ohm/square} \quad (3.51)$$

Substituting for R_s in Eq. (3.50), we get

$$Q_c = 0.63 h\sqrt{f_{GHz}/\sigma} \qquad (3.52)$$

where σ is the conductivity of the dielectric substrate board in mho per meter.

The conduction attenuation constant α_c for copper is $\alpha_c = 5.8 \times 10^7$ mho/m. Hence, the quality factor Q_c becomes

$$Q_c = 4780 h\sqrt{f_{GHz}} \qquad (3.53)$$

(ii) Quality factor Q_d

Similarly, the quality factor Q_d due to dielectric attenuation constant is given by

$$Q_d = 27.3/\alpha_d \qquad (3.54)$$

where α_d is in dB/λ_g. Substituting for α_d, we obtain

$$Q_d = \lambda_0 \sqrt{\varepsilon}\tan\theta \approx 1/\tan\theta \qquad (3.55)$$

where λ_0 is the free space wavelength in cm. Thus, the Q_d of a microstrip line is approximately equal to the reciprocal of the dielectric loss tangent and is fairly constant with frequency.

3.10 PARALLEL STRIP LINES

A parallel strip line is similar to a two-conductor transmission line. It consists of two perfectly parallel strips that are separated by a perfect dielectric slab of uniform thickness as shown in Fig. 3.20. It supports a

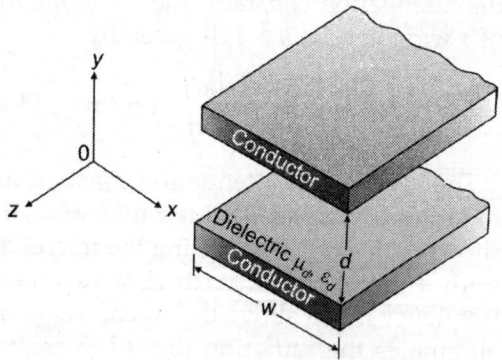

Fig. 3.20: Planar strip line

quasi-TEM mode. Its plate width is w, the distance of separation is d and the relative dielectric constant of the slab is ε_{rd}. In microwave integrated circuits, the microstrip line can be easily fabricated on a dielectric substrate by printed-circuit technique.

3.10.1 Distributed Parameters

Let us consider a **TEM** mode wave propagating through a loss-less strip line in the positive z-direction. The magnetic field is in the x-direction and the electric field is in the y-direction. The fringe capacitance of the strip line is negligible if the width w of the strip line is much larger than its separation distance.

The inductance along the two conducting strips is given by

$$L = \mu_r d/w \quad \text{H/m} \qquad (3.56)$$

where μ_r is the permeability of the conductor.

The capacitance between the two conducting strips is given by

$$C = \varepsilon_d w/d \quad \text{F/m} \qquad (3.57)$$

where ε_d is the permittivity of the dielectric slab.

The series resistance for both the strips is given by

$$R = \frac{2R_s}{w} = \left(\frac{2}{w}\right)\sqrt{\pi f \mu/\sigma_c} \quad \text{ohm/m} \quad (3.58)$$

where $R_s = \sqrt{\pi f \mu/\sigma}$ is the conductor surface resistance in ohm/m and σ_c is the conductivity of the conductor in mho/m.

The shunt conductance G of the strip line is given by

$$G = \sigma_c w/d \qquad (3.59)$$

σ_c is the conductivity of the dielectric constant.

3.10.2 Characteristic Impedance

The characteristic impedance of a loss-less parallel strip line is given by

$$Z_0 = \sqrt{\frac{L}{C}} = \left(\frac{d}{w}\right)\sqrt{\frac{\mu_d}{\varepsilon_{rd}}} \qquad (3.60a)$$

$$= \left(\frac{377}{\sqrt{\varepsilon_{rd}}}\right)\left(\frac{d}{w}\right) \quad \text{for } w \gg d \; (3.60b)$$

The phase velocity along the parallel strip line is given by

$$v_p = \frac{\omega}{\beta} = \frac{1}{\sqrt{LC}} \qquad (3.61a)$$

$$= \frac{1}{\sqrt{\mu_d \varepsilon_d}} = \frac{c}{\sqrt{\varepsilon_d}} \quad \text{m/s} \qquad (3.61b)$$

for $\qquad \mu_d = \mu_0$

At microwave frequencies, $\omega L \gg R$ and $\omega C \gg G$. The characteristic impedance of a lossy parallel strip line can be approximated to

$$Z_0 = \sqrt{\frac{L}{C}} = \left(\frac{377}{\sqrt{\varepsilon_{rd}}}\right)\left(\frac{h}{w}\right) \qquad (3.62)$$

3.10.3 Attenuation Losses

The propagation constant γ at microwave frequencies is given by

$$\gamma = \sqrt{(R + j\omega L)(G + j\omega C)}$$
$$\omega L \gg R \text{ and } \omega C \gg G \quad (3.63)$$

$$= \frac{1}{2} R\sqrt{\frac{C}{L}} + G\sqrt{\frac{L}{C}} + jw\sqrt{\frac{L}{C}} \quad (3.64)$$

Hence, the attenuation and phase constants are given by

$$\alpha = \frac{1}{2}\left(R\sqrt{\frac{C}{L}} + G\sqrt{\frac{L}{C}}\right) \quad \text{Np/m} (3.65)$$

$$\beta = \omega\sqrt{\frac{L}{C}} \quad \text{rad/m} \qquad (3.66)$$

The attenuation constant can be expressed as

$$\alpha = \alpha_c + \alpha_d = \frac{1}{2}\left(R\sqrt{\frac{C}{L}} + G\sqrt{\frac{L}{C}}\right) \quad (3.67)$$

Hence, the conduction attenuation constant α_c is given by

$$\alpha_c = \frac{1}{2}\left(R\sqrt{\frac{C}{L}}\right) = \left(\frac{1}{d}\right)\sqrt{\frac{\pi f \mu}{\sigma_c}} \quad \text{Np/m} \quad (3.68)$$

The dielectric attenuation constant α_d is given by

$$\alpha_d = \frac{1}{2}\left(G\sqrt{\frac{L}{C}}\right) = \frac{188\sigma_d}{\sqrt{\varepsilon_{rd}}} \text{ Np/m} \qquad (3.69)$$

3.11 SLOT LINES

Slot lines consist of two conductors separated in a single plane on the dielectric substrate as shown in Fig. 3.21. Since they are planar lines, they are used as transmission lines in microwave integrated circuits. Active and passive microwave devices can easily be mounted across the slot lines from the top. The electric fields are concentrated in the dielectric regions of the gap between the two conductors. The propagation mode is **TE** mode because the magnetic field has both longitudinal and transverse components. The magnetic field is circularly polarized at periodical locations. This is utilized in the design of ferrite isolators. The characteristic impedance of slot lines increases with the increase in width of the slot and varies rapidly with frequency compared to microstrip lines.

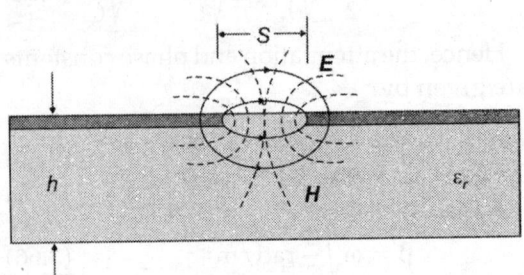

Fig. 3.21: Slot line

3.12 SHIELED STRIP LINES

A partially shielded strip line is one in which its strip conductor is embedded in a dielectric medium with its top and bottom ground planes having no connection as shown in Fig. 3.22.

The characteristic impedance Z_0 for a wide shielded strip is given by

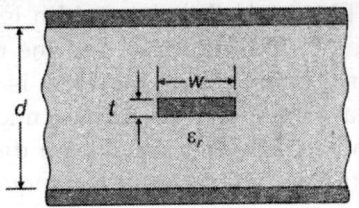

Fig. 3.22: Partially shielded strip line

$$Z_0 = \left(94.15\sqrt{\varepsilon_r}\right)\left[(w/d)K + C_f/8.854\varepsilon_r\right]^{-1} \qquad (3.70)$$

where $K = 1/[1 - (t/d)]$,

t is the thickness of the shielded strip,

d is the distance between the two ground planes,

$C_f = (8.854\,\varepsilon_r/\pi)\,[2K \ln(K+1) - (K-1)\ln(K^2 - 1)$ is the fringe capacitance in pF/m.

Fig. 3.23 shows the variation of Z_0 of a partially shielded strip line with t/d ratio.

3.13 COPLANAR STRIP LINES

A coplanar strip line, shown in Fig. 3.24, is a parallel three-conductor line consisting of a *thin* center strip of width w and two *thin* ground strips G on a dielectric substrate. Coplanar lines are very convenient for series mounting of the components across the gap in the center strip and shunt mounting across the slots between the conductors. The propagation mode is also **TE** mode and the magnetic field is circularly polarized. Therefore, they are used in the design of ferrite components.

The characteristic impedance Z_0 of a coplanar strip line is given by

$$Z_0 = 2P_{av}/I_0^2 \qquad (3.71)$$

The current I_0 is the total peak current in one strip and P_{av} is the average power flowing in the positive z-direction. The average power is expressed as

$$P_{av} = \frac{1}{2}\text{Re}\iint\left(E_x \times H_y^*\right)u_z\,dx\,dy \qquad (3.72)$$

where E_x is the electric field in the positive x-direction and H_y is the magnetic field intensity in the positive y-direction

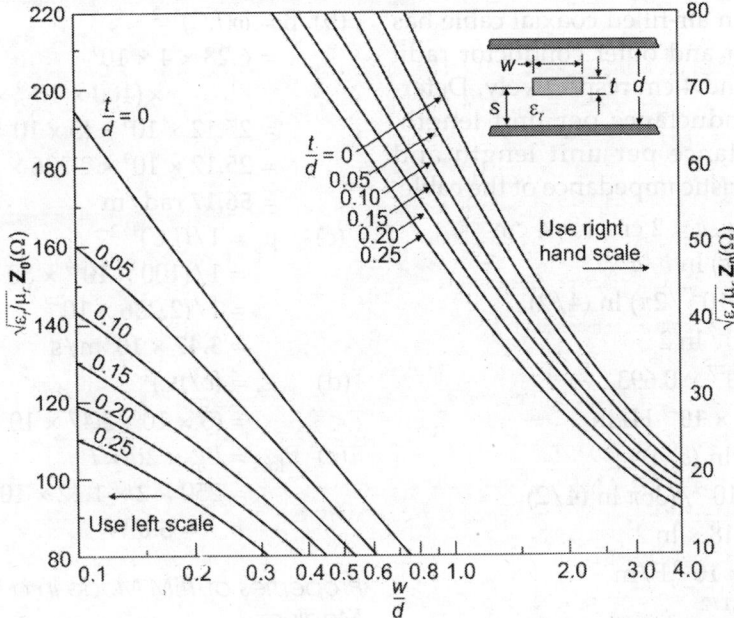

Fig. 3.23: Variation of Z_0 of a partially shielded strip line with t/d ratio

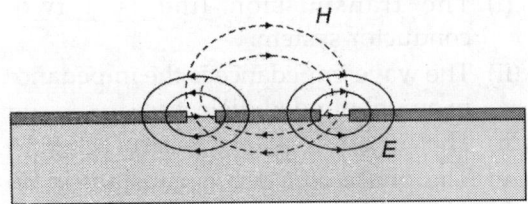

Fig. 3.24: Coplanar strip line

Advantages of Planar Strip Lines

The advantages of planar strip lines are:

(a) Small size and light in weight

(b) Flush mounting of components on a metallic body

(c) Easy access for component mounting

(d) Increased reliability

(e) Low cost

(f) Z_0 can be controlled by defining dimensions in a single plane

(g) Passive circuits can be designed easily by changing the dimensions of the line in a single plane

Disadvantages of Planar Strip Lines

The disadvantages of planar strip lines are:

(a) Low power handling capacity because of small size.

(b) Radiation losses from the open structures.

(c) Exact analysis is difficult because the field extends outside the dielectric.

The radiation loss can be reduced by confining the field lines more in the dielectric substrate of high dielectric constant such as Alumina with dielectric constant of 9 to 10 and sapphire with dielectric constant of 9.3 to 11.7.

The circuit design using the planar strip lines must be very accurate as matching devices such as tuning screws and short-circuit plungers cannot be used in these line circuits. The quality factor Q obtainable with these lines is low, in the order of 100. Hence, the design of some active devices is limited.

Example 3.1: An air-filled coaxial cable has inner conductor and outer conductor radii equal to 2 cm and 4 cm respectively. Determine (a) the inductance per unit length, (b) the capacitance per unit length and (c) the characteristic impedance of the cable.

Solution: Given: $a = 2$ cm, $b = 4$ cm

(a) $L = (\mu_0/2\pi) \ln b/a$

$= (4\pi \times 10^{-7}/2\pi) \ln (4/2)$

$= 2 \times 10^{-7} \ln 2$

$= 2 \times 10^{-7} \times 0.693$

$= \mathbf{1.386 \times 10^{-7}}$ **H/m.**

(b) $C = 2\pi\varepsilon_0/\ln (b/a)$

$= 2\pi \times 10^{-9}/(36\pi \ln (4/2))$

$= 10^{-9}/18 \times \ln 2$

$= \mathbf{0.08 \times 10^{-9}}$ **F/m**

(c) $Z_0 = (L/C)^{1/2}$

$= [(1.386 \times 10^{-7})/(0.08 \times 10^{-9})]^{1/2}$

$= (1732.5)^{1/2} = \mathbf{41.6}$ **ohm**

Example 3.2: The primary constants of a coaxial cable at 4 GHz are: $L = 100$ nH/m, $C = 50$ pF/m, $R = 0.1$ ohm/m and $G = 0$. Determine (a) the attenuation constant, (b) the phase constant, (c) the phase velocity, (d) the relative permittivity and (e) the power loss for a length of 10 m when the input power is 250 W.

Solution: Given: $f = 4$ GHz, $L = 100$ nH/m, $C = 50$ pF/m, $R = 0.1$ ohm/m, $G = 0$, $P_{in} = 250$ and $l = 10$.

$\omega L = 2\pi f L$

$= 2\pi \times 4 \times 10^9 \times 100 \times 10^{-9}$

$= 2513.3$ ohm

$\omega C = 2\pi f C$

$= 2\pi \times 4 \times 10^9 \times 50 \times 10^{-12}$

$= 1.257$ ohm

Since $G = 0$ and $\omega L \gg R$, the characteristic impedance is given by

$Z_0 = (L/C)^{1/2}$

$= 100 \times 10^{-9}/50 \times 10^{-12}$

$= 44.72$ ohm

(a) $\alpha = R/2Z_0$

$= 0.1/(2 \times 44.72) = \mathbf{1.12 \times 10^{-3}}$ Np/m

$= 1.12 \times 8.686 \times 10^{-3} = \mathbf{9.73 \times 10^{-3}}$ **dB/m**

(b) $\beta = \omega(LC)^{1/2}$

$= 6.28 \times 4 \times 10^9$

$\times (100 \times 10^{-9} \times 50 \times 10^{-12})^{1/.2}$

$= 25.12 \times 10^9 \times (5 \times 10^{-18})^{1/2}$

$= 25.12 \times 10^9 \times 2.236 \times 10^{-9}$

$= \mathbf{56.17}$ **rad/m**

(c) $\mu_p = 1/(LC)^{1/2}$

$= 1/(100 \times 10^{-9} \times 50 \times 10^{-12})^{1/.2}$

$= 1/(2.236 \times 10^{-9}$

$= \mathbf{3.47 \times 10^8}$ **m/s**

(d) $\varepsilon_r = (c/\mu_p)^2$

$= (3 \times 10^8/3.47 \times 10^8)^2 = \mathbf{0.75}$

(e) $P_{loss} = P_{in} \times 2\alpha \times l$

$= 250 \times 2 \times 1.12 \times 10^{-3} \times 10$

$= \mathbf{5.6}$ **W**

Properties of TEM Mode in a Lossless Medium

The important properties of TEM mode in a loss-less medium are summarized below:

(i) The transmission line is a two-conductor system.

(ii) The wave impedance is the impedance in an unbounded dielectric.

(iii) The cut-off frequency is zero.

(iv) The phase constant is constant in an unbounded dielectric.

(v) The phase velocity is the velocity of light in an unbounded dielectric.

3.14 ADDITIONAL EXAMPLES

Example 3.3: An air-filled coaxial cable has inner conductor and outer conductor radii equal to 3 cm and 5 cm respectively. Determine (a) the inductance per unit length, (b) the capacitance per unit length and (c) the characteristic impedance of the cable.

Solution: Given: $a = 3$ cm, $b = 5$ cm

(a) $L = (\mu_0/2\pi) \ln b/a$

$= (4\pi \times 10^{-7}/2\pi) \ln b/a$

$= \mathbf{1.022 \times 10^{-7}}$ **H/m.**

(b) $C = 2\pi\varepsilon_0/\ln (b/a)$

$= 2\pi \times 10^{-9}/(36\pi \ln 5/3)$

$= \mathbf{0.109 \times 10^{-9}}$ **F/m**

(c) $Z_0 = (L/C)^{1/2}$

$= (1.022 \times 10^{-7}/0.109 \times 10^{-9})^{1/2}$

$= \mathbf{30.62}$ **ohm**

Example 3.4: The primary constants of a coaxial cable at 1 GHz are: L = 200 nH/m, C = 100 pF/m, R = 0.1 ohm/m and G = 0. Determine (a) the attenuation constant, (b) the phase constant, (c) the phase velocity, (d) the relative permittivity and (e) the power loss for a length of 10 m when the input power is 500 W.

Solution: Given: f = 1 GHz, L = 200 nH/m, C = 100 pF/m, R = 0.1 ohm/m and G = 0, l = 10, P_{in} = 500.

$\omega L = 2\pi \times 1 \times 10^9 \times 200 \times 10^{-9} = 1256.6$ ohm

$\omega C = 2\pi \times 1 \times 10^9 \times 100 \times 10^{-12} = 0.628$ ohm

Since G = 0 and $\omega L \gg R$, the characteristic impedance is given by

$Z_0 = (L/C)^{1/2}$

$= 200 \times 10^{-9}/100 \times 10^{-12}$

$= 44.72$ ohm

(a) $\alpha = R/2Z_0 = 0.1/(2 \times 44.72)$

$= \mathbf{1.12 \times 10^{-3}}$ **Np/m**

$= 1.12 \times 8.686 \times 10^{-3}$

$= \mathbf{9.73 \times 10^{-3}}$ **dB/m**

(b) $\beta = w(LC)^{1/2}$

$= 6.28 \times 1 \times 10^9$

$\times (200 \times 10^{-9} \times 100 \times 10^{-12})^{1/.2}$

$= \mathbf{28.09}$ **rad/m**

(c) $\mu_p = 1/(LC)^{1/2}$

$= 1/(200 \times 10^{-9} \times 100 \times 10^{-12})^{1/.2}$

$= \mathbf{2.236 \times 10^8}$ **m/s**

(d) $\varepsilon_r = (c/\mu_p)^2$

$= (3 \times 10^8/2.236 \times 10^8)^2 = \mathbf{1.80}$

(e) $P_{loss} = P_{in} \times 2\alpha \times l$

$= 500 \times 2 \times 1.12 \times 10^{-3} \times 10$

$= \mathbf{11.2}$ **W**

Example 3.5: A zero thickness microstrip line of copper conductors on substrate having dielectric constant of 8.4 and tan δ of 0.0005 has thickness 2.5 mm. If the line width is 1 mm and operated at 10 GHz, calculate (a) the characteristic impedance, (b) the attenuation due to conductor and dielectric loss.

Solution: Given: ε_r = 8.4, tan δ = 0.0005, h = 2.5 mm, w = 1 mm, f = 10 GHz, t = 0

$\lambda = c/f = 30 \times 18/10^9 = 3$ cm

(a) $w/h = 1/2.5 = 0.40 < 1$.

$\varepsilon_{eff} = (\varepsilon_r+1)/2 + [(\varepsilon_r-1)/2] \times$

$[(1+12h/w)^{-1/2} + 0.04(1-w/h)^2]$

$= (8.4+1)/2 + [(8.4-1)/2] \times$

$[1 + 12/0.4)^{-1/2} + 0.04(1-0.4)^2$

$= 5.42$

$Z_0 = \left(\dfrac{60}{\sqrt{\varepsilon_{eff}}}\right)\ln(8h/w+w/4h)$

$= \left(\dfrac{60}{\sqrt{5.42}}\right)\ln[8/0.4+0.4/4]$

$= \mathbf{77.32}$ **ohm**

(b) $\alpha_c = 8.686\, R_s/Z_0 w$

$R_s = \sqrt{\pi f \mu/\sigma}$

$= \sqrt{\dfrac{(3.14\times10\times10^9\times4\pi\times10^{-7})}{5.8\times10^7}}$

$= 2.6 \times 10^{-2}$ ohm/sq.m

$\alpha_c = 8.686 \times 2.6 \times 10^{-2}/77.32 \times 1 \times 10^{-3}$

$= \mathbf{2.92}$ **dB/m**

$\alpha_d = 27.3[(\varepsilon_{eff}-1)/(\varepsilon_r-1)] \times$

$[(\varepsilon_r/\varepsilon_{eff})(\tan δ/\lambda_g)]$

$\lambda_g = \lambda/\varepsilon_{eff} = \dfrac{3}{\sqrt{5.42}} = 1.288$ cm

$\alpha_d = 27.3[(5.42-1)/(8.4-1)] \times$

$[(8.4/5.42)(0.0005/1.288 \times 10^{-2})]$

$= \mathbf{0.980}$ **dB/m**

Example 3.6: A microstrip line has ε_r = 5.23, h = 0.8 mils, t = 2.8 mils and w = 10 mils. Determine the characteristic impedance.

Solution: Given: ε_r = 5.23, h = 0.8 mils, t = 2.8 mils, w = 10 mils

$w/h = 10/0.8 = 12.5$

For $w/h \gg 1$, the effective dielectric constant is given by

$$\varepsilon_{eff} = (\varepsilon_r + 1)/2 + [(\varepsilon_r - 1)/2]$$
$$[(1 + 12h/w)^{-1/2}]$$
$$= (5.23 + 1)/2 + [5.23 - 1)/2]$$
$$[1 + 12 \times 0.8/10]^{-1/2}$$
$$= 6.076$$

The characteristic impedance is given by

$$Z_0 = \left(\frac{376.7}{\sqrt{\varepsilon_{eff}}}\right)\left(\frac{h}{w}\right) \text{ ohm}$$

$$= \left(\frac{376.7}{\sqrt{6.076}}\right)\left(\frac{0.8}{10}\right) = 12.23 \text{ ohms}$$

Example 3.7: A lossless parallel strip line has a relative dielectric constant $\varepsilon_{rd} = 6$ and a thickness $d = 5$ mm. Determine (a) the required w for $Z_0 = 50$ ohms, (b) the strip line capacitance, (c) the strip line inductance and (d) the phase velocity.

Solution: Given: $\varepsilon_{rd} = 6$ and a thickness $d = 5$ mm.

(a) The characteristic impedance of a lossless parallel strip line is given by

$$Z_0 = \sqrt{\frac{L}{C}} = \left(\frac{d}{w}\right)\sqrt{\frac{\mu_d}{\varepsilon_{rd}}}$$

$$= \left(\frac{377}{\sqrt{\varepsilon_{rd}}}\right)\left(\frac{d}{w}\right)$$

Hence, the width is given by

$$w = \left(\frac{377}{\sqrt{\varepsilon_{rd}}}\right)\left(\frac{d}{Z_0}\right)$$

$$= \left(\frac{377}{\sqrt{6}}\right)\left(\frac{5}{50}\right) = 15.39 \text{ mm}$$

(b) The capacitance of the strip line is given by

$$C = \varepsilon_d w/d \quad \text{F/m}$$
$$= 8.854 \times 10^{-12} \times 6 \times 15.39/5$$
$$= 163.5 \quad \text{pF/m}$$

(c) The inductance of strip line is given by

$$L = \mu_r \, d/w \quad \text{H/m}$$
$$= 4\pi \times 10^{-7} \times 5/15.39$$
$$= 0.41 \quad \text{mH/m}$$

(d) The phase velocity is given by

$$v_p = c/\sqrt{\varepsilon_{rd}}$$

$$= \frac{3 \times 10^{10}}{\sqrt{6}} = 1.22 \times 10^8 \quad \text{m/s}$$

Example 3.8: A partially shielded strip line has $\varepsilon_r = 2.56$, $t = 15$ mils, $d = 70$ mils and $w = 25$ mils. Determine (a) K, (b) the fringe capacitance and (c) the characteristic impedance.

Solution: Given:
$$\varepsilon_r = 2.56, t = 15 \text{ mils,}$$
$$d = 70 \text{ mils } w = 25 \text{ mils}$$

(a) The factor K is given by
$$K = 1/[1 - (t/d)]$$
$$= 1/[1 - (15/70)] = 1.27$$

(b) The fringe capacitance is given by
$$C_f = (8.854 \, \varepsilon_r/\pi) \, [2K \ln (K + 1)$$
$$- (K - 1) \ln (K^2 - 1)] \text{ pF/m}$$
$$= (8.854 \times 2.56/3.14) \, [2 \times 1.27 \times \ln$$
$$(1.27 + 1) - (1.27 - 1) \ln (1.27^2 - 1)]$$
$$= 15.61 \text{ pF/m}$$

(c) The characteristic impedance is given by

$$Z_0 = \left(\frac{94.15}{\sqrt{\varepsilon_r}}\right)\left[(w/d)K + C_f/8.854\varepsilon_r\right]^{-1}$$

$$= \left(\frac{94.15}{\sqrt{2.56}}\right)[25/70)(1.27)$$
$$+ 15.61/(8.854 \times 2.56)]^{-1}$$
$$= 51.48 \text{ ohms}$$

Example 3.9: A coaxial line filled with air is operating at $\lambda = 3$ cm in TEM mode. Assume $b/a = 3$ and $a = \lambda/4\pi$. Calculate the breakdown power for $E_d = 30$ kV/m.

Solution: Given:
$$\lambda = 3 \text{ cm, } b/a = 3, \ a = \lambda/4\pi,$$
$$E_d = 30 \text{ kV/m}$$

The breakdown power is given by

$$P_{bd} = a^2 E_d^2 \ln (b/a)/120$$
$$= (3/4\pi)^2 (30 \times 10^3)^2 (\ln 3)/120$$
$$= 0.057 \times 9 \times 10^8 \times 1.0986/120$$
$$= \mathbf{469.7} \ \text{kW}$$

KEY POINTS

- At microwave frequencies, conventional open-wire lines are not used because of high radiation losses.

- The microwave transmission lines are: (i) Multi-conductor lines, (ii) Single conductor lines and (iii) open-boundary structures.

- The mode of transmission is **TE**, **TM** or **TEM** mode.

- Ideal coaxial lines consist of an inner perfect conductor and an outer perfect conductor with negligible resistance.

- In symmetrical coaxial lines, the dominant mode of propagation is **TEM** wave. The coaxial lines with 50-ohm impedance are commonly used for microwave transmission with minimum attenuation.

- RF breakdown voltage or electric field intensity limits the maximum power that can be transmitted through a microwave transmission line.

- The value of breakdown voltage depends on the gas medium, gas pressure, extent of initial gas ionization and frequency of operation.

- Planar transmission lines are flat transmission lines with low profile and light in weight. They are therefore suitable for microwave integrated circuits.

- Four basic forms of planar transmission lines that are widely used in microwave integrated circuits are: (i) strip lines, (ii) microstrip lines, (iii) slot lines and (iv) coplanar strip lines.

- A strip line consists of a central thin conducting strip of width w that is very much greater than its thickness t. The propagation mode is nearly **TEM** mode.

- Coaxial lines with special launcher are used as interface to excite the strip lines. The launcher consists of a thin flat small center conductor.

- Microstrip lines consist of a single ground plane and a thin strip conductor on a dielectric substrate above the ground plane. The propagation mode is quasi-**TEM** mode.

- Microstrip lines are excited by coaxial line through a launcher.

- Microwave integrated circuits require very high-Q resonant circuits. The quality factor Q of a microstrip line is very high. Hence, it is used with microwave integrated circuits.

- However, the radiation losses of the substrate and the low dielectric constant limit its Q.

- Two quality factors are defined in microstrip line. They are (i) the quality factor Q_c related to the conductor attenuation constant and (ii) the quality factor Q_d related to the dielectric attenuation constant.

- A parallel strip consists of two perfectly parallel strips that are separated by a perfect dielectric slab of uniform thickness. It supports a quasi-**TEM** mode.

- In microwave integrated circuits, the strip line can be easily fabricated on a dielectric substrate by printed-circuit technique.

- Slot lines consist of two conductors separated in a single plane on the dielectric substrate. The propagation mode is **TE** mode.

- A coplanar line is a parallel three-conductor line consisting of a thin center strip of width w and two thin ground strips G on a dielectric substrate. The propagation mode is **TE** mode.

- A partially shielded strip line is one in which its strip conductor is embedded in a dielectric medium with its top and bottom ground planes having no connection.

- The advantages of planar transmission lines are (i) Small size and light in weight, (ii) Flush mounting of components on a metallic body, (iii) Easy access for component mounting, (iv) Increased reliability, (v) Low cost, (vi) Z_0 can be controlled by defining dimensions in a single plane and (vii)Passive circuits can be designed easily by changing the dimensions of the line in a single plane

- The disadvantages of planar transmission lines are (i) Low power handling capacity because of small size and (ii) Radiation losses from the open structures

- The radiation loss can be reduced by confining the field lines more in the dielectric substrate of high dielectric constant such as Alumina with dielectric constant of 9 to 10 and sapphire with dielectric constant of 9.3 to 11.7.

- The circuit design using the planar transmission lines must be very accurate as matching devices such as tuning screws and short-circuit plungers cannot be used in these line circuits.

- The quality factor Q obtainable with these lines is low, in the order of 100. Hence, the design of some active devices is limited.

FURTHER READING

1. Altman JL (1962). *Microwave Circuits*, Van Nostrand, NJ
2. Chodorov M and Susskind C (1964). *Fundamentals of Microwave Electronics*, McGraw-Hill, NY.
3. Collins RE (1996). *Foundations of Microwave Engineering*, McGraw Hill, NY
4. Pozar DM (1990). *Microwave Engineering*, Addison-Wesley, Mass.
5. Rizzi PA (1999). *Microwave Engineering: Passive Circuits*, PH, NJ

REVIEW QUESTIONS

3.1 Why are the conventional open wire transmission lines not used at microwave frequencies?

3.2 Mention the types of transmission lines used at microwave frequencies and give an example in each.

3.3 What is a coaxial line?

3.4 Derive expressions for attenuation constant and characteristic impedance in a low-loss coaxial line.

3.5 What are the factors that cause power loss in coaxial cables?

3.6 What is a strip line?

3.7 Mention the method of exciting strip line.

3.8 What is a microstrip line?

3.9 What are the losses in a microstrip line?

3.10 Mention the method of exciting microstrip line.

3.11 What is a parallel strip line?

3.12 What is a slot line?

3.13 What is a coplanar strip line?

3.14 What is a partially shielded strip line?

3.15 What are the advantages of planar transmission lines?

3.16 What are the disadvantages of planar strip lines?

3.17 Give expression for the characteristic impedance in a strip line.

3.18 Give expressions for attenuation constant and characteristic impedance in a microstrip line.

3.19 Define the breakdown power?

3.20 On what factors the breakdown power depends?

DESCRIPTIVE QUESTIONS

3.1 Describe the various types of microwave transmission line.

3.2 Derive expressions for attenuation constant and characteristic impedance in a low loss coaxial line.

3.3 Describe the strip line with sketches and give expression for characteristic impedance. Explain the method of excitation.

3.4 Describe the microstrip line with sketches and give expression for attenuation constant and characteristic impedance in a microstrip line. Explain the method of excitation.

3.5 What are the losses in a microstrip line? Explain the quality factors associated with it.

3.6 Describe the parallel strip line with sketches and give expressions for characteristic impedance, inductance, capacitance and series resistance.

3.7 Describe the coplanar and partially shielded strip lines with sketches and give expressions for characteristic impedance.

PRACTICE PROBLEMS

3.1 An air-filled coaxial cable has inner conductor and outer conductor radii equal to 3 cm and 6 cm respectively. Determine (a) the inductance per unit length, (b) the capacitance per unit length and (c) the characteristic impedance of the cable.
(**Ans:** 1.386×10^{-7} H/m, 0.08×10^{-9} F/m, 41.50 W)

3.2 The primary constants of a coaxial cable at 1 GHz are: $L = 200$ nh/m, $C = 100$ pF/m, $R = 0.1$ ohm/m and $G = 0$. Determine (a) the attenuation constant, (b) the phase constant, (c) the phase velocity, (d) the relative permittivity and (e) the power loss for a length of 10 m when the input power is 500 W.
(**Ans:** 5.08×10^{-3} dB/m, 30.6 rad/m, 2.05×10^{8} m/s, 2.14, 5.85 W)

3.3 A zero thickness microstrip line of copper conductors on substrate having dielectric constant of 8.4 and tan d of 0.0005 has thickness 2.4 mm. If the line width is 1 mm and operated at 10 GHz, calculate (a) the characteristic impedance, (b) the attenuation due to conductor and dielectric loss.

(**Ans:** 76.2 ohm, 0.98 dB/m)

3.4 A microstrip line has $\varepsilon_r = 5.23$, $h = 7$ mils, $t = 2.8$ mils and $w = 10$ mils. Determine the characteristic impedance.

(**Ans:** 46.74 ohms)

3.5 A loss-less parallel strip line has a relative dielectric constant $e_{rd} = 6$ and a thickness $d = 4$ mm. Determine (a) the required w for $Z_0 = 50$ ohms, (b) the strip line capacitance, (c) the strip line inductance and (d) the phase velocity.

(**Ans:** (a) 12.31 mm, (b) 163.5 pF/m, (c) 0.41 mH/m, (d) 1.22×10^8 m/s)

3.6 A partially shielded strip line has $e_r = 2.56$, $t = 14$ mils, $d = 70$ mils and $w = 25$ mils.

Determine (a) K, (b) the fringe capacitance and (c) the characteristic impedance.

(**Ans:** (a) 1.25, (b) 15.61 pF/m, (c) 50.29 ohms)

REFERENCE

1. Rizzi PA (2001). *Microwave Engineering: Passive Circuits*, PH, NJ.
2. Terman FE (1955). *Electronic and Radio Engineering*, McGraw-Hill, Intl.
3. Liao SY (2000). *Microwave Devices and Circuits*, PHI New Delhi.
4. Das A and Das SK (2004). *Microwave Engineering*, TMH, New Delhi.
5. Seeger JA (1988). *Microwave Theory Components and Devices*, PH, NJ.
6. Roddy D (1986). *Microwave Technology*, PH, NJ.
7. Ramo S, Whinnery JR and Van Duzer (1965). *Fields and Waves in Communication Electronics*, Wiely, NY.

Single Line and Open-Boundary Structures

Objectives

- Understand the propagation of EM waves through waveguides.
- Study the various types of multiconductor lines and their characteristics.
- Know the construction details and modes of operation.
- Explain the details of open-boundary structures.

4.1 INTRODUCTION

Waveguides are *metallic hallow tubes* of rectangular or circular shape and are used to guide the electromagnetic waves through them. Waveguides provide an alternative to coaxial cables for use at microwave frequencies. Waveguides are superior in terms of attenuation per unit length experienced by the wave propagating through them. The standard waveguides are made of brass, bronze or aluminum with the inner surface coated with silver to minimize ohmic loss.

Figure 4.1 shows rectangular and circular waveguide sections. We shall now study some practical aspects of these waveguides and open-boundary structures.

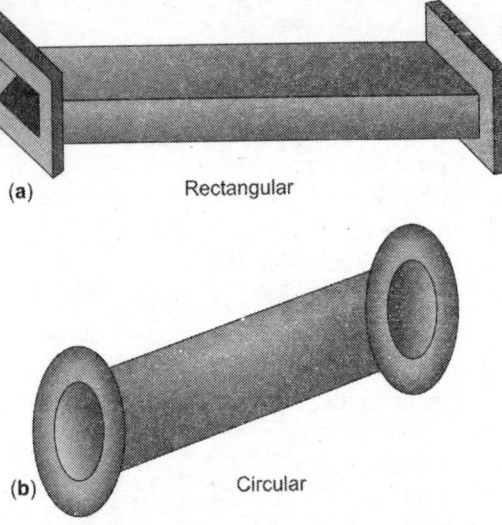

(a)   Rectangular

(b)   Circular

Fig. 4.1: Waveguide sections

4.2 WAVEGUIDES

Since waveguide is a hollow metallic tube, the electric and magnetic fields in the waveguide are confined inside the waveguide. Hence, no power is lost through radiation. As the waveguides are normally air-filled, the dielectric loss is negligible.

However, due to heat in the walls of the waveguides, some power loss occurs but it is negligible.

The electric and magnetic field configurations inside a waveguide that satisfies the Maxwell's equation is known as a *mode*. Within a waveguide, several modes of propagation are possible. For each allowed mode, the waveguide has a definite cut-off frequency f_c. The cut-off frequency is determined by the dimensions and geometry of the waveguide. For a given mode, if the permissible signal frequency is above the cut-off frequency, the electromagnetic energy can be transmitted through the waveguide without attenuation. If the signal frequency is below the cut-off frequency, the electromagnetic energy will be attenuated within a short distance to a negligible value and hence will not be transmitted through the waveguide. *The mode that has the lowest cut-off frequency is known as the dominant mode of the waveguide.* Therefore, the waveguide dimensions are chosen such that only the electromagnetic energy of the dominant mode is transmitted through the waveguide.

4.3 RECTANGULAR WAVEGUIDE

The most commonly used waveguide has a rectangular cross-section. Hence, it is known as rectangular waveguide. The standard rectangular waveguide WR-90 used in the X-band frequency range of 8 to 12 GHz has inner dimensions of 2.286 cm (0.9 in) × 1.016 cm (0.4 in) and its outside dimensions are 2.54 cm (1 in) × 1.27 cm (0.5 in).

The electromagnetic fields are confined inside the waveguide and are guided by conducting walls. Due to total internal reflection, the plane waves are reflected from the wall to wall as the wave travels down the waveguide longitudinally. This gives rise to a component of the electric or magnetic field in the direction of propagation of the resultant wave. Hence, it is no longer a transverse electromagnetic (**TEM**) wave. Any uniform plane wave in a loss-less waveguide can be resolved into transverse electric (**TE**) and transverse magnetic (**TM**) waves, as shown in Fig. 4.2. The wavelength λ is in the direction of propagation of the *incident wave*. It has two components: one component λ_n is along the direction that is

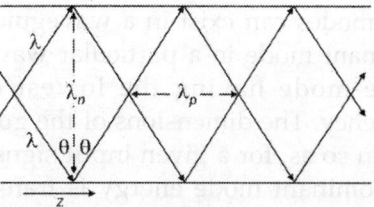

Fig. 4.2: Plane wave reflected in a waveguide

normal to the reflecting plane and is given by

$$\lambda_n = \lambda / \cos \theta \qquad (4.1)$$

Another component λ_p is along the direction that is parallel to the plane. This component is given by

$$\lambda_p = \lambda / \sin \theta \qquad (4.2)$$

θ is the angle of incidence and λ is the wavelength of the incident signal in unbounded medium.

Thus, a plane wave in a waveguide resolves into two components:

(i) A standing wave in the direction normal to the reflecting walls of the waveguide.

(ii) Another traveling wave in the direction parallel to the reflecting walls.

The modes in lossless waveguides are classified as either transverse electric (**TE**) mode or transverse magnetic (**TM**) modes. In rectangular waveguides, these modes are designated as **TE**$_{mn}$ or **TM**$_{mn}$. The subscript m denotes the number of half waves of the electric or magnetic intensity in the x-direction and the subscript n is the number of half waves of the electric or magnetic intensity in the y-direction and the wave propagation is in the positive z-direction.

4.3.1 Design Specifications

A rectangular waveguide is a hollow metallic section with rectangular cross-section. The sides are designated as a and b, $a > b$. The conducting walls of the guide confine the electromagnetic fields and thereby guide the electromagnetic wave. A number of distinct field modes can exist in a waveguide. The dominant mode in a particular waveguide is the mode having the lowest cut-off frequency. The dimensions of the guide are chosen so as, for a given input signal, only the dominant mode energy is transmitted through the guide.

The design requirements for the dominant mode are:

(i) Dominant mode energy transmission

(ii) Very low attenuation

(iii) Transmitted power less than the break-down power.

The successive higher order modes for a waveguide of dimension $2b < a$ are TE_{10}, TE_{20}, TE_{01} etc. Therefore, for dominant mode propagation, the cross-section dimensions are determined by the following restrictions.

(i) **For TE_{10} mode:**
$$\lambda_{max} < \hat{\lambda}_c = 2a \qquad (4.3a)$$

(ii) **For TE_{20} mode:**
$$\lambda_{min} > \lambda_c = a \qquad (4.3b)$$

(iii) **For TE_{01} mode:**
$$\lambda_{min} > \lambda_c = 2b \qquad (4.3c)$$

Therefore, the dimensions of the cross-section of the rectangular waveguides for dominant mode propagation are to be selected according to

$$0 < b < \lambda/2 \qquad (4.4a)$$
$$\lambda/2 < a < \lambda \qquad (4.4b)$$

The dimensions of the waveguide are chosen such that the power handling capability is adequate. The dimensions in terms of wavelength are:

$$b = 0.3\lambda \text{ to } 0.4\lambda \qquad (4.5a)$$
$$a = 0.7\lambda \text{ to } 0.8\lambda \qquad (4.5b)$$

For example, at X-band frequencies (8 to 12 GHz), the inside dimensions of a rectangular waveguide (WR 90) are 2.286 cm × 1.016 cm (0.9" × 0.4") and the outside dimensions are 2.54 cm × 1.27 cm (1" × 0.5").

4.3.2 Solutions of Wave Equations in Rectangular Waveguides

Each wave equation may be solved in time-domain and frequency-domain[4]. For sake of simplicity, only frequency-domain or sinusoidal steady-state solution is discussed here. Figure 4.3 shows the rectangular coordinate system.

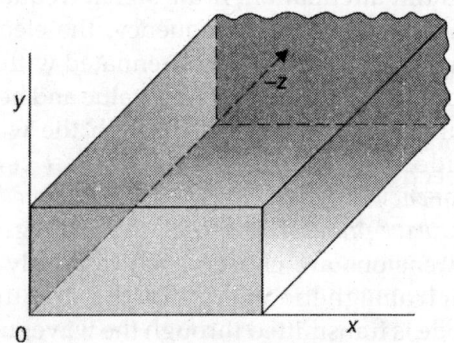

Fig. 4.3: Rectangular coordinates system

(i) Vector wave equations

In the frequency-domain, the electric and magnetic wave equations are known as *vector wave equations* and are given by

$$\nabla^2 E = \gamma^2 E \qquad (4.6)$$
$$\nabla^2 H = \gamma^2 H \qquad (4.7)$$

$$\gamma = \alpha + j\beta = \sqrt{j\omega\mu(\sigma + j\omega\varepsilon)}$$

is the propagation constant.

(ii) Helmholtz equation

The rectangular components of E and H satisfy the Helmholtz or complex scalar equation given by

$$\nabla^2 \psi = \gamma^2 \psi \qquad (4.8)$$

Assuming that the propagation of the wave is in the positive z-direction, the Helmholtz equation in rectangular coordinates is given by

$$\frac{\partial^2 \psi}{\partial x^2} + \frac{\partial^2 \psi}{\partial y^2} + \frac{\partial^2 \psi}{\partial z^2} = \gamma^2 \psi \qquad (4.9)$$

By method of separation, a solution of the above linear and inhomogeneous partial differential equation may be assumed to be

$$\psi = X(x)Y(y)Z(z) \qquad (4.10)$$

Substituting Eq. (4.10) in (4.9), we get

$$\frac{\partial^2 XYZ}{\partial x^2} + \frac{\partial^2 XYZ}{\partial y^2} + \frac{\partial^2 XYZ}{\partial z^2} = \gamma^2 XYZ \quad (4.11)$$

Dividing the above equation by Eq. (4.10), we obtain

$$\left(\frac{1}{X}\right)\frac{d^2 X}{dx^2} + \left(\frac{1}{Y}\right)\frac{dY}{d^2 y^2} + \left(\frac{1}{Z}\right)\frac{dZ}{d^2 z^2} = \gamma^2 \quad (4.12)$$

Each term on the left-hand side is independently variable and their sum is a constant. Hence, each term must be equal to a constant. Let them be $-k_x^2, -k_y^2$ and $-k_z^2$ respectively. Then, Eq. (4.12) becomes

$$k_x^2 + k_y^2 + k_z^2 = -\gamma^2 \quad (4.13)$$

The general solution of each differential equation in Eq. (4.12) is given by

$$d^2 X / dx^2 = -k_x^2 X \quad (4.14a)$$
$$d^2 Y / dy^2 = -k_y^2 Y \quad (4.14b)$$
$$d^2 Z / dz^2 = -k_z^2 Z \quad (4.14c)$$

The solution of the above equations is given below:

$$X = A \sin(k_x, x) + B \cos(k_x, x) \quad (4.15a)$$
$$Y = C \sin(k_y, y) + D \cos(k_y, y) \quad (4.15b)$$
$$Z = E \sin(k_z, z) + F \cos(k_z, z) \quad (4.15c)$$

Thus, the solution of the Helmholtz equation in the rectangular coordinates is

$$\psi = [A \sin(k_x, x) + B \cos(k_x, x)]$$
$$\times [C \sin(k_y, y) + D \cos(k_y, y)]$$
$$\times [E \sin(k_z, z) + F \cos(k_z, z)] \quad (4.16)$$

Assuming the propagation is in the positive z-direction, the propagation constant γ_g in the waveguide is different from the intrinsic propagation constant γ of the dielectric. It is given by

$$\gamma_g^2 = \gamma^2 + k_x^2 + k_y^2$$
$$= \gamma^2 + k_c^2 \quad (4.17a)$$

Here $k_c = \sqrt{k_x^2 + k_y^2}$ is known as the *cut-off wave number*. For a loss-less dielectric,

$$\gamma^2 = -\omega^2 \mu\varepsilon \quad (4.17b)$$

Then, the propagation constant in the waveguide is

$$\gamma_g = \pm \sqrt{\omega^2 \mu\varepsilon - k_c^2} \quad (4.18)$$

Depending on the value of k_c, γ_g may be zero, +ve or −ve. These three cases for the propagation constant in the waveguide are discussed below:

Case 1: When $\omega^2 \mu\varepsilon = k_c^2$

In this case, the propagation constant in the waveguide $\gamma_g = 0$. Hence, there will not be wave propagation (*evanescence*) in the guide. The cut-off frequency is given by

$$f_c = \frac{\sqrt{k_x^2 + k_y^2}}{2\pi\sqrt{\mu\varepsilon}} = \frac{k_c}{2\pi\sqrt{\mu\varepsilon}} \quad (4.19)$$

Case 2: When $\omega^2 \mu\varepsilon > k_c^2$

In this case, the propagation constant in the waveguide is given by

$$\gamma_g = \pm j\beta_g = \pm j\omega\sqrt{\mu\varepsilon - (k_c / \omega_c)^2}$$
$$= \pm j\omega\sqrt{\mu\varepsilon - (4\pi^2 \mu\varepsilon f_c^2 / 4\pi^2 f^2)}$$
$$= \pm j\omega\sqrt{\mu\varepsilon}\sqrt{1 - (f_c / f)^2} \quad (4.20)$$

Hence, there will be wave propagation in the guide provided the operating frequency is above the cut-off frequency.

Case 3: When $\omega^2 \mu\varepsilon < k_c^2$

In this case, the propagation constant in the waveguide is given by

$$\gamma_g = \pm\alpha_g = \pm\omega\sqrt{\mu\varepsilon - (k_c / \omega_c)^2}$$
$$= \pm w\sqrt{\mu\varepsilon - (4\pi^2 \mu\varepsilon f_c^2 / 4\pi^2 f^2)}$$
$$= \pm\omega\sqrt{\mu\varepsilon}\sqrt{(f_c / f)^2 - 1} \quad (4.21)$$

This above equation implies that if the operating frequency f is below the cut-off frequency f_c, the wave will be attenuated exponentially by $e^{-\alpha_g z}$. Hence, there will not be any wave propagation. Therefore, the solution of the Helmholtz equation in the rectangular coordinates is

$$\psi = [A \sin (k_x, x) + B \cos (k_x, x)] \psi \times$$

$$[C \sin (k_y, y) + D \cos (k_y, y)]e^{-j\beta_g z} \quad (4.22)$$

4.3.3 TE Mode Solution in Rectangular Waveguide

Figure 4.4 shows the coordinates of the rectangular waveguide with the assumption that the waves are propagating along the rectangular waveguide in the positive z-direction. For the $\mathbf{TE}_{mn}$ modes, $E_z = 0$. To have electromagnetic energy transmission in the rectangular waveguide, the z-component of the magnetic field, H_z must exist[5]. Therefore, the Helmholtz equation is given by

$$\nabla^2 H_z = \gamma^2 H_z, \quad (4.23)$$

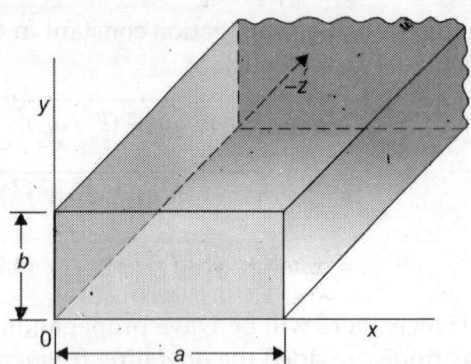

Fig. 4.4: Rectangular waveguide coordinates

The boundary condition to be satisfied is that the normal derivative of H_z is zero at the conducting walls; i.e., $\partial H_z / \partial n = 0$. Hence, the magnetic field in the z-direction satisfying the boundary conditions on the waveguide walls is given by

$$H_z = H_{0z} \cos (m\pi x/a) \cos (n\pi y/b) e^{-\beta_g z} \quad (4.24)$$

Here H_{0z} is the amplitude constant. The other $\mathbf{TE}_{mn}$ field equations are

$$E_x = E_{0x} \cos (m\pi x/a) \sin (n\pi y/b) e^{-\beta_g z} \quad (4.25)$$

$$E_y = E_{0y} \sin (m\pi y/a) \cos (n\pi y/b) e^{-\beta_g z} \quad (4.26)$$

$$E_z = 0 \quad (4.27)$$

$$H_x = H_{0x} \sin (m\pi x/a) \cos (n\pi y/b) e^{-\beta_g z} \quad (4.28)$$

$$H_y = H_{0y} \cos (m\pi x/a) \sin (n\pi y/b) e^{-\beta_g z} \quad (4.29)$$

$m = 0, 1, 2,.., n = 0, 1, 2,..,$ and $m = n = 0$ is excluded.

For $\mathbf{TE}_{mn}$ mode, the important parameters are:

(i) The cut-off wave number k_c for $\mathbf{TE}_{mn}$ modes is given by

$$k_c = \sqrt{(m\pi / a)^2 + (n\pi / b)^2} = \omega_c \sqrt{\mu\varepsilon} \quad (4.30)$$

The dimensions of a and b are in meters.

(ii) The cut-off frequency f_c for the $\mathbf{TE}_{mn}$ modes is given by

$$f_c = \sqrt{[(m/a)^2 + (n/b)^2]/(4\mu\varepsilon)} \quad (4.31)$$

(iii) The phase or propagation constant β_g is given by

$$\beta_g = \omega\sqrt{\mu\varepsilon} \sqrt{1 - (f_c / f)^2} \quad (4.32)$$

(iv) The guide velocity v_g in the positive z-direction is given by

$$v_g = \omega / \beta_g = v_p / \sqrt{1 - (f_c / f)^2} \quad (4.33)$$

(v) The phase velocity v_p in an unbounded dielectric is given by $v_p = 1/\sqrt{\mu\varepsilon}$

(vi) The characteristic wave impedance Z_g of $\mathbf{TE}_{mn}$ modes in the waveguide is defined as

$$Z_g = E_x/H_y = -E_y/H_x$$

Since $\beta_g E_x = \omega\mu H_y$ and $\beta_g E_y = -\omega\mu H_z$, we obtain

$$Z_g = \omega\mu/\beta_g$$

Substituting for β_g from Eq. (4.32), we get

$$Z_g = \omega\mu / \beta_g = \eta / \sqrt{(1 - (f_c / f)^2}$$

$$= 377 \lambda_g/\lambda_0 \text{ ohm} \quad (4.34)$$

Here η is the intrinsic impedance in an unbounded dielectric and is given by $\eta = \sqrt{\mu/\varepsilon}$.

(vii) The wavelength l_g in the waveguide is given by

$$\lambda_g = \lambda / \sqrt{1 - (f_c / f)^2} \qquad (4.35)$$

Here λ is the wavelength in an unbounded dielectric and is given by $\lambda = v_p/f$.

Example 4.1: A rectangular waveguide has a broad wall dimension of 2.5 cm and is fed by a 10 GHz signal from a coaxial cable. Determine whether a $\mathbf{TE_{10}}$ will be propagated and, if so, its guide wavelength, phase velocity and group velocity.

Solution: Given: $a = 2.5$ cm,

$$f = 10 \text{ GHz}, \text{ mode} = \mathbf{TE_{10}}$$

For $\mathbf{TE_{10}}$ mode,

$$\lambda_c = 2a = 2 \times 2.5 = 5 \text{ cm}$$
$$\lambda = c/f = 3 \times 10^{10}/10^{10} = 3 \text{ cm}$$

Since $\lambda_c > \lambda$, $\mathbf{TE_{10}}$ will propagate.

From Eq. (4.34), the guide wavelength is given by

$$\lambda_g = \frac{\lambda}{\sqrt{1 - (f_c / f)^2}}$$

$$= \frac{\lambda}{\sqrt{1 - (\lambda / \lambda_c)^2}}$$

$$= \frac{3}{\sqrt{1 - (3/5)^2}} = 3.75 \text{ cm}$$

The phase velocity is given by

$$v_p = c\lambda_g/\lambda = 3 \times 10^8 \times 3.75/3$$
$$= 3.75 \times 10^8 \text{ m/sec.}$$

The group velocity is given by

$$v_g = c\lambda/\lambda_g = 3 \times 10^8 \times 3/3.75$$
$$= 2.40 \times 10^8 \text{ m/sec.}$$

4.3.4 Degenerate Modes

The cut-off frequency given by Eq. (4.31) is a function of the modes and waveguide dimensions. Therefore, the physical size of the waveguide will determine the propagation modes. Whenever two or more modes have the same cut-off frequency, they are said to be degenerate modes. In a rectangular waveguide, the $\mathbf{TE_{mn}}$ and $\mathbf{TM_{nm}}$ modes are degenerative modes.

4.3.5 Dominant Modes

The dimensions of rectangular waveguides are such that $a = 2b$. In a waveguide, the mode with the lowest cut-off frequency is known as *dominant mode*. In a rectangular waveguide with $a > b$, *the dominant mode is the* $\mathbf{TE_{10}}$ *mode*. Fig. 4.5 shows the specific field pattern of each mode. In a waveguide, all modes exist simultaneously. However, the higher modes are attenuated rapidly near the sources or discontinuities and only the dominant mode propagates. The ratio of cut-off frequency of higher order modes normalized with respect to that of the dominant $\mathbf{TE_{10}}$ mode is shown in Table 4.1.

4.3.6 TM Mode Solution in Rectangular Waveguide

For the $\mathbf{TM_{mn}}$ modes in rectangular waveguides, $H_z = 0$. To transmit electromagnetic energy in the rectangular waveguide, the z-component of the electric field, E_z must exist[6]. Therefore, the Helmholtz equation is

$$\nabla^2 E_z = \gamma^2 E_z \qquad (4.36)$$

The boundary condition to be satisfied is that the tangent component of the electric

Table 4.1: Modes of $(f_c)_{mn}/(f_c)_{TE_{10}}$ for $a > b$

a/b	TE_{10}	TE_{01}	TE_{11} TM_{11}	TE_{20}	TE_{02}	TE_{21} TM_{21}	TE_{12} TM_{12}	TE_{22} TM_{22}	TM_{30}
1	1	1	1.414	2	2	2.236	2.236	2.828	3
1.5	1	1.5	1.803	2	3	2.500	3.162	3.606	3
2	1	2	2.236	2	4	2.828	3.123	3.472	3
3	1	3	3.162	2	6	3.606	6.083	6.325	3

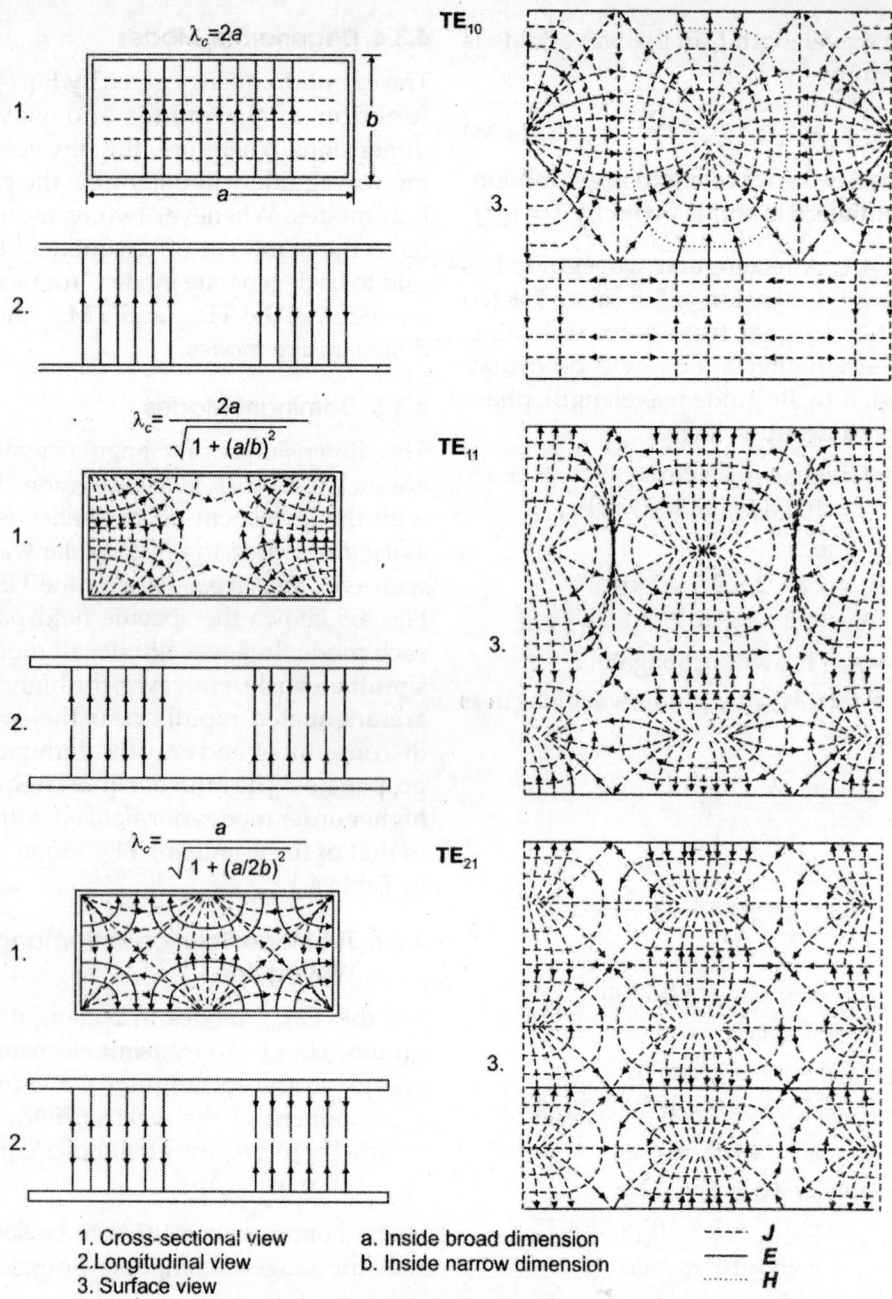

1. Cross-sectional view
2. Longitudinal view
3. Surface view

a. Inside broad dimension
b. Inside narrow dimension

```
----- J
——— E
......... H
```

Fig. 4.5: TE mode field configurations

field E_z is zero at the conducting wall. The electric field in the positive z-direction satisfying the boundary conditions on the waveguide walls is given by

$$E_z = E_{0z} \sin (m\pi x/a) \sin (n\pi y/b) e^{-j\beta_g z} \quad (4.37)$$

E_{0z} is the amplitude constant. The other TM_{mn} field equations are:

$$E_x = E_{0x} \cos (m\pi x/a) \sin (n\pi y/b) e^{-j\beta_g z} \quad (4.38)$$

$$E_y = E_{0y} \sin (m\pi x/a) \cos (n\pi y/b) e^{-j\beta_g z} \quad (4.39)$$

$$H_x = H_{0x} \sin (m\pi x/a) \cos (n\pi y/b) e^{-j\beta_g z} \quad (4.40)$$

$$H_y = H_{0y} \cos{(m\pi x/a)} \sin{(n\pi y/b)} e^{-j\beta_g z} \quad (4.41)$$
$$H_z = 0 \quad (4.42)$$
$$m = 1, 2, \ldots \text{and} \quad n = 1, 2, \ldots$$

If $m = 0$ or $n = 0$, the field intensities become zero. This means that the TM_{01} and TM_{10} modes do not exist in a rectangular waveguide. Hence, TE_{10} mode is the dominant mode in a rectangular waveguide for $a > b$.

The important parameters of the TM_{mn} modes are:

(i) The cut-off wave number k_c for TM_{mn} modes is given by

$$k_c = \sqrt{(m\pi/a)^2 + (n\pi/b)^2} = \omega_c \sqrt{\mu\varepsilon}$$

(ii) The cut-off frequency f_c is given by

$$f_c = \sqrt{(m/a)^2 + (n/b)^2/(4\mu\varepsilon)} \quad (4.43)$$

(iii) The phase or propagation constant β_g is given by

$$\beta_g = \omega\sqrt{\mu\varepsilon}\sqrt{1-(f_c/f)^2} \quad (4.44)$$

(iv) The guide velocity in the positive z-direction is given by

$$v_g = w/\beta_g = v_p/\sqrt{1-(f_c/f)^2} \quad (4.45)$$

(v) The phase velocity v_p in an unbounded dielectric is given by $v_p = 1/\sqrt{\mu\varepsilon}$

(vii) The characteristic wave impedance Z_g of TM_{mn} modes in the waveguide is given by

$$Z_g = E_x/H_y = -E_y/H_x$$

Since
$$E_x = (-j\beta_g/k_c^2)\,(\partial E_z/\partial x)$$
$$E_y = (-j\beta_g/k_c^2)\,(\partial E_z/\partial x)$$
$$H_x = (j\omega\varepsilon/k_c^2)\,(\partial E_z/\partial x)$$
$$H_y = (-j\omega\varepsilon/k_c^2)\,(\partial E_z/\partial x)$$
$$Z_g = \beta_g/\omega\varepsilon$$

$$= \frac{\omega\sqrt{\mu\varepsilon\left[1-(f_c/f)^2\right]}}{\omega\varepsilon}$$

$$= \sqrt{\mu/\varepsilon\left[1-(f_c/f)^2\right]}$$

$$= \eta\sqrt{[1-(f_c/f)^2]}$$

$$= 377\,\lambda_g/\lambda_0 \text{ ohm} \quad (4.46)$$

Figure 4.6 shows the field configuration of different **TM** modes in rectangular waveguides.

4.3.7 Power Transmission in Rectangular Waveguides

To calculate the power transmitted through a rectangular waveguide, it is assumed that there is no reflection from the receiving end. This is possible if (i) the waveguide is infinitely long compared to the wavelength or, (ii) the waveguide is match-terminated at the load end.

The power transmitted through the waveguide is given by

$$P_{tr} = \oint P ds = \oint \frac{1}{2}(E \times H^*)ds \quad (4.47)$$

If the dielectric is loss-less, the average power-flow in the rectangular waveguide in terms of electric and magnetic field intensities is

$$P_{tr} = \left(\frac{1}{2Z_g}\right)\int\!\!\int_a |E|^2\, da$$

$$= \left(\frac{Z_g}{2}\right)\int\!\!\int_a |H|^2\, da \quad (4.48)$$

The guide impedance
$$Z_g = E_x/H_y = -E_y/H_x;$$
$$|E|^2 = |E_x|^2 + |E_y|^2$$
and $|H|^2 = |H_x|^2 + |H_y|^2$

(i) *For TE_{mn} modes:* The average power transmitted through the rectangular waveguide is

$$P_{tr} = \frac{\sqrt{1-(f_c/f)^2}}{2\eta} \times$$
$$\int_0^b\int_0^a (|E_x|^2 + |E_y|^2)dx\,dy \quad (4.49)$$

(ii) *For TM_{mn} modes:* The average power transmitted through the rectangular waveguide is given by

$$P_{tr} = \frac{1}{\left[2\eta\sqrt{1-(f_c/f)^2}\right]} \times$$
$$\int_0^b\int_0^a (|E_x|^2 + |E_y|^2)dx\,dy \quad (4.50)$$

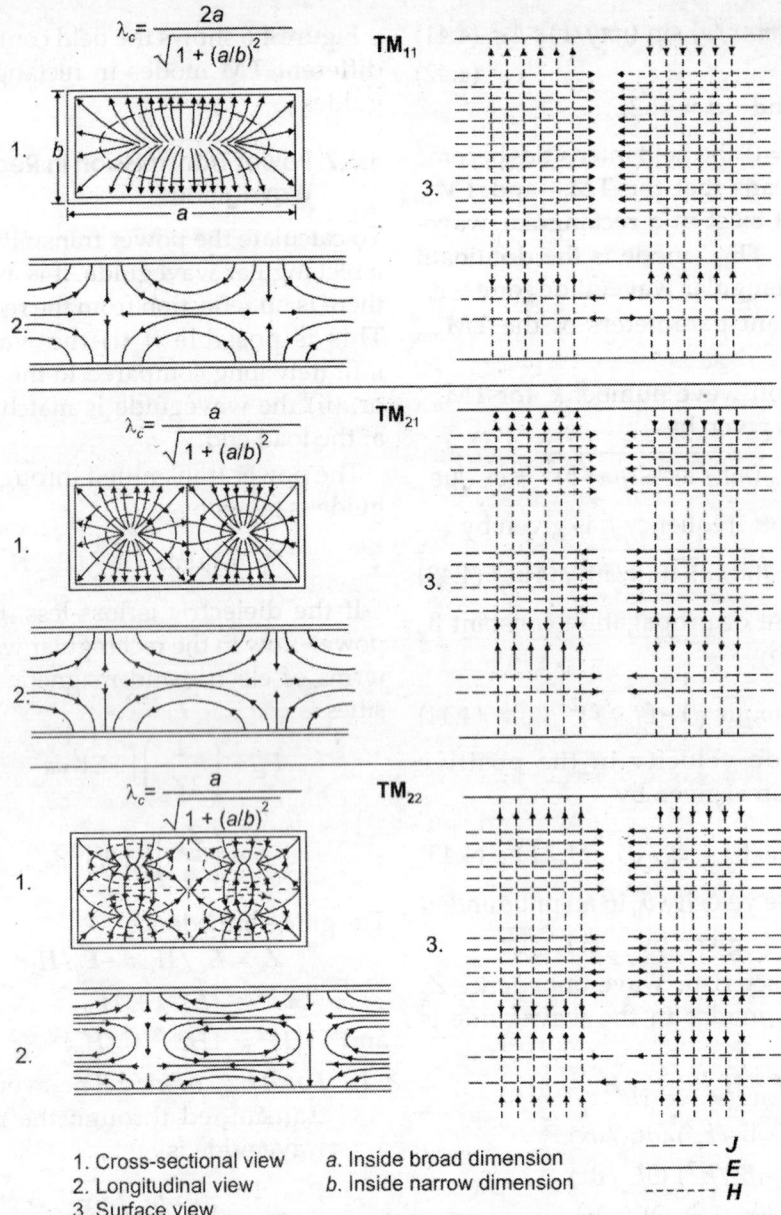

1. Cross-sectional view   *a.* Inside broad dimension
2. Longitudinal view   *b.* Inside narrow dimension
3. Surface view

Fig. 4.6: TM mode field configurations

η is the intrinsic impedance in an unbounded dielectric and is given by

$$\eta = \sqrt{\mu/\varepsilon}.$$

4.3.8 Power Losses in Rectangular Waveguides

As the power is transmitted through the waveguide, power loss occurs in the wave-guide walls. Two types of power loss occur in a rectangular waveguide. They are: (i) Dielectric losses (ii) Waveguide wall losses

(a) Power loss due to dielectric attenuation:
For a plane wave traveling in an unbounded low-loss dielectric ($\sigma \ll \mu\varepsilon$), the attenuation constant is given by

$$\alpha_0 = (\sigma/2)\sqrt{\mu/\varepsilon} = \eta\sigma/2 \qquad (4.51)$$

The low-loss dielectric in the rectangular waveguide attenuates TE_{mn} or TM_{mn} modes.

The attenuation constant in the waveguide is given by

(i) *For TE mode:*

$$\alpha_g = \frac{\alpha_0}{\sqrt{1-(f_c/f)^2}} \qquad (4.52)$$

(ii) *For TM mode:*

$$\alpha_g = \alpha_0 \sqrt{1-(f_c/f)^2} \qquad (4.53)$$

If the operating frequency $f \gg f_c$, the attenuation constant α_g in the rectangular waveguide approaches α_0, the attenuation constant for the unbounded dielectric.

(b) Power loss due to guide walls: The magnitudes of the electric and magnetic field intensities propagating through a lossy waveguide are given by

$$|E| = |E_{0z}| \, e^{-\alpha_g z} \qquad (4.54)$$

$$|H| = |H_{0z}| e^{-\alpha_g z} \qquad (4.55)$$

E_{0z} and H_{0z} are the electric and magnetic field intensities respectively at $z = 0$. For a low-loss dielectric, the average power-flow decreases exponentially. Therefore the transmitted power P_{tr} is given by

$$P_{tr} = P_{inc}e^{-2\alpha_g z} = (P_{tr} + P_{loss})e^{-2\alpha_g z} \quad (4.56)$$

Since $2\alpha_g z$ is $\ll 1$, $e^{-2\alpha_g z} \approx 1 - 2\alpha_g z$. Hence, Eq. (4.56) becomes

$$P_{tr} = (P_{tr} + P_{loss}) (1 - 2\alpha_g z)$$

$P_{loss} 2\alpha_g z$ is negligibly small. Hence,

$$P_{tr} \approx P_{tr} + P_{loss} - 2\alpha_g z \, P_{tr}$$

Dividing both sides of the above equation by P_{tr} and simplifying, we obtain

$$P_{loss}/P_{tr} = 2\alpha_g z \qquad (4.57)$$

The power loss P_l per unit length of the waveguide is given by

$$P_l = 2\alpha_g P_{tr}$$

4.3.9 Attenuation in Rectangular Waveguides

The attenuation constant in a rectangular waveguide is given by

$$\alpha_g = P_l /2P_{tr} \qquad (4.58)$$

Thus, the attenuation constant of the waveguide walls is the ratio of the power loss per unit length to twice the power transmitted through the waveguide.

As the waves progress into the low-loss waveguide, the electric and magnetic field intensities at the wall surface decrease exponentially with respect to the skin depth. Hence, the surface resistance of the waveguide walls is given by

$$R_s = \rho/\delta = 1/\sigma\delta$$

$$= \alpha_g /\sigma = \sqrt{\pi f \mu/\sigma} \ \ \Omega/\text{square} \quad (4.59)$$

ρ is the resistivity of the conducting wall in ohm-meter, δ is the skin depth or depth of penetration in meters and σ is the conductivity in mhos /meter. The power loss per unit length of the waveguide is given by

$$P_l = (R_s/2)\int_s |H_t|^2 \, ds \ \ \text{W/unit length} \ (4.60)$$

H_t is the tangential component of the magnetic field intensity at the waveguide walls.

The attenuation constant in the waveguide is given by

$$\alpha_g = \left(\frac{R_s}{2Z_g}\right)\frac{\int_s |H_t|^2 \, ds}{\int_a |H|^2 \, da} \qquad (4.61)$$

$$|H|^2 = |H_z|^2 + |H_y|^2$$

and $\quad |H_t|^2 = |H_{tz}|^2 + |H_{ty}|^2 \qquad (4,62)$

It can be shown that the attenuation constant is

$$\alpha_g = 8.686 \, R_s \left[1+(2b/a)(f_c/f)^2\right]\lambda$$

$$\left[b\sqrt{\mu/\varepsilon} \sqrt{(1-(f_c/f)^2}\right] \ \text{dB/m} \ (4.63)$$

Because of finite conductivity of the waveguide walls, the attenuation for the

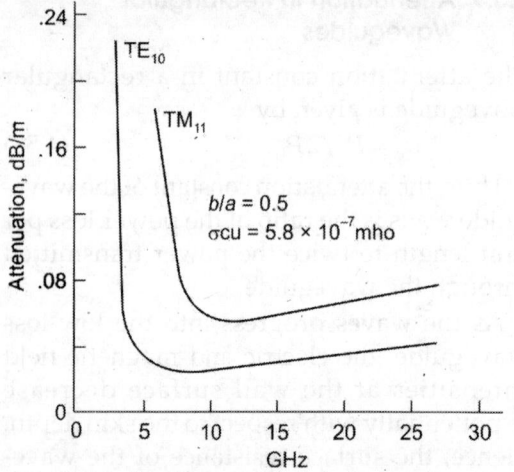

Fig. 4.7: Attenuation of dominant modes in rectangular waveguides

dominant mode varies as a function of frequency and is shown in Fig. 4.7. The attenuation is very high at $f = f_c$ and decreases with increase in frequency to a low value and then increases with increase in frequency.

4.3.10 Modes of Excitation in Rectangular Waveguides

The device used to excite the desired mode in the waveguides is known as *probe*. The probe is also known as the coupling loop, the loop antenna or monopole antenna. In rectangular waveguides, the probe may be a coaxial cable with the center conductor acting as a probe or loop-coupling device. The probe should be so located as to excite the electric field intensity of the desired mode. The coupling loop is located in such a way as to generate the magnetic field intensity for the desired mode. When more than one probe is used, it should be ensured that the proper phase relationship exists between the currents in various probes. This is accomplished by inserting additional lengths of transmission line in one or more of the antenna feeders. Impedance matching is achieved (i) by varying the position and the depth of the probe in the waveguide, or,

(ii) by using impedance matching stubs on the coaxial lines that feed the guide. The probe exciting a given mode in the waveguide can also be used reciprocally as the collector or receiver of the energy of that mode. Figure 4.8 shows the methods of excitation for various modes in the rectangular waveguides.

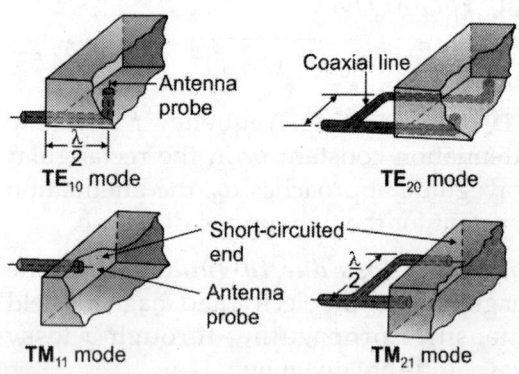

Fig. 4.8: Excitation modes in rectangular waveguide

Two probes are used to excite TE_{10} mode in one direction of the waveguide. The two exciting probes are positioned in such a way that the field intensities reinforce in one direction and cancel each other in the other direction. Such an arrangement for launching TE_{10} mode in one direction only is shown in Fig. 4.9. The two probes are placed a quarter-wavelength apart and their phases are in time quadrature. An additional quarter-wavelength section of the line is used for phase compensation. The field intensities radiated by the two probes are in phase to the right of the antennas and reinforce each

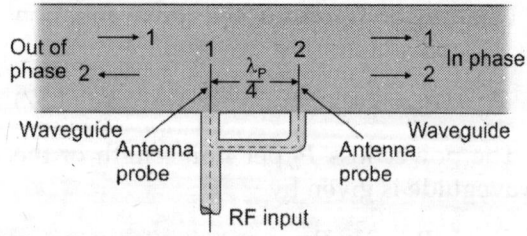

Fig. 4.9: Launching of TE_{10} mode in one direction

other whereas the field intensities to the left of the antennas are in opposition and cancel each other. Thus, the resulting wave propagates to the right in the waveguide.

The presence of obstacles, bends and loads form the discontinuities. At discontinuities, higher-order modes are generated. They are, however, heavily attenuated. As the attenuation of the dominant mode is less, even though the waveguide dimensions are large enough to support higher order modes, the dominant mode tends to remain as the dominant mode

4.3.11 Rectangular Waveguides Characteristics

At microwave frequencies rectangular waveguides are widely used for power transmission. Their physical dimensions are determined by the transmitted signal frequency. For example, a standard rectangular waveguide WR 90, has an outer dimensions of 2.54 cm × 1.27 cm (1″ × 0.5″) at X-band frequencies (8 GHz to 12 GHz) and its inner dimensions are 2.286 cm × 1.016 cm. The characteristics of the standard rectangular waveguides are given in Table 4.2[8].

Table 4.2: Characteristics of standard rectangular waveguides

EIA[a] designation WR[b]	Physical dimensions Inside, in cm (inch)		Outside, in cm (inch)		Cutoff frequency for air-filled waveguide in GHz	Recommended frequency range for TE_{10} mode in GHZ
	Width	Height	Width	Height		
2300	58.420 (23.000)	29.210 (11.500)	59.055 (23.250)	29.845 (11.750)	0.257	0.32–0.49
2100	53.340 (21.000)	26.670 (10.500)	53.973 (21.250)	27.305 (10.750)	0.281	0.35–0.53
1800	45.720 (18.000)	22.860 (9.000)	46.350 (18.250)	23.495 (9.250)	0.328	0.41–062
1500	38.100 (15.000)	19.050 (7.500)	38.735 (15.250)	19.685 (7.750)	0.394	0.49–0.75
1150	29.210 (11.500)	14.605 (5.750)	29.845 (11.750)	15.240 (6.000)	0.514	0.64–0.98
975	24.765 (9.750)	12.383 (4.875)	25.400 (10.000)	13.018 (5.125)	0.606	0.76–1.15
770	19.550 (7.700)	9.779 (3.850)	20.244 (7.970)	10.414 (4.100)	0.767	0.96–1.46
650	16.510 (6.500)	8.255 (3.250)	16.916 (6.660)	8.661 (3.410)	0.909	1.14–1.73
510	12.954 (5.100)	6.477 (2.500)	13.360 (5.260)	6.883 (2.710)	1.158	1.45–2.20
430	10.922 (4.300)	5.461 (2.150)	11.328 (4.460)	5.867 (2.310)	1.373	1.72–2.61
340	8.636 (3.400)	4.318 (1.700)	9.042 (3.560)	4.724 (1.860)	1.737	2.17–3.30
284	7.214 (2.840)	3.404 (1.340)	7.620 (3.000)	3.810 (1.500)	2.079	2.60–3.95
229	5.817 (2.290)	2.908 (1.145)	6.142 (2.418)	3.233 (1.273)	2.579	3.22–4.90

(Contd.)

Table 4.2: Characteristics of standard rectangular waveguides (Contd.)

EIA[a] designation WR[b]	Physical dimensions Inside, in cm (inch)		Outside, in cm (inch)		Cutoff frequency for air-filled waveguide in GHz	Recommended frequency range for TE_{10} mode in GHZ
	Width	Height	Width	Height		
187	4.755 (1.872)	2.215 (0.872)	5.080 (2.000)	2.540 (1.000)	3.155	3.94–5.99
159	4.039 (1.590)	2.019 (0.795)	4.365 (1.718)	2.344 (0.923)	3.714	4.64–7.05
137	3.485 (1.372)	1.580 (0.622)	3.810 (1.500)	1.905 (0.750)	4.304	5.38–8.17
112	2.850 (1.122)	1.262 (0.497)	3.175 (1.250)	1.588 (0.625)	5.263	6.57–9.99
90	2.286 (0.900)	1.016 (0.400)	2.540 (1.000)	1.270 (0.500)	6.562	8.20–12.50
75	1.905 (0.750)	0.953 (0.375)	2.159 (0.850)	1.207 (0.475)	7.874	9.84–15.00
62	1.580 (0.622)	0.790 (0.311)	1.783 (0.702)	0.993 (0.391)	9.494	11.90–18.00
51	1.295 (0.510)	0.648 (0.255)	1.499 (0.590)	0.851 (0.335)	11.583	14.50–22.00
42	1.067 (0.420)	0.432 (0.170)	1.270 (0.500)	0.635 (0.250)	14.058	17.60–26.70
34	0.864 (0.340)	0.432 (0.170)	1.067 (0.420)	0.635 (0.250)	17.361	21.70–33.00
28	0.711 (0.280)	0.356 (0.140)	0.914 (0.360)	0.559 (0.220)	21.097	26.40–40.00
22	0.569 (0.224)	0.284 (0.112)	0.772 (0.304)	0.488 (0.192)	26.362	32.90–50.10
19	0.478 (0.188)	0.239 (0.094)	0.681 (0.268)	0.442 (0.174)	31.381	39.20–59.60
15	0.376 (0.148)	0.188 (0.074)	0.579 (0.228)	0.391 (0.154)	39.894	49.80–75.80
12	0.310 (0.122)	0.155 (0.061)	0.513 (0.202)	0.358 (0.141)	48.387	60.50–91.90
10	0.254 (0.100)	0.127 (0.050)	0.457 (0.180)	0.330 (0.130)	59.055	73.80–112.00
8	0.203 (0.080)	0.102 (0.040)	0.406 (0.160)	0.305 (0.120)	73.892	92.20–140.00
7	0.165 (0.065)	0.084 (0.033)	0.343 (0.135)	0.262 (0.103)	90.909	114.00–173.00
5	0.130 (0.051)	0.066 (0.026)	0.257 (0.101)	0.193 (0.076)	115.385	145.00–220.00
4	0.109 (0.043)	0.056 (0.022)	0.211 (0.083)	0.157 (0.062)	137.615	172.00–261.00
3	0.086 (0.034)	0.043 (0.017)	0.163 (0.064)	0.119 (0.047)	174.419	217.00–333.00

Example 4.2: An air-filled coaxial cable has inner conductor and outer conductor radii equal to 2 cm and 4 cm respectively. Determine (a) the inductance per unit length, (b) the capacitance per unit length and (c) the characteristic impedance of the cable.

Solution: Given: $a = 2$ cm, $b = 4$ cm

(a) $L = (\mu_0/2\pi) \ln b/a$

$\quad = (4\pi \times 10^{-7}/2\pi) \ln (4/2)$

$\quad = 2 \times 10^{-7} \ln 2$

$\quad = 2 \times 10^{-7} \times 0.693$

$\quad = \mathbf{1.386 \times 10^{-7}}$ H/m.

(b) $C = 2\pi\varepsilon_0/\ln (b/a)$

$\quad = 2\pi \times 10^{-9}/(36\pi \ln (4/2))$

$\quad = 10^{-9}/(18 \times \ln 2)$

$\quad = \mathbf{0.08 \times 10^{-9}}$ F/m

(c) $\mathbf{Z_0} = (L/C)^{1/2}$

$\quad = (1.386 \times 10^{-7})/(0.08 \times 10^{-9})^{1/2}$

$\quad = (1732.5)^{1/2}$

$\quad = \mathbf{41.6}$ ohm

Example 4.3: An air-filled rectangular copper waveguide with dimensions 1.27 cm × 2.5 cm and a length of 25 cm is operated in the dominant mode at 12 GHz. Determine (a) the cut-off frequency, (b) guide wavelength, (c) phase velocity, (d) the characteristic impedance and (e) the power loss.

Solution: Given: $a = 2.5$ cm, $b = 1.27$ cm, $l = 25$ cm, $f = 12$ GHz, TE_{10} dominant mode.

(a) $\lambda = \dfrac{30}{12} = 2.5$ cm

$f_c = \dfrac{c}{2a} = \dfrac{300 \times 10^8}{(2 \times 2.5)} = \mathbf{6.0}$ GHz

(b) $\lambda_g = \dfrac{\lambda}{\sqrt{1 - (f_c/f)^2}}$

$\quad = \dfrac{2.5}{\sqrt{1 - (6/12)^2}}$

$\quad = \dfrac{2.5}{\sqrt{0.75}} = \mathbf{2.887}$ cm

(c) $u_p = \dfrac{c}{\sqrt{1 - (f_c/f)^2}}$

$\quad = \dfrac{3 \times 10^8}{\sqrt{1 - (6/12)^2}} = \dfrac{3 \times 10^8}{\sqrt{0.75}}$

$\quad = \mathbf{3.46 \times 10^8}$ m/sec

(d) $Z_0 = \dfrac{377}{\sqrt{[1 - (f_c/f)^2]}} = \dfrac{377}{\sqrt{[1 - (6/12)^2]}}$

$\quad = \dfrac{377}{\sqrt{0.75}} = \mathbf{435.3}$ ohm

4.4 CIRCULAR WAVEGUIDES

Figure 4.10 shows a circular waveguide. It is a hollow metallic circular tube or pipe with uniform cross-section and a finite radius a. The propagation of a plane wave through a circular waveguide is either in transverse electric (**TE**) mode or transverse magnetic (**TM**) mode. The general properties of the modes in circular waveguides are similar to those in rectangular waveguides.

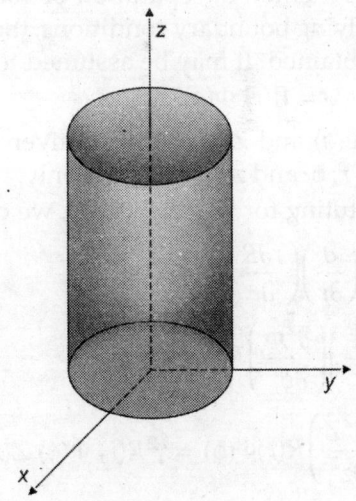

Fig. 4.10: Circular waveguide

4.4.1 Solutions of Wave Equations in Circular Waveguides

In this case also, we shall discuss the frequency-domain or the sinusoidal steady-

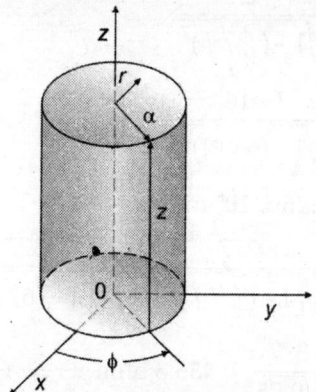

Fig. 4.11: Cylindrical coordinate system

state solution[3,7] Fig. 4.11 shows the cylindrical coordinate system.

(i) Helmholtz equation

The scalar Helmholtz equation in cylindrical coordinates is given by

$$\left(\frac{1}{r}\right)\left(\frac{\partial}{\partial r}\right)\left(\frac{r\partial\psi}{\partial r}\right)+\left(\frac{1}{r^2}\right)\left(\frac{\partial^2\psi}{\partial\phi^2}\right)+\left(\frac{\partial^2\psi}{\partial z^2}\right)=\gamma^2\psi \tag{4.64}$$

By the method of separation of variables and applying boundary conditions, the solution is obtained. It may be assumed to be

$$\psi = R(r)\,\Phi(\phi)Z(z) \tag{i}$$

$R(r)$, $\Phi(\phi)$ and $Z(z)$ are respectively functions of r, ϕ and z coordinates only.

Substituting for ψ in Eq. (4.64), we obtain

$$\left(\frac{1}{r}\right)\left(\frac{\partial}{\partial r}\right)\left(\frac{r\partial R}{\partial r}\right)\Phi(\phi)Z(z)$$

$$+\left(\frac{1}{r^2}\right)\left(\frac{\partial^2\Phi}{\partial\phi^2}\right)R(r)Z(z)$$

$$+\left(\frac{\partial^2 Z}{\partial z^2}\right)R(r)\Phi(\phi)=\gamma^2 R(r)\,\Phi(\phi)\,Z(z) \tag{ii}$$

Dividing both sides by $\psi = R(r)\,\Phi(\phi)\,Z(z)$, we have

$$\left(\frac{1}{Rr}\right)\left(\frac{d}{dr}\right)\left(\frac{r dR}{dr}\right)+\left(\frac{1}{\Phi r^2}\right)\left(\frac{d^2\Phi}{d\phi^2}\right)$$

$$+\left(\frac{1}{Z}\right)\left(\frac{d^2 Z}{dz^2}\right)=\gamma^2 \tag{iii}$$

Each term on the left-hand side is independently variable and their sum is a constant. Hence, each term must be equal to a constant. Setting the third term to a constant γ_g^2, where γ_g is the propagation constant, we have

$$\frac{d^2 Z}{dz^2}=\gamma_g^2 Z \tag{iv}$$

or, $$Z = Ae^{-\gamma_g z}+Be^{\gamma_g z} \tag{v}$$

Replacing $\left(\frac{1}{Z}\right)\left(\frac{d^2 Z}{dz^2}\right)=\gamma_g^2$ in Eq. (iii), we get

$$\left(\frac{1}{Rr}\right)\left(\frac{d}{dr}\right)\left(\frac{r dR}{dr}\right)+\left(\frac{1}{\Phi r^2}\right)\left(\frac{d^2\Phi}{d\phi^2}\right)+\gamma_g^2=\gamma^2 \tag{vi}$$

Substituting $k_c^2=\gamma_g^2-\gamma^2$, we obtain

$$\left(\frac{1}{Rr}\right)\left(\frac{d}{dr}\right)\left(\frac{r dR}{dr}\right)+\left(\frac{1}{\Phi r^2}\right)\left(\frac{d^2\Phi}{d\phi^2}\right)+k_c^2=0 \tag{vii}$$

Multiplying the above equation by r^2, we have

$$\left(\frac{r}{R}\right)\left(\frac{d}{dr}\right)\left(\frac{r dR}{dr}\right)+\left(\frac{1}{\Phi}\right)\left(\frac{d^2\Phi}{d\phi^2}\right)+k_c^2 r^2=0 \tag{viii}$$

Let the second term be a constant $(-n^2)$. Thus,

$$\frac{d^2\Phi}{d\phi^2}=-n^2\Phi \tag{ix}$$

Solving for ϕ, we obtain
$$\Phi = A_n\sin(n\phi)+B_n\cos(n\phi)$$
$$= F_n\cos(n\phi+\theta) \tag{x}$$

Replacing $(1/\Phi)(d^2\Phi/d\phi^2)=-n^2$ in Eq. (viii), we have

$$\left(\frac{r}{R}\right)\left(\frac{d}{dr}\right)\left(\frac{r dR}{dr}\right)-n^2+k_c^2 r^2=0 \tag{xi}$$

(ii) Bessel's equation of order n

Multiplying both sides by R, we get the Bessel's equation of order n. Thus,

$$\left(\frac{r d}{dr}\right)\left(\frac{r dR}{dr}\right)+(k_c^2 r^2-n^2)R=0 \tag{xii}$$

(iii) Characteristic equation of the Bessel's equation

The characteristic equation of the Bessel's equation is given by

$$k_c^2 + \gamma^2 = \gamma_g^2 \qquad (4.65)$$

The solution of Eq. (xii) yields

$$R = C_n J_n(k_c r) + D_n N_n(k_c r) \qquad (xiii)$$

Since $r = 0$ on the z-axis, $D_n = 0$, Hence,

$$R = C_n J_n(k_c r) \qquad (xiv)$$

Therefore, the final solution of the scalar Helmholtz equation is

$$\psi = C_n J_n(k_c r) \times F_n \cos(n\phi + \theta) Z e^{\pm j \beta_g z}$$

Since Z contributes to the magnitude only, we have

$$\psi = \psi_0 J_n(k_c r) \cos(n\phi) e^{-j \beta_g z} \qquad (4.66)$$

$\psi_0 = C_n F_n Z \cdot J_n(k_c r)$ is the nth order Bessel function of the first kind. For $r < a$, it represents a standing wave of $\cos(n\phi)$ as shown in Fig. 4.12.

(iv) Phase constant β_g

For loss-less line, $\gamma^2 = -\omega^2 \mu\varepsilon$ and $\gamma_g^2 = -\beta_g^2$. Substituting these values in Eq. (4.65), the phase constant β_g is given by

$$\beta_g = \pm\sqrt{\omega^2 \mu\varepsilon - k_c^2} \qquad (4.67)$$

4.4.2 TE Modes in Circular Waveguides

Generally, the electromagnetic waves in circular waveguides are assumed to be propagating in the positive z-direction. In circular waveguide, the TE_{np} modes are characterized by $E_z = 0$. This implies that, for transmission of electromagnetic energy in the circular waveguide, the z-component of the magnetic field H_z must exist[9].

(i) Helmholtz equation

The Helmholtz equation in a the circular waveguide is given by

$$\nabla^2 H_z = \gamma^2 H_z \qquad (4.68)$$

Its solution obtained after satisfying the boundary condition is

$$H_z = H_{0z} J_n(k_c r) \cos(n\phi) e^{-j\beta_g z} \qquad (4.69)$$

(ii) Boundary conditions

The boundary conditions to be satisfied are:
(i) The tangential electric field $E_\phi = 0$ at the inner surface of the circular waveguide.
(ii) The normal magnetic field $H_r = 0$ at the inner surface of the circular waveguide.

Since $H_r = 0$ at $r = a$, $\partial H_z / \partial r = 0|_{r=a}$

or

since $E_\phi = 0$ at $r = a$, $\partial H_z / \partial r = 0|_{r=a}$

Therefore, from Eq. (4.69), we get

$$\partial H_z / \partial r = H_{0z} J_n'(k_c r)|_{r=a} \cos(n\phi) e^{-j\beta_g z} = 0$$
$$(i)$$

The above equation implies that

$$J_n'(k_c r) = 0 \qquad (ii)$$

J_n' is the derivative of J_n.

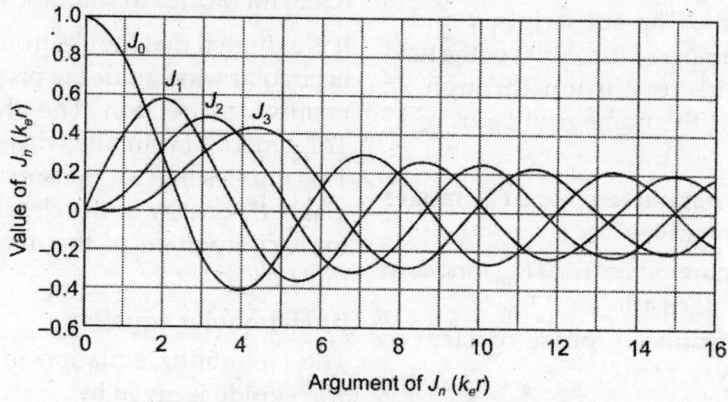

Fig. 4.12: Bessel function of the first kind

J_n is an oscillatory function. Hence, its derivative J_n' is also an oscillatory function. X'_{np} are the numerous roots of J_n' $(k_c a)$ and correspond to the maxima and minima of the curves J_n' $(k_c a)$ as shown in Fig. 4.12. A few roots of J_n' $(k_c a)$ are give in Table 4.3 for lower order n.

Table 4.3: p^{th} zeros of J_n' $(k_c a)$ for TE_{np} modes

$p \, n$	0	1	2	3	4	5
1	3.832	1.841	3.054	4.201	5.317	6.416
2	7.016	5.331	6.706	8.015	9.282	10.520
3	10.173	8.536	9.969	11.346	12.682	13.987
4	13.324	11.706	14.170			

(iii) Circular waveguide field equations for the TE_{np} modes

The complete field equations for the TE_{np} modes in circular waveguides are:

$$H_r = -(E_{0\phi}/Z_g) J_n(X'_{np} r/a) \cos (n\phi) e^{-j\beta_g z}$$
$$(4.70)$$

$$H_\phi = (E_{0r}/Z_g) J_n(X'_{np} r/a) \sin (n\phi) e^{-j\beta_g z}$$
$$(4.71)$$

$$H_z = H_{0z} J_n(k_c r) \cos (n\phi) e^{-j\beta_g z} \quad (4.72)$$
$$E_r = E_{0r} J_n(X'_{np} r/a) \sin (n\phi) e^{-j\beta_g z} \quad (4.73)$$
$$E_\phi = E_{0\phi} J_n'(X'_{np} r/a) \cos (n\phi) e^{-j\beta_g z} \quad (4.74)$$
$$E_z = 0 \quad (4.75)$$
$$n = 0, 1, 2,... \text{ and } p = 1, 2, 3,...$$

The permissible value of k_c is $k_c = X'_{np}/a$. $Z_g = E_r/H_\phi = -E_\phi/H_r$ has been used in the above equations. The subscripts n and p represent the number of full cycles of the field variation in one revolution through 2π radians of ϕ and the number of zeros of E_ϕ respectively.

(iv) Important parameters for TE_{np} modes in circular waveguides

The important parameters for TE_{np} modes in circular waveguides are:

(a) The propagation or phase constant β_g is given by

$$\beta_g = \sqrt{\omega^2 \mu \varepsilon - k_c^2} \quad (4.76)$$

(b) The cut-off wave number of a mode is that for which the propagation constant vanishes. Substituting $\beta_g = 0$ in Eq. (4.76), the cut-off wave number is given by

$$k_c = \omega_c \sqrt{\mu \varepsilon} = X'_{np}/a \quad (4.77)$$

(c) The cut-off frequency obtained from the above equation is given by

$$f_c = X'_{np}/(2\pi a \sqrt{\mu \varepsilon}) \quad (4.78)$$

(d) The guide velocity is given by

$$v_g = \frac{\omega}{\beta_g} = \frac{v_p}{\sqrt{1-(f_c/f)^2}} \quad (4.79)$$

(e) The phase velocity v_p in an unbounded dielectric is given by

$$v_p = 1/\sqrt{\mu \varepsilon} = c/\sqrt{\mu_g \varepsilon_r}$$

(f) The characteristic wave impedance Z_g is given by

$$Z_g = \frac{\omega \mu}{\beta_g} = \frac{\eta}{\sqrt{1-(f_c/f)^2}} \text{ ohm } (4.80)$$

Here $\eta = \sqrt{\mu/\varepsilon}$ is the intrinsic impedance in an unbounded dielectric.

(g) The wavelength λ_g in the waveguide is given by

$$\lambda_g = \frac{\lambda}{\sqrt{1-(f_c/f)^2}} \quad (4.81)$$

Here $\lambda = v_p/f$ is the wavelength in an unbounded dielectric.

4.4.3 TM Modes in Circular Waveguides

It is assumed that the electromagnetic waves in circular waveguide are propagating in the positive z-direction. The characteristic of TM_{np} modes in circular waveguide is $H_z = 0$. This implies that for transmission of electromagnetic energy in the circular waveguide, the z-component of the magnetic field H_z must exist.

(i) Helmholtz equation

The Helmholtz equation in a the circular waveguide is given by

$$\nabla^2 E_z = \gamma^2 E_z \quad (4.82)$$

Solving the above equation after satisfying the boundary conditions yields

$$E_z = E_{0z} J_n(k_c r) \cos(n\phi) e^{-j\beta_g z} \quad (4.83)$$

(ii) Boundary condition

The boundary condition to be satisfied is that the tangential component of the electric field E_r at the inner surface of the waveguide is zero, i.e. $E_z = 0$ at $r = a$. Hence,

$$J_n(k_c r) = 0 \qquad (i)$$

J_n is an oscillatory function. Hence, its derivative J'_n is also an oscillatory function. X_{np} are the numerous roots of $J_n(k_c a)$ and they correspond to the maxima and minima of the curves $J_n'(k_c a)$ as shown in Fig. 4.12. A few roots of $J_n(k_c a)$ are given in Table 4.4 for lower order n.

Table 4.4: p^{th} zeros of $J_n'(k_c a)$ for TM_{np} modes

p n	0	1	2	3	4	5
1	2.405	3.582	5.136	6.380	7.588	8.771
2	5.520	7.106	8.417	9.761	11.065	12.339
3	8.645	10.173	11.620	13.015	14.372	
4	11.792	13.324	14.796			

(iii) Circular waveguide field equations for the TM_{np} modes

The complete field equations for the TM_{np} modes in circular waveguides are:

$$E_r = -E_{0r} J'_n (X_{np} r/a) \cos(n\phi) e^{-j\beta_g z} \quad (4.84)$$

$$E_\phi = E_{0\phi} J_n (X_{np} r/a) \sin(n\phi) e^{-j\beta_g z} \quad (4.85)$$

$$E_z = E_{0z} J_n (X_{np} r/a) \cos(n\phi) e^{-j\beta_g z} \quad (4.86)$$

$$H_r = (E_{0\phi}/Z_g) J_n(X_{np} r/a) \sin(n\phi) e^{-j\beta_g z} \quad (4.87)$$

$$H_\phi = (E_{0r}/Z_g) J'_n(X_{np} r/a) \cos(n\phi) e^{-j\beta_g z}$$

$$H_z = 0 \qquad (4.88)$$

$$n = 0, 1, 2,... \text{ and } p = 1, 2, 3,...$$

The permissible value of k_c is $k_c = X_{np}/a$. $Z_g = E_r/H_\phi = -E_\phi/H_r$ has been used in the above equations. The subscripts n and p represent the number of full cycles of the field variation in one revolution through 2π

radians of ϕ and the number of zeros of E_ϕ respectively.

(iv) Important parameters for TM_{np} modes in circular waveguides

The important parameters for TM_{np} modes in circular waveguides are:

(a) The mode of propagation or phase constant β_g is given by

$$\beta_g = \sqrt{\omega^2 \mu\varepsilon - k_c^2} \qquad (4.90)$$

(b) The cut-off wave number of a mode is that for which the propagation constant vanishes. Substituting $\beta_g = 0$ in Eq. (4.90), the cut-off wave number is given by

$$k_c = \omega_c \sqrt{\mu\varepsilon} = X_{np}/a \qquad (4.91)$$

(c) The cut-off frequency obtained from the above equation is given by

$$f_c = X_{np}/(2\pi a \sqrt{\mu\varepsilon}) \qquad (4.92)$$

(d) The guide velocity is given by

$$v_g = \frac{\omega}{\beta_g} = \frac{v_p}{\sqrt{1-(f_c/f)^2}} \qquad (4.93)$$

(e) The phase velocity v_p in an unbounded dielectric is given by

$$v_p = 1/\sqrt{\mu\varepsilon}$$

(f) The characteristic wave impedance Z_g is given by

$$Z_g = \frac{\beta_g}{\omega\mu} = \eta\sqrt{1-(f_c/f)^2} \text{ ohm} \quad (4.94)$$

Here η is the intrinsic impedance in an unbounded dielectric and is given by

$$\eta = \sqrt{\mu/\varepsilon}$$

(g) The wavelength λ_g in the waveguide is given by

$$\lambda_g = \frac{\lambda}{\sqrt{1-(f_c/f)^2}} \qquad (4.95)$$

Here $\lambda = v_p/f$ is the wavelength in an unbounded dielectric.

Fig. 4.13 shows the field configuration of different **TE** modes in a circular waveguide.

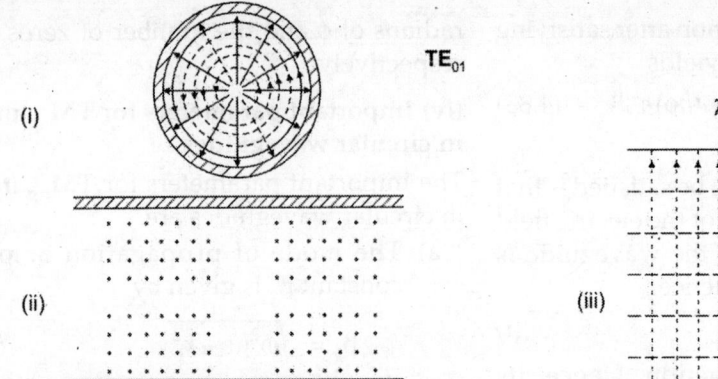

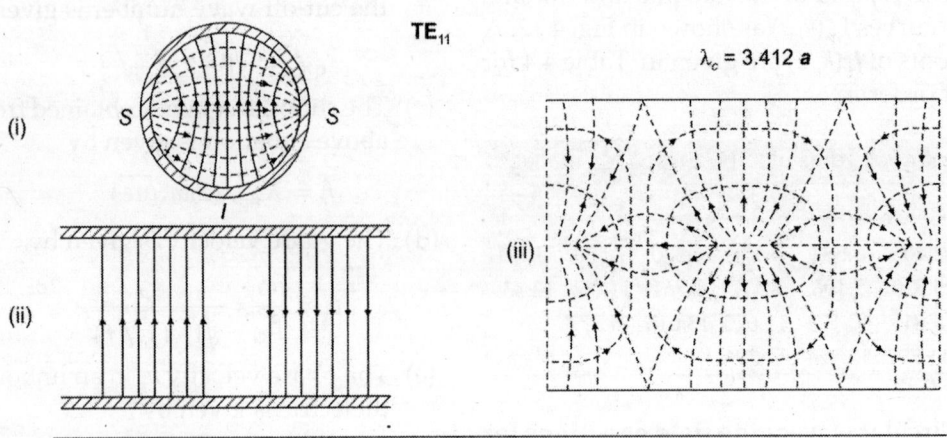

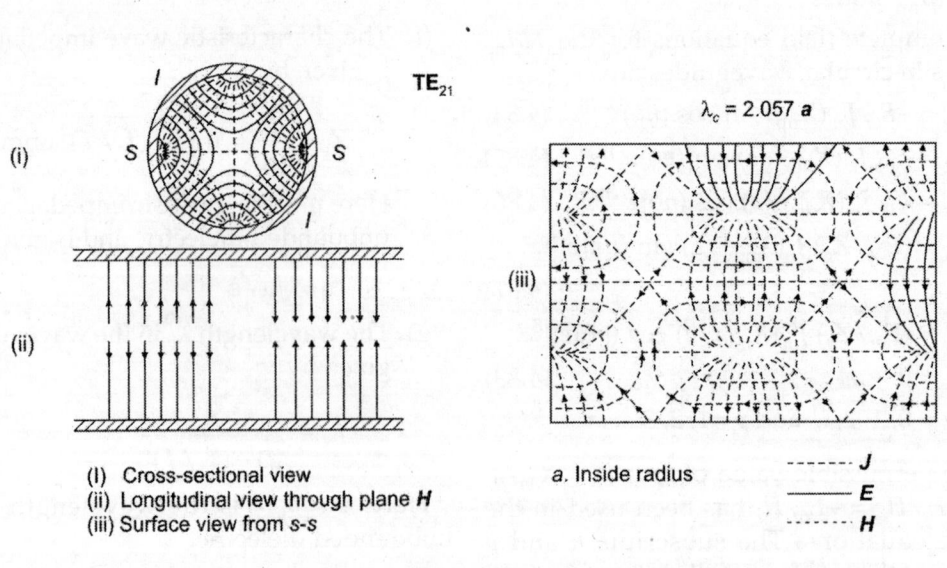

(I)   Cross-sectional view
(ii) Longitudinal view through plane **H**
(iii) Surface view from s-s

a. Inside radius

------- J
——— E
- - - - H

(a)

TM modes in circular wavwguide

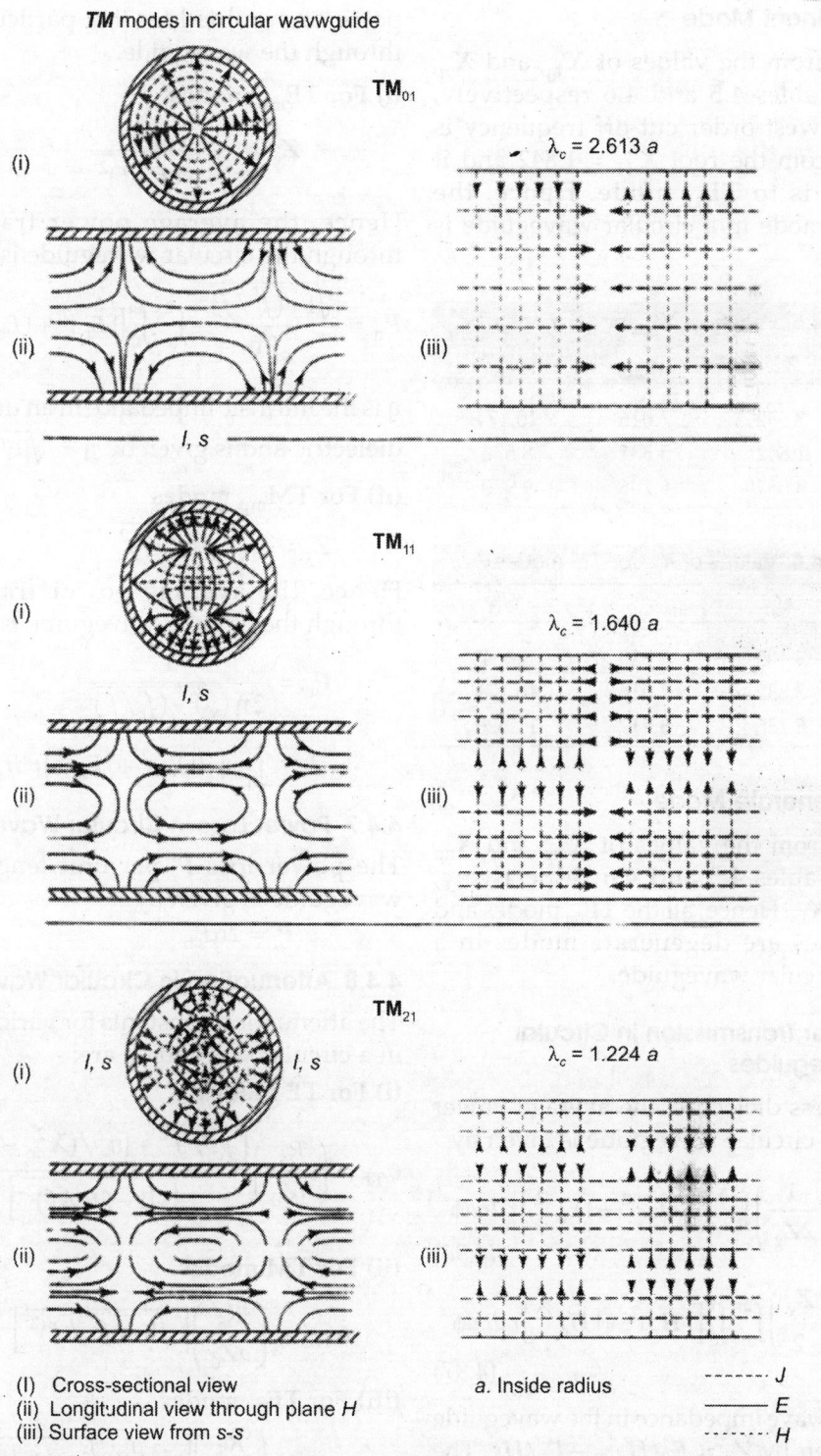

(I) Cross-sectional view
(ii) Longitudinal view through plane *H*
(iii) Surface view from *s-s*

a. Inside radius

------- *J*
——— *E*
·------ *H*

(b)

Fig. 4.13: Mode field configurations (a) **TE** and (b) **TM** modes of field configuration

4.4.4 Dominant Mode

It is seen, from the values of X'_{op} and X_{op} given in Tables 4.5 and 4.6 respectively, that the lowest-order cut-off frequency is obtained from the root $X'_{11} = 1.842$ and it corresponds to TE_{11} mode. Hence, the dominant mode in a circular waveguide is TE_{11} mode.

Table 4.5: Values of X'_{np} for TE modes

n	X'_{n1}	X'_{n2}	X'_{n3}
0	3.832	7.016	10.174
1	1.842	5.331	8.536
2	3.054	6.706	9.970

Table 4.6: Values of X_{np} for TM modes

n	X'_{n1}	X'_{n2}	X'_{n3}
0	2.405	5.520	8.654
1	3.832	7.016	10.174
2	5.135	8.417	11.620

4.4.5 Degenerate Mode

It is seen from the values of X'_{np} and X_{np} given in Tables 4.5 and 4.6 respectively, that $X'_{0p} = X_{1p}$. Hence, all the TE_{0p} modes and TM_{1p} modes are degenerate modes in a uniform circular waveguide.

4.4.6 Power Transmission in Circular Waveguides

For a lossless dielectric, the average power flow in the circular waveguide is given by

$$P_{tr} = \left(\frac{1}{2Z_g}\right)\int_0^{2\pi}\int_0^a \left[|E_r|^2 + |E_\phi|^2\right] r\, dr\, d\phi$$
(4.96)

or $\quad P_{tr} = \left(\frac{Z_g}{2}\right)\int_0^{2\pi}\int_0^a \left[|H_r|^2 + |H_\phi|^2\right] r\, dr\, d\phi$
(4.97)

Z_g is the wave impedance in the waveguide and is given by $Z_g = E_r/H_\phi = -E_\phi/Hr$. The radius of the circular waveguide is a. Substitution of Z_g in Eq. (4.96) yields the power transmitted for that particular mode through the waveguide.

(i) For TE_{mp} modes

$$Z_g = \frac{\eta}{\sqrt{1-(f_c/f)^2}}$$

Hence, the average power transmitted through the circular waveguide is given by

$$P_{tr} = \frac{\sqrt{1-(f_c/f)^2}}{2\eta}\int_0^{2\pi}\int_0^a \left(|E_r|^2 + |E_\phi|^2\right) r\, dr\, d\phi$$
(4.98)

η is the intrinsic impedance in an unbounded dielectric and is given by $\eta = \sqrt{\mu/\varepsilon}$

(ii) For TM_{mp} modes

$$Z_g = \eta\sqrt{1-(f_c/f)^2}$$

Hence, the average power transmitted through the circular waveguide is given by

$$P_{tr} = \frac{1}{2\eta\left(\sqrt{1-(f_c/f)^2}\right)} \times$$
$$\int_0^{2\pi}\int_0^a \left(|E_r|^2 + |E_\phi|^2\right) r\, dr\, d\phi \quad (4.99)$$

4.4.7 Power Loss in Circular Waveguides

The power loss P_l per unit length of the waveguide is given by

$$P_l = 2\alpha P_{tr}$$
(4.11)

4.4.8 Attenuation in Circular Waveguides

The attenuation constants for various modes in a circular waveguide are:

(i) For TE modes

$$\alpha_{TE} = \left(\frac{R_S}{aZ_0}\right)\frac{\left[f_c^2/f^2 + \{n^2/(X_{np}^2 - n^2)\}\right]}{\left[\sqrt{1-(f_c/f)^2}\right]}$$
(4.101)

(ii) For TM modes

$$\alpha_{TM} = \left(\frac{R_S}{aZ_0}\right)\left[\sqrt{1-(f_c^2/f)^2}\right]^{-1/2}$$ (4.102)

(iii) For TE_{0p} modes

$$\alpha = \left(\frac{R_S}{aZ_0}\right)\left[f_c^2/\left(f\sqrt{1-(f_c/f)^2}\right)\right]$$
(4.103)

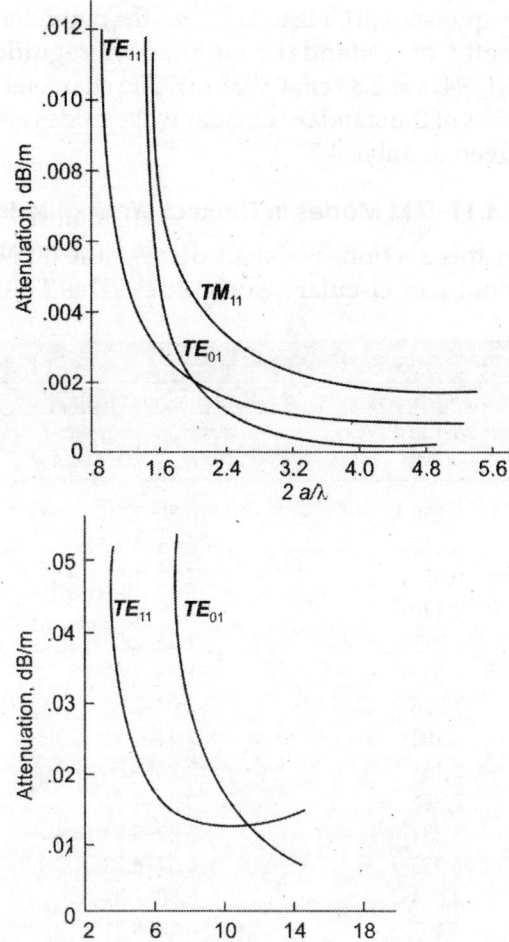

Fig. 4.14: Circular waveguide attenuation characteristics

For TE_{0p} modes, the attenuation decreases as $f^{-3/2}$ as shown in Fig. 4.14. Because of rapid decrease in attenuation with increasing frequency, the circular waveguides are used in TE_{01} for very long distance communication links. However, at any small discontinuities, the TE_{01} mode is converted into higher modes and, after a sufficient distance from the discontinuities, these additional higher modes are again converted into the TE_{01} mode leading to distortion of signal.

4.4.9 Mode of Excitation in Circular Waveguides

In the TE modes, the z-component of the electric field $E_z = 0$ and in TM modes, the

z-component of the magnetic field $H_z = 0$. Therefore, if a probe inserted in a circular waveguide excites only z-component of electric field intensity, then the wave propagating through the circular waveguide will be **TM** mode. On the other hand, if the probe excites only z-component of magnetic field intensity, the wave propagating through the circular waveguide will be **TE** mode. Fig. 4.15 shows the methods of excitation of modes in circular waveguides.

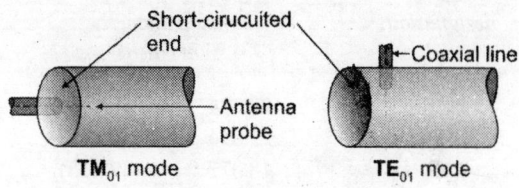

Fig. 4.15: Excitation methods in circular waveguides

Coaxial lines may also be used as probes. Figure 4.16 shows a common method of exciting **TM** modes in a circular waveguide using coaxial line. The large magnetic field existing at the end of coaxial line in the φ-direction of the wave propagation will excite the **TM** modes in the circular waveguide. However, a discontinuity exists at the junction of the circular waveguide and a coaxial line. This increases the standing wave

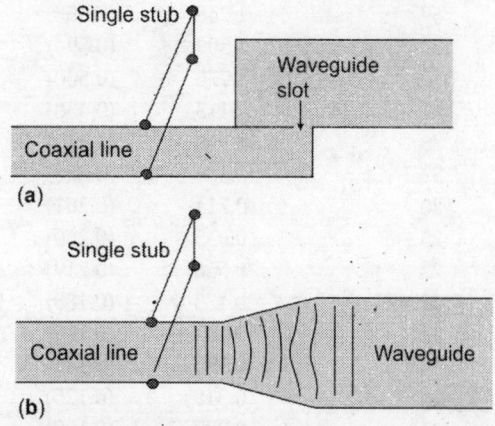

Fig. 4.16: Excitation of **TM** modes in circular waveguide coaxial line (a) with a slotted WG (b) in series with a circular WG

ratio on the line and the transmitted power is decreased due to reflection. Therefore, to suppress the reflection, a tuning device is used around the junction.

4.4.10 Circular Waveguide Characteristics

The frequency of the signal that is being transmitted determines the inner diameter of the circular waveguides. At X-band

frequencies (8 GHz to 12 GHz), the inner diameter of a standard circular waveguide WC 94, are 2.83 cm (0.938 in). The characteristics of the standard circular waveguides are given in Table 4.7.

4.4.11 TEM Modes in Circular Waveguides

In this section, we shall discuss the **TEM** modes in circular waveguides. The **TEM**

Table 4.7: Characteristics of standard circular waveguides

EIA_a-designation WC_b	Inside diameter cm (inch)		Cutoff frequency for air-filled WG GHz	Recommended frequency range for TE_{11} mode GHz
992	25.184	(9.915)	0.698	0.80–1.10
847	21.514	(8.470)	0.817	0.94–1.29
724	18.377	(7.235)	0.957	1.10–1.51
618	15.700	(6.181)	1.120	1.29–1.76
528	13.411	(5.280)	1.311	1.51–2.07
451	11.458	(4.511)	1.534	1.76–2.42
385	9.787	(3.853)	1.796	2.07–2.83
329	8.362	(3.292)	2.102	2.42–3.31
281	7.142	(2.812)	2.461	2.83–3.88
240	6.104	(2.403)	2.880	3.31–4.54
205	5.199	(2.047)	3.381	3.89–5.33
175	4.445	(1.750)	3.955	4.54–6.23
150	3.810	(1.500)	4.614	5.30–7.27
128	3.254	(1.281)	5.402	6.21–8.51
109	2.779	(1.094)	6.326	7.27–9.97
94	2.383	(0.938)	7.377	8.49–11.60
80	2.024	(0.797)	8.685	9.97–13.70
69	1.748	(0.688)	10.057	11.60–15.90
59	1.509	(0.594)	11.649	13.40–18.40
50	1.270	(0.500)	13.842	15.90–21.80
44	1.113	(0.438)	15.794	18.20–24.90
38	0.953	(0.375)	18.446	21.20–29.10
33	0.833	(0.328)	21.103	24.30–33.20
28	0.714	(0.281)	24.620	28.30–38.80
25	0.635	(0.250)	27.683)	31.80–43.60
22	0.556	(0.219)	31.617	36.40–49.80
19	0.478	(0.188)	36.776	42.40–58.10
17	0.437	(0.172)	40.227	46.30–63.50
14	0.358	(0.141)	49.103	56.60–63.50
13	0.318	(0.125)	55.280	63.50–77.50
11	0.277	(0.109)	63.462	72.70–99.70
9	0.239	(0.094)	73.552	84.80–116.00

a. Electronic Industry Association b. Circular waveguide

mode is also known as transmission-line mode. The **TEM** mode is characterized by

$$E_z = 0 \text{ and } H_z = 0. \qquad (4.104)$$

This implies that the electric and magnetic fields are completely transverse to the direction of propagation. Since the propagation of TEM mode requires two conductors, it is propagated in coaxial cables and two-open-wire transmission lines. Figure 4.17 shows the coordinates of a coaxial line.

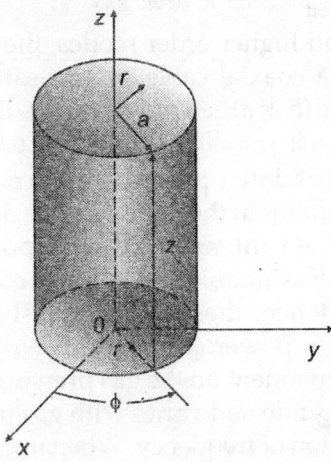

Fig. 4.17: Cylindrical coordinates for **TEM** mode

The Maxwell's equations in cylindrical coordinates are

$$\nabla \times E = -j\omega\mu H \qquad (4.105)$$
$$\nabla \times H = j\omega\varepsilon E \qquad (4.106)$$

These equations reduce to

$$\beta_g E_r = \omega\mu H_\phi \qquad (4.107)$$
$$\beta_g E_\phi = \omega\mu H_r \qquad (4.108)$$
$$\partial(rE_\phi)/\partial r - \partial E_r/\partial\phi = 0 \qquad (4.109)$$
$$\beta_g H_r = -\omega\varepsilon E_\phi \qquad (4.110)$$
$$\beta_g H_\phi = \omega\varepsilon E_r \qquad (4.111)$$
$$\partial(rH_\phi)/\partial r - \partial H_r/\partial\phi = 0 \qquad (4.112)$$

where $\qquad \partial/\partial r = -j\beta_g.$

Thus, From Eq. (4.109), we get

$$H_\phi = \beta_g E_r/\omega\mu \qquad (4.113)$$

The phase constant β_g of the **TEM** mode in coaxial lines is obtained by substituting Eq. (4.113) into Eq. (4.111) for H_r.

$$\beta_g \beta_g E_\phi/\omega\mu = \omega\varepsilon E_r \qquad (4.114)$$
$$\therefore \qquad \beta_g = \omega\sqrt{\mu\varepsilon} \qquad (4.115)$$

Thus, β_g is the phase constant of the **TEM** mode in a lossless transmission line with a dielectric.

The characteristic equation of Helmholtz equation in cylindrical coordinates is given by

$$\beta_g = \sqrt{\omega^2\mu\varepsilon - k_c^2} \qquad (4.116)$$

Comparing Eqs (4.115) and (4.116), it is evident that

$$k_c = 0 \qquad (4.117)$$

This implies that the cut-off frequency of the **TEM** mode in coaxial lines is zero.

From Eq. (4.115), the phase velocity of the **TEM** mode in coaxial lines is given by

$$v_p = \omega/\beta_g = 1/\sqrt{\mu\varepsilon} = c \qquad (4.118)$$

c is the velocity of light in an unbounded dielectric.

The wave impedance of the **TEM** mode in coaxial lines is given by

$$\eta_{\mathbf{TEM}} = \beta_g/\omega\varepsilon = \omega\sqrt{\mu\varepsilon}/\omega\varepsilon = \sqrt{\mu/\varepsilon} \qquad (4.119)$$

This is the wave impedance of in a loss-less transmission line with a dielectric.

According to Ampere's law, the line integral of H about any closed path is exactly equal to the current enclosed by that path. Thus,

$$\oint H \cdot dl = I_0 e^{-j\beta_g z} = 2\pi r H_\phi \qquad (4.120)$$

where I is the complex current through the center conductor of the coaxial line.

Equation (4.120) proves beyond doubt that the propagation of **TEM** mode requires two conductors. Hence, **TEM** mode cannot exist in a hollow waveguide since it is a single conductor system.

4.4.12 Properties of TEM Mode in Lossless Medium

The important properties of **TEM** mode in a loss-less medium are summarized below:
  (i) The transmission line is a two-conductor system.
 (ii) The wave impedance is the impedance in an unbounded dielectric.
(iii) The cut-off frequency is zero.
 (iv) The phase constant is the constant in an unbounded dielectric.
  (v) The phase velocity is the velocity of light in an unbounded dielectric.

4.5 POWER HANDLING CAPABILITIES

RF breakdown voltage or electric field intensity limits the maximum power that can be transmitted through a microwave transmission line. This occurs in the region where the electric intensity E_{bd} is at its maximum in the line or the waveguide. The breakdown is in the form of a spark discharge with a loud sound at atmospheric pressure and as a glow discharge at low pressures. At this discharge point, the waveguide or the conductor of the line is oxidized or burnt out. At the discharge locations, reflections will be very high. This affects the sending end signal source and may even damage. The value of breakdown voltage depends on the gas medium, gas pressure, extent of initial gas ionization and frequency of operation.

4.5.1 Coaxial Lines

The breakdown field strength E_{bd} is determined by the dielectric breakdown. The peak break down voltage is given by

$$V_{peak} = 2aE_{bd} \ln (b/a) \qquad (4.121)$$

V_{peak} is the peak breakdown voltage and a and b are the diameters of the inner and outer conductor respectively. From Eq. (3.7), $\ln (b/a) = Z_0\sqrt{\varepsilon_r}/60$, we get

$$V_{peak} = 2aE_{bd}Z_0\sqrt{\varepsilon_r}/60$$

Assume that a sinusoidal voltage of peak value V_{peak} is applied to the input of the matched coaxial line so that the input impedance is also Z_0. Therefore the average input power is given by

$$
\begin{aligned}
P_{bd} &= (V_{peak}/\sqrt{2})^2/Z_0 \\
&= [2aE_{bd}Z_0\sqrt{\varepsilon_r}/\sqrt{2}]^2/Z_0 \\
&= a^2E_{bd}^2Z_0\varepsilon_r/1800 \text{ W} \qquad (4.122)
\end{aligned}
$$

The breakdown power for an air-filled coaxial cable ($\varepsilon_r = 1$ and $Z_0 = 77\ \Omega$) for **TEM** mode for a breakdown field intensity of $E_{bd} = 30$ kV/cm, is given by

$$P_{bd} = 38.5 \times 10^3 a^2 \text{ kW} \qquad (4.123)$$

To avoid higher order modes, the dimensions of a coaxial cable should satisfy the condition $(b + a) < \lambda/\pi$. For a 50-ohm line with $b/a = 2.3$, $a = 0.3\lambda/\pi$ and $b = 0.7\lambda/\pi$.

The breakdown power is reduced at the discontinuities in the cable because of higher electric field intensity at these points. In practice, discontinuities exist at the connector points. Hence, these connectors limit the breakdown power. The breakdown field is highly dependent on the gas pressure inside the waveguide and varies with gas pressure as a function of frequency. When microwave equipment is to be operated at high altitudes where the pressure is low, the waveguide is usually pressurized to increase the breakdown voltage.

4.5.2 Rectangular Waveguides

The dominant mode in rectangular waveguides is **TE$_{01}$** mode. The normalized electric and magnetic field equations for the dominant **TE$_{10}$** mode are given by

$$
\begin{aligned}
E_y &= E_0 \sin (\pi x/a) & (4.124) \\
H_x &= -E_0/Z_g \sin (\pi x/a) & (4.125) \\
H_z &= (jk_c/\omega\mu) \cos (\pi x/a) & (4.126) \\
E_x &= H_y = E_z = 0 & (4.127)
\end{aligned}
$$

For the dominant mode **TE$_{10}$**, the average power flow through the rectangular waveguide is given by

$$
\begin{aligned}
P_{10} &= (E_0^2 ab/4Z_g)(\beta/k_c)^2 & (4.128) \\
&= (E_0^2 ab/4\eta)\,[1 - (f_c/f)^2]^{1/2} & (4.129)
\end{aligned}
$$

η is the intrinsic impedance of the free space and is given by $\eta = \sqrt{\mu_0/\varepsilon_0}$. Z_g is the characteristic wave impedance for the dominant mode. The breakdown power for the dominant TE_{10} mode corresponding to the breakdown field of 30 kV/m, is given by

$$P_{bd} = 597\, ab\sqrt{[1-(\lambda_0/2a)^2]}\ \text{kW} \qquad (4.130)$$

The dimensions of a, b and λ_0 are in cm.

Example 4.4: For an air-filled rectangular waveguide of dimension 2.3 cm × 1.0 cm, calculate the breakdown power in the dominant TE_{10} mode at 9.375 GHz.

Solution: Given:

$$a = 2.3\ \text{cm} \quad b = 1.0\ \text{cm,}$$
$$f = 9.375\ \text{GHz}$$
$$\lambda_0 = 3 \times 10^{10}/9.375 \times 10^9 = 3.2\ \text{cm}$$

From Eq. (4.130), the breakdown power is given by

$$P_{bd} = 597\, ab\sqrt{[1-(\lambda_0/2a)^2]}\ \text{kW}$$
$$= 597 \times 2.3 \times 1.0\sqrt{[1-(3.2/4.6)^2]}$$
$$= 597 \times 2.3 \times 1.0\sqrt{[1-0.484]}$$
$$= 1373.1 \times \sqrt{0.516}$$
$$= 1373.1 \times 0.718 = \mathbf{986}\ \text{kW}$$

4.5.3 Circular Waveguides

The dominant mode in circular waveguides is TE_{11} mode. The minimum attenuation mode is TE_{01} mode. Assuming a breakdown field of 30 kV/m, the breakdown powers for these modes are given by

(i) For TE_{11} mode

$$P_{bd} = 1790a^2\sqrt{[1-(f_{c11}/f)^2]}\ \text{kW}\quad (4.131)$$

(ii) For TE_{01} mode

$$P_{bd} = 1805a^2\sqrt{[1-(f_{c01}/f)^2]}\ \text{kW}\quad (4.132)$$

The radius of the circular waveguide a is in cm. f_{c01} and f_{c11} are the cut-off frequencies for TE_{01} and TE_{11} modes respectively.

Example 4.5: A circular waveguide has a radius of 3 cm and contains air dielectric. The mode of propagation is TE_{11} mode. Find: (a) the cut-off frequency, (b) the wavelength in the waveguide for an operating frequency of 10 GHz, (c) the wave impedance and (d) the bandwidth.

Solution: Given: $a = 3$ cm, $f = 10$ GHz, TE_{11} mode

(a) From the Table 4.5, for $n = 1$ and $p = 1$,
$$x'_{11} = 1.841 = k_c a$$
The cut-off frequency is given by
$$f_c = c\, x'_{11}/2\pi a$$
$$= 3 \times 10^{10} \times 1.841/(2 \times 3.14 \times 3)$$
$$= \mathbf{2.93}\ \text{GHz}$$

(b) The wavelength in the waveguide is
$$\lambda = c/f = 300 \times 10^8/10 \times 10^9 = 3\ \text{cm}$$
$$\lambda_g = \frac{\lambda}{\sqrt{[1-(f_c/f)^2]}}$$
$$= \frac{3}{\sqrt{[1-(2.93/10)^2]}}$$
$$= \frac{3}{\sqrt{0.914}} = \mathbf{3.14}\ \text{cm}$$

(c) The wave impedance in the guide is
$$Z_g = 377\, \lambda_g/\lambda$$
$$= 377 \times 3.14/3 = \mathbf{394.6}\ \text{ohm}$$

(d) The bandwidth for the dominant mode is given by
$$B = f_c \text{ the next higher order } TM_{01} \text{ mode}$$
$$- f_c \text{ of } TE_{11} \text{ mode}$$
$$= (c \times x'_{11}/2\pi a) - f_c \text{ of } TE_{11} \text{ mode}$$
$$= (3 \times 10^{10} \times 2.405/2 \times 3.14 \times 3)$$
$$\qquad\qquad - (2.93 \times 10^9)$$
$$= (7.215 \times 10^{10}/18.84) - (2.93 \times 10^9)$$
$$= 3.83 \times 10^{10} - 2.93 \times 10^9 = \mathbf{0.9}\ \text{GHz}$$

4.6 SOME SPECIAL CONFIGURATIONS OF WAVEGUIDES

Special waveguide configurations are sometimes required for many applications. We shall discuss now some common types, such as capacitive-loaded waveguide, Ridge waveguide, dielectric-loaded waveguide etc.

4.6.1 Capacitively loaded Rectangular Waveguide

The useful bandwidth of a rectangular wave guide is limited to 40%. When larger bandwidth is required, ridge waveguide is often used. Since the ridge waveguide is a form of capacitively-loaded waveguide, let us first consider a capacitively-loaded waveguide shown in Fig. 4.18. C_p' is the shunt capacitance per unit length. If $C_p' = 0$, it reduces to an ordinary rectangular waveguide whose TE_{10} and TE_{20} cut-off wavelengths are $2a$ and a respectively. These wavelengths may be interpreted in terms of transverse **TEM** resonance in the waveguide. At cut-off, $\theta = 0^0$ and the two **TEM** waves propagate transverse to the guide axis. Hence, at the

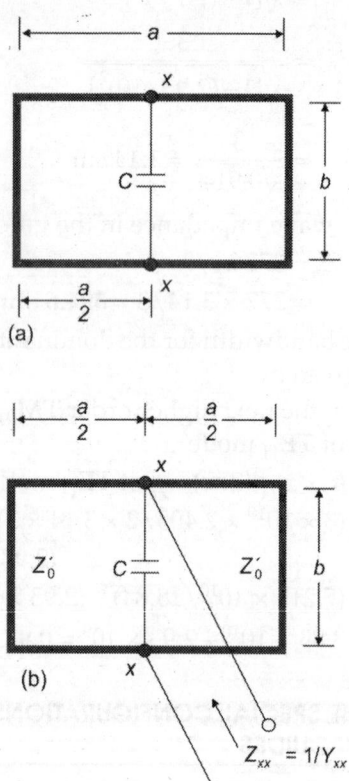

(a)

(b)

$Z_{xx} = 1/Y_{xx}$

Fig. 4.18: Capacitively-loaded rectangular waveguide

cut-off frequency f_c, the waveguide may be considered as two shorted parallel-plane lines of length $a/2$ connected across the center of the waveguide axis. This is shown in Fig. 4.19 for a one-meter length of the waveguide with the centerline denoted as x–x.

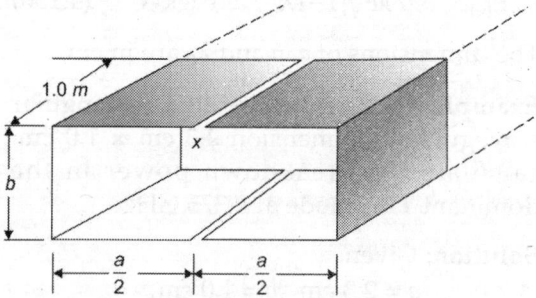

Fig. 4.19: Equivalent circuit for Fig. 4.18

For TE_{10} mode: The cut-off wavelength $\lambda_c = 2a$. Hence, the line length l is $a/2 = \lambda_c/4$. This implies that the impedance of the two quarter-wave shorted lines is infinite. Their parallel combination is $Z_{xx} = \infty$ or $Y_{xx} = 0$.

For TE_{20} mode: The cut-off wavelength $\lambda_c = a$. Hence, the line length l is $a/2 = \lambda_c/2$. This implies that the impedance of the two quarter-wave shorted lines is zero. Their parallel combination is $Z_{xx} = 0$ or $Y_{xx} = \infty$ since line lengths are each half wavelength long.

This result may be generalized for all symmetric structures so as to include all **TE**$_{m0}$ modes.

For m is odd, $Z_{xx} = \infty$ or $Y_{xx} = 0$ at f_c.

For m is even, $Z_{xx} = 0$ at f_c.

The method of determining the cut-off frequencies for various modes by applying the above condition is known as *transverse-resonance method.*

The above method may be applied to determine the TE_{10} and TE_{20} cut-offs for the capacitively-loaded rectangular waveguide. Due to capacitive loading, the field patterns for these modes are distorted versions of **TE** modes in ordinary rectangular waveguides as shown in Fig. 4.20.

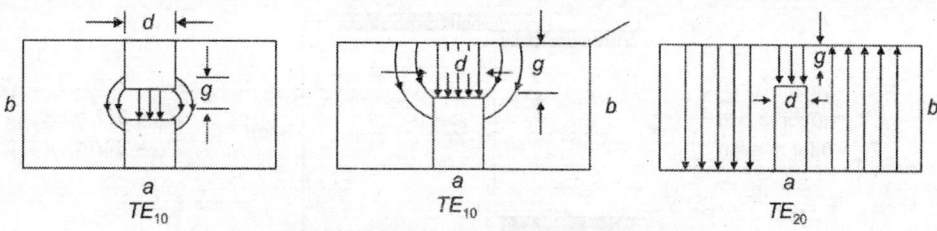

Fig. 4.20: E-field pattern in ridge waveguide

For TE_{m0} mode (m is odd): The transverse-resonance condition is Y_{xx} is zero at f_c. Hence, the admittance equation is given by

$$-j\,2Y_0' \cot\left[(2\pi/\lambda_c)\,(a/2)\right] + j\,2\pi f_c\,C_p' = 0$$

i.e., $\quad Y_0' \cot(\pi a/\lambda_c) = \pi f_c C_p'$

or, $\quad\tan(\pi \alpha/\lambda_c) = Y_0'/\pi f_c C_p' \quad$ (4.133)

$Y_0'\,(=1/Z_0')$ is the characteristic admittance of a 1 m wide parallel line. With $w = 1$, the impedance Z_0' is given by

$$Z_0' = 1/Y_0' = 377b\sqrt{\mu_r/\varepsilon_r} \quad (4.134)$$

Substituting Eqs (4.134) in (4.133), we get

$$\tan(\pi a/\lambda_c) = \frac{1}{(377b\sqrt{\mu_r/\varepsilon_r}\,\pi f_c C_p')} \quad (4.135)$$

Since $f_c = c/(\mu_r/\varepsilon_r)$, the above equation becomes

$$\tan(\pi \alpha/\lambda_c) = (\varepsilon_r/377\,\pi bc)\,(\lambda_c/C_p') \quad (4.136)$$

The above equation is known as cut-off equation.

For ordinary rectangular waveguide, $C_p' = 0$. Hence

$$\tan(\pi a/\lambda_c) = \infty$$

or, $\quad \pi a/\lambda_c = n\pi/2,\ (n = 1, 3, 5,...)$

$\therefore \qquad \lambda_c = 2a/n \quad (n = 1, 3, 5,...) \quad (4.137)$

For a capacitively-loaded waveguide, C_p' is finite. Hence,

$$\tan(p\,a/\lambda_c) < \infty$$

or, $\quad \pi a/\lambda_c < n\pi/2,\ (n = 1, 3, 5,...)$

$\therefore \qquad \lambda_c < 2a/n \quad (n = 1, 3, 5,...) \quad (4.138)$

Thus, λ_c is increased for finite values of C_p' and hence the cut-off frequency f_c increased. This is because the electric field is the maximum at the center and the presence of capacitance C_p' changes the cut-off frequency f_c significantly.

For TE_{m0} mode (m is even): The transverse-resonance condition is Z_{xx} is zero at f_c. Hence, the impedance equation is given by

$$j(Z_0/2) \tan\left[(2\pi/\lambda_c)\,(a/2)\right] = 0 \quad (4.139)$$

The above equation simplifies that $Z_{xx} = 0$ when the input impedance of the two line shunt stub is zero. The capacitance C_p' is in parallel with the stub. Hence, the resonance condition is independent of C_p'. From Eq. (4.139), we get

$$\tan(\pi a/\lambda_c) = 0$$
$$\pi a/\lambda_c = n\pi$$
$$\lambda_c = a/n \quad n = 1, 2, 3,... \quad (4.140)$$

Hence, the cut-off wavelength λ_c for TE_{20}, TE_{40}, TE_{60}, etc. are $a, a/2, a/3$ etc.. Thus, they are identical to the corresponding modes in the ordinary rectangular waveguide. Since the TE_{10} cut-off frequency is decreased while TE_{20} cut-off frequency is unchanged because the electric field at the center is zero. Therefore, the bandwidth with the capacitance loading is increased.

4.6.2 Ridge Waveguide

One form of capacitively-loaded waveguide is the ridge waveguide shown in Fig. 4.21.

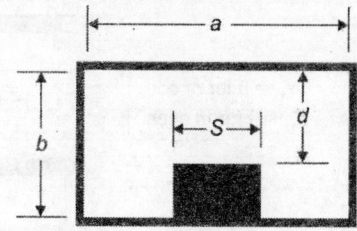

Fig. 4.21: Single-ridge waveguide (cross-sectional view)

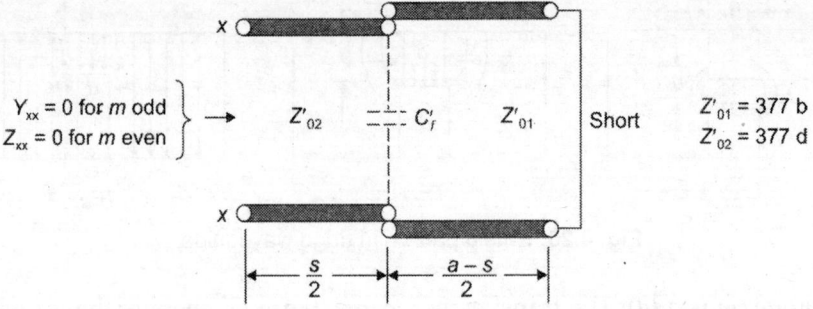

Fig. 4.22: Equivalent circuit for Fig. 4.21

The shunt capacitance is contributed by a small section of a low-loss impedance line. In this case, the low-loss impedance line is the reduced height portion of the air-filled rectangular guide (d). By applying the trans-verse-resonance method, to the equivalent circuit shown in Fig. 4.22, the cut-off wavelengths are obtained. C_f' is due to the fringing fields at the step-discontinuities between d and b. Cohn[10] and Hofer[11] have solved this problem for both single and double ridge configurations. For large ridges (i.e. for small d/b), the TE_{10} cut-off frequency is reduced significantly while TE_{20} cut-off frequency is unchanged. Hence, greater bandwidth of the order of an octave or more can easily be obtained.

The advantages of ridge waveguide are:
(i) Greater bandwidth
(ii) Reduced size for a given operating frequency

The disadvantages are:
(i) Higher conduction loss
(ii) Lower power handling capacity.

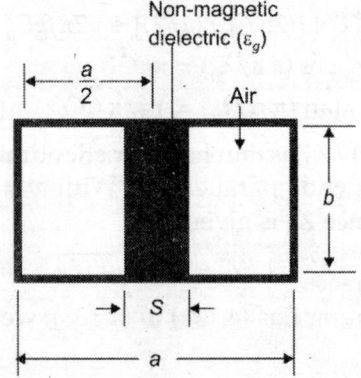

Fig. 4.23: Dielectric-loaded rectangular waveguide

4.6.3 Dielectric-Loaded Waveguide

Rectangular waveguide can be capacitively-loaded by placing a slab of dielectric material across the narrow walls of the waveguide as shown in Fig. 4.23. For the TE_{m0} cut-off wavelengths, the following equations are obtained by the application transverse-resonance condition at the center line as shown in Fig. 4.24.

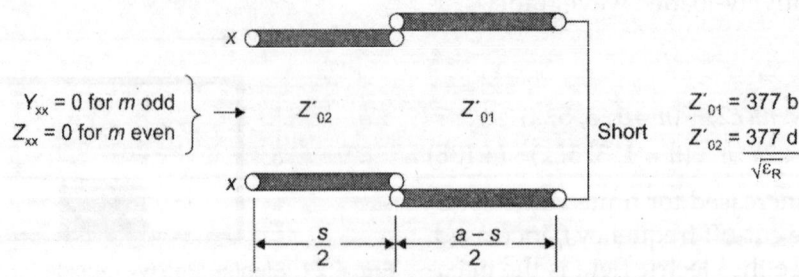

Fig. 4.24: Equivalent circuit for Fig. 4.23

For TE$_{m0}$ mode (m is odd)

$$\cot[\pi(a-s)/\lambda_c] = \sqrt{\varepsilon_r} \tan \pi \sqrt{\varepsilon_r}(s/\lambda_c) \quad (4.141)$$

For TE$_{m0}$ mode (m is even)

$$\tan \pi \sqrt{\varepsilon_r}(s/\lambda_c) = -\tan(\pi(a-s)/\lambda_c) \quad (4.142)$$

where $\lambda_c = c/f_c$. It can easily be shown that the bandwidth of this waveguide is substantially greater than that of an ordinary rectangular waveguide. This is clearly brought out in the following example.

The disadvantages of the dielectric-loaded waveguide are:

(i) Cross-mode (TE$_{01}$ mode) cut-off frequency is reduced.

(ii) Conduction loss is increased.

(iii) Power handling capacity is reduced.

4.7 OPEN-BOUNDARY STRUCTURES OR SURFACE WAVEGUIDES

The rectangular and circular waveguides so far discussed are closed boundary structures in which the transmitted EM energy is guided through a hollow metallic enclosure with very good conducting walls that prevent radiations of EM energy from the transmission line. The waveguides in which the EM energy is not confined within the conducting walls and the EM field extends outside the boundaries are known as open-boundary structures or surface waveguides. These are dielectric rod, dielectric-coated conducting wire, dielectric sheet on a metal plane, corrugated conducting plane. They are shown in Fig. 4.25. They guide EM waves in the longitudinal direction with a propagation function $e^{-j\beta z}$. However, the field strength decays from the surface exponentially in the transverse direction.

The characteristics of these waveguides are:

(i) Finite number of discrete modes at a given frequency together with continuous eigen value spectrum.

(ii) Hybrid mode HE$_{mn}$ of propagation (TE$_{mn}$ + TM$_{mn}$) except axisymmetric pure TE$_{0n}$ or TM$_{0n}$ modes.

(iii) Zero frequency cut-off for nonaxisymmetric dominant hybride mode HE$_{11}$.

4.8 DIELECTRIC ROD WAVEGUIDES

A dielectric rod or slap can be used to completely guide the electromagnetic waves[11,12]. The TE$_{10}$ mode propagation in a rectangular waveguide takes place with zigzag waves being reflected by narrow walls of the rectangular guide. A wave

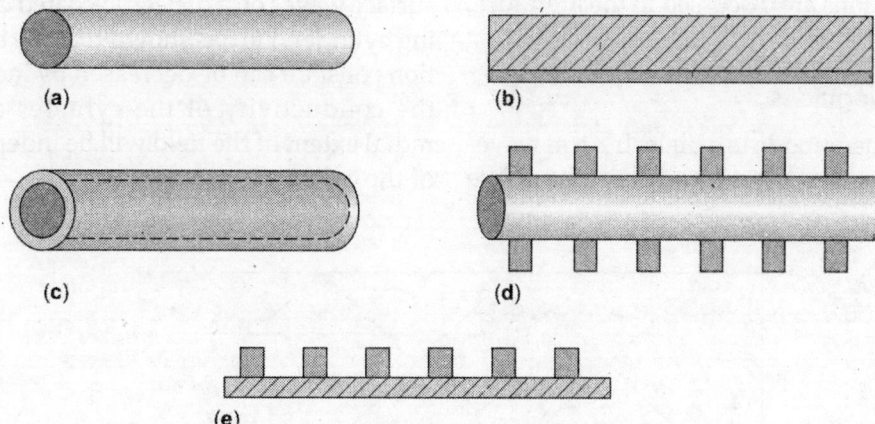

(a)

(b)

(c)

(d)

(e)

Fig. 4.25: Open-boundary structures (a) Dielectric rod (b) Dielectric sheet on conducting plane (c) Dielectric-coated conducting rod (d) Corrugated dielectric cylinder (e) Corrugated dielectric plane

traveling from high to low refractive index region can be completely reflected at the interface under certain conditions. If the dielectric is surrounded by air, complete reflection takes place when the angle of incidence θ_i is greater than a critical angle θ_c. This critical angle θ_c is given by

$$\theta_c = \sin^{-1} \sqrt{(1/\mu_r \varepsilon_r)} \qquad (4.143)$$

where μ_r and ε_r represent dielectric rod or slab properties. The angle of incidence θ_i is a function of frequency and guide dimensions. When the guide size is fixed, θ_c is equal to θ_i at some frequency f_c. At frequencies below this critical frequency f_c, $\theta_i < \theta_c$. This causes a part of the waves to be transmitted into the air region whenever they strike the dielectric boundary and hence, the transmission loss of the dielectric waveguide is high. For frequencies greater than the critical frequency f_c, $\theta_i > \theta_c$. The zigzag waves are totally contained by the dielectric resulting in low-loss transmission along the dielectric rod or slab. This is shown in Fig. 4.26. These results have been verified by theoretical analysis[14].

Since the precise fabrication of an ordinary rectangular waveguide is extremely difficult at millimeter wavelengths, the dielectric-rod waveguide is used as a low-loss transmission line at these frequencies. Many other special configurations are discussed in the literature.

4.8.1 Excitation of Dielectric Rod Waveguides

The dominant mode in a dielectric rod waveguides is excited by using a dielectric surface waveguide. The propagation of obliquely incident wave at the interface between the dielectric and outside air medium takes place by total internal reflection. The rod is tapered inside the waveguide for impedance matching. The launching efficiency is given by

$$\eta_L = \frac{\text{Surface power}}{\text{Input power} - \text{Reflected power}} \qquad (4.144)$$

4.9 DIELECTRIC SHEET ON CONDUCTING PLANE

Attwood has investigated the problem of propagation of surface waves along a conducting plane coated with a thin layer of dielectric. He has shown that a thin film of dielectric on a conducting plane surface increases the concentration of the field near the surface. The attenuation in such cases is less than that in rectangular waveguides. The attenuation in the z-direction of a copper plane coated with a thin film of polystyrene is found to be 3.1×10^{-3} neper/m.

4.10 DILECTRIC-COATED CONDUCTING CYLINDER OR GOUBAU LINE

Goubau has studied the propagation of surface waves on a dielectric-coated conducting cylinder. He has shown that the attenuation constant can be decreased by increasing the conductivity of the cylinder and the radial extent of the field will be independent of the cylinder conductivity.

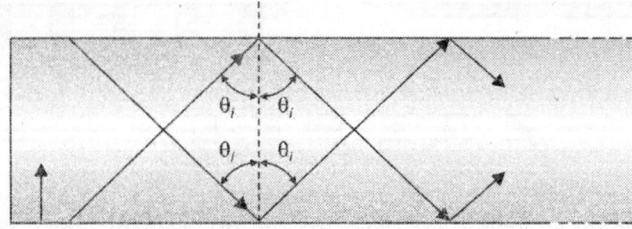

Fig. 4.26: Total reflection of waves in a dielectric waveguide for $\theta_i > \theta_c$

Advantages of Waveguides

Compared to coaxial lines, the waveguides have the following advantages:
1. A simpler low cost mechanical structure.
2. Higher power handling capacity
3. Lower loss per unit length.

4.11 COMPARISON BETWEEN COAXIAL LINES AND WAVEGUIDES

Waveguides are used for transmission of power upto wavelengths of 10 cm with low attenuation or high power carrying capability. The power losses in waveguides are one-third of that in coaxial lines. The power carrying capability of waveguides is three to ten times that of the coaxial lines. Waveguide size at short wavelengths, such as 1 cm, is a reasonable fraction of a wavelength whereas that of coaxial line is prohibitively small. At wavelengths greater than 10 cm, the size of the wavelength is large. The waveguides have an advantage in mechanical simplicity.

The comparison of waveguides with coaxial lines are presented below:

Waveguide	Coaxial line
1. Useful up to 10 cm or less	Useful for 10 cm and above
2. For λ > 10 cm, size is large	Size is not so large
3. For λ = 1cm, size is practical	Size is prohibitively small.
4. Low attenuation	High attenuation (3 times that of WG)
5. High power carrying capability	Low power carrying capability (1/3 of WG)
6. Construction is simple	Construction is a little complex

4.12 COMPARISON OF VARIOUS TRANSMISSION LINES

The characteristics of various MW transmission lines are shown in Table. 4.8.

4.13 ADDITIONAL EXAMPLES

Example 4.6: An air-filled rectangular copper waveguide with dimensions 1.27 cm × 2.5 cm and a length of 25 cm is operated in the dominant mode at 12 GHz. Determine (a) the cut-off frequency, (b) guide wavelength, (c) phase velocity, (d) the characteristic impedance and (e) the power loss.

Solution: Given: $a = 2.5$ cm, $b = 1.27$ cm, $l = 25$ cm, $f = 12$ GHz, TE_{10} mode.

(a) $\lambda = \dfrac{30}{12} = 2.5$ cm

$f_c = \dfrac{c}{2a} = 300 \times 10^8/(2 \times 2.5) = \mathbf{6.0\ GHz}$

(b) $\lambda_g = \dfrac{\lambda}{\sqrt{[1-(f_c/f)^2]}}$

$= \dfrac{2.5}{\sqrt{[1-(6/12)^2]}}$

$= \dfrac{2.5}{\sqrt{0.75}} = \mathbf{2.887\ cm}$

Table 4.8: Characteristics of transmission lines

Type	Frequency range	Usable BW	Losses	Power handling capability	Physical size	Modes of operation
Open wire	Low to VHF (500 MHz)	Lowest	Very high	Very high	Small	**TEM**
Coaxial lines	Low to MW (18 GHz)	High	Medium	Medium	Medium	**TEM**
Waveguides	MW (300 GHZ)	High	Low	Very high	Large	**TE, TM**
Strip and micro-strip lines	MW (30 GHz)	High	High	Low	Small	

(c) $u_p = \dfrac{c}{\sqrt{[1-(f_c/f)^2]}}$

$= \dfrac{3\times10^8}{\sqrt{[1-(6/12)^2]}}$

$= \dfrac{3\times10^8}{\sqrt{0.75}} = 3.46 \times 10^8 \text{ m/sec}$

(d) $Z_0 = \dfrac{377}{\sqrt{[1-(f_c/f)^2]}}$

$= \dfrac{377}{\sqrt{[1-(6/12)^2]}}$

$= \dfrac{377}{\sqrt{0.75}} = 435.3 \text{ ohm}$

Example 4.7: An air-filled rectangular waveguide with inside dimension 6 × 3 cm operates in $\mathbf{TE_{10}}$ mode. Determine (a) the cut-off frequency, (b) the phase velocity of the wave in the waveguide at a frequency of 3.0 GHz and (c) the guided wavelength at the same frequency.

Solution: Given: $a = 7$ cm, $b = 3.5$ cm, $\mathbf{TE_{10}}$ mode, $f = 3$ GHz.

(a) $f_c = \dfrac{c}{2a} = \dfrac{3\times10^8}{2\times6\times10^{-2}} = 2.5 \text{ GHz}$

(b) $v_g = \dfrac{c}{[1-(f_c/f)^2]^{1/2}}$

$= \dfrac{3\times10^8}{[1-(2.5/3)^2]^{1/2}} = 5.43 \times 10^8 \text{ m/s}$

(c) $\lambda_g = \dfrac{\lambda_0}{[1-(f_c/f^2)]^{1/2}}$

$= \dfrac{(3\times10^8/3\times10^9)}{[1-(2.5/3)^2]^{1/2}} = 18.1 \text{ cm}$

Example 4.8: A rectangular waveguide has dimension 6 cm × 3 cm and is used to propagate $\mathbf{TM_{11}}$ mode at 10 GHz. Determine the cut-off wavelength and the characteristic impedance.

Solution: Given: $a = 6$ cm, $b = 3$ cm,
mode = $\mathbf{TM_{11}}$, $f = 10$ GHz.

(a) $\lambda_c = \dfrac{2}{\sqrt{[(m/a)^2+(n/b)^2]}} = \dfrac{2ab}{\sqrt{(a^2+b^2)}}$

$= \dfrac{2\times6\times3}{\sqrt{6^2+3^2}} = 5.37 \text{ cm}$

(b) $Z_0 = 120\pi\sqrt{[1-(\lambda/\lambda_c)^2]}$

$= 120\pi\sqrt{[1-(3/5.37)^2]}$

$= 454.52 \text{ ohm}$

Example 4.9: An air-filled rectangular copper waveguide with dimensions 1 cm × 2 cm and a length of 30 cm is operated in the dominant mode at 10 GHz. Determine (a) the cut-off frequency, (b) guide wavelength, (c) phase velocity, (d) the characteristic impedance and (e) the power loss.

Solution: Given: $a = 2$ cm, $b = 1$ cm, $l = 30$ cm, $f = 10$ GHz, $\mathbf{TE_{10}}$ mode

(a) $\lambda = \dfrac{30}{10} = 3 \text{ cm}$

$f_c = \dfrac{c}{2a} = \dfrac{300\times10^8}{(2\times2)} = 7.5 \text{ GHz}$

(b) $\lambda_g = \dfrac{\lambda}{\sqrt{[1-(f_c/f)^2]}}$

$= \dfrac{3}{\sqrt{[1-(7.5/10)^2]}}$

$= \dfrac{3}{\sqrt{0.4375}} = 4.536 \text{ cm}$

(c) $u_p = \dfrac{c}{\sqrt{[1-(f_c/f)^2]}}$

$= \dfrac{3\times10^8}{\sqrt{[1-(7.5/10)^2]}}$

$= \dfrac{3\times10^8}{\sqrt{0.4375}} = 4.536 \times 10^8 \text{ m/sec}$

(d) $Z_0 = \dfrac{377}{\sqrt{[1-(f_c/f)^2]}}$

$= \dfrac{377}{\sqrt{[1-(7.5/10)^2]}}$

$$= \frac{377}{\sqrt{0.4375}} = \textbf{570 ohm}$$

(e) $\alpha_c = R_s \left[1 + (2b/a)\, (f_c/f)^2\right]$

$$\left[b\sqrt{\mu/\varepsilon}\,\sqrt{1-(f_c/f)^2}\,\right]$$

$$R_s = \sqrt{\pi f \mu/\sigma}$$

$$= \sqrt{\frac{3.14 \times 10 \times 10^9 \times 4\pi \times 10^{-7}}{5.8 \times 10^7}}$$

$$= 2.6 \times 10^{-2}\ \text{ohm}$$

$\therefore \qquad \alpha_c = 2.6 \times 10^{-2}\,[(1 + (2 \times 1/2)\,(7.5/10)^2)]$

$$\left(1 \times 377 \sqrt{(1-(7.5/10)^2}\,\right)$$

$$= 1.488 \times 10^{-4}\,\text{Np/m}$$

The attenuation for 30 cm length is

$$\alpha = 1.488 \times 10^{-4} \times 30$$
$$= 3.464 \times 10^{-3}\ \text{Np}$$
$$= 8.686 \times 3.464 \times 10^{-3}\ \text{dB}$$
$$= \textbf{0.0388 dB}$$

Example 4.10: A circular waveguide has a radius of 4 cm and contains air dielectric. The mode of propagation is **TE$_{11}$** mode. Find (a) the cut-off frequency, (b) the wavelength in the waveguide for an operating frequency of 3 GHz and (c) the wave impedance.

Solution: Given: $a = 4$ cm, $f = 3$ GHz, **TE$_{11}$** mode

(a) $\lambda = c/f = 3 \times 10^{10}/3 \times 10^9 = 10$ cm

From the Table 4.5, for $n = 1$ and
$$p = 1,\ x'_{11} = 1.841$$

The cut-off frequency is given by
$$f_c = c\, x'_{11}/2\pi a$$
$$= 3 \times 10^{10} \times 1.841/(2 \times 3.14 \times 4)$$
$$= \textbf{2.2 GHz}$$

(b) The wavelength in the waveguide is

$$\lambda_g = \frac{\lambda}{\sqrt{1-(f_c/f)^2}}$$

$$= \frac{10}{\sqrt{1-(2.2/3)^2}} = \textbf{14.71 cm}$$

(c) The wave impedance in the guide is

$$Z_g = 377\,\lambda_g/\lambda$$
$$= 377 \times 14.71/10$$
$$= \textbf{554.57 ohm}$$

Example 4.11: A circular waveguide has a radius of 2 cm and contains air dielectric. The mode of propagation is **TE$_{11}$** mode. Find (a) the cut-off frequency, (b) the wavelength in the waveguide for an operating frequency of 10 GHz, (c) the wave impedance and (d) the bandwidth.

Solution: Given: $a = 2$ cm, $f = 10$ GHz, **TE$_{11}$** mode

(a) From the Table 4.5, for $n = 1$ and
$$p = 1,\ x'_{11} = 1.841 = k_c a$$

(b) The cut-off frequency is given by
$$f_c = c\, x'_{11}/2\pi a$$
$$= 3 \times 10^{10} \times 1.841/2 \times 3.14 \times 2$$
$$= \textbf{4.397 GHz}$$

(c) The wavelength in the waveguide is

$$\lambda_g = \sqrt{\lambda/[1-(f_c/f)^2]}$$

$$= \frac{3}{\sqrt{[1-(4.397/10)^2]}}$$

$$= \textbf{3.34 cm}$$

(d) The wave impedance in the guide is
$$Z_g = 377\,\lambda_g/\lambda$$
$$= 377 \times 3.34/3 = \textbf{419.73 ohm}$$

(e) The bandwidth for the dominant mode is given by

$B = f_c$ the next higher order **TM$_{01}$** mode $-f_c$ of **TE$_{11}$** mode

$$= (c \times x'_{11}/2\pi a) - f_c \text{ of } \textbf{TE}_{11} \text{ mode}$$
$$= (3 \times 10^{10} \times 2.405/2 \times 3.14 \times 2)$$
$$- (4.397 \times 10^9)$$
$$= \textbf{1.347 GHz}$$

Example 4.12: A circular waveguide with air as dielectric has a radius of 2.5 cm and carries energy at a frequency of 10 GHz. Determine all the **TE$_{np}$** and **TM$_{np}$** modes for which energy transmission is possible.

Solution: Given: $a = 2.5$ cm, $f = 10$ GHz.

The physical dimensions of the waveguide and the frequency of the wave remain **constant. Hence, the product** $k_c a$ is a constant. Thus,

$$k_c a = \left(\omega\sqrt{\mu_0\varepsilon_0}\right)a = (2\pi \times 10 \times 10^9)$$
$$\sqrt{4 \times 3.14 \times 10^{-7} \times 8.854 \times 10^{-12}}$$
$$(2.5 \times 10^{-2}) = 5.23$$

Any mode having the product of $(k_c a)$ greater than or equal to 5.23 will not propagate the wave with a frequency of 10 GHz. From Tables 3.4 and 3.5, the possible modes are:

TE_{11} (1.841)

TE_{21} (3.054)

TE_{01} (3.832)

TM_{01} (2.045)

TM_{11} (3.832)

TM_{21} (5.136)

Example 4.13: An air-filled rectangular waveguide with dimensions 2 × 1 cm, shown in Fig. 4.27, operates in the TE_{10} mode at the rate of 1.0 hp. The signal frequency is 30 GHz. What is the peak value of the electric field occurring in the waveguide?

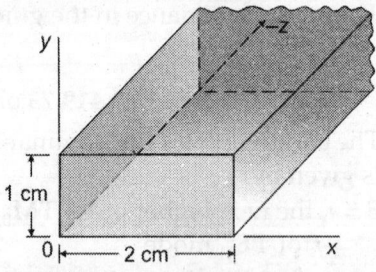

Fig. 4.27: Diagram for Example 4.17

Solution: Given: $a = 2$ cm, $b = 1$ cm,

$f = 30$ GHz,

$$\beta_g = \sqrt{\omega^2\mu_0\varepsilon_0 - (\pi/a)^2}$$
$$= \pi\sqrt{(2f/c)^2 - (1/a)^2}$$
$$= \pi\sqrt{(2 \times 30 \times 10^9/3 \times 10^8) - (1/2 \times 10^{-2})^2}$$

The power delivered by the waveguide in the z-direction is given by

$$P = \frac{1}{4}E_{0y}^2 \, \beta_g \, ab/\omega\mu_0$$

$$1 \times 746 = \frac{\frac{1}{4}E_{0y}^2 193.5\pi(2 \times 10^{-2})(1 \times 10^{-2})}{(2\pi \times 30 \times 10^9 \times 4\pi \times 10^{-7})}$$

$$E_{oy} = 76.23 \text{ kV/m}$$

Example 4.14: A rectangular waveguide with dimension 1 cm × 2 cm is excited in dominant mode at 10 GHz. Find the breakdown power.

Solution: Given: $a = 2$ cm, $b = 1$ cm, $f = 10$ GHz, $\lambda = (3 \times 10^{10})/(10 \times 10^9) = 3$ cm

Assuming the breakdown field to be 30 kV/cm, the breakdown power is given by

$$P_{bd} = 597ab\sqrt{1 - (\lambda/2a)^2}$$
$$= 597 \times 2 \times 1 \times \sqrt{1 - [3/(2 \times 2)]^2}$$
$$= 789.8 \text{ kW}$$

KEY POINTS

- Waveguides are metallic hallow tubes of rectangular or circular shape. Waveguides are mainly used in the microwave frequency range.

- The dominant mode in a particular waveguide is the mode that has the lowest cut-off frequency.

- In rectangular waveguides, the modes are designated as TE_{mn} or TM_{mn}.

- For the TE_{mn} modes in rectangular waveguides, $E_z = 0$ and the z-component of the magnetic field, H_z must exist in order to have energy transmission in the rectangular waveguide.

- The physical size of the waveguide determines the propagation modes. Whenever two or more modes have the same cut-off frequency, they are known degenerate modes.

- Rectangular waveguides ordinarily have dimensions of $a = 2b$ ratio. The mode with the lowest cut-off frequency in a particular waveguide is known as dominant mode. The dominant mode in a rectangular waveguide with $a > b$ is the TE_{10} mode.

- In a rectangular waveguide, the corresponding TE_{mn}, TE_{nm}, TM_{mn} and TM_{nm} modes form a foursome of degeneracy

- In rectangular waveguides, the field intensities of the desired mode can be established by means of a coaxial cable with the center conductor acting as a probe or loop-coupling device.
- Circular waveguides are metallic hollow circular tubes or pipes with uniform cross-section of a finite radius. The propagation is **TE** mode or **TM** mode.
- The dominant mode in a circular waveguide is TE_{11} mode.

FURTHER READING

1. **Altman L (1962).** *Microwave Circuits*, Van Nostrand, NJ.

2. Chodorov M and Susskind C (1964). *Fundamentals of Microwave Electronics*, McGraw Hill, NY.

3. Collins RE (1996). *Foundations of Microwave Engineering*, McGraw Hill, NY.

4. Wheeler GJ (1963). *Introduction to Microwaves*, Englewood Cliffs, NJ.

5. Edminister JA (2001). *Electromagnetics*, TMH, New Delhi.

6. Liao SY (1988). *Engineering Applications of Electromagnetic Theory*, West, Minn, USA.

7. Kraus HL (1949). *Transmission Line Charts, Elec. Eng.*, vol. 68, p 767, Sept.

8. Liboff RL and Dalman GC (1985). *Transmission Lines, Wave Guides and Smith Charts*, MacMillan, NY.

REVIEW QUESTIONS

4.1 What is a waveguide?

4.2 What are the types of waveguides?

4.3 What are the modes of propagation in rectangular waveguides?

4.4 What is the dominant mode?

4.5 Which mode is dominant mode in rectangular waveguides?

4.6 Which mode is dominant mode in circular waveguides?

4.7 Which mode is degenerate mode in rectangular waveguides?

4.8 Which mode is degenerate mode in circular waveguides?

4.9 What are higher order modes in circular waveguides and their effects?

4.10 What is the lowest order mode in circular waveguide?

4.11 How is the propagation mode excited in rectangular waveguides?

4.12 Give expressions for attenuation constant and characteristic impedance in a rectangular waveguide.

DESCRIPTIVE QUESTIONS

4.1 Obtain the **TE** wave solution for a rectangular waveguide.

4.2 Obtain the **TM** wave solution for a rectangular waveguide.

4.3 Obtain the **TE** wave solution for a circular waveguide.

4.4 Obtain the **TM** wave solution for a circular waveguide.

4.5 Explain the excitation methods used in microwave transmission line.

4.6 Describe any two special configurations of waveguides.

PRACTICE PROBLEMS

4.1 A rectangular waveguide has dimension 5 cm × 2 cm and is used to propagate TM_{11} mode at 10 GHz. Determine the cut-off wavelength and the characteristic impedance.
(**Ans:** 3.174 cm, 222.24 ohm)

4.2 An air-filled rectangular waveguide with inside dimension 7 × 3.5 cm operates in TE_{10} mode as shown in Fig. 4.25. Determine (a) the cut-off frequency, (b) the phase velocity of the wave in the waveguide at a frequency of 3.5 GHz and (c) the guided wavelength at the same frequency.
(**Ans:** 2.14 GHz, 3.78×10^8 m/s, 10.8 cm)

4.3 An air-filled rectangular copper waveguide with dimensions 2.28 cm × 1.01 cm and a length of 30.48 cm is operated in the dominant mode at 9.2 GHz. Determine (a) the cut-off frequency, (b) guide wavelength, (c) phase velocity, (d) the characteristic impedance and (e) the power loss.
(**Ans:** 6.579 GHz, 4.664 cm, 4.29×10^8 m/s, 539.3 ohm, 0.036 dB)

4.4 A circular waveguide has a radius of 1 cm and contains air dielectric. The mode of propagation is TE_{11} mode. Find (a) the cut-off frequency, (b) the wavelength in the waveguide for an operating frequency of 10 GHz, (c) the wave impedance and (d) the bandwidth.
(**Ans:** 8.795 GHz, 6.303 cm, 792 ohm, 2.695 GHz).

4.5 A circular waveguide has a radius of 5 cm and contains air dielectric. The mode of propagation is TE_{11} mode. Find (a) the cut-off frequency, (b) the wavelength in the waveguide for an operating frequency of 3 GHz and (c) the wave impedance.
(**Ans:** 1.758 GHz, 12.3 cm, 465 ohm)

4.6 A circular waveguide with air as dielectric has a radius of 2 cm and carries energy at a frequency of 10 GHz. Determine all the TE_{np} and TM_{np} modes for which energy transmission is possible.
(**Ans:** TE_{01}, TE_{11}, TE_{21}, TM_{01} TM_{11})

4.7 A rectangular waveguide with dimension 1 cm × 2.3 cm is excited in dominant mode at 9.375 GHz. Find the breakdown power.
(**Ans:** 986.4 kW)

4.8 A coaxial line filled with air is operating at $\lambda = 3.2$ cm in **TEM** mode. Assume $b/a = 3$ and $a = \lambda/4\pi$. Calculate the breakdown power.
(**Ans:** 256.5 kW)

4.9 In air-filled rectangular waveguide with dimensions 2 × 1 cm, shown in Fig. 4.16, operates in the TE_{10} mode at the rate of 0.5 hp. The signal frequency is 30 GHz. What is the peak value of the electric field occurring in the waveguide?
(**Ans:** 53.87 kV/m)

REFERENCES

1. Argence E and Hahan T (1967). *Theory of Waveguides and Cavity Resonators,* Blackie and Sons, London.
2. Gandhi OP (1981). *Microwave Engineering and Applications,* Pergamon, NY.
3. Ghose RN (1963). *Microwave Circuit Theory and Analysis,* McGraw Hill, NY.
4. Kennedy G and Davis B (1999). *Electronic Communication Systems,* TMH, New Delhi.
5. Lebedev I (1973). *Microwave Engineering,* MIR Publications, Moscow.
6. Liao SY (2000). *Microwave Devices and Circuits,* PHI, New Delhi.
7. Malherbe JAG (1979). *Microwave Transmission Line Filters,* Aptech, Dedham, Mass.
8. Montogomery CG et al (1948). *Principles of Microwave Circuits,* McGraw-Hill, N.Y.
9. Pozar DM (1990). *Microwave Engineering,* Addison-Wesley, Mass.
10. Reich HJ et al (1953). *Microwave Theory and Techniques,* Van Nostrand, NJ.
11. Reich HJ (1978). *Microwave Principles,* East-West, New Delhi.
12. Roddy D (1999). *Microwave Technology,* PH, N.J.
13. Ryder, JD (1997). *Networks, Lines and Fields,* PHI, New Delhi.
14. Skilling HH (1951). *Electrical Transmission Lines,* McGraw Hill, NY.
15. Slater JC (1950). *Microwave Electronics,* Van Nostrand, NJ.
16. Soohoo RF (1971). *Microwave Electronics,* Addison-Wesley, Mass.
17. Thomas EH (1976). *Handbook of Microwave Techniques,* PH, NJ.
18. Van Valkenberg NE (2005). *Network Analysis,* PHI, New Delhi.
19. Veley VF (1987). *Modern Microwave Technology,* PH, NJ.
20. Wolff EA and Kaul R (1988). *Microwave Engineering and Systems,* John Wiley, NY.
21. Pramanik A (2003). *Electromagnetism: Theory and Applications,* PHI, New Delhi.
22. Ramo S, Whinnery JR and Van Duzer (1965). *Fields and Waves in Communication Electronics,* Wiley, NY.
23. Terman FE (1955). *Electronic and Radio Engineering,* McGraw Hill, NY.
24. Liboff RL and Dalman GC (1985). *Transmission Lines, Wave Guides and Smith Charts,* MacMillan, NY.
25. Marcavitz N (1951). *Wave Guide Handbook, MIT Rad. Lab.,* Vol. 10, McGraw Hill, NY.
26. Cohn SB (1947). *Properties of Ridge Waveguides,* Proc. IRE, Vol. 35, pp. 783–788.
27. Hopfer S (1955). *The Design of Ridged Waveguides,* IRE Trans. MTT-3, pp. 20–29.
28. Vartanian PH, Ayres WP and Helgesson AL (1958). *Propagation in Dielectric Slab Loaded Rectangular Waveguide,* IRE Trans. MTT-6, pp. 215–222.
29. Gardiol FE (1968). *Higher –Order Modes in Dielectrically Loaded Rectangular Waveguides,* IEEE, Trans. MTT-16. pp. 919–924.
30. Tisher FJ (1959). *Properties of the H guide at microwaves and millimeter Waves,* Proc. IEE (London), B106 (13).
31. King DD (1955). *Properties of Dielectric Image Lines,* IRE Trans. MTT-3, pp. 75–81.
32. Goubau G (1951). *Single Conductor Surface-Wave Transmission Lines,* Proc. IRE, pp. 62, 19–624.
33. Das A and Das SK (2004). *Microwave Engineering,* Tata-McGraw Hill, New Delhi.

Microwave Network Theory

* Review the Z, Y, h and $ABCD$ parameters of electrical networks.
* Understand the need for S-matrix.
* Study the properties of the S-matrix.
* Derive S-matrix for two and multi-port MW networks.
* Describe relationship between S-matrix and Z, Y, h and $ABCD$ parameters.

5.1 INTRODUCTION

In microwave frequency range of 1 to 100 GHz, we use transmission lines or wave-guide components instead of lumped circuit elements. Thus, the term microwave engineering, in general, refers to the engineering and design of information handling systems in the frequency range of 1 GHz to 100 GHz. The characteristic feature of microwave engineering is the short wave lengths involved. These wavelengths are of the same order of magnitude as the microwave circuit elements and devices employed. As a result of this, the conventional low frequency circuit analysis is not applicable at microwave frequencies. For this reason, a successful microwave engineer must have a good working knowledge of electromagnetic field theory.

In this chapter, we shall first review the low frequency circuit analysis, then deal with microwave network analysis, discuss the properties of microwave circuits, derive the S-matrix and its relationship with network parameters.

5.2 ELECTRICAL NETWORK PARAMETERS

An electric network is a combination of several electrical devices and components such as sources, resistors, inductors and capacitors, etc. that are connected together so as to achieve the desired transmission of electrical signal. The point of interconnection of two or more devices or components is known as a *junction*. A *port* is a pair of two terminals.

A two-port network is shown in Fig. 5.1. The behavior of a 2-port network is described by two independent equations relating the four variables V_1, I_1, V_2 and I_2 at the port terminals. Any two variables are taken as independent and the remaining two as the dependent. The currents entering the ports

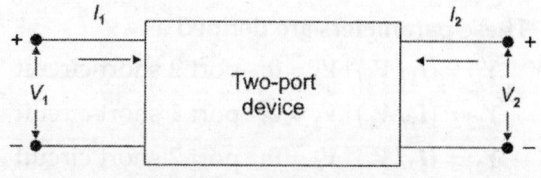

Fig. 5.1: Two-port network

are taken as positive. These may be described by parameter sets such as *Z, Y, h* and *ABCD* parameters[1]. These are defined below.

5.2.1 Z-Parameters or Open Circuit Parameters

Considering the currents as independent parameters, the voltages V_1 and V_2 are expressed as

$$V_1 = Z_{11}I_1 + Z_{12}I_2 \qquad (5.1a)$$
$$V_2 = Z_{21}I_1 + Z_{22}I_2 \qquad (5.1b)$$

In matrix form

$$\begin{pmatrix} V_1 \\ V_2 \end{pmatrix} = \begin{pmatrix} Z_{11} & Z_{12} \\ Z_{21} & Z_{22} \end{pmatrix} \begin{pmatrix} I_1 \\ I_2 \end{pmatrix} \qquad (5.2a)$$

or, $\qquad V = ZI \qquad (5.2b)$

These parameters are defined as

$Z_{11} = (V_1/I_1) | I_2 = 0$; port 2 open circuit
$Z_{12} = (V_1/I_2) | I_1 = 0$; port 1 open circuit
$Z_{21} = (V_2/I_1) | I_2 = 0$; port 2 open circuit
$Z_{22} = (V_2/I_2) | I_1 = 0$; port 1 open circuit

Since port 1 or 2 is open circuited for defining the *Z*-parameters, they are also known as *open-circuit parameters*.

5.2.2 Y-Parameters or Short Circuit Parameters

Considering the voltages as independent variables, I_1 and I_2 are expressed as

$$I_1 = Y_{11}V_1 + Y_{12}V_2 \qquad (5.3a)$$
$$I_2 = Y_{21}V_1 + Y_{22}V_2 \qquad (5.3b)$$

In matrix form,

$$\begin{pmatrix} I_1 \\ I_2 \end{pmatrix} = \begin{pmatrix} Y_{11} & Y_{12} \\ Y_{21} & Y_{22} \end{pmatrix} \begin{pmatrix} V_1 \\ V_2 \end{pmatrix}$$

or $\qquad I = YV \qquad (5.4b)$

These parameters are defined as

$Y_{11} = (I_1/V_1) | V_2 = 0$; port 2 short circuit
$Y_{12} = (I_1/V_2) | V_1 = 0$; port 1 short circuit
$Y_{21} = (I_2/V_1) | V_2 = 0$; port 2 short circuit
$Y_{22} = (I_2/V_2) | V_1 = 0$; port 1 short circuit

Since the port 1 or 2 is shorted for defining the *Y*-parameters, they are also known as *short circuit parameters*.

5.2.3 h-Parameters or Hybrid Parameters

Consider V_1 and I_2 as independent variables. They are expressed as

$$V_1 = h_{11}I_1 + h_{12}V_2 \qquad (5.5a)$$
$$I_2 = h_{21}I_1 + h_{22}V_2 \qquad (5.5b)$$

In matrix form,

$$\begin{pmatrix} V_1 \\ I_2 \end{pmatrix} = \begin{pmatrix} h_{11} & h_{12} \\ h_{21} & h_{22} \end{pmatrix} \begin{pmatrix} I_1 \\ V_2 \end{pmatrix} \qquad (5.6)$$

These parameters are defined as

$h_{11} = (V_1/I_1) | V_2 = 0$; port 2 short circuit
$h_{12} = (V_1/V_2) | I_1 = 0$; port 1 open circuit
$h_{21} = (I_2/I_1) | V_2 = 0$; port 2 short circuit
$h_{22} = (I_2/V_2) | I_1 = 0$; port 1 open circuit

Since these parameters correspond to voltage gain, current gain, impedance or admittance, they are known as *hybrid* or *mixed parameters*.

5.2.4 ABCD Parameters or Transmission Parameters

Considering V_2 and I_2 as independent variables, V_1 and I_I are expressed as

$$V_1 = AV_2 - BI_2 \qquad (5.7a)$$
$$I_1 = CV_2 - DI_2 \qquad (5.7b)$$

In matrix form,

$$\begin{pmatrix} V_1 \\ I_1 \end{pmatrix} = \begin{pmatrix} A & -B \\ C & -D \end{pmatrix} \begin{pmatrix} V_2 \\ I_2 \end{pmatrix} \qquad (5.8)$$

These parameters are defined as

$A = (V_1/V_2) | I_2 = 0$; port 2 open circuit
$B = (-V_1/I_2) | V_2 = 0$; port 1 short circuit
$C = (I/V_2) | I_2 = 0$; port 2 open circuit
$D = (-I_1/I_2) | V_2 = 0$; port 1 short circuit

Since these parameters are mainly used for transmission lines, they are known as *transmission parameters*.

5.3 SYMMETRICAL PROPERTY OF RECIPROCAL NETWORK

An important property of a reciprocal network is its impedance and the admittance matrices are symmetrical[2]. The junction media are characterized by the scalar parameters μ and ε.

Proof: For an N-port network, let the incident wave amplitude be V_n. It is so chosen that the total voltage $V_n (= V_n^+ + V_n^-)$ is zero at all ports except the ith port where the electric and magnetic fields are E_i and H_i respectively. Similarly, let V_n be zero at all ports except the jth port where the electric and magnetic fields are E_j and H_j respectively. According to the Lorenz reciprocity theorem, with no sources in the closed surfaces,

$$\oint_s (E_i \times H_j - E_j \times H_i) \cdot n \, ds = 0 \qquad (5.9)$$

S is the closed surface area of the conducting walls enclosing the junction and the N ports. As the conducting walls are perfect conductors, the integral over the wall surface vanishes. The non-zero integrals are those over the terminal port. Thus

$$\sum_{n-1}^{N} \int_{t_n} (E_i \times H_j - E_j \times H_i) \cdot n \, ds = 0 \qquad (5.10)$$

All V_n except V_i and V_j are zero. Hence, Eq. (5.10) reduces to

$$\int_{t_i} E_i \times H_j \cdot n \, ds = \int_{t_j} E_j \times H_i \cdot n \, ds \qquad (5.11)$$

i.e.,
$$V_i (I_i)_j = V_j (I_j)_i \qquad (5.12)$$

$(I_i)_j$ is the current at the terminal port i due to an input voltage at port j. Similarly, $(I_j)_i$ is the current at the terminal port j due to an input voltage at port i.

Substituting, $[I] = [Y][V]$, Eq. (5.12) becomes

$$V_i V_j Y_{ij} = V_j V_i Y_{ji} \qquad (5.13)$$

or,
$$Y_{ij} = Y_{ji} \qquad (5.14)$$

$\therefore$
$$Z_{ij} = Y_{ji} \qquad (5.15)$$

Thus the symmetry of impedance and admittance matrices is proved.

5.4 SCATTERING MATRIX OF A MULTI-PORT NETWORK

A microwave circuit or network consists of several microwave components such as sources, attenuators and resonators that are connected together in such a way as to achieve the desired transmission of microwave signals. The point of interconnection of two or more devices/components is called a *microwave junction*. The commonly used microwave junctions are *waveguides*, *tees*, *hybrid rings*, *directional couplers* and *circulators* shown in Fig. 5.2.

5.4.1 Why S-Matrix

The Z, Y, h and *ABCD* parameters cannot be used to describe a microwave network because, at microwave frequencies,

(i) The physical length of microwave components is comparable to or much longer than the wavelength.

(ii) Voltage and current cannot be measured directly.

(iii) Short and open circuits are difficult to achieve for a wide range.

(iv) Microwave active devices are unstable for short and open circuits.

Because of the above limitations, a new method of characterization of microwave circuits is required. The new method should be based on direct measurable quantities. The directly measurable quantities are the amplitudes and phase angles of the waves *reflected* or *scattered* from a microwave junction relative to the incident wave amplitude and phase angles. Moreover, the scattered wave amplitudes are linearly related to the amplitudes of incident waves. The parameter that describes the relationship between these two is known as *S-parameters*[3-5].

5.4.2 Scattering Matrix

Since voltages, currents and impedances cannot be measured easily and directly at

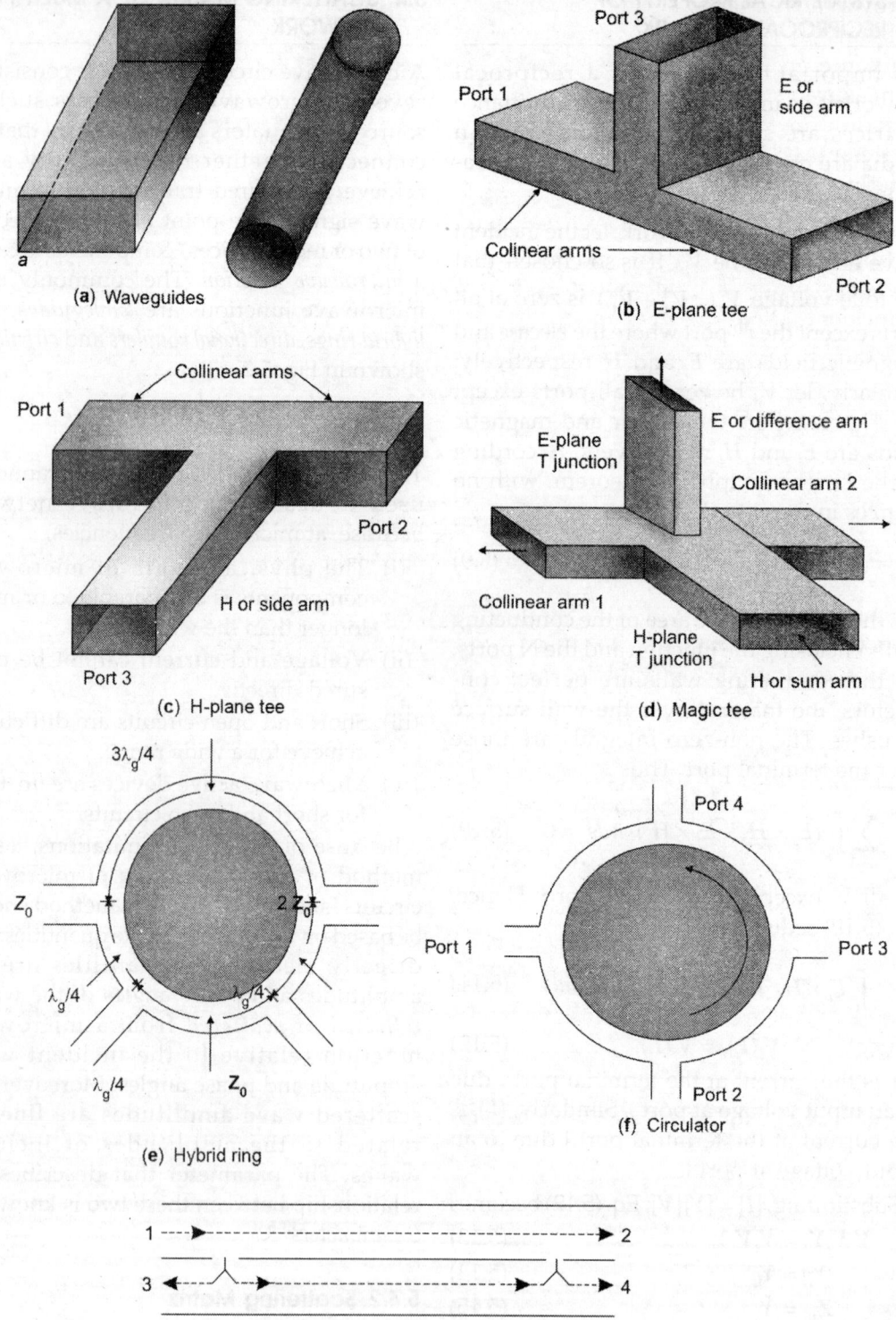

(a) Waveguides

(b) E-plane tee

Port 3

Port 1

E or side arm

Colinear arms

Port 2

Collinear arms

Port 1

Port 2

H or side arm

Port 3

(c) H-plane tee

E-plane T junction

E or difference arm

Collinear arm 2

Collinear arm 1

H-plane T junction

H or sum arm

(d) Magic tee

$3\lambda_g/4$

Z_0

$2 Z_0$

$\lambda_g/4$

$\lambda_g/4$

$\lambda_g/4$

Z_0

(e) Hybrid ring

Port 4

Port 1

Port 3

Port 2

(f) Circulator

1 ——▶ 2

3 ◀—— ▶ 4

Fig. 5.2: Microwave hybrid junctions

microwave frequencies, microwave networks are not represented by impedance or admittance matrix. The quantities that may be measured in a direct manner are the reflection coefficients and transmission coefficients. They form the basis of the scattering matrix formulation.

Definition: A scattering matrix represents the linear relationship between the parameters $a_n's$ and $b_n's$ that are proportional to the incident and the reflected waves at the nth port. The $a_n's$ and $b_n's$ are defined as

$$a_n = \frac{V_n^+}{\sqrt{Z_{on}}} \qquad (5.16a)$$

$$b_n = \frac{V_n^-}{\sqrt{Z_{on}}} \qquad (5.16b)$$

Here V_n^+ and V_n^- represent the incident and reflected waves along the transmission line connected to the nth port and Z_{on} is the characteristic impedance of the line.

5.4.3 Two-Port Microwave Network

Let us consider a two-port microwave network shown in Fig. 5.3. The relationship between $b_n's$ and $a_n's$ for a two-port network are given below:

$$b_1 = S_{11} a_1 + S_{12} a_2 \qquad (5.17a)$$

$$b_2 = S_{21} a_1 + S_{22} a_2 \qquad (5.17b)$$

In matrix form,

$$\begin{pmatrix} b_1 \\ b_2 \end{pmatrix} = \begin{pmatrix} S_{11} & S_{12} \\ S_{21} & S_{22} \end{pmatrix} \begin{pmatrix} a_1 \\ a_2 \end{pmatrix} \qquad (5.18a)$$

$$[b] = [S] [a] \qquad (5.18b)$$

The matrix $[S]$ is known as scattering matrix of the microwave network. S_{11} is the input reflection coefficient, S_{22} is the output reflection coefficient, S_{12} is the reverse transmission coefficient and S_{21} is the forward transmission coefficient.

5.4.4 Definition of S-Parameters

The S-parameters are defined as:

$$S_{11} = b_1/a_1 \,|\, a_2 = 0 = \Gamma_1;$$

the input reflection coefficient at Port 1 with Port 2 terminated with matched load.

$$S_{12} = b_1/a_2 \,|\, a_1 = 0;$$

the attenuation or reverse transmission coefficient of the wave traveling from Port 2 to Port 1.

$$S_{21} = b_2/a_1 \,|\, a_2 = 0;$$

the attenuation or forward transmission coefficient of the wave traveling from Port 1 to Port 2.

$$S_{22} = b_2/a_2 \,|\, a_1 = 0 = \Gamma_2;$$

the output reflection coefficient at Port 2 with Port 1 terminated with matched load.

Since the incident and reflected waves have both amplitude and phase, the S-parameters are in general complex quantities.

At microwave frequencies, the S-parameters are related to measurable power ratios[6,7]. Thus,

$$|S_{11}|^2 = \frac{\text{Power reflected from the input port}}{\text{Power incident on the input port}} \bigg|_{Z_L = Z_0}$$

$$|S_{22}|^2 = \frac{\text{Power reflected from the output port}}{\text{Power incident on the output port}} \bigg|_{\substack{Z_g = Z_0 \\ V_g = 0}}$$

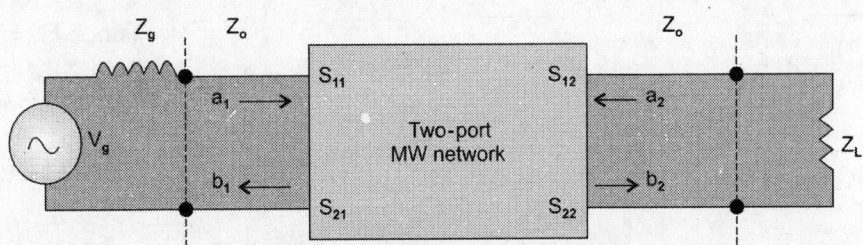

Fig. 5.3: Two-port microwave network

$$|S_{12}|^2 = \frac{\text{Power delivered to matched}}{\text{Power incident on the output port}}\Bigg|_{\substack{Z_G = Z_0 \\ V_g = 0}}$$

$$|S_{21}|^2 = \frac{\text{Power delivered to matched load}}{\text{Power incident on the output port}}\Bigg|_{Z_L = Z_0}$$

Since the incident power is equal to the available power of the generator when $Z_G = Z_0$, $|S_{21}|^2$ will represent the forward transducer gain ratio.

5.4.5 Multiport Network

Let us consider the N-Port microwave network shown in Fig. 5.4. Assume that a microwave with an associated equivalent voltage a_1 is incident at terminal plane t_1 or port 1. It produces a reflected wave $S_{11}a_1 = b_1$ on line 1. S_{11} is the reflection or scattering co-efficient for line 1. In addition, waves will be transmitted or scattered to the other junctions due to the incident wave at port 1 with proportional to a_2. These may be expressed as $b_n = S_{n1}a_1$, $n = 2, 3, ... N$. S_{n1} is the transmission coefficient of port n from port 1. When waves are incident on all ports, the scattered wave at each port has contributions from all other incident waves. Hence, we may write

$$b_n = \sum S_{ni}\, a_i; \quad n = 1 \text{ to } N, i = 1 \text{ to } N \quad (5.19a)$$

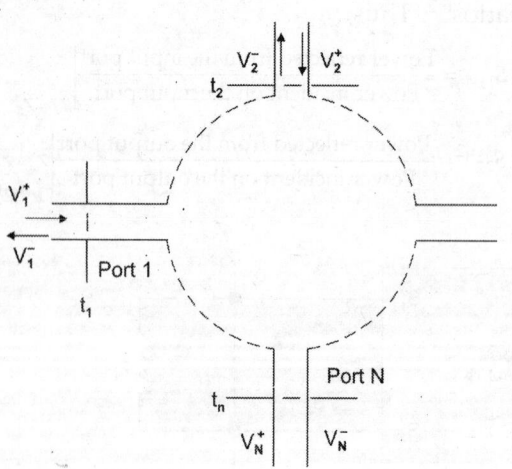

Fig. 5.4: N-port microwave junction

In matrix form, it can be expressed as

$$\begin{pmatrix} b_1 \\ b_2 \\ \vdots \\ b_n \end{pmatrix} = \begin{pmatrix} S_{11} & S_{12} & S_{13} & \cdots & S_{1N} \\ S_{21} & S_{22} & S_{23} & \cdots & S_{2N} \\ \cdots & \cdots & \cdots & \cdots & \cdots \\ S_{N1} & S_{N2} & S_{N13} & \cdots & S_{NN} \end{pmatrix} \begin{pmatrix} a_1 \\ a_2 \\ \vdots \\ a_n \end{pmatrix}$$

$$(5.19b)$$

$$\text{or} \qquad [b] = [S]\,[a] \qquad (5.19c)$$

Here [S] is the scattering matrix for multi-port network.

5.4.6 Power Relations

The amplitudes of the incident and reflected waves at any point are normalized so that the square of any of these variables gives the average power in that wave.

The incident or input power P_{in} at the nth port is given by

$$P_{in} = \left(V_n^+ / \sqrt{2}\right) \cdot \left(I_n^{+*} / \sqrt{2}\right)$$

$$= \left(V_n^+ / \sqrt{2}\right)\left(V_n^{+*} / \sqrt{2}\right) / Z_{on}$$

$$\text{(since } I_n^{+*} = V_n^{+*} / Z_{on})$$

$$= \frac{1}{2}\left(V_n^+ / \sqrt{Z_{on}}\right)\left(V_n^{+*} / \sqrt{Z_{on}}\right)$$

$$= \frac{1}{2} a_n a_n^* \quad \text{(since } a_n = V_n^+ / \sqrt{Z_{on}})$$

$$= \frac{1}{2} |a_n|^2 \qquad (5.20)$$

Similarly, the reflected power P_{rn} at the nth port is given by

$$P_{rn} = \left(V_n^- / \sqrt{2}\right)\left(I_n^{-*} / \sqrt{2}\right)$$

$$= \left(V_n^- / \sqrt{2}\right)\left(V_n^{-*} / \sqrt{2}\right) Z_{on}$$

$$\text{(since } I_n^{-*} = V_n^{-*} / Z_{on})$$

$$= \frac{1}{2}\left(V_n^- / \sqrt{Z_{on}}\right)\left(V_n^{-*} / \sqrt{Z_{on}}\right)$$

$$= \frac{1}{2} b_n b_n^* \quad \text{(since } b_n = V_n^- / \sqrt{Z_{on}})$$

$$= \frac{1}{2} |b_n|^2 \qquad (5.21)$$

5.5 LOSSES IN MICROWAVE CIRCUITS

The several losses that occur in a microwave circuit are usually expressed in terms of S-parameters when ports are terminated with matched loads. In a two-port network, let P_i be the power incident at port 1 and P_r be the power reflected at the same port and P_0 be the output power or the transmitted power at port 2. Then the insertion loss is given by

Insertion loss (dB)

$$= 10 \log (P_i/P_0)$$

$$= 10 \log \left(\frac{1}{2} |a_1|^2 \right) \Big/ \left(\frac{1}{2} |b_2|^2 \right)$$

$$= 10 \log |1/(|b_2|^2/|a_1|^2|$$

$$= \mathbf{20 \log [1/|S_{21}|]} \text{ (since } b_2/a_2 = S_{21})$$

$$= \mathbf{20 \log [1/|S_{12}|]} \text{ (since } S_{21} = S_{12}) \quad (5.22)$$

The transmission loss or attenuation is given by

Transmission loss or attenuation (dB)

$$= 10 \log [(P_i - P_r)/P_0]$$

$$= 10 \log \frac{1}{2} \Big[|a_1|^2 - |b_1|^2 \Big] \Big/ \left(\frac{1}{2} |b_2|^2 \right)$$

$$= 10 \log [|a_1|^2/|b_2|^2] \cdot [1 - |b_1|^2/|a_1|^2|]$$

$$= 10 \log [1/|S_{12}|^2] [1 - |S_{11}|^2]$$

$$= \mathbf{10 \log [1 - |S_{11}|^2]/|S_{12}|^2} \quad (5.23)$$

The reflection loss is given by

Reflection loss (dB)

$$= 10 \log [P_i/(P_i - P_r)]$$

$$= 10 \log \left[\frac{1}{2} |a_1|^2 \right] \Big/ \left[\frac{1}{2} (|a_1|^2 - |b_1|^2) \right]$$

$$= 10 \log \{1/[1 - (|b_1|^2/|a_1|^2)]\}$$

$$= \mathbf{10 \log [1/(1 - |S_{11}|^2)]} \quad (5.24)$$

The return loss is given by

Return loss (dB)

$$= 10 \log (P_i/P_r)$$

$$= 10 \log \left[\frac{1}{2} |a_1|^2 \right] \Big/ \left[\frac{1}{2} |b_1|^2 \right]$$

$$= 20 \log 1/[|b_1|/|a_1|]$$

$$= \mathbf{20 \log [1/|S_{11}|]} \quad (5.25)$$

Example 5.1: A certain two-port network has $S_{11} = 0.26 - j0.16$, $S_{12} = S_{21} = 0.42$ and $S_{22} = 0.36 - j0.57$. Compute the insertion loss (a) when $Z_g = Z_l = Z_0$ and (b) when $Z_g = Z_0$ and $Z_l = 3Z_0$.

Solution: Given: $S_{11} = 0.26 - j0.16$, $S_{12} = S_{21} = 0.42$ and $S_{22} = 0.36 - j0.57$.

(a) $Z_g = Z_l = Z_0$

Hence, $\Gamma_g = \Gamma_l = 0$.

From Eq. (5.23), the insertion loss is

$IL = 20 \log (1/|S_{12}|) = 20 \log (1/0.42)$

$= 20 \log 2.381 = \mathbf{7.54 \text{ dB}}$

(b) $Z_g = Z_0$ and $Z_l = 3Z_0$.

Hence, $\Gamma_g = 0$

and $\Gamma_l = (Z_l - Z_0)(Z_l + Z_0)$

$$= \frac{2Z_0}{4Z_0} = \frac{1}{2}$$

In this case the insertion loss is given by

$IL = 10 \log (1 - S_{22}\Gamma_l)^2/[|S_{12}|^2(1 - |\Gamma_l|^2)]$

$$= \frac{10 \log \left[1 - (0.36 - j0.57) \times \frac{1}{2} \right]^2}{\left[(0.42)^2 \times \left(1 - \frac{1}{4} \right) \right]}$$

$= 10 \log [0.82 + j0.285]^2/[0.1764 \times 0.75]$

$= 10 \log 0.7536/0.1323 = 10 \log 5.7$

$= \mathbf{7.6 \text{ dB}}$

5.6 PROPERTIES OF S-MATRIX

The scattering parameters are complex quantities and have the following properties.

(i) Uniqueness of S-matrix for perfectly matched loads $S_{ii} = 0$.

(ii) Symmetrical property of scattering matrix $S_{ij} = S_{ji}$.

(iii) Unitary property of S-matrix for loss-less junction $\sum_{n=1}^{N} S_{ni}S_{ni}^x = 1$.

(iv) Null or zero property of S-matrix for a lossless junction

5.6.1 Uniqueness of S-Matrix for Perfectly Matched Loads

For a perfect matched loads or terminations, the diagonal elements of the S-matrix, S_{ii} are zero, since there is no reflection from any port.

5.6.2 Symmetrical Property of Scattering Matrix

For a reciprocal junction, the scattering matrix is symmetrical, $S_{ij} = S_{ji}$.

Proof: A reciprocal network has the same transmission characteristics in either direction of a pair of ports. The relationship between the scattering matrix and the impedance matrix is given by

$$[V] = [Z] [I] \qquad (5.26)$$

The total voltage is given by

$$V = V^+ + V^- \qquad (5.27a)$$

Using Eq. (5.27a) and assuming that lines or wave guides connected to various ports, have equal characteristic impedance Z_0, we have

$$I = [V^+ - V^-]/Z_0 \qquad (5.27b)$$

Hence, $V = [V^+] + [V^-]$

$$= [Z] (1/Z_0) [(V^+) - (V^-)] \qquad (5.28)$$

$$= [Z'] ([(V^+) - (V^-)]) \qquad (5.29)$$

Here $[Z'] = [Z]/Z_0$

Rearranging Eq. (5.29), we get

$$[(Z') + (U)] (V^-) = [(Z') - (U)] (V^+) \qquad (5.30)$$

Here $[U]$ is the unit matrix in which all diagonal elements of $[U]$ are unity.

From Eq. (5.19b), $[V^-] = [S] [V^+]$ since $[b]$ is proportional to the reflected wave amplitude V^- and $[a]$ is the incident wave amplitude V^+.

From Eq. (5.30),

$$[V^-] = ([Z'] + [U])^{-1} ([Z'] - [U]) [V^+] \qquad (5.31)$$

Hence the S-matrix is given by

$$[S] = [V^-]/[V^+] = ([Z'] + [U])^{-1} ([(Z'] - [U]) \qquad (5.32)$$

Alternative Proof: An alternative form of deriving the S-matrix is as follows. Since

$$V_n = V_n^+ + V_n^-$$

and $Z_0 I_n = V_n^+ - V_n^- \qquad (5.33)$

We may write

$$V = [V^+] + [V^-] \qquad (5.34)$$

$$Z_0 [I] = [V^+] - [V^-] \qquad (5.35)$$

From the above two equations, we get

$$[V^+] = \frac{1}{2} ([V] + Z_0[I])$$

$$= \frac{1}{2} ([Z] + Z_0 [U]) [I] \qquad (5.36)$$

Similarly,

$$[V^-] = \frac{1}{2} ([V] - Z_0 [I])$$

$$= \frac{1}{2} ([Z] - Z_0 [U]) [I] \qquad (5.37)$$

From Eq. (5.36), we have

$$[I] = 2([Z] + Z_0 [U])^{-1} [V^+] \qquad (5.38)$$

Substituting for $[I]$ in Eq. (5.37), we get

$$[V^-] = ([Z] - Z_0 [U]) [I] ([Z] + Z_0 [U])^{-1} [V^+]$$

$$= ([Z'] - [U]) ([Z'] + [U])^{-1} \qquad (5.39)$$

From Eq. (5.32), the S-matrix is given by

$$[S] = ([Z'] + [U])^{-1} ([Z'] - [U]) \qquad (5.40)$$

The transpose of the matrix is

$$[S]_t = ([Z'] + [U])_t^{-1} ([Z'] + [U])_t \qquad (5.41)$$

Since (Z') and (U) are symmetrical matrix for a reciprocal network,

$$([Z'] + [U])_t^{-1} = ([Z'] + [U])^{-1} \qquad (5.42)$$

$$([Z'] - [U])_t = ([Z'] - [U]) \qquad (5.43)$$

Therefore,

$$[S] = [S]_t \qquad (5.44)$$

or $\qquad S_{ij} = S_{ji} \qquad (5.45)$

Thus, the scattering matrix $[S]$ is symmetrical.

5.6.3 Unitary Property of S-Matrix for Lossless Junction

For a lossless junction, the unitary property of *S*-matrix states that the *sum of the products of any row or column of the S-matrix with the conjugate of that row or column is equal to unity.* Thus,

$$\sum_{n=1}^{N} S_{ni} \cdot S_{ni}^* = 0$$

Proof: According to the law of conservation, for a loss-less junction, the total power leaving all the N ports must be equal to the sum of the incident powers. Mathematically expressed, we get

$$\sum_{n=1}^{N} |b_n|^2 = \sum_{n=1}^{N} |a_n|^2 \qquad (5.46)$$

The parameter b_n is given by

$$b_n = \sum_{i=1}^{N} S_{ni} a_i \quad n = 1, 2,..., N \qquad (5.47)$$

Therefore Eq. (5.46) may be expressed as

$$\sum_{i=1}^{N} \sum_{i=1}^{N} |S_{ni} a_i|^2 = \sum_{i=1}^{N} |a_i|^2 \qquad (5.48)$$

Assuming that only the ith port is excited and all other ports are terminated with matched loads (i.e., $a_n = 0$ except a_i), we have

$$\sum_{n=1}^{N} |S_{ni} a_i|^2 = |a_i|^2 \qquad (5.49)$$

or $\quad \displaystyle\sum_{n=1}^{N} |S_{ni}|^2 |a_i|^2 = |a_i|^2$

or $\quad \displaystyle\sum_{n=1}^{N} |S_{ni}|^2 = 1 = \sum_{n=1}^{N} S_{ni} S_{ni}^* \qquad (5.50)$

Since the index i is arbitrary,

$$\sum_{n=1}^{N} S_{ni} S_{ni}^* = 1 \qquad (5.51)$$

Eq. (5.51) is valid for all values of i. Hence for a loss-less network, the product of any row or column of the S-matrix with the conjugate of that row or column is equal to unity.

5.6.3 Null or Zero Property of S-matrix for Loss-Less Junctions

The null or zero property of the S-matrix sates that the sum of the products of any row

or column of the S-matrix with the conjugate of any other row or column is equal to zero.

$$\sum_{n-1}^{N} S_{ni} S_{nk}^* = 0; \ i \neq k$$

Proof: If all $a_n = 0$ except a_i and a_k, then from Eq. (5.48), we get

$$\sum_{n-1}^{N} |S_{ni} a_i + S_{nk} a_k|^2$$

$$= \sum_{n-1}^{N} (S_{ni} a_i + S_{nk} a_k)(S_{ni} a_i + S_{nk} a_k)$$

$$= |a_i|^2 + |a_k|^2$$

Expanding the left hand side, we obtain

$$\sum_{n-1}^{N} |S_{ni} a_i|^2 + \sum_{n-1}^{N} |S_{nk} a_k|^2$$

$$+ \sum_{n-1}^{N} S_{ni} S_{nk}^* a_i a_k^* + \sum_{n-1}^{N} S_{nk} a_i^* a_k$$

$$= |a_i|^2 + |a_k|^2 \qquad (5.52)$$

In view of the independence of a_i and a_k, let us choose $a_i = j a_k$. Then from the above equation, we get

$$\sum_{n=1}^{N} (S_{nk} S_{nk}^* - \Sigma S_{ni}^* S_{nk}) = 0 \qquad (5.53)$$

This states that for a lossless network, the sum of the product of any row or column of the S-matrix with the conjugate of any other row or column is equal to zero.

5.6.4 Phase Shift Property of S-matrix

The S-matrix of a phase-shifted network is equal to

$$[S'] = [\phi_1] [S] [\phi_2]$$

Here $[\phi]$ is the phase shift diagonal matrix with diagonal elements only.

Proof: Let us consider a two-port network for the sake of simplicity shown in Fig. 5.5. For this network, let [S] be the S-matrix with respect to plane 1 and 2. The S-parameters are complex quantities and they differ with respect to port positions or reference planes.

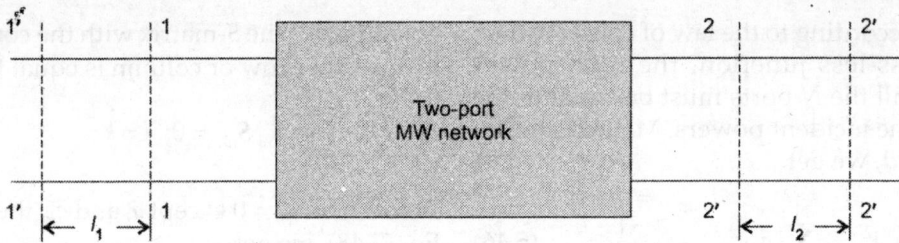

Fig. 5.5: Phase shift property of *S*-matrix

If the reference planes are shifted outward to 1' and 2', the corresponding phase shifts are $\phi_1 = \beta_1 l_1$ and $\phi_2 = \beta_2 l_2$, where β_1 and β_2 are phase constants of port 1 and 2 respectively. Hence the new *S*-parameters are

$$[S'] = \begin{pmatrix} e^{-j\phi_1} & 0 \\ e^{-j\phi_2} & 0 \end{pmatrix} [S] \begin{pmatrix} e^{-j\phi_1} & 0 \\ 0 & e_2^{-j\phi_2} \end{pmatrix} \quad (5.54)$$

This property is known as phase shift property and valid for any number of ports.

5.7 S-MATRIX OF A TWO-PORT NETWORK WITH MISMATCHED LOAD

When a two-port network is formed there is discontinuity between the input port and the output port of a transmission line. Figure 5.6 shows a two-port configurations. When microwave signal is propagated through the junction, at each discontinuity evanescent modes are excited. These modes, containing reactive energy, decay very fast and become negligible after a distance of one wavelength from the junction. The terminal reference planes 1 and 2 are usually located beyond this distance. The equivalent voltage and current are proportional to the total transverse electric and magnetic fields respectively.

Let us consider a two-port network with characteristic impedance Z_0 and load impedance Z_L. At the load end, the total line voltage must be equal to the voltage across the load, and the current must be continuous through the load. Therefore we have,

$$V = V^+ + V^- = V_L \quad (5.55a)$$

$$I = I^+ - I^- = I_L \quad (5.55b)$$

Since $I = V/Z_0$, $I^+ = V^+/Z_0$, and $I^- = -V^-/Z_0$, we get from Eq. (5.55b)

$$V/Z_0 = V^+/Z_0 - V^-/Z_0 = V_L/Z_L$$

or, $\quad V_L = V^+ Z_L/Z_0 - V^- Z_L/Z_0 \quad (5.56)$

The normalized load impedance z_L is Z_L/Z_0. Equating Eqs (5.55a) and (5.56), we obtain

$$V^+ + V^- = V^+ Z_L/Z_0 - V^- Z_L/Z_0$$

or, $\quad V^-(1 + Z_L/Z_0) = V^+(Z_L/Z_0 - 1) \quad (5.57)$

The load reflection coefficient Γ_2 is the ratio of the reflected wave amplitude to the incident wave amplitudes. Therefore,

$$\Gamma_2 = V^-/V^+$$
$$= [(Z_L/Z_0) - 1]/[(Z_L/Z_0) + 1]$$
$$= (Z_L - Z_0)/(Z_L + Z_0) = a_2/b_2 \quad (5.58)$$

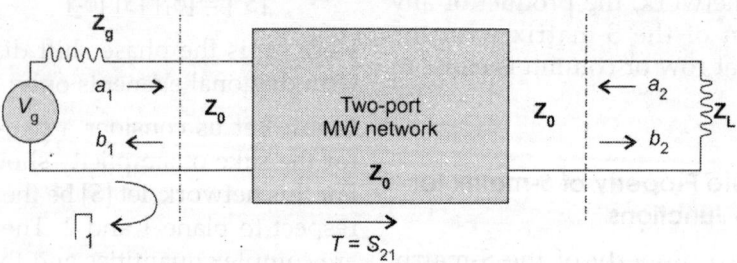

Fig. 5.6: Two-port network with mismatched load

For a two-port network, we know that

$$b_1 = S_{11}a_1 + S_{12}a_2$$
$$b_2 = S_{21}a_1 + S_{22}a_2$$

Substituting $a_2 = b_2 \Gamma_2$ in the above two equations, we get

$$b_1 = S_{11}a_1 + S_{12}b_2\Gamma_2 \qquad (5.59)$$
and $\qquad b_2 = S_{21}a_1 + S_{22}b_2\Gamma_2 \qquad (5.60)$

Dividing Eq. (5.59) by a_1 and substituting $b_1/a_1 = \Gamma_1$, we obtain

$$b_1/a_1 = \Gamma_1 = S_{11} + S_{12}(b_2/a_1)\Gamma_2 \qquad (5.61)$$

From Eq. (5.60), we get

$$b_2(1 - S_{22}\Gamma_2) = S_{21}a_1$$
or, $\qquad b_2/a_1 = S_{21}/(1 - S_{22}\Gamma_2) \qquad (5.62)$

Substitution of Eq. (5.62) in Eq. (5.61) yields

$$\Gamma_1 = S_{11} + (S_{12}S_{21})\,\Gamma_2/(1 - S_{22}\Gamma_2) \qquad (5.63)$$

Thus, for a mismatched load, $\Gamma_1 \neq S_{11}$ whereas for a matched load, $\Gamma_1 = S_{11}$.

For a reciprocal network, $S_{12} = S_{21}$. Hence

$$\Gamma_1 = S_{11} + [S_{12}^2\,\Gamma_2/(1 - S_{22}\Gamma_2)] \qquad (5.64)$$

Equation (5.64) is useful for computing S-matrix. By measuring Γ_1 for values of $\Gamma_2 = 0, -1$ and $+1$, a set of simultaneous equations is obtained. The solution of these equations gives the S-parameters of the lossless reciprocal junction with a mismatched load.

For a lossless junction, from the unitary and zero-properties from Eq. (5.51) and Eq. (5.53)], we obtain

$$S_{11}S_{11}^* + S_{12}S_{12}^* = 1 \qquad (5.65a)$$
$$S_{22}S_{22}^* + S_{12}S_{12}^* = 1 \qquad (5.65b)$$
$$S_{11}S_{12}^* + S_{12}S_{22}^* = 0 \qquad (5.65c)$$

Hence, for a loss-less reciprocal network terminated with mismatched load, we get from Eqs (5.65a) and (5.65b),

$$S_{11}S_{11}^* + S_{12}S_{12}^* = S_{22}S_{22}^* + S_{12}S_{12}^*$$
$$\therefore \qquad |S_{11}| = |S_{22}| \qquad (5.66)$$

Substituting $|S_{11}| = |S_{22}|$ in Eqs (5.65a) and (5.65b), we have

$$|S_{12}| = \sqrt{(1 - |S_{11}|^2)} = \sqrt{(1 - |S_{22}|^2)} \qquad (5.67)$$

Example 5.2: A certain two-port network has $S_{11} = 0.26 - j0.16$, $S_{12} = S_{21} = 0.42$ and $S_{22} = 0.36 - j0.57$. Compute the input reflection coefficient (a) when $Z_g = Z_l = Z_0$ and (b) when $Z_g = Z_0$ and $Z_l = 3Z_0$.

Solution: Given: $S_{11} = 0.26 - j0.16$, $S_{12} = S_{21} = 0.42$ and $S_{22} = 0.36 - j0.57$.

(a) $Z_g = Z_l = Z_0$

Hence, $\Gamma_g = \Gamma_l = 0$.

From Eq. (5.63) the input reflection coefficient is given by

$$\Gamma_{l\,in} = S_{11} + [S_{12}S_{21}\,\Gamma_l/(1 - S_{22}\Gamma_l)] = S_{11}$$
$$= 0.26 - j0.16 = \mathbf{0.305\ \angle -31.6°}$$

(b) $Z_g = Z_0$ and $Z_l = 3Z_0$

Hence, $\Gamma_g = 0$.

$$\Gamma_l = (Z_l - Z_0)/(Z_l + Z_0)$$
$$= (3Z_0 - Z_0)/(3Z_0 + Z_0) = 1/2$$

From Eq. (5.63) the input reflection coefficient is given by

$$\Gamma_{l\,in} = S_{11} + [S_{12}S_{21}\,\Gamma_l/(1 - S_{22}\Gamma_l)]$$

$$= \frac{0.26 - j0.16 + \left[(0.42)^2 \times \dfrac{1}{2}\right]}{\left[1 - (0.28 - j0.56) \times \dfrac{1}{2}\right]}$$

$$= 0.26 - j0.16 + [0.0882/(0.86 + j0.28)]$$
$$= 0.26 - j0.16 + 0.882/0/904\ \angle 18°$$
$$= 0.26 - j0.16 + 0.0973\ \angle -18°$$
$$= 0.26 - j0.16 + 0.0925 - j0.0301$$
$$= 0.3525 - j1901 = \mathbf{0.4\ \angle -28.34°}$$

5.8 COMPARISON BETWEEN S, Z AND Y PARAMETERS

S, Z and Y matrices represent unique intrinsic characteristics of the device at a given frequency. The S-matrix may be expressed in terms of Z and Y. In terms of Z, it is given by

$$[S] = ([Z]/Z_0 - [U])\,([Z]/Z_0 + [U])^{-1} \qquad (5.68)$$

In terms of Y, it is given by

$$[S] = ([U] - [Y]/Y_0)\,([Y]/Y_0 + [U])^{-1} \qquad (5.69)$$

The properties common to them are:

(i) They are of the same dimensions.

(ii) For reciprocal networks, they satisfy reciprocity property.

i.e., $Y_{ij} = Y_{ji}$; $Z_{ij} = Z_{ji}$; $S_{ij} = S_{ji}$

(iii) [S] is symmetrical if [Z] or [Y] is symmetrical.

5.9 ADVANTAGES OF S-MATRIX OVER Z AND Y MATRICES

The advantages of S-matrix over Z and Y matrices are enumerated below.

(a) Measurement of VSWR, power and phase are essentially measurement of (b/a), $|a|^2$ and $|b|^2$. Such direct correspondence does not exist in Z and Y representation.

(b) For loss-less structures, the unitary property of [S] can be used as a quick check of the power balance. Such immediate check is not possible with Z and Y representation.

(c) In microwave measurements, the S-matrix is defined for a set of reference planes. Only the phase of the S-parameters vary when the reference planes are changed. In the case of Z and Y representations, both the magnitude and phase change since the voltage and current are functions of the complex impedance.

5.10 DERIVATION OF RELATIONSHIP BETWEEN S, Z, Y AND ABCD PARAMETERS

In this section, we shall derive the relationships between S-parameters and Z, Y and ABCD parameters.

5.10.1 S–Parameters in Terms of Z-Parameters

This relationship can be derived from Eq. (5.68) that is reproduced below:

$$[S] = \{[Z]/Z_0 - [U]\}\{[Z]/Z_0 + [U]\}^{-1}$$

$$= (1/Z_0)\begin{pmatrix} Z_{11} - Z_0 & Z_{12} \\ Z_{21} & Z_{22} - Z_0 \end{pmatrix} \times$$

$$(1/Z_0)^{-1}\begin{pmatrix} Z_{11} + Z_0 & Z_{12} \\ Z_{21} & Z_{22} + Z_0 \end{pmatrix}^{-1}$$

$$= \frac{\begin{pmatrix} Z_{11} - Z_0 & Z_{12} \\ Z_{21} & Z_{22} - Z_0 \end{pmatrix}\begin{pmatrix} Z_{22} + Z_0 & -Z_{12} \\ -Z_{21} & Z_{11} + Z_0 \end{pmatrix}}{\Delta_z}$$

$$= (1/\Delta_z) \times$$

$$\begin{pmatrix} (Z_{11} - Z_0)(Z_{22} + Z_0) - Z_{12}Z_{21} & 2Z_{12}Z_0 \\ 2Z_{21}Z_0 & (Z_{11} + Z_0)(Z_{22} - Z_0) - Z_{12}Z_{21} \end{pmatrix}$$

Hence

$$S_{11} = \frac{[(Z_{11} - Z_0)(Z_{22} + Z_0) - Z_{12}Z_{21}]}{\Delta_z} \quad (5.70a)$$

$$S_{12} = 2Z_{12}Z_0/\Delta_z \quad (5.70b)$$

$$S_{21} = 2Z_{21}Z_0/\Delta_z \quad (5.70c)$$

$$S_{22} = \frac{[(Z_{11} + Z_0)(Z_{22} - Z_0) - Z_{12}Z_{21}]}{\Delta_z} \quad (5.70d)$$

$$\Delta_z = (Z_{11} + Z_0)(Z_{22} + Z_0) - Z_{12}Z_{22} \quad (5.70e)$$

Example 5.3: The normalized impedance matrix of a simple device is given by $\begin{pmatrix} 2 & 4 \\ 4 & 2 \end{pmatrix}$.

Find its S-matrix.

Solution: Given: $z_{11} = 2$, $z_{12} = z_{21} = 4$, $z_{22} = 2$

From Eq. (5.70a), S_{11} is given by

$$S_{11} = [(Z_{11} - Z_0)(Z_{22} + Z_0) - Z_{12}Z_{21}]/\Delta_z$$

$$= [(z_{11} - 1)(z_{22} + 1) - z_{12}z_{21}]/\Delta_z$$

$$\Delta_z = (Z_{11} + Z_0)(Z_{22} + Z_0) - Z_{12}Z_{22}$$

$$= (z_{11} + 1)(z_{22} + 1) - z_{12}z_{21}$$

$$= 3 \times 3 - 4 \times 4 = -7$$

$$S_{11} = [(z_{11} - 1)(z_{22} + 1) - z_{12}z_{21}]/\Delta_z$$

$$= [1 \times 3 - 16]/[-7] = 13/7$$

$$S_{12} = 2z_{12}z_0/\Delta_z = 2z_{12}/\Delta_z$$

$$= 2 \times 4/-7 = -8/7$$

Because of symmetry,

$$S_{11} = S_{22}, S_{12} = S_2$$

$$\therefore \quad S = \begin{pmatrix} 13/7 & -8/7 \\ -8/7 & 13/7 \end{pmatrix}$$

5.10.2 Z-Parameters in Terms of S-Parameters

This relationship can be derived from Eq. (5.68) that is reproduced below:

$$[S] = \{[Z]/Z_0 - [U]\}\{[Z]/Z_0 + [U]\}^{-1}$$

$$= [Z]/Z_0 - [U]/[Z]/Z_0 + [U]$$

Multiplying both sides by the denominator, we get

$$\{[Z]/Z_0 + [U]\} [S] = [Z]/Z_0 - [U]$$

Rearranging, we obtain

$$[Z]/Z_0 - [Z]/Z_0 [S] = [U] + [S]$$

$$[Z]/Z_0 \{[U] - [S]\} = [U] + [S]$$

$$\therefore \qquad [Z]/Z_0 = \{[U] - [S]\}^{-1} \{[U] + [S]\}$$

It can be shown that

$$Z_{11} = [(1 + S_{11})(1 - S_{22}) + S_{12}S_{21}]/\Delta_s \quad (5.71a)$$

$$Z_{22} = [(1 - S_{11})(1 + S_{22}) + S_{12}S_{21}]/\Delta_s \quad (5.71b)$$

$$Z_{12} = 2S_{12}/\Delta_s \quad (5.71c)$$

$$Z_{21} = 2S_{21}/\Delta_s \quad (5.71d)$$

$$\Delta_s = (1 - S_{11})(1 - S_{22}) - S_{12}S_{21}] \quad (5.71e)$$

Example 5.4: The S-matrix of a simple device is given by $S_{11} = 0.5 + j0.5$, $S_{12} = S_{21} = j0.5$ and $S_{22} = 0.5 - j0.5$. Find its Z-matrix.

Solution: Given: $S_{11} = 0.5 + j0.5$, $S_{12} = S_{21} = j0.5$ and $S_{22} = 0.5 - j0.5$.

$$Z_{11} = [(1 + S_{11})(1 - S_{22}) + S_{12} S_{21}]/\Delta_s$$

$$\Delta_s = [(1 - S_{11})(1 - S_{22}) - S_{12} S_{21}]$$

$$= (0.5 - j0.5)(0.5 + j0.5) + 0.25$$

$$= [0.25 + j0.25 - j0.25 + 0.25 + 0.25] = \mathbf{0.75}$$

$$Z_{11} = [(1.5 + j0.5)(0.5 + j0.5) - 0.25]/0.75$$

$$= [(0.75 + j0.75 + j0.25 - 0.25 - 0.25]/0.75$$

$$= (0.25 + j1)/0.75 = \mathbf{(1 + j4)/3}$$

$$Z_{22} = [(1 - S_{11})(1 + S_{22}) + S_{12} S_{21}]/\Delta_s$$

$$= [(0.5 - j0.5)(1.5 - j0.5) + 0.25]/0.75$$

$$= [0.75 + j0.25 + j0.75 + 0.25 + 0.25]/0.75$$

$$= (0.25 - j1)/0.75 = (1 - j4)/3$$

$$Z_{12} = Z_{21} = 2 S_{12}/\Delta_s$$

$$= 2 \times j0.5/0.75 = j\mathbf{4}/\mathbf{3}$$

$$\therefore \ Z = \frac{1}{3}\begin{pmatrix} 1 + j4 & j4 \\ j4 & 1 - j4 \end{pmatrix}$$

5.10.3 S–Parameters in Terms of Y-Parameters

This relationship can be derived from Eq. (5.69) that is reproduced below:

$$[S] = \{[U] - [X]/Y_0\} \{[U] + [X]/X_0\}^{-1}$$

$$= (1/Y_0)\begin{pmatrix} Y_0 - Y_{11} & -Y_{12} \\ -Y_{21} & Y_0 - Y_{22} \end{pmatrix} \times$$

$$(1/Y_0)^{-1}\begin{pmatrix} Y_0 - Y_{22} & -Y_{12} \\ -Y_{21} & Y_0 + Y_{11} \end{pmatrix}$$

$$= \frac{\begin{pmatrix} Y_0 - Y_{11} & -Y_{12} \\ -Y_{21} & Y_0 - Y_{22} \end{pmatrix}\begin{pmatrix} Y_0 + Y_{22} & -Y_{12} \\ -Y_{21} & Y_0 + Y_{11} \end{pmatrix}}{\Delta_y}$$

$$= (1/\Delta_y) \times$$

$$\begin{pmatrix} (Y_0 - Y_{11})(Y_0 + Y_{22}) - Y_{12}Y_{22} & -2Y_{12}Y_0 \\ -2Y_{21}Y_0 & (Y_{11} + Y_0)(Y_0 - Y_{22}) - Y_{12}Y_{21} \end{pmatrix}$$

Hence

$$S_{11} = \frac{[(Y_0 - Y_{11})(Y_0 + Y_{22}) - Y_{12}Y_{21}]}{\Delta_y} \quad (5.72a)$$

$$S_{12} = -2Y_{12}Y_0/\Delta_y \quad (5.72b)$$

$$S_{21} = -2Y_{21}Y_0/\Delta_y \quad (5.72c)$$

$$S_{22} = \frac{[(Y_0 + Y_{11})(Y_0 - Y_{22}) + Y_{12}Y_{21}]}{\Delta_y} \quad (5.72d)$$

$$\Delta_y = (Y_{11} + Y_0)(Y_{22} + Y_0) - Y_{12}Y_{22} \quad (5.72e)$$

5.10.4 Y-Parameters in Terms of S-Parameters

This relationship can be derived from Eq. (5.69) that is reproduced below:

$$[S] = \{[U] - [Y]/Y_0\} \{[U] + [Y]/Y_0\}^{-1}$$

$$= \{[U] - [Y]/Y_0\}/\{[U] + [Y]/Y_0\}$$

Multiplying both sides by the denominator, we get

$$\{[U] + [Y]/Y_0\}[S] = \{[U] - [Y]/Y_0\}$$

Rearranging, we obtain

$$[Y]/Y_0 - [Y]/Y_0 [S] = [U] + [S]$$

$$[Y]/Y_0 \{[U] - [S]\} = [U] + [S]$$

$$\therefore \qquad [Y]/Y_0 = [U] - [S] \{[U] + [S]\}^{-1}$$

It can be shown that

$$Y_{11} = [(1 - S_{11})(1 + S_{22}) + S_{12}S_{21}]/\Delta_s \quad (5.73a)$$

$$Y_{22} = [(1 + S_{11})(1 - S_{22}) + S_{12}S_{21}]/\Delta_s \quad (5.73b)$$

$$Y_{12} = -2 S_{12}/\Delta_s \quad (5.73c)$$

$$Y_{21} = -2 S_{21}/\Delta_s \quad (5.73d)$$

$$\Delta_s = (1 + S_{11})(1 + S_{22}) - S_{12}S_{21} \quad (5.73e)$$

5.10.5 S-Parameters in Terms of ABCD-Parameters

To derive this relationship, first we derive the relationship between ABCD and Z parameters and then use these to derive the S-parameters

The ABCD parameter equations of a two-port passive network is given by

$$V_1 = AV_2 - BI_2 \quad (5.74a)$$

$$I_1 = CV_2 - DI_2 \quad (5.74b)$$

The Z-parameter equations of a two-port passive network is given by

$$V_1 = Z_{11}I_1 - Z_{12}I_2 \quad (5.75a)$$

$$V_2 = Z_{21}I_1 - Z_{22}I_2 \quad (5.75b)$$

We have to express Eq. (5.75b) with I_1 as the independent variable for comparing with Eq. (5.74b). From Eq. (5.75b), I_1 is given by

$$I_1 = (V_2 + Z_{22}I_2)/Z_{21}$$
$$= (1/Z_{21}) V_2 + (Z_{22}/Z_{21})I_2 \quad (5.76a)$$

Substituting this in Eq. (5.75a), we get

$$V_1 = Z_{11}[(1/Z_{21}) V_2 + (Z_{22}/Z_{21})] I_2 - Z_{12}I_2$$
$$= (Z_{11}/Z_{21}) V_2 + \{(Z_{11}Z_{22} - Z_{12}Z_{21})/Z_{21}\}I_2 \quad (5.76b)$$

Comparing Eqs (5.74a) and (5.74b) with Eqs (5.76b) and (5.76a), we obtain

$$A = Z_{11}/Z_{21};$$
$$B = -(Z_{11}Z_{22} - Z_{12}Z_{21})/Z_{21};$$
$$C = 1/Z_{21};$$
$$D = -Z_{22}/Z_{21} \quad (5.77)$$

Therefore, we now derive the S-parameters in terms of ABCD parameters using these relationships.

$$S_{11} = \frac{[(Z_{11} - Z_0)(Z_{22} + Z_0) - Z_{12}Z_{21}]}{[(Z_{11} + Z_0)(Z_{22} + Z_0) - Z_{12}Z_{21}]}$$

$$= \frac{[Z_{11}Z_{22} + Z_0(Z_{11} - Z_{22}) - Z_0^2 - Z_{12}Z_{21}]}{[Z_{11}Z_{22} + Z_0(Z_{11} + Z_{22}) + Z_0^2 - Z_{12}Z_{21}]}$$

$$= \frac{[(Z_{11}Z_{22} - Z_{12}Z_{21}) + Z_0(Z_{11} - Z_{22}) - Z_0^2]}{[(Z_{11}Z_{22} - Z_{12}Z_{21}) + Z_0(Z_{11} + Z_{22}) + Z_0^2]}$$

Expressing them in terms of ABCD parameters, we get

$$Z_{11}Z_{22} - Z_{12}Z_{21} = -B/C$$
$$Z_{11} + Z_{22} = (A - D)/C$$
$$Z_{11} - Z_{22} = (A - D)/C$$
$$Z_{12} = B - (AD/C)$$

Substituting these in S_{11}, we obtain

$$S_{11} = \frac{[(-B/C) + Z_0(A + D)/C - Z_0^2]}{[(-B/C) + Z_0(A - D)/C + Z_0^2]}$$

$$= \frac{[AZ_0/C - (B/C) + DZ_0/C - Z_0^2]}{[AZ_0/C - (B/C) + Z_0^2 - DZ_0/C]}$$

$$= \frac{[AZ_0 - B - CZ_0^2 + DZ_0]}{[AZ_0 - B + CZ_0^2 - DZ_0]} \quad (5.78)$$

Similarly, S_{22} is given by

$$S_{22} = \frac{[(Z_{11} + Z_0)(Z_{22} - Z_0) - Z_{12}Z_{21}]}{[(Z_{11} + Z_0)(Z_{22} + Z_0) - Z_{12}Z_{21}]}$$

$$= \frac{[Z_{11}Z_{22} - Z_0(Z_{11}Z_{22}) - Z_0^2 - Z_{12}Z_{21}]}{[Z_{11}Z_{22} + Z_0(Z_{11} + Z_{22}) + Z_0^2 - Z_{12}Z_{21}]}$$

$$= \frac{[(Z_{11}Z_{22} - Z_{12}Z_{21}) - Z_0(Z_{11} - Z_{22}) - Z_0^2]}{[(Z_{11}Z_{22} - Z_{12}Z_{21}) + Z_0(Z_{11} + Z_{22}) + Z_0^2]}$$

$$= \frac{[(-B/C) - Z_0(A + D)/C - Z_0^2]}{[(-B/C) + Z_0(A - D)/C + Z_0^2]}$$

$$= \frac{[-AZ_0/C - (B/C) - DZ_0/C - Z_0^2]}{[AZ_0/C + (-B/C) + Z_0^2 - DZ_0/C]}$$

$$= \frac{[-AZ_0 - B - CZ_0^2 - DZ_0]}{[AZ_0 - B + CZ_0^2 - DZ_0]} \quad (5.79)$$

$$S_{12} = \frac{2Z_{12}Z_0}{[(Z_{11} + Z_0)(Z_{22} + Z_0) - Z_{12}Z_{21}]}$$

$$= \frac{2[B - (AD/C)]Z_0}{[AZ_0/C - B/C + Z_0^2 - DZ_0]}$$

$$= \frac{2Z_0[BC - AD]}{[AZ_0 - B + CZ_0^2 - DZ_0]} \quad (5.80)$$

$$S_{21} = \frac{2Z_{21}Z_0}{[(Z_{11} + Z_0)(Z_{22} + Z_0) - Z_{12}Z_{21}]}$$

$$= \frac{(2Z_0/C)}{[AZ_0/C - B/C + Z_0^2 - DZ_0]}$$

$$= \frac{2Z_0}{[AZ_0 - B + CZ_0^2 - DZ_0]} \quad (5.81)$$

5.10.6 ABCD–Parameters in Terms of S–Parameters

From Eq. (5.77),

$$A = Z_{11}/Z_{21};$$
$$B = -(Z_{11}Z_{22} - Z_{12}Z_{21})/Z_{21};$$
$$C = 1/Z_{21};$$
$$D = -Z_{22}/Z_{21}$$

Substituting for Z-parameters from Eq. (5.79), we obtain

$$A = Z_{11}/Z_{21}$$
$$= [(1 + S_{11})(1 - S_{22}) + S_{12}S_{21}]/2S_{21} \quad (5.82)$$

$$B = -(Z_{11}Z_{22} - Z_{12}Z_{21})/Z_{21} \quad (5.83)$$
$$= \{[(1 + S_{11})(1 - S_{22}) + S_{12}S_{21}] \times$$
$$[(1 - S_{11})(1 + S_{22}) + S_{12}S_{21}] - 2S_{12}2S_{21}]\} \quad (5.84)$$

$$C = 1/Z_{21} = \Delta_s/2S_{21}$$
$$= (1 - S_{11})(1 - S_{22}) - S_{12}S_{21}]/2S_{21} \quad (5.85)$$

$$D = -Z_{22}/Z_{21}$$
$$= -[(1 - S_{11})(1 + S_{22}) + S_{12}S_{21}]/2S_{21} \quad (5.86)$$

5.11 ADDITIONAL EXAMPLES

In this section, we solve some typical problems pertaining to the microwave network theory discussed.

Example 5.5: Derive the S-matrix of a section of a microwave transmission line of length L as shown in Fig. 5.7.

Solution: The microwave transmission line of length L may be considered as a two-port network. The incident waves are a_1, a_2 and the outgoing waves are b_1, b_2 at port 1 and 2

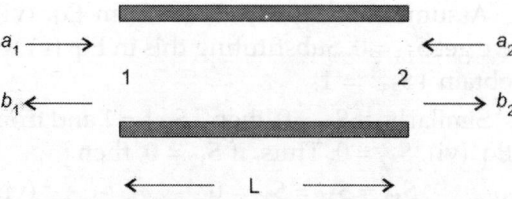

Fig. 5.7: Section of transmission line

respectively. Since no junction is formed, there are no reflections at the two ports as i_1 and a_2 are transmitted to ports 2 and 1 respectively. Hence

$$S_{11} = S_{22} = 0.$$

Therefore, we have

$$b_1 = a_2 = e^{-j\beta_L} \quad \text{(i)}$$
$$b_2 = a_1 = e^{-j\beta_L} \quad \text{(ii)}$$

Hence the S-matrix is given by

$$[S] = \begin{pmatrix} b_1 \\ b_2 \end{pmatrix} \begin{pmatrix} 0 & e^{-j\beta_L} \\ e^{-j\beta_L} & 0 \end{pmatrix} \begin{pmatrix} a_1 \\ a_2 \end{pmatrix} \quad \text{(iii)}$$

Here β is the phase constant.

Example 5.6: Derive the S-matrix of a perfectly matched three-port microwave network. Show that a 3-port network cannot be matched al all ports simultaneously.

Solution: As the three ports are perfectly matched,

$$S_{11} = S_{22} = S_{33} = 0 \quad \text{(i)}$$

Hence the S-matrix is given by

$$[S] = \begin{pmatrix} 0 & S_{12} & S_{13} \\ S_{21} & 0 & S_{23} \\ S_{31} & S_{32} & 0 \end{pmatrix} \quad \text{(ii)}$$

If the junction is loss-less, conservation of power theorem requires that the S-matrix satisfy the unitary and null properties. Applying the conditions, we obtain

$$S_{12}S_{12}^* + S_{22}S_{22}^* = 1 \quad \text{(iii)}$$
$$S_{21}S_{21}^* + S_{31}S_{31}^* = 1 \quad \text{(iv)}$$
$$S_{13}S_{13}^* + S_{23}S_{23}^* = 1 \quad \text{(v)}$$
$$S_{12}S_{13}^* = S_{21}S_{23}^*$$
$$= S_{31}S_{32}^* = 0 \quad \text{(vi)}$$

Assume that $S_{12} \neq 0$. Then from Eq. (vi), we get $S_{13} = 0$. Substituting this in Eq. (v) we obtain $|S_{23}| = 1$.

Similarly, if $S_{21} = 0$, then $|S_{31}| = 1$ and from Eq. (vi), $S_{32} = 0$. Thus, if $S_{12} \neq 0$, then

$$S_{13} = S_{21} = S_{32} = 0 \qquad \text{(vii)}$$

Equation (vii) states that there exists perfect transmission from port 2 to port 1, from port 3 to port 2 and from port 1 to port 3. Also, there is no transmission in the reverse direction. The resultant scattering matrix of any three-port network that is matched, loss-less and non-reciprocal is of the form

$$[S] = \begin{pmatrix} 0 & S_{12} & 0 \\ 0 & 0 & S_{23} \\ S_{31} & 0 & 0 \end{pmatrix} \qquad \text{(viii)}$$

Alternatively, it may have the following form:

$$[S] = \begin{pmatrix} 0 & 0 & S_{13} \\ S_{21} & 0 & 0 \\ 0 & S_{32} & 0 \end{pmatrix} \qquad \text{(ix)}$$

If we properly choose the locations of the terminal planes or ports, the phase angles of S_{13}, S_{21} and S_{32} can be made zero and hence $S_{13} = S_{21} = S_{32} = 1$.

If the above junction is perfectly matched, loss-less and reciprocal, then, according to the reciprocity theorem,

$$S_{13} = S_{21} = S_{32} = 0 \qquad \text{(x)}$$

Since S_{13}, S_{21} and S_{32} are zero, the resultant matrix would vanish. This states that it is not possible to construct a perfectly matched, loss-less, reciprocal three-port network. At least, one of the reflection coefficients must be present in the reciprocal case.

Example 5.7: Derive the S-matrix of the junction of two transmission lines with characteristic impedances Z_1 and Z_2 respectively shown in Fig. 5.8.

Solution: Assume that the output line is matched, i.e. $a_2 = 0$. Then the input impe-

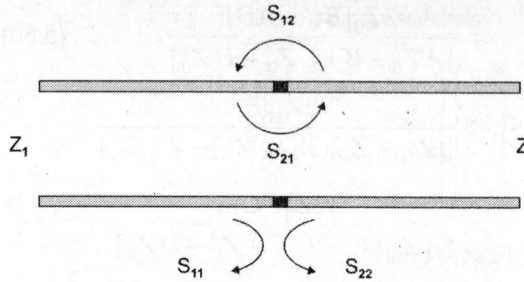

Fig. 5.8: Junction of two transmission lines

dance Z_{in} at the junction = Z_2 = load on line Z_2. Therefore

$$S_{11} = (Z_2 - Z_1)/(Z_2 + Z_1)$$

Similarly, with $a_1 = 0$, we have

$$S_{22} = (Z_1 - Z_2)/(Z_1 + Z_2)$$

For a lossless line with $a_2 = 0$, Z_{in} at the junction = Z_2, a shunt element. Therefore

$$b_2 = a_1 + b_1 = a_1 + S_{11}a_1 = a_1(1 + S_{11})$$
$$b_2/a_1 = S_{21} = 1 + S_{11}$$
$$= 1 + (Z_2 - Z_1)/(Z_2 + Z_1)$$
$$= 2Z_2/(Z_2 + Z_1)$$

Similarly,

$$b_1 = a_2 + b_2 = a_2 + S_{22} a_2 = a_2(1 + S_{22})$$
$$b_{21} a_2 = S_{12} = 1 + S_{22}$$
$$= 1 + (Z_1 - Z_2)/(Z_1 + Z_2)$$
$$= 2Z_1/(Z_2 + Z_1)$$

Therefore the S-matrix is given by

$$[S] = \begin{pmatrix} (Z_2 - Z_1)/(Z_2 + Z_1) & 2Z_1/(Z_2 + Z_1) \\ 2Z_2/(Z_2 + Z_1) & (Z_1 - Z_2)/Z_1 + Z_2 \end{pmatrix}$$

Example 5.8: The S-parameters of a certain two-port network are $S_{11} = 0.26 - j0.16$, $S_{12} = S_{21} = 0.42$ and $S_{22} = 0.36 - j0.57$. Calculate the four losses.

Solution: Insertion loss
$$IL = 20 \log |1/S_{12}|$$
$$= 20 \log (1/0.42) = \textbf{7.54 dB}$$

Transmission loss
$$= TL = 10 \log [(1 - |S_{11}|^2)/|S_{12}|^2]$$
$$= 20 \log [(1 - 0.305^2)/0.42^2 = \textbf{7.11 dB}$$

Reflection loss

$$= 10 \log [1/(1 - |S_{11}|^2)]$$
$$= 10 \log [1/(1 - 0.305^2)] = \textbf{0.42 dB}$$

Return loss

$$= RL = 20 \log [1/|S_{11}|]$$
$$= 10 \log [1/0.305] = \textbf{10.31 dB}$$

KEY POINTS

- Microwave frequency range is from 1 GHz to 100 GHz.
- The microwave circuit elements and devices at microwave frequencies are of the same order of magnitude as the wavelengths. Hence, the conventional low frequency circuit analysis is not applicable at microwave frequencies.
- The behavior of a 2-port network is described by Z, Y, h and $ABCD$ parameters.
- In a reciprocal network, its impedance and the admittance matrices are symmetrical.
- A microwave network consists of microwave sources, attenuators, resonators etc. connected together to achieve the desired transmission of microwave signals.
- A microwave junction is the point of interconnection of two or more devices/components. Wave-guides, tees, hybrid rings, directional couplers and circulators are the commonly used microwave junctions.
- The Z, Y, h and $ABCD$ parameters cannot be used to describe a microwave network.
- At microwave frequencies, (i) the physical length of microwave components is comparable to the wavelength, (ii) voltage and current cannot be measured directly, (iii) short and open circuits are difficult to achieve for a wide range of microwave frequencies, (iv) voltage, current and impedance cannot be measured directly, (v) short and open circuits are difficult to achieve for a wide frequency range and (vi) microwave active devices are unstable for short and open circuit.
- The parameters that describe the relationship between the scattered wave amplitudes and the amplitudes of incident waves are known as S-parameters.

FURTHER READING

1. Collins RE (1996). *Foundations of Microwave Engineering*, McGraw Hill, NY.
2. Das A and Das SK (2004). *Microwave Engineering*, TMH, New Delhi.
3. Gandhi OP (1981). *Microwave Engineering and Applications*, Pergamon, NY.
4. Liao SY (2000). *Microwave Devices and Circuits*, PHI, New Delhi.

REVIEW QUESTIONS

5.1 Mention the four parameter sets used to describe a two-port electrical network.

5.2 Define the Z-parameters of a two-port network.

5.3 Define the Y-parameters of a two-port network.

5.4 Define the h-parameters of a two-port network

5.5 Define the $ABCD$-parameters of a two-port network.

5.6 Define a reciprocal network.

5.7 Define a microwave network.

5.8 Why is S-matrix used to describe a microwave circuit?

5.9 Define the S-parameters.

5.10 State the properties of S-matrix.

5.11 Write an expression for the S-matrix of a two-port microwave network.

5.12 Write down an expression for the S-matrix of a N-port microwave network.

5.13 Express the input and reflected powers in terms of incident and reflected wave amplitudes.

5.14 Mention the four losses that occur in a microwave network.

5.15 Give expressions for the four losses in a microwave network in terms of S-parameters.

5.16 Compare S, Z and Y matrices.

5.17 Mention the advantages of S-matrix over Z and Y matrices.

5.18 Express S-parameters in terms of Z-parameters.

5.19 Express S-parameters in terms of Y-parameters.

5.20 Express S-parameters in terms of $ABCD$-parameters.

5.21 Express S-parameters in terms of Z-parameters when normalized.

5.22 Write down the S-matrix of a microwave transmission line of length L.

5.23 Write down the S-matrix for perfectly matched 3-port microwave network.

5.24 Write down the S-matrix for the junction of two microwave transmission lines of characteristic impedances Z_1 and Z_2.

DESCRIPTIVE QUESTIONS

5.1 Show that Z and Y parameters are symmetrical for a reciprocal network.

5.2 Derive the S-matrix of a two-port microwave network.

5.3 Derive the power relations of a two-port microwave network.

5.4 Derive the expressions for the losses that occur in a two-port microwave network in terms of S-parameters.

5.5 Prove the unitary property of the S-matrix.

5.6 Prove the null property of the S-matrix.

5.7 Prove the symmetry property of the S-matrix.

5.8 Prove the phase shift property of the S-matrix.

5.9 Derive the S-matrix of a two-port microwave network with mismatched load.

5.10 Prove that it is not possible to construct a perfectly matched, loss-less reciprocal 3-port network.

5.11 Derive the relationship between S and Z parameters.

5.12 Derive the relationship between S and Y parameters.

5.13 Derive the relationship between S and $ABCD$ parameters

5.14 Derive the relationship between $ABCD$ and Z parameters.

PRACTICE PROBLEMS

5.1 A series element of impedance Z is connected to a transmission line of characteristic impedance Z_0. Find the S-matrix at the junction so formed.

$$[\text{Ans: } S_{11} = S_{22} = Z/(Z + 2Z_0);$$
$$S_{12} = S_{21} = 2Z_0/(Z + 2Z_0)]$$

5.2 A shunt element of impedance Z is connected across a transmission line of characteristic impedance Z_0. Find the S-matrix at the junction so formed.

$$[\text{Ans: } S_{11} = S_{22} = -Z_0 Y/(2 + Z_0 Y);$$
$$S_{12} = S_{21} = 2/(2 + Z_0 Y)]$$

5.3 The S-parameters of a certain two-port network are $S_{11} = 0.26 - j0.16$, $S_{12} = S_{21} = 0.42$ and $S_{22} = 0.36 - j0.57$. Calculate the four losses and Γ_L.

(**Ans:** $IL = 5.04$ dB, $TL = 4.68$ dB, Refl. $L = 0.35$ dB and $RL = 15.07$ dB, $\Gamma_L = 0.67 \angle{-57.7°}$)

5.4 The S-parameters of a certain two-port network are $S_{11} = S_{22} = -j0.54$, $S_{12} = S_{21} = 0.84$. Calculate the four losses and Γ_L.

(**Ans:** $IL = 5.51$ dB, $TL = 0.017$ dB, Ref. $L = 5.5$ dB and $RL = 5.35$ dB, $G_L = 0.54 \angle{-90°}$)

5.5 A reciprocal two-port device has a VSWR of 5.5 and insertion loss of 2 dB. Calculate the magnitudes of S-parameters.

(**Ans:** $S_{11} = S_{22} = 0.2$, $S_{12} = S_{21} = 0.7943$)

REFERENCE

1. Ryder JD (1997). *Networks, Lines and Fields*, PHI, New Delhi.

2. Liao SY (2000). *Microwave Devices and Circuits*, PHI, New Delhi.

3. Chodorov M and Susskind C (1964). *Fundamentals of Microwave Electronics*, McGraw-Hill, NY.

4. Harvey AF (1963). *Microwave Engineering*, Acad. Press, NY.

5. Montogomery CG et al (1948). *Principles of Microwave Circuits*, McGraw Hill, NY.

6. Roddy D (1986). *Microwave Technology*, PH, NJ.

7. Reich HJ (1978). *Microwave Principles*, East-West, New Delhi.

8. Rizzi PA (1999). *Microwave Engineering: Passive Circuits*, PH, NJ.

9. Seeger JA (1988). *Microwave Theory Components and Devices*, PH, NJ.

10. Pozar DM (1990). *Microwave Engineering*, Addison-Wesley, Massachusetts.

6
■ Microwave Passive Components

Objectives

• Familiarize with the construction of waveguide flanges, matched terminations and short-circuit plungers.
• Study the waveguide transitions, corners, bends, twists and waveguide adaptors.
• Understand the principle of waveguide apertures, couplers, attenuators and phase shifters.
• Gain knowledge of *E, H* and magic tees, their *S*-matrices and their applications.

6.1 INTRODUCTION

The MW passive components are:
  i. Transmission line, waveguide and coaxial line stub
  ii. Waveguide windows
  iii. Tuning screws
  iv. Matched terminations
  v. Inductive and capacitive posts
  vi. Single and multisection quarter-wave transformers
  vii. Tapered transmission lines
  viii. Waveguide choke flanges
  ix. Short-circuit plunger
  x. Wageguide transition
  xi. Waveguide corners, bands and twists
  xii. Adaptors
  xiii. Coupling loops
  xiv. Coupling apertures
  xv. Altenuators
  xvi. Phase shifters
  xvii. Waveguide tees

Of these, stubs, waveguide windows, tuning screws and inductive and capacitive posts have been discussed in Section 2.12. In this chapter, we shall describe other MW passive components.

The commonly used passive components in MW communication and radar systems are waveguide choke flanges, matched terminations, short-circuit plunger, attenuators, phase shifters, T-junctions and hybrids. These components can be considered as one-port or multiport networks. They are characterized by the basic parameters such as VSWR, reflection coefficients and various losses under matched output conditions. We shall now study the basic operating principles of these components.

6.2 WAVEGUIDE CHOKE FLANGES

Waveguides are fitted with flanges at the ends so that they can be connected with other waveguides or devices by using the nut-bolt

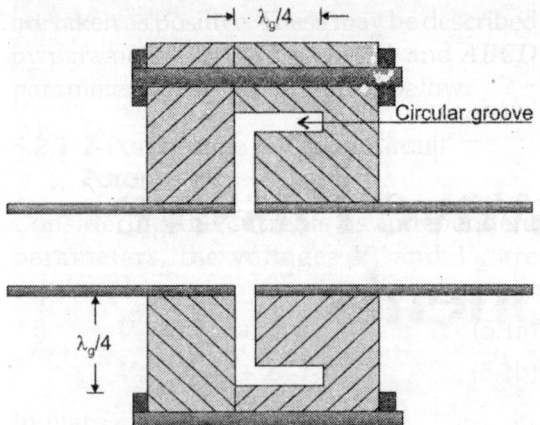

Fig. 6.1: Waveguide choke flange

arrangement as shown in Fig. 6.1. The choke flanges are used to avoid leakage of high power signals between the two flange joints. They consist of a circular groove of depth d in the flange such that the depth d plus the distance to the waveguide joint on the wide wall is one half of the wavelength. This arrangement results in an ideal short-circuited half-wavelength line and it provides zero resistance contact between inner walls of the two waveguide sections at the joint. Improper contact at the joint will cause power loss due to leakage of power, heating and partial reflection of waves. In high power applications, improper contact may burn out the contacts.

One of the two waveguides is fitted with a choke flange and the other with a plane flange so that the choke provides a low characteristic impedance line. The choke flange is frequency sensitive. The frequency sensitivity is minimized by choosing the low impedance line to be half wavelength. Low VSWR of the order of 1.02 to 1.05 can be achieved at the edge of the 10–15% bandwidth. The choke flanges are used in MW oscillator and amplifier tubes and rotary joints.

6.3 SHORT CIRCUIT PLUNGER

The simplest form of adjustable variable short circuit plunger is a sliding block of

copper or any other good conductor that makes a snag fit in the guide, as shown in Fig. 6.2. The position of the block is varied by a micrometer drive. This simple form is not very satisfactory because of erratic contact resulting power leakage and a reflection coefficient less than unity. These problems may be overcome by using a choke-type plunger.

The main requirements of a short circuit plunger are:

1. Low contact resistance at guide walls
2. Constant contact resistance along the line.

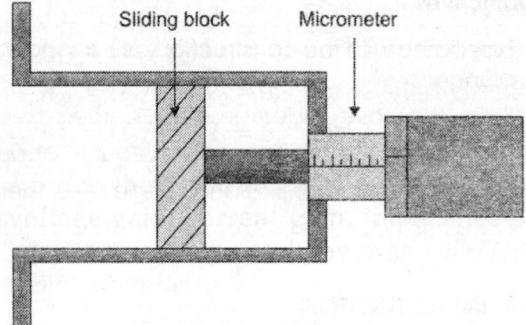

Fig. 6.2: Short circuit plunger

These are achieved in the choke-type plunger. It uses the impedance transformation properties of a quarter wave transformer. It is shown in Fig. 6.3. In this type, the front choke and the second section are both quarter guide wavelength long. The width of the plunger is uniform and slightly less than the interior guide width. However, the height of the plunger is non-uniform. The front one is less than the guide height b by an amount $2b_1$. The gap b_1 is made as small as practicable without touching the upper and lower waveguide walls. The second is less by an amount $2b_2$. It is as large as possible consistent with mechanical strength of the plunger. The final back section makes a sliding fit in the guide. In this arrangement, the contact resistance is in a current antinode

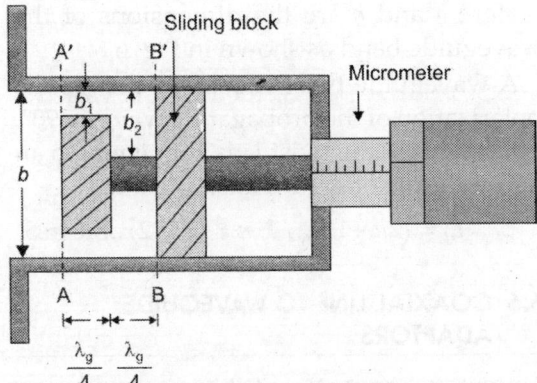

Fig. 6.3: Choke-type plunger

and the output impedance is zero at the plane of reflection. The two quarter-wave sections have equivalent characteristic impedances, Z_1 and Z_2 proportional to $b - 2b_1/b - 2b_2$ respectively relative to that of the input guide. Therefore, the input impedance Z'_{in} is given by

$$\mathbf{Z}_{in} = (\mathbf{Z}_1/\mathbf{Z}_2)^2 \, \mathbf{Z}'_i$$
$$= (b_1/b_2)^2 \, \mathbf{Z}'_I \qquad (6.1)$$

Here Z'_i is the normalized input impedance at the second section plane BB. $\mathbf{Z}_{in}$ tends to 0 if $b_2 \gg b_1$. By a good mechanical design, it is possible to achieve $b_1/b_2 = 10$. The improvement in the short circuit effect is 100 times than that of non-choke type.

A different short circuit plunger used frequently is shown in Fig. 6.4. Two-section

folded quarter-wave transformer is used. The inner line transforms the short circuit impedance to an ideal open circuit at the plane *aa*. At the open circuit or infinite impedance point, the axial current is zero. Therefore, there is no current flow across the gap between the waveguide wall and the plunger at the contact point *aa*. The outer quarter-wave transformer transforms the open circuit impedance at *aa* into a short-circuit impedance at the front end of the plunger at plane *bb*. This type of short-circuit plungers give very satisfactory performance.

The application of quarter-wave transformers is also used in the construction of choke joints, in rotary joints and in plungers used to tune cavity resonators.

6.4 RECTANGULAR TO CIRCULAR WAVEGUIDE TRANSITION

Figure 6.5 shows a rectangular to circular waveguide transition section. It is used to convert the dominant $\mathbf{TE}_{10}$ mode in the rectangular waveguide to $\mathbf{TE}_{11}$ dominant mode in circular waveguide and vice versa. The minimum length of the section is $2\lambda_g$, where λ_g is the wavelength in the waveguide. Thus, avoid abrupt changes in the dimension and suppress higher order modes, the minimum length of the transition should be $\lambda_g/4$.

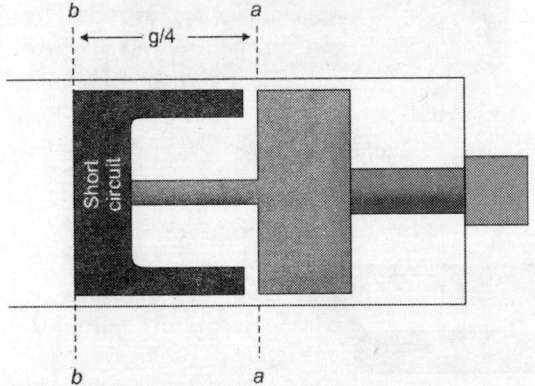

Fig. 6.4: Quarter-wave transformer plunger

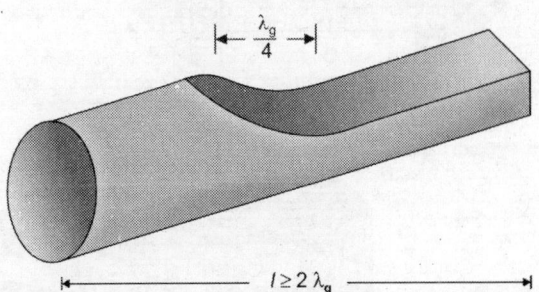

Fig. 6.5: Rectangular to circular waveguide transition

6.5 WAVEGUIDE CORNERS, BENDS AND TWISTS

Figure 6.6 shows the waveguide corner, bend and twist. These components are normally used to change the direction of the guide to any convenient angle. Such arrangement produces discontinuities. As a result of this, reflection takes place at the discontinuities. To minimize the reflections, the wavelength corner is designed such that the mean length L between the corner junctions is equal to an odd multiple of $\lambda_g/4$. Thus,

$$L = (2n + 1)\, \lambda_g/4, \quad n = 0, 1,... \quad (6.2)$$

If $L = (2n + 1)\lambda_g/4$, then the reflected waves from both ends of the waveguide section are completely cancelled. For a waveguide bend, the reflections are minimized by keeping the radius of curvature to the minimum.

$$R = 1.5b \quad \text{for } E\text{-bend} \quad (6.3)$$
$$R = 1.5a \quad \text{for } H\text{-bend} \quad (6.4)$$

Here a and b are the dimensions of the waveguide bend as shown in Fig. 6.6.

A waveguide twist is used to change the polarization of the propagating wave by 90°. The length of the twist L_t is kept equal to an odd multiple of $\lambda_g/4$. Thus,

$$L_t = (2n + 1)\, \lambda_g/4, \quad n = 0, 1, 2, ... \quad (6.5)$$

6.6 COAXIAL LINE TO WAVEGUIDE ADAPTORS

Numerous arrangements have been devised for coupling a coaxial line to a waveguide so that power may flow from coaxial line to the waveguide. Figure 6.7 shows a typical arrangement of a coaxial line delivering energy to a waveguide. The extension *ef* of the center conductor extends from the bottom to the top of the waveguide. When the coaxial line is excited, the current in *ef* generates a magnetic field in the guide which

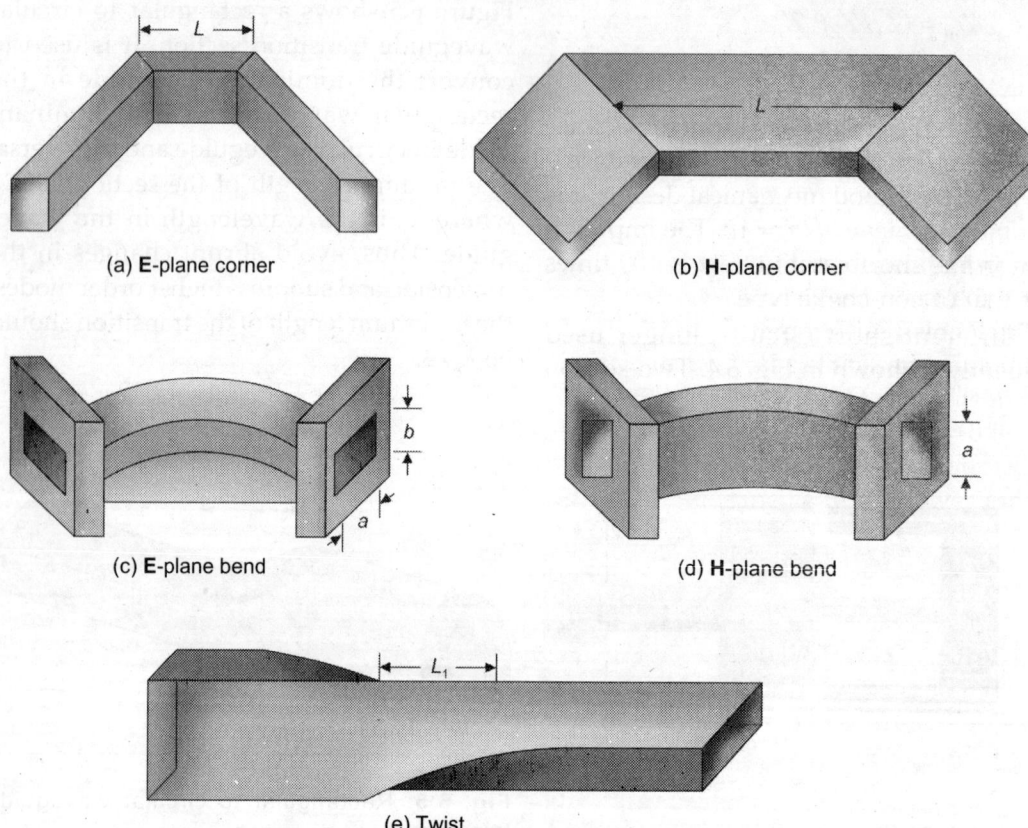

(a) **E**-plane corner

(b) **H**-plane corner

(c) **E**-plane bend

(d) **H**-plane bend

(e) Twist

Fig. 6.6: Waveguide corners, bends and twist

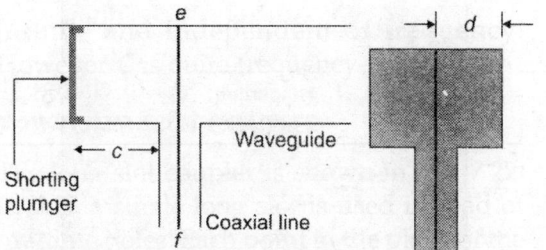

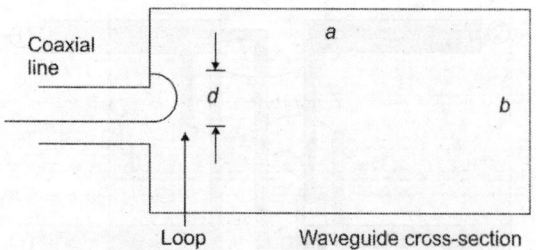

Fig. 6.7: (a) Coaxial to waveguide adapter (b) End view

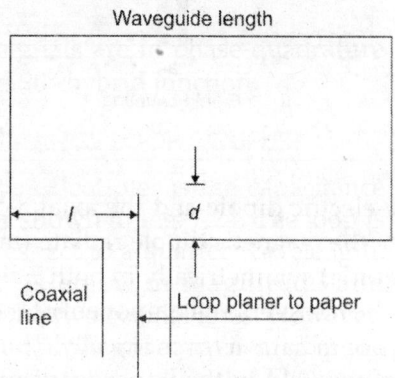

Fig. 6.8: Coupling loop

lies in planes parallel to the top and bottom sides of the guide. At the same time, the voltage drop along *ef* and the consequent differences in voltage thereby produced between the top and bottom of the guide result in electric fields being produced. This configuration suggests the **TE$_{10}$** mode in that the magnetic field lies in planes parallel to the top and bottom of the guide, while the electric field is vertical and is maximum midway between the sides of the guide. Thus the **TE$_{10}$** is the predominant mode. Since the coupling element *ef* is located midway between the sides, the system is symmetrical with respect to the center of the guide. Hence unsymmetrical modes, such as **TE$_{20}$, TE$_{40}$** cannot exist.

Thus, to obtain impedance match between the coaxial line and the waveguide such that power will flow from the coaxial line to the waveguide without producing a reflected wave, the characteristic impedance of the coaxial line should be properly matched. In addition, a compensating reactance must be introduced at the coupling point. A simple method of producing the required neutralizing effect is to adjust the distance *d* in Fig. 6.7(b) so that the shunt reactance observed by the coaxial line when looking towards the short-circuited end of the waveguide is equal and opposite of the shunt reactance associated with the coupling system.

6.7 COUPLING LOOPS

EM fields can also be coupled in waveguides using a coupling loop as shown in Fig. 6.8.

The loop is placed midway between the top and bottom walls of the guide with its plane being transverse to the waveguide. This arrangement couples maximum H-field for **TE$_{10}$** mode. For propagation of the wave in one direction only, a short circuit plate is placed at a distance *l* on the backside. The input impedance is made purely resistive and equal to **Z$_0$** of the coaxial line by adjusting the diameter *d* of the loop and *l* such that

$$d < \lambda_0/10 \tag{6.6}$$

$$\lambda_g/4 < l < \lambda_g/2 \tag{6.7}$$

6.8 COUPLING APERTURES

EM energy can be coupled from one waveguide to another by means of a small aperture of radius $r_0 \ll \lambda_g$ in the common wall as shown in Fig. 6.9. For the dominant **TE$_{10}$** mode of propagation, the aperture is excited by a *y*-directed electric dipole and *x*- and *z*-directed magnetic poles. The normal

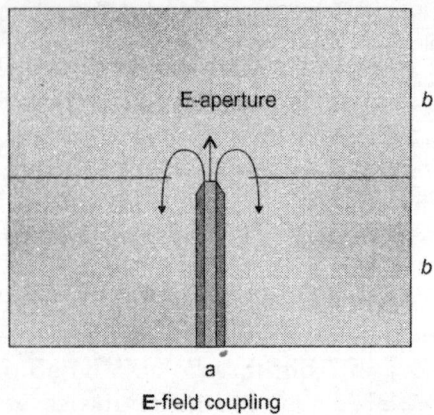

E-field coupling   H-field coupling

Fig. 6.9: Coupling apertures

y-electric dipole and the axial z-component of the magnetic dipole radiate (in the upper guide) symmetrically in both $\pm z$-directions. The transverse x-component of the magnetic pole radiates asymmetrically. The amplitude of the field in the upper waveguide can be controlled by adjusting the angle between the two waveguides or by adjusting the aperture position in the transverse direction.

6.9 ATTENUATORS

Attenuators are passive devices that are used to control power levels in MW systems by partial absorption of the transmitted signal power. The two common types of attenuators are

1. Fixed type
2. Variable or adjustable type

Both attenuators are constructed using resistance aquadag films.

The fixed type is used when a fixed amount of attenuation is to be provided. The variable type is used to measure transmission coefficients.

6.9.1 Fixed Type Attenuator

Figure 6.10 shows a fixed type attenuator used in coaxial cables. It consists of a thin dielectric strip coated with resistive aquadag film. It is placed at the center of the waveguide parallel to the maximum E-field. Incident waves induce current in the resistive film. This results in power dissipation or loss, leading to attenuation of MW energy. To reduce reflections, the dielectric strip is tapered at both ends for a length greater than $\lambda_g/2$.

The resistance vane is supported by two dielectric rods that are separated by an odd multiple of $\lambda_g/4$ and perpendicular to the electric field.

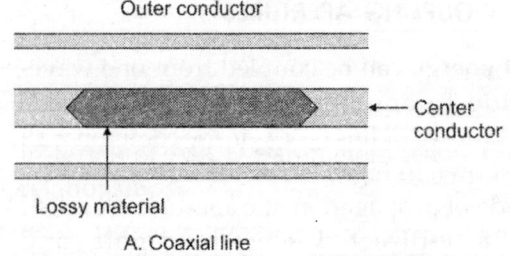

A. Coaxial line

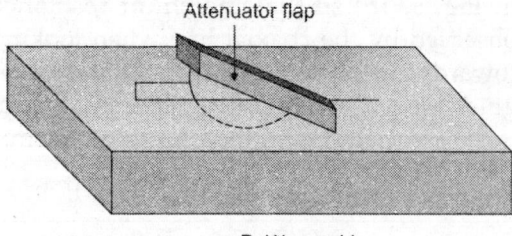

B. Waveguide

Fig. 6.10: Microwave attenuators

6.9.2 Precision Type Variable Attenuator

The most satisfactory precision variable attenuator developed to date is the rotary attenuator shown in Fig. 6.11. It consists of two rectangular to circular waveguide tapered transitions RC_1 and RC_2 and an intermediate section of circular waveguide C containing a very thin tapered resistive card R_2. This center resistive card is free to rotate. Two thin tapered resistive cards R_1 and R_3 are placed at the output end of each transition section and oriented parallel to the broad walls of the rectangular waveguide as shown in Fig. 6.11. The incoming TE_{10} mode in the rectangular guide is transformed into the TE_{11} mode in the circular guide with negligible reflection by the tapered transition. The polarization of the TE_{11} mode is such that the E-field is perpendicular to the resistive card R_1 at the transition section. Hence, this resistive card has negligible effect on the TE_{11} mode. As the center resistive card R_2 is rotated, its orientation with respect to the E-field of the incoming TE_{11} mode can be varied. Therefore, the power absorbed varies leading to variable attenuation. If the angle of rotation is θ, the horizontal component of the electric field $E\cos\theta$ is absorbed and the vertical component $E\sin\theta$ is transmitted without attenuation. This component appears as $E\sin^2\theta$ at the output. Hence, the attenuation α is proportional to $\sin^2\theta$ and is given by

$$\alpha = E/E\sin^2\theta$$
$$= 1/\sin^2\theta = 1/|S_{21}| \tag{6.8}$$
$$\alpha(dB) = -40\log\sin\theta$$
$$= -20\log|S_{21}| \tag{6.9}$$

Here θ is the orientation of R_2 relative to E-field. Thus the variable attenuation depends on θ only.

Since attenuators are normally matched reciprocal devices, we have

$$|S_{12}| = |S_{21}| \tag{6.10}$$

$$|S_{11}| = |S_{22}| = \frac{(VSWR-1)}{(VSWR+1)} \ll 0.1 \tag{6.11}$$

Here VSWR is measured at the port concerned. The S-matrix of an ideal precision type rotary attenuator is given by

$$[S] = \begin{pmatrix} 0 & \sin^2\theta \\ \sin^2\theta & 0 \end{pmatrix} \tag{6.12}$$

6.10 PHASE SHIFTERS

Phase shifter is a two-port passive MW device in which the phase shift of the signal traveling from one port to the other is varied. It should be matched at both ends and pass the signal without attenuation. The two types of phase shifters are

1. Continuously variable analogue phase shifter
2. Incremental or digital phase shifter

The analogue phase shifters are used in MW measurements and instruments. The digital phase shifters are extensively used in phased array antennas.

A phase shifter consists of a lossless dielectric slab placed within a waveguide parallel to and at the location of maximum

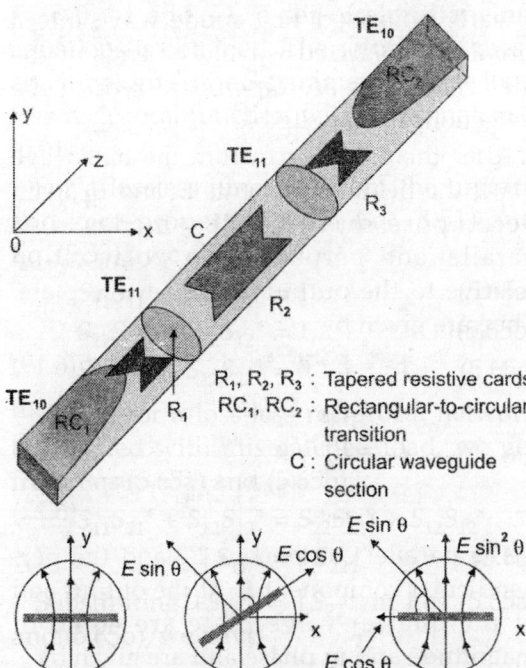

Fig. 6.11: Precision variable attenuator

E-field. Because of change of wave velocity through the dielectric slab, a differential phase change $\Delta\varphi$ given by

$$\Delta\varphi = (\beta_1 - \beta_2)l \qquad (6.13)$$

is produced. Here β_1 and β_2 are phase constants of waveguide and the dielectric slab respectively and l is the length of the slab. By adjusting the length of the slab, the phase shift can be varied.

The S-matrix of an ideal phase shifter is given by

$$[S] = \begin{pmatrix} 0 & e^{-j\Delta\varphi} \\ e^{-j\Delta\varphi} & 0 \end{pmatrix} \qquad (6.14)$$

6.10.1 Analogue or Rotary Phase Shifter

Figure 6.12 shows a precision rotary phase shifter. It consists of two rectangular to circular waveguide tapered transition sections RC_1 and RC_2 and a middle section of circular waveguide C. The center circular section consists of a half-wave plate that is free to rotate. Two quarter-wave dielectric plates are placed at the output end of the each transition section as shown in Fig. 6.12. Each quarter-wave plate converts a linearly polarized TE_{11} mode into a circularly polarized mode and *vice versa*. The half-wave plate at

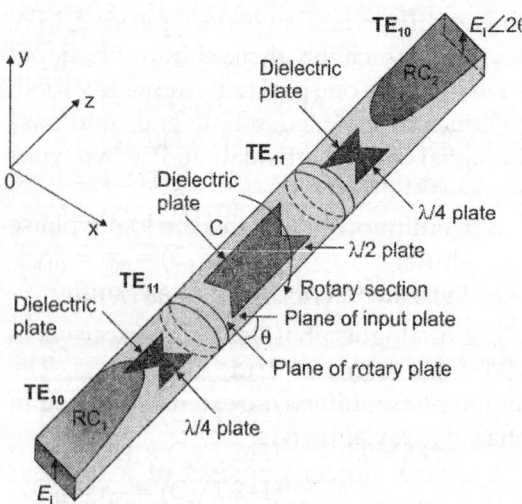

Fig. 6.12: Precision rotary phase shifter

the center, when rotated by an angle θ produces a phase shift equal to 2θ. The quarter wave plates are oriented at an angle of 45° relative to the broad wall of the rectangular guide.

The TE_{11} incident field E_i in the input quarter-wave plate is decomposed into transverse components E_1 and E_2. E_1 field is polarized parallel and E_2 is polarized perpendicular to quarter wave plate. The length l of the quarter-wave plate is adjusted such that these two fields have equal magnitude but a differential phase change $(\beta_2 - \beta_1)\,l = 90°$ where β_1 is the phase constant for parallel polarization and β_2 for perpendicular polarization. Hence the two fields are

$$E_1 = E_0 e^{-j\beta_1 l} \qquad (6.15)$$
$$E_2 = E_0 e^{-j\beta_2 l} \qquad (6.16)$$
$$= E_0 e^{-j(\beta_1 l - \frac{\pi}{2})} \qquad (6.17)$$
$$= E_0 e^{-j\beta_1 l} \cdot e^{j\frac{\pi}{2}} = jE_1 \qquad (6.18)$$

The fields E_1 and E_2 form a circularly polarized field. Thus, $\lambda/4$ plate converts a linearly polarized TE_{11} mode wave into a circularly polarized wave. The ends of the dielectric slabs are tapered to reduce the reflections to a negligible value.

After the emergence from the half wave plate, the field components E_3 and E_4 again decompose into two TE_{11} modes with parallel and perpendicular polarization relative to the output quarter-wave plate. They are given by

$$E_3 = E_1 e^{-j\theta - j2\beta_1 l} \qquad (6.19)$$
$$= E_0 e^{-j\theta - j3\beta_1 l} \qquad (6.20)$$
$$E_4 = E_2 e^{-j\theta} e^{-j2\beta_2 l} \qquad (6.21)$$
$$= E_0 e^{-j\left(\theta + \frac{\pi}{2}\right)} e^{-j3\beta_1 l} \qquad (6.22)$$

The parallel component E_5 and the perpendicular component E_6 at the output end of the quarter-wave plate are equal in magnitude and in phase and are given by

$$E_5 = E_6 = E_0 e^{-j2\theta} e^{-j4\beta_1 l}$$

This produces a resultant linearly polarized $\mathbf{TE}_{11}$ wave given by $E_0 = E_i\, e^{-j2\theta}\, e^{-j4\beta_1 l}$. This wave has the same polarization as the incident field E_i with a change in phase of $(2\theta + 4\beta_1 l)$. For a given frequency and structure, $4\beta_1 l$ is fixed. Hence a phase shift of 2θ can be obtained by rotating the half wave plate precisely through an angle θ relative to quarter wave plate.

6.10.2 Digital Phase Shifter

There are several basic designs used to construct a digital or electronically controlled phase shifter. In all these designs, PIN diodes are used to switch the circuit elements in and out of the transmission path. Each switching operation adds or subtracts a finite phase shift such as $\pm 11.25°$, $\pm 22.5°$, $\pm 45°$, $\pm 90°$ etc.

The simplest digital phase shifter is shown in Fig. 6.13. It consists of four PIN diode switches to switch one of the two alternate transmission line lengths l_1 or l_2 into the transmission path of the signal. The bias current is supplied by connections at the midpoint of a half-wave open-circuited stub as shown in Fig. 6.13. The first quarter wave section is a low impedance stub. It transforms the open circuit impedance to a low impedance or short circuit at the point where the

bias line is connected. The second quarter wave section uses a high impedance line and transforms the low impedance of the mid point into high impedance that produces negligible loading of the main transmission line. The dc return for the bias current is obtained by connecting the input and output lines to the ground plane through a short circuited high impedance quarter wave line sections as shown in Fig. 6.13.

If the lengths of the two transmission lines are l_1 and l_2, then the incremental phase change when line 2 is switched in to replace line 1 is $\Delta\varphi = \beta\,(l_2 - l_1)$ where β is the phase constant. β is a function of frequency. Hence $\Delta\varphi$ depends on the frequency. At a specified frequency, this type of phase shifter produces incremental changes in phase that is proportional to the difference in length of the two transmission paths. By cascade transmission paths, a full range from $0°$ to $180°$ phase shift can be obtained.

6.11 WAVEGUIDE TEES

A tee junction in MW network is a waveguide or a coaxial line junction with three independent ports. It is characterized by a 3×3 S'-matrix containing 9 elements. Six of them are independent. A three port junction characteristics can be explained by the three theorems of the tee junction.

Theorem:

1. If a short circuit is placed in one of the arms of a 3-port junction, no power is transmitted through the other two arms.

2. If the junction is symmetric about one of its arms and a short circuit is placed in that arm, no reflections occur between the other two arms. This implies that the two arms present matched impedances.

3. A general 3-port junction of arbitrary symmetry cannot be matched at all the three ports.

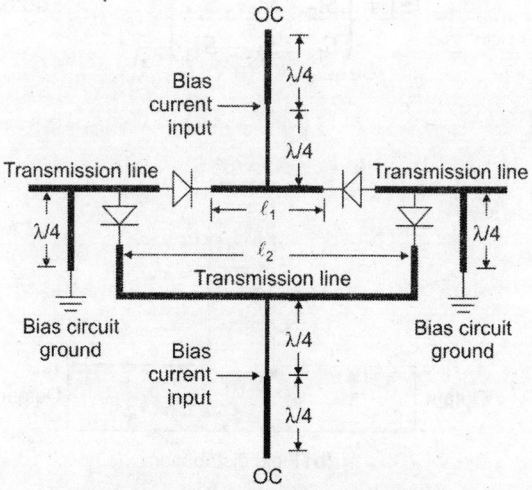

Fig. 6.13: Digital phase shifter

Most commonly used waveguide tees are E-plane or series tee, H-plane or shunt tee and hybrid or magic tee. These are used to split the line power or combine them.

6.11.1 E-Plane Tee or Series Tee

Figure 6.14(a) shows an E-plane tee. It is known as E-plane tee because the axis of the side arm is parallel to the E-field of the waveguide. The coupling from collinear arms to sidearm is by means of electric field. When EM waves in TE_{10} mode enter the junction from the side arm, the field is split and bent as it leaves the side arm and causes fields of opposite polarity to be setup in the collinear arms as shown in Fig. 6.14(b). If the junction is completely symmetrical, the waves of opposite polarity in the collinear arms are equal in magnitude.

When the **EM** waves in TE_{10} mode enters the junction through the collinear arms, the fields are split and bent as they approach the entrance of the side arm and cause fields of opposite polarity to be setup in the side arm as shown in Fig. 6.14(b). Fields of the same polarity, approaching the junction from opposite sides, setup fields of opposite polarity. If the instantaneous fields, entering the side arm from opposite directions are of equal magnitude and the same polarity, the net field in the side arm becomes zero. The resulting field is proportional to the difference between the two instantaneous fields entering the junction from opposite directions. Hence, the side arm is called difference arm. Therefore the E-plane tee is also known as *subtractor* or *differencer*. Since high energy delivery takes place to a branch line connected to a transmission line at a point of low voltage and high current if the branch line is connected in series with main line. Hence, the E-plane tee is known as *series tee*.

6.11.1.1 S-Matrix of E-Plane Tee

We derive below the S-matrix of E-plane tee using the properties of the tee.

1. From the *symmetry property* of the E-plane tee, we get

$$S_{12} = S_{21} \tag{6.23a}$$
$$S_{13} = S_{31} \tag{6.23b}$$
$$S_{23} = S_{32} \tag{6.23c}$$

2. From the *phase property* of the output waves, we have

$$S_{23} = -S_{13} \tag{6.24}$$

since the output at ports 1 and 2 are equal but out of phase

3. If the port 3 is perfectly matched,

$$S_{33} = 0 \tag{6.25}$$

Therefore, the S–matrix becomes

$$[S] = \begin{pmatrix} S_{11} & S_{12} & S_{13} \\ S_{12} & S_{22} & S_{23} \\ S_{13} & S_{23} & S_{33} \end{pmatrix} \tag{6.26}$$

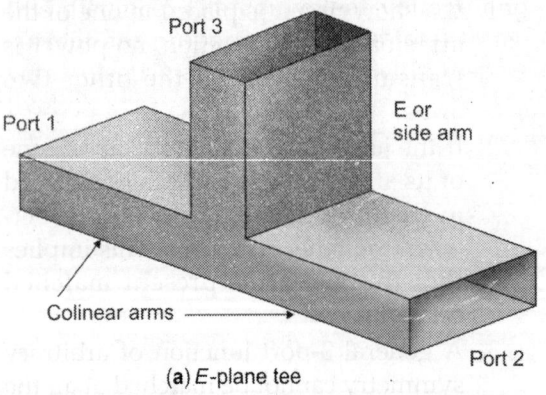

(a) *E*-plane tee

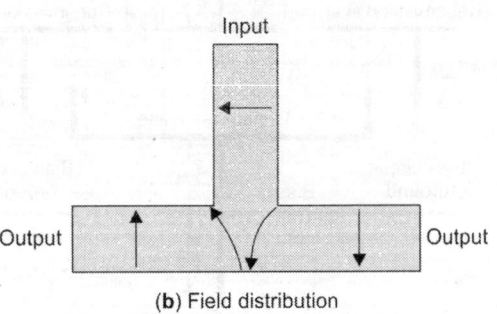

(b) Field distribution

Fig. 6.14: (a) **E**-plane tee (b) Field distribution

4. From the *unitary property*, we obtain

$$|S_{11}|^2 + |S_{12}|^2 + |S_{13}|^2 = 1 \quad (6.27)$$

$$|S_{12}|^2 + |S_{22}|^2 + |S_{13}|^2 = 1 \quad (6.28)$$

$$|S_{13}|^2 + |S_{13}|^2 = 1 \quad (6.29)$$

From Eq. (6.29), we get

$$2|S_{13}|^2 = 1$$

$$|S_{13}| = \frac{1}{\sqrt{2}} \quad (6.30)$$

Subtracting Eq. (6.28) from Eq. (6.27), we get

$$|S_{11}| = |S_{22}| \quad (6.31)$$

5. From *zero or null property*, we have from row 1 and row 3

$$S_{11}S_{13}^* - S_{12}S_{13}^* = 0 \quad (6.32)$$

Hence $\qquad S_{11} = S_{12} \quad (6.33)$

Substituting Eq. (6.29) in Eq. (6.27), we get

$$|S_{11}|^2 + |S_{11}|^2 + |1/\sqrt{2}|^2 = 1$$

$$|S_{11}| = \frac{1}{2} \quad (6.34)$$

Therefore, the **S** matrix of the **E**-plane tee with port 3 matched is given by

$$[S] = \begin{pmatrix} 1/2 & 1/2 & 1/\sqrt{2} \\ 1/2 & 1/2 & -1/\sqrt{2} \\ 1/\sqrt{2} & -1/\sqrt{2} & 0 \end{pmatrix} \quad (6.35)$$

Because of mismatch at any one of the ports, the VSWR at the mismatch is very high and is given by

$$\text{VSWR} = \frac{(1+S_{11})}{(1-S_{11})} = \frac{\left(1+\dfrac{1}{2}\right)}{\left(1-\dfrac{1}{2}\right)} = 3.0 \quad (6.36)$$

6.11.2 H-Plane Tee or Shunt Tee

Figure 6.15(a) shows the H-plane tee. It is so called because the axis is parallel to the H-field of the main transmission line and the coupling from the collinear arm to the side arm is by means of magnetic fields. If two EM waves of equal magnitude and same phase are fed into the collinear arms or ports 1 and 2, they will be added together in the side arm or **H**-arm (port 3).

Therefore, the side arm is known as *sum arm* and the **H**-plane tee as *adder*. In the H-plane tee, high-energy delivery takes place to a branch line is connected to a transmission line at a point of high voltage and low current if the branch line is connected in shunt with the main line. Hence, the H-plane tee is also known as *parallel* or *shunt tee*.

When the EM wave in TE_{10} mode enters the junction through the side arm, it is equally divided into collinear arms and in

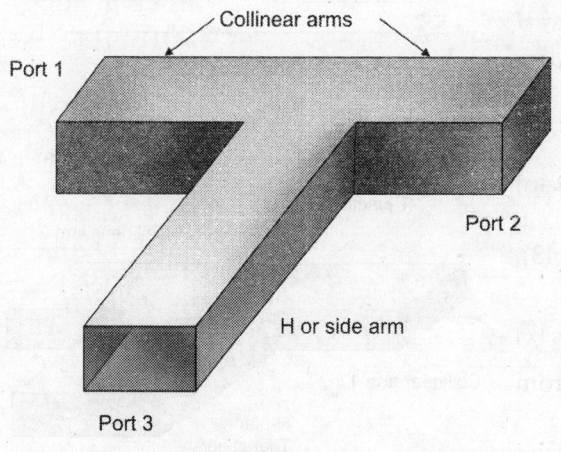

Collinear arms

Port 1

Port 2

H or side arm

Port 3

(a) **H**-plane tee

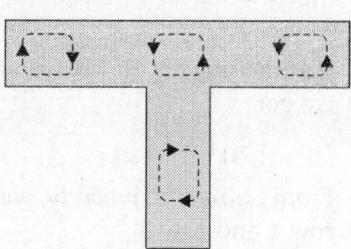

(b) Field distribution

Fig. 6.15: (a) **H**-plane tee (b) Field distribution

phase. The magnetic field gets divided into two collinear arms, similar to current division between branches in a parallel circuit. Hence, the *H*-plane tee is known as *shunt tee*. The *H*-field distribution is shown in Fig. 6.15.

6.14.2.1 S-Matrix of H-Plane Tee

We derive below the *S*-matrix of *H*-plane tee using the properties of the tee.

1. From the *symmetry property*, we get

$$S_{12} = S_{21} \quad (6.37)$$
$$S_{13} = S_{31} \quad (6.38)$$
$$S_{23} = S_{32} \quad (6.39)$$

2. From the *phase property* of the output waves, we have

$$S_{23} = S_{13} \quad (6.40)$$

since the outputs at ports 1 and 2 are equal and in phase

3. If the port 3 is perfectly matched,

$$S_{33} = 0 \quad (6.41)$$

Therefore, the S–matrix becomes

$$[S] = \begin{pmatrix} S_{11} & S_{12} & S_{13} \\ S_{12} & S_{22} & S_{13} \\ S_{13} & S_{13} & 0 \end{pmatrix} \quad (6.42)$$

4. From the *unitary* property, we obtain

$$|S_{11}|^2 + |S_{12}|^2 + |S_{13}|^2 = 1 \quad (6.43)$$
$$|S_{12}|^2 + |S_{22}|^2 + |S_{13}|^2 = 1 \quad (6.44)$$
$$|S_{13}|^2 + |S_{13}|^2 = 1 \quad (6.45)$$

From Eq. (6.45), we get

$$[S_{13}] = \frac{1}{\sqrt{2}} \quad (6.46)$$

Subtracting Eq. (6.44) from Eq. (6.43), we get

$$|S_{11}| = |S_{22}| \quad (6.47)$$

5. From *zero or null property*, we have from row 1 and row 3

$$S_{11} S_{13}^* + S_{12} S_{13}^* = 0 \quad (6.48)$$

Hence $\quad S_{11} = -S_{12} \quad (6.49)$

Substituting Eq. (6.49) in Eq. (6.43), we get

$$|S_{11}|^2 + |S_{11}|^2 + |1/\sqrt{2}|^2 = 1$$

$$|S_{11}| = \frac{1}{2} \quad (6.50)$$

Therefore, the **S**-matrix of the **H**-plane tee with port 3 matched is given by

$$[S] = \begin{pmatrix} 1/2 & -1/2 & 1/\sqrt{2} \\ -1/2 & 1/2 & 1/\sqrt{2} \\ 1/\sqrt{2} & 1/\sqrt{2} & 0 \end{pmatrix} \quad (6.51)$$

Because of mismatch at any one of the ports, the VSWR at the mismatch is very high and is given by

$$\text{VSWR} = \frac{(1+S_{11})}{(1-S_{11})} = \frac{\left(1+\dfrac{1}{2}\right)}{\left(1-\dfrac{1}{2}\right)} = 3 \quad (6.52)$$

6.11.3 Hybrid or Magic Tee

A hybrid circuit in general form is shown in Fig. 6.16 Its characteristics are such that if power enters the circuit through arm A or

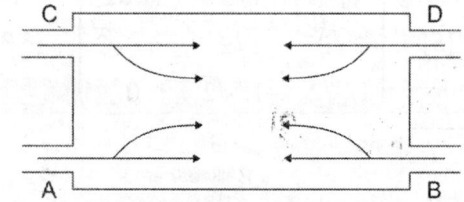

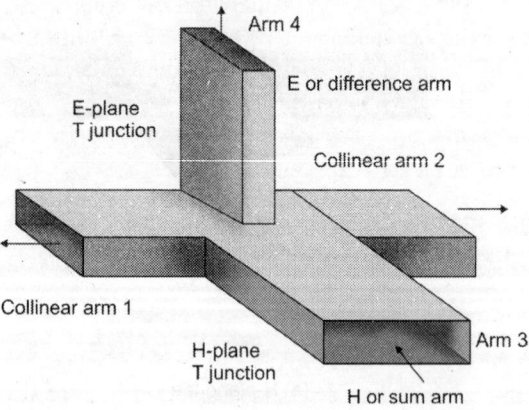

Fig. 6.16: (a) A general hybrid circuit (b) Magic tee

C, the power is delivered entirely to arms B and D, with no transmission from A to C or C to A. similarly, power entering from arm B or arm D is delivered entirely to arms A and C with no transmission between B and D.

The most commonly used hybrid waveguide junction is the *magic tee*. It is a combination of E-plane tee and H-plane tee as shown in Fig. 6.16. Arm 3 is called H-arm and forms the H-plane tee. Arm 4 is called E-arm and forms an E-plane tee in combination with arms 1 and 2.

The characteristics of magic tee are:

1. All ports are perfectly matched.
2. **E** and **H** arms as well as the two collinear arms are decoupled.
3. A signal fed into a collinear arm divides equally between **E-** and **H-**arms.
4. If power is fed into arm 1 or 2, no power is coupled to arm 2 or 1. This is because E-arm causes phase delay while **H-**arm causes phase advance.
5. If power is fed into arm 3 (**H-**arm), the power is equally divided between arms 1 and 2 and no power is coupled to arm 4.
6. Similarly, if power is fed into arm 4 (E-arm), the power is equally divided between arms 1 and 2 and no power is coupled to arm 3. Hence, ports 3 and 4 are isolated.
7. If power is fed from arms 1 and 2, it is added in **H-**arm while it is subtracted in E-arm. Hence E-arm is known as *difference arm* and H-arm as sum arm.

6.14.6.1 S-Matrix of Magic Tee

Since the magic tee has four ports, the S matrix is a 4×4 matrix.

1. From the *symmetry property*, we get

$$S_{12} = S_{21} \qquad (6.53)$$
$$S_{13} = S_{31} \qquad (6.54)$$
$$S_{14} = S_{41} \qquad (6.55)$$

$$S_{23} = S_{32} \qquad (6.56)$$
$$S_{24} = S_{42} \qquad (6.57)$$
$$S_{34} = S_{43} \qquad (6.58)$$

2. From the *phase property* of the output waves, we have

$$S_{23} = S_{13} \quad \text{(due to H-plane tee)} \quad (6.59)$$
$$S_{24} = -S_{14} \quad \text{(due to E-plane tee)} \quad (6.60)$$

3. Because of the *isolation property*,

$$S_{34} = S_{43} = 0 \qquad (6.61)$$

4. If the port 3 and 4 are perfectly matched,

$$S_{33} = S_{44} = 0 \qquad (6.62)$$

Therefore, the S–matrix becomes

$$[S] = \begin{pmatrix} S_{11} & S_{12} & S_{13} & S_{14} \\ S_{12} & S_{22} & S_{13} & -S_{14} \\ S_{13} & S_{13} & 0 & 0 \\ S_{14} & -S_{14} & 0 & 0 \end{pmatrix} \qquad (6.63)$$

5. From the *unitary property*, we obtain

$$|S_{11}|^2 + |S_{12}|^2 + |S_{13}|^2 + |S_{14}|^2 = 1 \quad (6.64)$$
$$|S_{12}|^2 + |S_{22}|^2 + |S_{13}|^2 + |S_{14}|^2 = 1 \quad (6.65)$$
$$|S_{13}|^2 + |S_{13}|^2 = 1 \quad (6.66)$$
$$|S_{14}|^2 + |S_{14}|^2 = 1 \quad (6.67)$$

From Eq. (6.66) and (6.67), we get

$$S_{13} = 1/\sqrt{2} \qquad (6.68)$$
$$S_{14} = 1/\sqrt{2} \qquad (6.69)$$

Subtracting Eq. (6.65) from Eq. (6.64), we get

$$|S_{11}| = |S_{22}| \qquad (6.70)$$

Substituting Eqs (6.68), (6.69) in Eq. (6.64), we get

$$|S_{11}|^2 + |S_{12}|^2 + \frac{1}{2} + \frac{1}{2} = 1$$

i.e. $$|S_{11}|^2 + |S_{12}|^2 = 0$$

or $$S_{11} = S_{12} = 0 \qquad (6.71)$$

Therefore $$S_{11} = S_{22} = 0 \qquad (6.72)$$

Equation (6.72) states that, in any 4-port junction, if 2-ports are perfectly matched to the junction, then the remaining 2-ports are automatically matched to the junction. Thus, in a hybrid or magic tee, all the 4 ports are perfectly matched.

Therefore, the S-matrix of the magic tee with any 2-ports perfectly matched is given by

$$[S] = \begin{pmatrix} 0 & 0 & 1/\sqrt{2} & 1/\sqrt{2} \\ 0 & 0 & 1/\sqrt{2} & -1/\sqrt{2} \\ 1/\sqrt{2} & 1/\sqrt{2} & 0 & 0 \\ 1/\sqrt{2} & -1/\sqrt{2} & 0 & 0 \end{pmatrix}$$

$$(6.73)$$

6.12 APPLICATIONS OF MAGIC TEE

Magic tee finds extensive applications in MW measurement systems. It is commonly used as a balanced mixer in MW superheterodyne receiver, and as an antenna duplexer, as an E–H tuner for impedance measurement and as a balanced phase detector.

6.12.1 Balanced Mixer

Figure 6.17 shows a balanced mixer using a magic tee. It balances out the local oscillator noise at the input of the IF amplifier. The arrangement shown in Fig. 6.17 can be used for IF frequencies from 1 MHz to 100 MHZ.

The local oscillator signal from **H**-arm arrives at the crystal diodes in phase whereas the incoming signal from E-arm arrives at the diodes out of phase. These signals are mixed at the non-linear crystal diodes and generate IF signals in the collinear arms that are out of phase by 180°. Since the local oscillator noise is in phase at the diodes, it gets cancelled at the balanced IF input. However the IF signals are added up in phase. Further, the local oscillator and antenna are isolated due to the magic tee properties of **E** and **H** arms.

6.15.2 Antenna Duplexer

A duplexer couples two circuits to the same load but avoids mutual coupling. A typical duplexer arrangement is shown in Fig. 6.18. The same antenna is used for the transmitter and the receiver but the transmitter and receiver are uncoupled. The matched receiver and the matched transmitter are connected to arms 1 and 2 respectively. Arm 3 (**H**-arm) is terminated in a matched load and arm 4 (**E**-arm) is connected to the matched antenna. Based on the coupling properties of magic tee, power received and power transmitted by the antenna remains isolated.

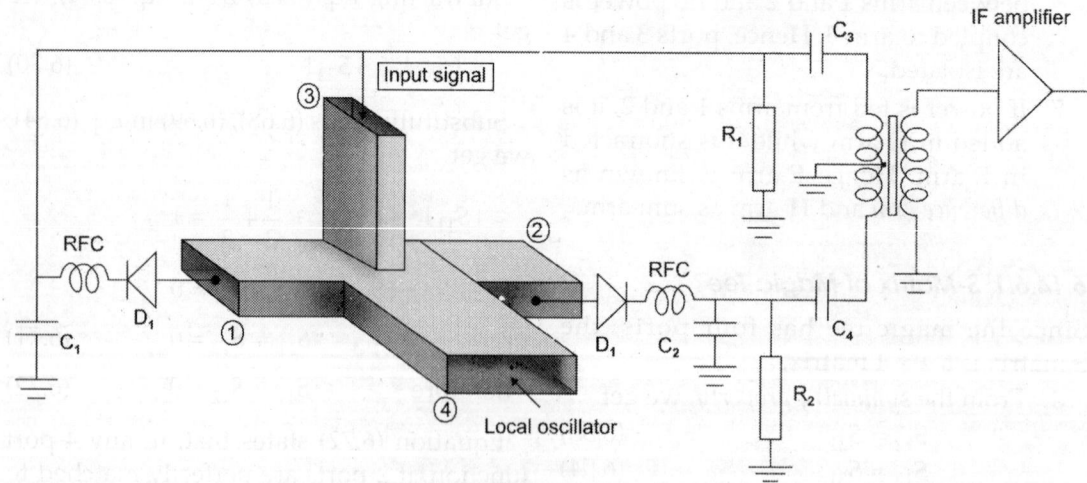

Fig. 6.17: Balanced mixer

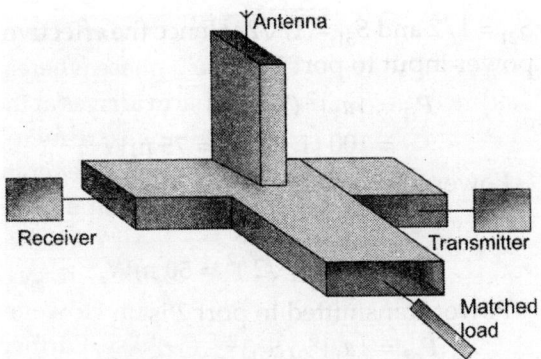

Fig. 6.18: Antenna duplexer

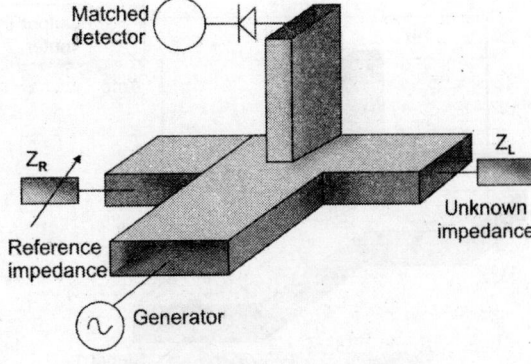

Fig. 6.20: Impedance bridge

6.12.3 E–H Tuner

Figure 6.19 shows an **E-H** tuner. In this, both **E** and **H** arms are terminated with movable shorts that act as **E**-plane and **H**-plane stubs. The position of the stubs can be adjusted so that a wide range of load impedance is matched to reduce the VSWR of a waveguide system connected through the collinear arms.

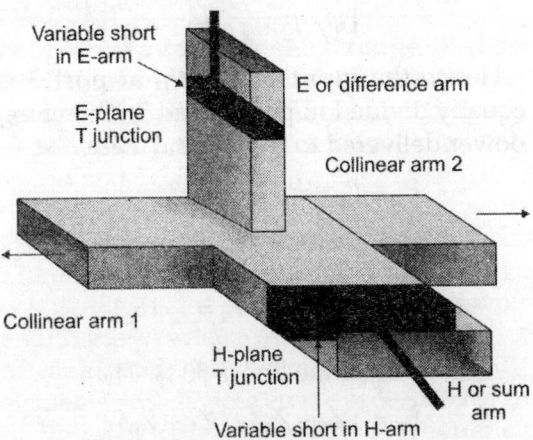

Fig. 6.19: E–H tuner

6.12.4 Impedance Bridge

A magic tee is frequently employed in MW impedance measuring bridges. Figure 6.20 shows a typical MW impedance bridge using a magic tee. Standard variable impedance is connected to port 1 as reference impedance and the impedance to be measured to the port 2. Power from a matched source is fed

in the **H**-arm or port 3 of the magic tee. A matched detector is connected to port 4 or **E**-arm to receive power reflected from arms 1 and 2. These powers are out of phase by 180°.

The reference impedance Z_R is adjusted so that no signal is received at the detector. Under this condition, the power reflected from the reference impedance and reaching the detector (half of the reflected power) equals the power reflected from the unknown impedance Z_L reaching the detector. Because the two powers are out of phase by 180° and the lengths of the two ports are equal, i.e. when the bridge is balanced, the reflection coefficient of the reference impedance z_R is equal to the reflection coefficient of the unknown impedance z_L. Thus

$$z_R = z_L \qquad (6.74)$$

or $$\frac{(z_R - 1)}{(z_R + 1)} = (z_L - 1)(z_L + 1) \qquad (6.75)$$

z_R and z_L are the normalized impedances of the reference impedance and unknown impedance respectively. Equation (6.75) is used to determine the unknown impedance z_L in terms of z_R.

6.15.5 Balanced Phase Detector

Figure 6.21 shows a balanced phase detector arrangement using a magic tee. The two signals whose relative phase has to be measured are fed from **E**- and **H**-arms. The power

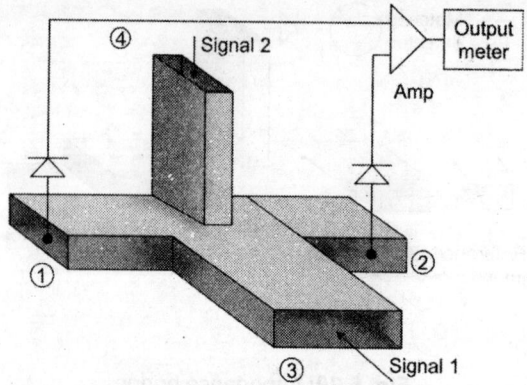

Fig. 6.21: Balanced phase shifter

detected by matched MW crystals at ports 1 and 2 are fed to the differential amplifier. Since the power fed at ports 1 and 2 are equal, then the output power of the differential amplifier is given by

$$P_0 = G\cos\theta \qquad (6.76)$$

Thus the phase angle θ may be detected with calibrated meter to indicate the phase difference directly.

6.13 NUMERICAL EXAMPLES

Example 6.1: Find the reflected power in a waveguide transmission with VSWR = 1.2 and the input power of 1W.

Solution: The reflection coefficient Γ is given by

$$\Gamma = (S-1)/(S+1)$$
$$= (1.2-1)/(1.2+1)$$
$$= 0.2/2.1 = \mathbf{0.091}$$

The reflected power P_r is

$$P_r = |\Gamma|^2 P_i$$
$$= 0.091^2 \times 1 = \mathbf{0.828\ W}$$

Example 6.2: A 100 mW signal is fed into the collinear ports of a loss-less **H-plane T**. Calculate the power delivered to each port when other ports are matched.

Solution: Let the power is incident in port 1. Ports 2 and 3 are matched. Hence $a_2 = a_3 = 0$. From the S-matrix of H-plane T, $S_{11} = 1/2$,

$S_{21} = 1/2$ and $S_{31} = 1/\sqrt{2}$. Hence the effective power input to port 1 is

$$P_{i1} = |a_1|^2 (1 - S_{11})$$
$$= 100\ (1 - 0.5^2) = \mathbf{75\ mW}$$

Power transmitted to port 3 is

$$P_{o3} = |a_1|^2 |S_{31}|^2$$
$$= 100\ (1/\sqrt{2})^2 = \mathbf{50\ mW}$$

Power transmitted to port 2 is

$$P_{o2} = |a_1|^2 |S_{21}|^2$$
$$= 100\ (1/2)^2 = \mathbf{25\ mW}$$

(*Check:* $P_{i1} = P_{o2} + P_{o3} = 50 + 25 = \mathbf{75\ mW}$)

Example 6.3: In an **H-plane** T, 10 mW is delivered to matched port 3. Calculate the power delivered to 60 Ω and 75 Ω connected to ports 1 and 2.

Solution: The S-matrix of **H-plane T** with port 3 matched is

$$[S] = \begin{pmatrix} 1/2 & 1/2 & 1/\sqrt{2} \\ -1/2 & 1/2 & 1/\sqrt{2} \\ 1/\sqrt{2} & 1/\sqrt{2} & 0 \end{pmatrix}$$

Hence the input power P_{i3} at port 3 is equally divided in ports 1 and 2. Therefore, power delivered to ports 1 and 2 are

$$P_1 = P_2 = P_i/2 = 10/2$$
$$= 5\ mW = \frac{1}{2}|b_1|^2 = \frac{1}{2}|b_2|^2$$
$$P_1 = \frac{1}{2}|b_1|^2; \quad P_2 = \frac{1}{2}|b_2|^2$$

Assume Z_0 of the line is 50 Ω. Then

$$\Gamma_1 = |Z_1 - Z_0| / |Z_1 + Z_0|$$
$$= |60 - 50| / |60 + 50| = \mathbf{1/11}$$
$$\Gamma_2 = |Z_2 - Z_0| / |Z_2 + Z_0|$$
$$= |75 - 50| / |75 + 50| = \mathbf{1/5}$$

$$\therefore \quad P_{21} = \frac{1}{2}|b_1|^2 - \frac{1}{2}|b_2|^2$$
$$= \frac{1}{2}|b_1|^2 (1 - \Gamma_1^2)$$
$$= 5[1 - (1/11)^2] = \mathbf{4.9586\ mW}$$

$$\therefore \qquad P_{z2} = \frac{1}{2}|b_2|^2(1 - \Gamma_2^2)$$

$$= 5[1 - (1/5)^2] = \textbf{4.8 mW}$$

Example 6.4: In a magic T, ports 1, 2 and 4 are terminated with impedances of reflection coefficients $\Gamma_1 = 0.6$, $\Gamma_2 = 0.7$ and $\Gamma_4 = 0.8$ respectively. If 1 W power is fed at ports, find the reflected power at port 3 and transmitted powers to other ports.

Solution: The S-matrix of a magic T is given by

$$[S] = \frac{1}{\sqrt{2}}\begin{pmatrix} 0 & 0 & 1 & 1 \\ 0 & 0 & 1 & -1 \\ 1 & 1 & 0 & 0 \\ 1 & -1 & 0 & 0 \end{pmatrix}$$

Let a_1, a_2, a_3 and a_4 be the normalized input voltages and b_1, b_2, b_3 and b_4 are the corresponding output voltages at respective ports. Then

$$a_1 = \Gamma_1 b_1 = 0.6\,b_1$$
$$a_2 = \Gamma_2 b_1 = 0.7 b_2$$
$$a_4 = \Gamma_4 b_4 = 0.8 b_4$$

The input power P_i is given by

$$P_i = |a_3|^3 = 1 \text{ W}$$

$$\therefore \qquad a_3 = 1$$

Hence, we have

$$\begin{pmatrix} b_1 \\ b_2 \\ b_3 \\ b_4 \end{pmatrix} = \frac{1}{\sqrt{2}}\begin{pmatrix} 0 & 0 & 1 & 1 \\ 0 & 0 & 1 & -1 \\ 1 & 1 & 0 & 0 \\ 1 & -1 & 0 & 0 \end{pmatrix}\begin{pmatrix} 0.6b_1 \\ 0.7b_1 \\ 1.0 \\ 0.8b_4 \end{pmatrix}$$

Expanding and rearranging, we get

$$\sqrt{2}\cdot b_1 + 0 + 0 - 0.8b_4 = 1$$

$$0 + \sqrt{2}\cdot b_2 + 0 + 0.8b_4 = 1$$

$$-0.6b_1 - 0.7b_2 + \sqrt{2}\cdot b_3 + 0 = 0$$

$$-0.6b_1 + 0.7b_2 + 0 + \sqrt{2}\cdot b_4 = 0$$

The above simultaneous equation may be solved using Cramer's rule $b_i = \Delta_i/\Delta$.

$$\Delta = \begin{vmatrix} \sqrt{2} & 0 & 0 & -0.8 \\ 0 & \sqrt{2} & 0 & 0.8 \\ -0.6 & -0.7 & \sqrt{2} & 0 \\ -0.6 & 0.7 & 0 & \sqrt{2} \end{vmatrix}$$

$$= 2[2 - 0.8\,(0.6 + 0.7)] = 1.92$$

$$b_1 = \frac{\begin{vmatrix} 1 & 0 & 0 & -0.8 \\ 1 & \sqrt{2} & 0 & 0.8 \\ 0 & -0.7 & \sqrt{2} & 0 \\ 0 & 0.7 & 0 & \sqrt{2} \end{vmatrix}}{\Delta}$$

$$= 2\sqrt{2}\,(1 - 0.7 \times 0.8)]/1.92$$

$$= 1.2443/1.92 = \textbf{0.6480}$$

Similarly,

$$b_2 = \Delta_2/\Delta = 2\sqrt{2}\,(1 - 0.6 \times 0.8)]/1.92$$
$$= 1.4706/1.92 = \textbf{0.7659};$$

$$b_3 = \Delta_3/\Delta$$
$$= 2(0.6 + 0.70 - 2 \times 0.6 \times 0.7 \times 0.8)/1.92$$
$$= 1.256/1.92 = \textbf{0.6542}$$

$$b_4 = \Delta_4/\Delta = 2\,(-0.7 + 0.6)/1.92$$
$$= -0.2/1.92 = \textbf{-0.1042}$$

Hence

$$P_{o1} = |b_1|^2 = |0.6480|^2 = \textbf{0.4200 W}$$
$$P_{o2} = |b_2|^2 = |0.7659|^2 = \textbf{0.5866 W}$$
$$P_{o3} = |b_3|^2 = |0.6542|^2 = \textbf{0.4280 W}$$
$$P_{o4} = |b_4|^2 = |-0.1042|^2 = \textbf{0.01086 W}$$

KEY POINTS

- The passive MW components are WG flanges, connectors and adapters, matched terminations, attenuators, phase shifters, T-junctions and hybrids.
- To change the direction of EM waves along any convenient direction, wave guide bends, corners and twists are used. These produce discontinuities and reflections.

- Apertures and coupling loops are used to couple the EM waves.
- Attenuators are passive devices that absorb MW power. They are used to control the MW power flow.
- Phase shifters are two-port MW devices that are used to shift the phase of the travelling signal from one port to the other.
- T-junctions are wave guides with three independent ports. It is characterized by 3 × 3 S-matrix of which 6 elements are independent.
- Hybrid circuits have four ports: *A, B, C* and *D*. MW power entering *A* or *C* is entirely delivered to *B* and *D* only. No power is transmitted from *A* to *C* or *C* to *A*.
  Similarly, MW power entering *B* or *D* is entirely delivered to *A* and *C* only. No power is transmitted from *B* to *D* or *D* to *B*.
- Magic-T is the combination of *E* and *H* plane tees with matched four ports. It is commonly used in balanced mixer, antenna duplexer, *E-H* tuner, balanced phase detector and impedance measurements.

FURTHER READING

1. Collins RE (1996). *Foundations of Microwave Engineering*, McGraw Hill, NY.
2. Das A and Das SK (2004). *Microwave Engineering*, TMH, New Delhi.
3. Gandhi OP (1981). *Microwave Engineering and Applications*, Pergamon, NY.
4. Liao SY (2000). *Microwave Devices and Circuits*, PHI New Delhi.

REVIEW QUESTIONS

6.1 Mention the commonly used MW passive devices.

6.2 What are the basic parameters of MW passive devices?

6.3 What devices are used for joining with other waveguides?

6.4 Mention the ideal parameters of a matched load.

6.5 Mention the basic requirements of a short circuit plunger.

6.6 How do you convert the dominant TE_{10} mode to TE_{11} dominant mode?

6.7 Why should the minimum length of a rectangular to circular transition be $\lambda_g/4$?

6.8 Mention the use of WG bends, corners and twists.

6.9 What is an attenuator? Mention the types.

6.10 Give the S-matrix of an attenuator.

6.11 Mention the active MW devices used in electronic attenuators.

6.12 What is a phase shifter? Mention the types.

6.13 Give the S-matrix of a phase shifter.

6.14 Mention the active device used in digital phase shifters.

6.15 What is a T-junction?

6.16 How many ports are there in a T-junction?

6.17 What happens if a short circuit is placed in one arm of a T-junction?

6.18 Can a T-junction be matched at all the three ports? Explain.

6.19 Mention the most commonly used waveguide tees.

6.20 Mention the purpose of WG-tee.

6.21 What is a series-Tee? Why is it so called?

6.22 What is a shunt-Tee? Why is it so called?

6.23 Give the S-matrix of a E-plane T.

6.24 What is the value of VSWR in E-plane T?

6.25 Give the S-matrix of a **H**-plane T.

6.26 What is the value of VSWR in H-plane T?

6.27 Explain the unitary property of an S-matrix.

6.28 Explain the null property of an S-matrix.

6.29 Explain the reciprocity of an S-matrix.

6.30 What is a magic-T?

6.31 What are the characteristics of a magic-T?

6.32 Give the S-matrix of an magic-T.

6.33 What is the phase property of E-plane T?

6.34 What is the phase property of **H**-plane T?

6.35 Mention the applications of magic-T.

DESCRIPTIVE QUESTIONS

6.1 What are the scattering coefficients of a MW device? Discuss the scattering properties of a multi-port junction.

6.2 Obtain the scattering matrix of a magic-T. What are the uses of magic-Tee? Explain its use as a duplexer, a mixer for a super-heterodyne receiver.

6.3 Explain the construction and working of a two choke-type movable short-circuit used in MW measurements.

6.4 Distinguish between **E**-plane and **H**-plane Tees. Hence discuss the construction and working of a magic-Tee.

6.5 Explain the construction and working of a wave-guide phase shifter.

6.6 Explain the construction and working of a precision variable attenuator. Discuss its frequency response and reflection loss.

6.7 Explain the 4-port circulator using magic tees.

6.8 Write short notes on: (i) Rotary attenuator, (ii) Rotary phase shifter.

PRACTICE PROBLEMS

6.1 A 40 mW signal is fed into the collinear ports of a loss-less **H**-plane T. Calculate the power delivered to each port when other ports are matched.

[**Ans:** P_{i1} = 30 mW, P_{o3} = 20 mW, P_{o2} = 10 mW]

6.2 In an **H**-plane T, 10 mW is delivered to matched port 3. Calculate the power delivered to 40 Ω and 75 Ω connected to ports 1 and 2.

[**Ans:** P_{z1} = 4.9383 mW, P_{z2} = 4.9586 mW]

6.3 In an **H**-plane T, 20 mW is delivered to matched port 3. Calculate the power delivered to 50 Ω and 60 Ω connected to ports 1 and 2.

[**Ans:** P_{z1} = 9.922 mW, P_{z2} = 9.9 mW]

6.4 In a magic T, ports 1, 2 and 4 are terminated with impedances of reflection coefficients Γ_1 = 0.5, Γ_2 = 0.6 and Γ_4 = 0.8 respectively. If 1W power is fed at ports, find the reflected power at port 3 and transmitted powers to other ports.

[**Ans:** P_{o1} = 0.4309 W, P_{o2} = 0.5738 W, P_{o3} = 0.3065 W and P_{o4} = 0.00797 W]

6.5 Show that the S-matrix of a series T-junction matched at arm 3 is given by

$$[S] = \frac{1}{2}\begin{pmatrix} 1 & 1 & \sqrt{2} \\ \sqrt{2} & 1 & -\sqrt{2} \\ \sqrt{2} & -\sqrt{2} & 0 \end{pmatrix}$$

6.6 Show that the S-matrix of a shunt T-junction matched at arm 3 is given by

$$[S] = \frac{1}{2}\begin{pmatrix} -1 & 1 & \sqrt{2} \\ 1 & -1 & \sqrt{2} \\ \sqrt{2} & \sqrt{2} & 0 \end{pmatrix}$$

6.7 Show that the S-matrix of a hybrid ring-junction is given by

$$[S] = -\frac{1}{2}\begin{pmatrix} 0 & 0 & 1 & 1 \\ 0 & 0 & 1 & -1 \\ 1 & 1 & 0 & 0 \\ 1 & -1 & 0 & 0 \end{pmatrix}$$

6.8 A matched·attenuator has S_{11} = S_{22} = 0 and S_{-12} = S_{21} = 0.5 ∠90°. Find $|S_{21}|$ if the measured loss of the attenuator is 6 dB and both the generator and the load are perfectly matched. [**Ans:** 0.5]

6.9 A reciprocal 2-port MW device has a VSWR of 1.5 and an insertion loss of 2 dB. Find the S-matrix.

[**Ans:** S_{11} = S_{22} = 0.2 and S_{12} = S_{21} = 0.7943]

6.10 The input power to the sum arm of an ideal matched magic-T is 1 W. Calculate the output powers in other arms.

[**Ans:** P_1 = P_2 = 0.5W, P_3 = 0]

6.11 An E-plane tee is match terminated at all the ports with an input power of 5 mW fed at the E-arm. (a) Calculate the power flow through the junction. (b) What changes will occur in power distribution if the power is fed at the collinear arm.

[**Ans:** 1.9025 mW, 96.25 Ω, 22.5 Ω]

6.12 A rectangular waveguide has the dimensions a = 3 cm and b = 1.5 cm. Calculate the guide wavelength at 8 GHz. [**Ans:** 4.80 cm]

6.13 For an electronically controlled attenuator, the return loss is 10 dB. Calculate the VSWR, R_1 and R_3.

[**Ans:** VSWR = 1.925, R_1 = 96.25 ohms and R_3 = 22.5 ohms]

REFERENCE

1. Montogomery CG et al (1948). *Principles of Microwave Circuits*, McGraw Hill, NY.

2. Roddy D (1986). *Microwave Technology*, PH, NJ.

3. Reich HJ (1978). *Microwave Principles*, East-West, New Delhi.

4. Rizzi PA (1999). *Microwave Engineering*: Passive Circuits, PH, NJ.

5. Seeger JA (1988). *Microwave Theory Components and Devices*, PH, NJ.

6. Pozar DM (1990). *Microwave Engineering*, Addison-Wesley, Mass.

7. Wheeler GJ (1963). *Introduction to Microwave*, Englewood Cliffs, NJ.

8. Wolff EA and Kaul R (1988), *Microwave Engineering and Systems*, John Wiley, NY.

9. Terman FE (1955). *Electronic and Radio Engineering*, McGraw Hill Intl.

10. Reich HJ (1978). *Microwave Principles*, East-West, New Delhi

11. Rizzi PA. *Microwave Engineering*, Passive Circuits, PH, NJ.

12. Soohoo RF (1971). *Microwave Electronics*, Addison-Wesley, Masschusetts.

Microwave Isolators, Circulators and Directional Couplers

Objectives

- Classify the types of isolators, circulators, directional couplers and power dividers.
- Design Binomial and Tchebyshev couplers.
- Appreciate the simple and unique procedure presented for the design of binomial and Tchebyshev couplers.

7.1 INTRODUCTION

In the previous chapter, we have studied the various microwave components that are commonly used in microwave systems. In this chapter, we shall discuss the constructional details of microwave passive devices such as microwave isolators, circulators, directional couplers and power dividers, their S-matrices and applications.

7.2 ISOLATOR OR UNILINE

An isolator is a two-port nonreciprocal microwave transmission device. It is used to isolate one component from loading the other component in the transmission line. *An ideal isolator completely absorbs the power propagated in one direction and transmits the signal power without any attenuation in the opposite direction.* Therefore the isolator is also known as *uniline*[1].

Isolators are very useful components for avoiding the interaction between various parts of a microwave system. An isolator placed between a microwave signal generator

and the load prevents the reflected power from the unmatched load reaching the generator. This eliminates the source power variations and frequency pulling due to load variations. The arrangement is shown in Fig. 7.1.

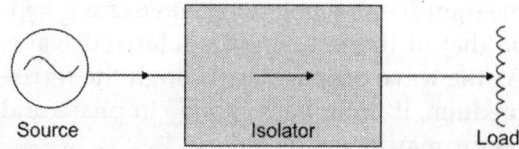

Fig. 7.1: Isolator

Isolators can be constructed in many ways. We shall now discuss Faraday rotation and resonance isolators.

7.2.1 Microwave Faraday Rotation

Consider a lossless ferrite medium magnetized in the positive z-direction and a plane wave traveling through this ferrite medium. In a magnetized ferrite medium, the normal mode of propagation is *circularly polarized waves*. Therefore, the plane wave traveling through this ferrite medium is decomposed into two *circularly polarized waves*. One wave undergoes *right-handed polarization* and the other *left-handed polarization*. The sum of these two waves constitutes the plane wave.

Let the propagation constants of the right- and left-handed circularly polarized waves be β_- and β_+ respectively; $\beta_- \neq \beta_+$. As the wave propagates through the magnetized ferrite medium, the plane of polarization is rotated by an angle θ with respect to the original plane of polarization (x-axis). This rotation is known as *microwave Faraday rotation*. The propagation constant β_- and β_+ are *dependent on the magnitude and direction of the magnetization*. They *do not depend on the direction of propagation*.

In order to find out the magnitude and direction of the magnetization, a linearly polarized wave is decomposed into right-handed polarization and the other left-handed polarizes waves. The plane wave is their sum. Thus,

$$E = (a_x + ja_y)\, E_0/2 + (a_x - ja_y)\, E_0/2,\ z = 0 \quad (1)$$

where a_x and a_y are x and y components of the electric field.

Let $\gamma_+ = j\beta_+$ be the propagation constant of the right-handed polarized wave and $\gamma_- = j\beta_-$ be that of the left-handed polarized wave. As the wave propagates through the ferrite medium, it undergoes change in phase and hence, may be expressed as

$$E = (a_x + ja_y)\left(\frac{E_0}{2}\right)e^{-j\beta_- z}$$
$$+ (a_x - ja_y)\left(\frac{E_0}{2}\right)e^{-j\beta_+ z}$$

At $z = l$, the above equation becomes

$$E = (a_x - ja_y)\,(E_0/2)e^{-j\beta_- l}$$
$$+ (a_x - a_y)\,(E_0/2)e^{-j\beta_+ l}$$

After some mathematical manipulations, the above equation reduces to

$$E = E_0\,[e^{-j(\beta_- + \beta_+)l/2}] \times$$
$$[a_y \cos(\beta_+ - \beta_-)l/2 - a_y \sin(\beta_+ - \beta_-)l/2]$$

A close examination of the above equation reveals

(i) The resultant wave is linearly polarized.
(ii) The wave has undergone a phase delay of $(\beta_+ + \beta_-)l/2$.
(iii) The new plane of polarization makes an angle of θ with the x-axis and is given by $\theta = -(\beta_+ - \beta_-)\,l/2$

The negative sign indicates phase delay.

Let the new plane polarized wave propagate in the negative direction. The plane of polarization rotates in the same direction as before by an angle θ Thus, if a plane polarized wave propagates in the positive z-direction from $z = 0$ to $z = l$, its plane of polarization rotates by an angle θ with respect to the x-axis and, then, if it propagates in the negative z-direction from $z = l$ to $z = 0$, it undergoes an angle θ in the same direction. Thus, the net angle of rotation is 2θ. Hence, the original direction of polarization is not restored. This is because of the fact that β_+ and β_- are independent of direction of propagation. Therefore, the resultant wave is rotated with respect to x-axis by an angle of 2θ. It is given by

$$2\theta = -(\beta_+ - \beta_-)\,l$$

Hence, the phase of the propagating wave is delayed by angle $\theta = (\beta_+ - \beta_-)\,l/2$ rad/m regardless of direction of propagation.

7.2.2 Faraday Rotation Isolator

Figure 7.2 shows a Faraday rotation isolator. The main part of the isolator is a circular wave-guide section C. A ferrite rod of smaller diameter is placed along its axis. The circular wave-guide is tapered to rectangular sections at both ends. The input rectangular wave-guide section has a 45° twist. The ferrite rod is magnetized with a static magnetic field along the axis of the waveguide. The length and the diameter of the ferrite rod and the magnitude of the static magnetic field determine the angle of rotation. They are selected such that the electric field vector of

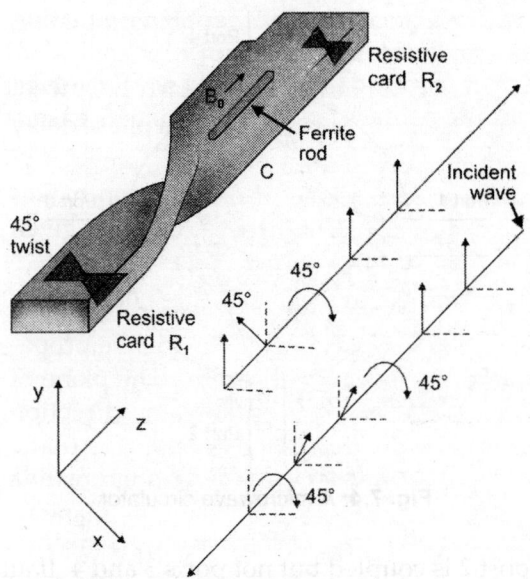

Fig. 7.2: Faraday rotation isolator

the wave, because of Faraday rotation, rotates by 45° clockwise at the desired operating frequency. In addition, two resistive cards R_1 and R_2 are also placed inside the wave-guide, one at each end. These cards are placed parallel to the broad walls of the rectangular wave-guides. The input resistive card R_1 is in the x–z plane and the output resistive card R_2 is displaced 45° with respect to the input card.

Principle of Operation

Let a wave be incident at the input port of the isolator with dominant TE_{10} mode. The TE_{10} mode is perpendicular to the input resistive card R_1. Hence, it does not get attenuated during transmission but its polarization is rotated 45° by the twist section. After passing theough the rectangular to circular waveguide transition, it enters the circular waveguide as TE_{11} mode. The electric field of this TE_{11} mode is parallel to the electric field of the incident wave. Thus, it is perpendicular to the resistive card R_1 near the input end. Therefore, the power incident at the input port is not attenuated by the resistive card near the input end. This

wave now passes through the magnetized ferrite rod. The electric field vector gets rotated by 45° clockwise. After this rotation, the electric field vector becomes perpendicular to the resistive card R_2 near the output end and hence, not attenuated by it. Thus, the incident power is transmitted without attenuation from the input port to the output port.

Let us consider a wave incident at the output port. In this case, the electric field direction is such that the wave is not affected by the resistive card R_2. While propagating through the ferrite rod, it encounters a static magnetic field in the reverse direction. Hence, the Faraday rotator rotates the electric field vector counter-clockwise by 45° as shown. After this rotation, the electric field becomes parallel to the resistive card R_1 and the power is completely absorbed. The edge of the card is tapered to reduce any reflection towards output port. Thus, a nonreciprocal isolation action takes place. Practical isolators of this type have forward attenuation of 1 dB and reverse isolation more than 20 dB.

7.2.3 Resonance Isolator

At and near the resonance frequency of the ferrite, the attenuation constant for TE_{10} mode with negative or clockwise circular polarization is always very small compared to that for positive or counterclockwise circular polarization. This property of TE_{10} mode is utilized in the resonance isolators. Fig. 7.3 shows a resonance isolator. It consists of a rectangular wave-guide operating in the dominant TE_{10} mode. One (or two) thin ferrite slab is located in the rectangular wave-guide at a position $x = x_1$ where the RF magnetic field is circularly polarized. The ferrite is magnetized by a static magnetic field H along the y-direction. For propagation in the forward or $+z$ direction, the magnetic field is negative circularly polarized and the wave passes without being attenuated. When it passes in the reverse direction, it is positive

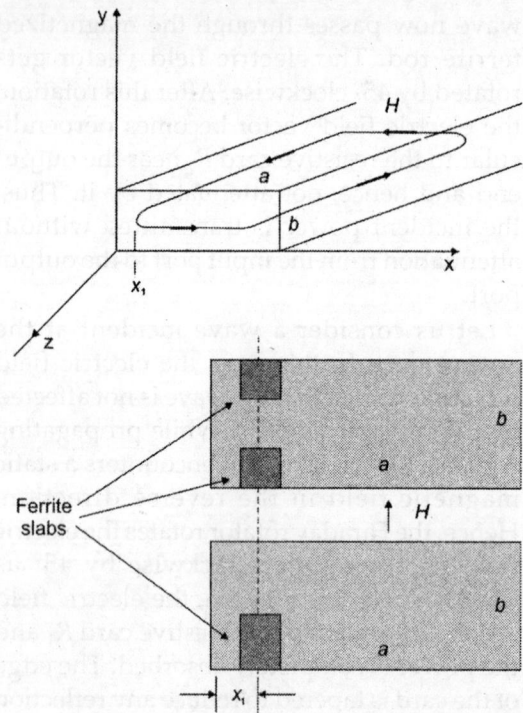

Fig. 7.3: Resonance of waveguide isolator

circularly polarized. This wave undergoes heavy attenuation and is absorbed in the ferrite. Practical isolators of this type have forward attenuation of 0.5 dB and reverse isolation more than 20 dB. The VSWR in the forward direction is about 1.1.

7.2.4 *S*-Matrix of Isolators

For an ideal loss-less, matched isolator,

$$|S_{21}| = 1,$$
$$|S_{12}| = |S_{11}| = |S_{22}| = 0 \quad (7.1)$$

Therefore the *S*-matrix of an ideal loss-less matched isolator is given by

$$[S] = \begin{pmatrix} 0 & 0 \\ 1 & 0 \end{pmatrix} \quad (7.2)$$

7.3 CIRCULATORS

A microwave circulator is a multi-port device in which the wave can flow from the *i*-th port to $(i + 1)$-*th* port in one direction as shown in Fig. 7.4. Thus, if power is incident in port 1,

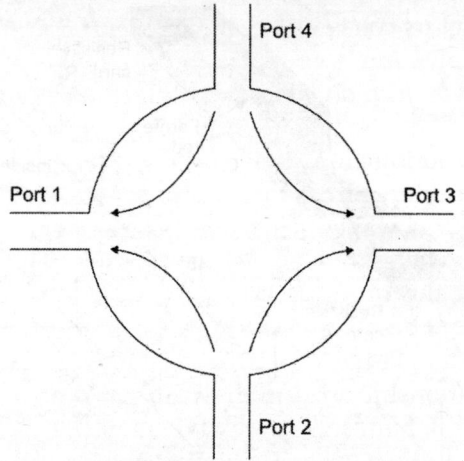

Fig. 7.4: A microwave circulator

port 2 is coupled but not ports 3 and 4. If all ports except one port are terminated in matched loads, the input impedance of the remaining port is equal to the characteristic impedance of the input line and hence, presents a matched load. Therefore, an ideal circulator is a matched device.

Although there is no restriction on the number of ports, the 4-port microwave circulator is the most common. Many types of microwave circulators are in use today. We shall discuss 4-port and 3-port circulators.

7.3.1 Four-port Circulator Using Magic Tees

Figure 7.5 shows a 4-port circulator. It is constructed with two magic tees and a phase shifter. The phase shifter provides a phase shift of 180° for propagation in the direction from *a* to *b*. The electrical path lengths are same for propagation from *b* to *a*, *c* to *d* and *d* to *c*.

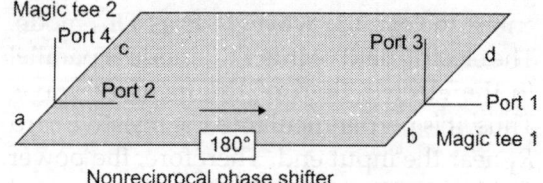

Fig. 7.5: Four-port circulator

Let us consider a wave incident in port 1. It splits into two equal amplitude in-phase waves in collinear arms b and d of the magic tee. They propagate in the side arms of the hybrid junction, arrive at a and c in phase, and emerge from the adder arm or port 2 of tee-2. A wave incident in port 2 splits into two waves, one arrives at d with a phase ϕ and the other arrives at b with a phase $(\phi + \pi)$ because of the presence of the phase shifter. These waves have the right phase relationship to combine and emerge from port 3. Similarly, a wave incident in port 3 splits into two equal amplitude out-of-phase waves. Hence, they arrive at the other hybrid junction to combine and emerge from port 4. In a similar way, a wave incident in port 4 splits into two equal amplitude out-of-phase waves. However, the phase shifter restores the phase equality so that the waves combine and emerge from port 1.

Principle of Operation

Let us consider a wave incident in port 1. The first 3 dB coupler splits the wave into two waves. Because of the transmission properties of an aperture, the wave in the upper waveguide undergoes a 90° change in phase. The upper guide wave arrives at the second coupler with a relative phase of 180° and the lower guide wave arrives with a relative phase of 90°. The second coupler splits these waves as illustrated in Fig. 7.5 Hence, the resultant waves are in phase at port 2 but out of phase in port 4. Thus transmission takes place from port 1 to 2. Similarly, a wave incident in port 2 emerges at port 3. In general, the sequence followed is $1 \rightarrow 2 \rightarrow 3 \rightarrow 4 \rightarrow 1$.

7.3.2 Four-port Circulator Using Directional Coupler

A compact 4-port circulator may be constructed using 3 dB side-hole directional couplers (discussed in Secton 7.4) and rectangular waveguide with two non-reciprocal phase shifters.

A nonreciprocal phase shifter consists of a thin ferrite slab of length l. It is located in a rectangular waveguide at $x = x_1$ where the magnetic field of TE_{10} mode is circularly polarized. It is biased with a y-direction magnetic field B_0 as shown in Fig. 7.6. For one direction of propagation, the ac magnetic field is clockwise circularly polarized at x_1 and for the opposite direction, counter clockwise circularly polarized. The two circular polarizations have different propagation phase constants β_+ and β_-. By selecting the length l of the ferrite slab so that $(\beta_+ - \beta_-)$. $l = \pi/2$, a differential phase shift of 90° for the both directions of propagation is obtained.

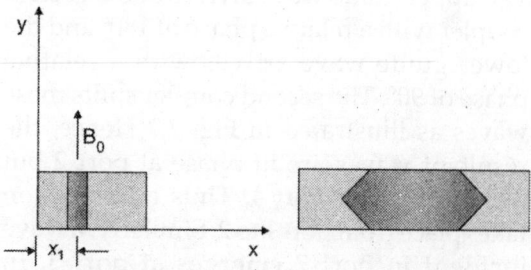

Fig. 7.6: Nonreciprocal phase shifter

7.3.3 Four-Port Circulator Using Phase Shifters

Figure 7.7 shows a 4-port circulator using two 90° nonreciprocal phase shifters. The two

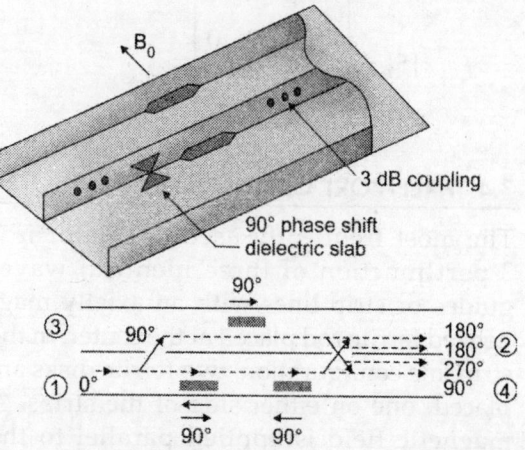

Fig. 7.7: A compact 4-port circulator

phase-shifters are biased in opposite directions with permanent magnets. A dielectric slab is inserted in one waveguide to provide an additional phase shift of 90°. The coupling holes are arranged to provide 3 dB of coupling. The wave coupled through the apertures undergoes a 90° change in phase. This phase change is important for proper operation of the circulator.

Principle of Operation

Let us consider a wave incident in port 1. The first 3-dB coupler splits the wave into two waves. Because of the transmission properties of an aperture, the wave in the upper wave-guide undergoes a 90° change in phase. The upper guide wave arrives at the second coupler with a relative phase of 180° and the lower guide wave arrives with a relative phase of 90°. The second coupler splits these waves as illustrated in Fig. 7.7 Hence, the resultant waves are in phase at port 2 but out of phase in port 4. Thus transmission takes place from port 1 to 2. Similarly, a wave incident in port 2 emerges at port 3. In general, the sequence followed is $1 \rightarrow 2 \rightarrow 3 \rightarrow 4 \rightarrow 1$.

7.3.4 S-Matrix of 4-port Circulator

The S-matrix of a perfectly matched, loss-less non-reciprocal 4-port circulator is given by

$$[S] = \begin{pmatrix} 0 & 0 & 0 & 1 \\ 1 & 0 & 0 & 0 \\ 0 & 1 & 0 & 0 \\ 0 & 0 & 1 & 0 \end{pmatrix} \qquad (7.3)$$

7.4 THREE-PORT CIRCULATOR

The most frequently used circulator is a 3-port junction of three identical wave-guides or strip lines with an axially magnetized ferrite rod placed at the center. In the strip line configuration, two ferrite disks are placed, one on either side of the strips. A magnetic field is applied parallel to the axis of the ferrite rod or disks. The magnetic

field gives the junction the required non-reciprocal property.

Principle of Operation

Figure 7.8 shows the 3-port circulator. Microwave power incident at one port divides equally in other two ports but the ferrite rod causes phase variations in waves such that the two waves are added in port 2 while they are subtracted in port 3 and so on.

In addition, the 3-port circulator can also be used as (i) an isolator by terminating one of the ports in a matched load or (ii) a switch by reversing the static magnetic field.

7.4.1 S-matrix of 3-port Circulator

The S-matrix of a perfectly matched loss-less non-reciprocal 3-port circulator is given by

$$[S] = \begin{pmatrix} 0 & 0 & S_{13} \\ S_{12} & 0 & 0 \\ 0 & S_{32} & 0 \end{pmatrix} \qquad (7.4)$$

If the terminal planes are properly chosen so as to make the phase angles of S_{13}, S_{21} and S_{32} zero, then

$$S_{13} = S_{21} = S_{32} = 1 \qquad (7.5)$$

The S-matrix then becomes

$$[S] = \begin{pmatrix} 0 & 0 & 1 \\ 1 & 0 & 0 \\ 0 & 1 & 0 \end{pmatrix} \qquad (7.6)$$

The junctions may be matched by placing suitable tuning elements in each arm. In practical circulators, losses are always present. Typical values are: insertion loss is less than 1 dB; isolation loss is from 30 dB to 40 dB and the VSWR is less than 1.5

7.5 DIRECTIONAL COUPLERS

Figure 7.9 shows a directional coupler. It is a four-port waveguide junction. It is used to couple a fraction of the microwave power to a port in the secondary waveguide, called a *coupled port*, while, in the primary line, free

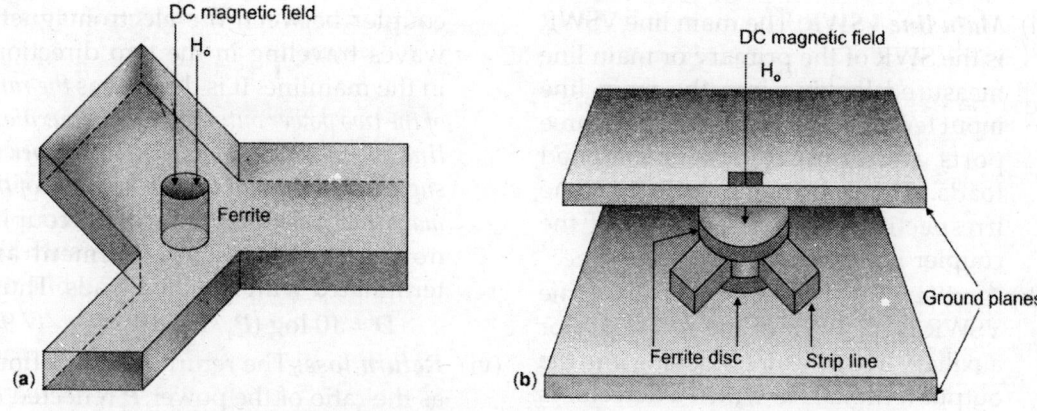

Fig. 7.8: Three-port circulator (a) Waveguide type (b) Strip line type

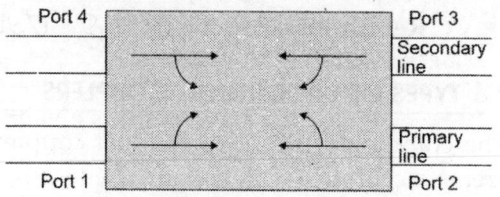

Fig. 7.9: A directional coupler

transmission of power takes place from the input port to the output port. No power reaches the fourth port, called *isolated port*. All ports of the directional couplers are matched; i.e if three ports are matched, the fourth port appears terminated in a matched load. An incident wave at this port suffers no reflection. The coupled power in the coupled port is used for measurement and power monitoring in microwave circuits.

7.5.1 Ideal Directional Coupler

The characteristics of an ideal directional coupler are:

(i) If power is fed into port 1, the power flows to port 2; a fraction of the power is coupled to port 3 and none to port 4. Thus, the power flows in the forward direction of the secondary waveguide. Port 3 is the *coupled port* and port 4 is the *isolated port*.

(ii) Similarly, if power is fed into port 2, the power flows to port 1, a fraction is coupled in port 4 and none in port 3.

(iii) If power is fed into port 3, the power flows into port 4, a fraction is coupled to port 1 and none to port 2

(iv) If power is fed into port 4, the power flows into port 3, a fraction is coupled to port 2 and none to port 1.

7.5.2 Forward and Backward Directional Couplers

In all the above cases, power flows in the forward direction in the secondary wave-guide. Such directional couplers are known as *forward directional couplers*. In a backward directional coupler, the coupled and isolated ports are interchanged. Therefore, power flows in the reverse or backward direction in the secondary waveguide. Hence they are known as *backward directional couplers*. Coaxial, strip and micro-strip couplers are backward directional couplers.

7.5.3 Directional Coupler Parameters

The important parameters of directional couplers are:

(i) Main line VSWR

(ii) Auxiliary line VSWR

(iii) Coupling coefficient

(iv) Main line insertion loss

(v) Directivity

(vi) Return loss

(i) *Main line VSWR:* The main line VSWR is the SWR of the primary or main line measured looking into the main line input terminals when all the other three ports are terminated with matched loads. This parameter will be same irrespective of the orientation of the coupler in the transmission line.

(b) *Auxiliary line VSWR:* The auxiliary line VSWR is the SWR of the secondary or auxiliary line measured looking into the output terminals to which a detector is normally connected when all other ports are terminated with matched loads.

(iii) *Coupling coefficient:* Coupling coefficient is the ratio of power P_1 incident at port 1 of the main line to the coupled power P_3 at port 3 of the auxiliary output. The coupling coefficient C is usually expressed in dB.

$$C = 10 \log (P_1/P_3) \text{ dB} \qquad (7.7)$$

(iv) *Main line insertion loss:* The main line insertion loss is the attenuation introduced in a transmission line by the insertion loss of the directional coupler (Fig. 7.10). The auxiliary line of the coupler is perfectly terminated with matched load. The main line insertion loss IL is given by

$$IL = 10 \log (P_1/P_2) \text{ dB} \qquad (7.8)$$

(v) *Directivity:* The directivity D of a directional coupler is a measure of the discrimination property of a directional coupler between the electromagnetic waves traveling in the two directions in the mainline. It is defined as *the ratio of the two power outputs from the auxiliary line when a given amount of power is successively applied to each terminal of the main line.* The other ports of the coupler not used for the measurement are terminated with matched loads. Thus,

$$D = 10 \log (P_4/P_3) \text{ dB} \qquad (7.9a)$$

(vi) *Return loss:* The return loss is defined as the ratio of the power P, reflected or returned to port 1 to the incident power P_1 at port 1 of the main line. Thus

$$\textbf{Return loss} = 10 \log (P_r/P_1) \qquad (7.9b)$$

7.6 TYPES OF DIRECTIONAL COUPLERS

The common types of directional couplers are:

(a) Single-hole or Bethe-hole couplers
(b) Two-hole couplers
(c) Multi-hole couplers
(d) Coupled transmission line couplers
(e) Multi-section coupler
(f) Branch line coupler
(g) Hybrid or rat race coupler
(h) Schwinger reversed phase coupler
(i) Long slot coupler
(j) Lange coupler
(k) Capacitance loop coupler

7.7 SINGLE -HOLE OR BETHE-HOLE COUPLER

Single-hole or Bethe-hole coupler consists of two rectangular waveguides coupled by means of a small circular aperture located at the center of the common broad wall. Depending on the location of the hole, it is classified as

(i) Center hole couplers
(ii) Offset hole couplers

7.8 CENTER-HOLE COUPLER

It consists of two rectangular waveguides placed one over the other with the common

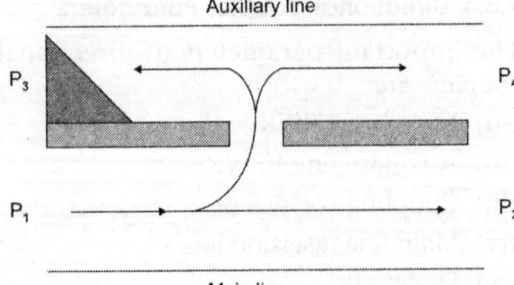

Auxiliary line

P_3 P_4

P_1 P_2

Main line

Fig. 7.10: Power coupling in a coupler

broad side. To achieve maximum directivity, the axis of the two waveguides must be at an angle θ. The electric and magnetic couplings are made equal by rotating the auxiliary guide relative to the main guide about the coupling hole as shown in Fig 7.11(a). The magnetic coupling is a function of the angle θ, whereas the electric coupling is essentially independent of the angle. Therefore, there exists an optimum angle at which the directivity is maximum. This is achieved by rotating the auxiliary guide relative to the main guide about the coupling hole such that the electric and magnetic couplings are equal.

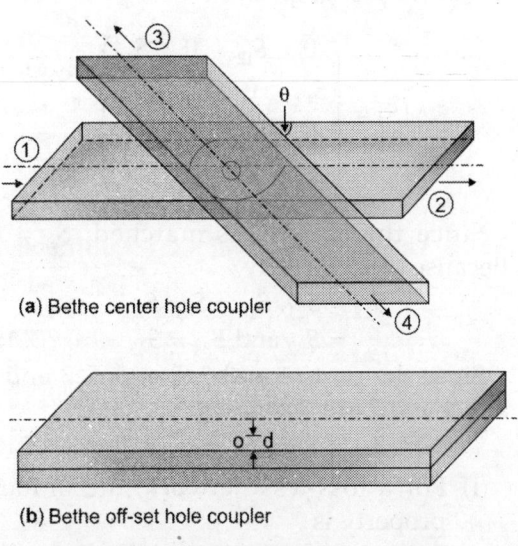

(a) Bethe center hole coupler

(b) Bethe off-set hole coupler

Fig. 7.11: Bethe single hole coupler

The coupling coefficient and directivity of the center-hole coupler are given by

$$C = 20 \log [1/(x \cos \theta)] \text{ dB} \qquad (7.10)$$

$$D = C + 20 \log [2 \cos \theta/(1 + \cos \theta)] \text{ dB} \qquad (7.11)$$

$x = 16\pi r_0^3/(3ab\lambda_g)$. r_0 is the radius of the center hole, $\lambda_g = \sqrt{\lambda_0/[(1-(\lambda_0/2a)^2]}$. a and b are the dimensions of the waveguide. For $P_4 = 0$, the optimum angle θ_{opt} is a function of λ_g and λ_0 and is given by $\theta_{opt} = \cos^{-1}(\lambda_g^2/2\lambda_0^2)$.

7.9 OFFSET-HOLE COUPLER

In the second type of Bethe-hole coupler, the angle $\theta = 0$ but with an offset aperture as shown in Fig. 7.11(b). In this case, the spacing d should be chosen such that $\sin (\pi d/a) = \lambda_0/(\sqrt{6}a)$. With $P_4 = 0$, the maximum coupling and the directivity are given by

$$C = 20 \log [(1 + x^2)/x] \qquad (7.12)$$

$$D = 10 \log (1/x) \qquad (7.13)$$

Here $x = (16\pi r_0^3/3ab\lambda_g) \sin^2 (\pi d/a)$ where d is the offset distance.

The coupling and the directivity of a Bethe-hole coupler are sensitive to changes in frequency and dimensions of the waveguides.

7.10 TWO-HOLE COUPLER

In a two-hole coupler, the two rectangular wave-guides are coupled by two identical apertures spaced a quarter wavelength, $\lambda_g/4$ apart as shown in Fig. 7.12. Let a wave of unit amplitude be incident at port 1, the field coupled into the second wave-guide be an amplitude of B_f in the forward direction and B_b in the backward direction. B_f and B_b are known as forward and backward aperture coupling coefficients respectively because they are the amplitudes of the coupled fields of unit-amplitude incident wave. The first aperture couples only a small amount of incident power. Hence, the amplitude of the incident wave at the second aperture is almost unity. The field that travels back to the first hole from the second hole is 180° out of phase and hence they cancel in

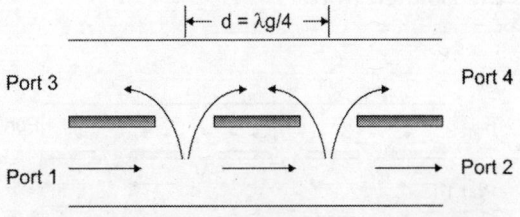

Fig. 7.12: Two-hole directional coupler

the backward direction. The fields in the forward direction are in phase and hence they add together. If the distance between the two holes is other than $\lambda_g/4$, the above characteristics of coupling and directivity cannot be achieved. Therefore, this is a narrow-band coupler. The coupling and directivity are given by

$$C = 20 \log (2/|B_f|) \tag{7.14}$$

$$D = 20 \log [|B_f/B_b|] + 20 \log |\sec \beta d| \tag{7.15}$$

Here $\sec \beta d$ is the array factor. Thus the directivity is the sum of the inherent directivity of a single aperture and directivity associated with the array of two holes.

7.11 MULTI-HOLE COUPLER

Multi-hole couplers are used to achieve good directivity over a band of frequencies. Figure 7.13 shows the structure of a multi-hole coupler that is symmetrical with respect to a transverse plane. The spacing between successive apertures is quarter wavelength. The coupled waves traveling back to port 3 will be out of phase and cancel out. The forward waves are in phase and thus reinforce each other. Hence, port 3 is the *isolated port* and matched terminated so that it absorbs any coupled power flowing in that port under practical situations. As power flows in the forward direction, from port 1 to port 2, it is known as *forward coupler*. If the power is incident at port 2, power flows to port 1 and the coupled power is absorbed at port 3. No power flows into Port 4 and it is the isolated port.

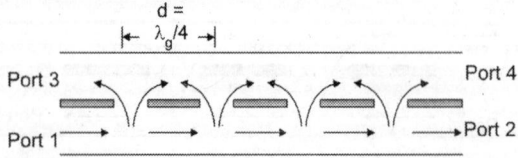

Fig. 7.13: Multi-hole directional coupler

The coupling and directivity are given by

$$C = -20 \log \left| \sum_{n=1}^{N} C_n \right| \, \mathrm{dB} \tag{7.16}$$

$$D = -C - 20 \log \left| \sum_{n=1}^{N} D_n e^{-j2(n-1)\beta d} \right| \, \mathrm{dB} \tag{7.17}$$

Depending on the size and location of the holes in the common wall, the coupling coefficient C varies from 3 dB to 30 dB and the directivity D from 30 dB to 40 dB.

7.12 S-MATRIX OF A DIRECTIONAL COUPLER

The S-matrix of a reciprocal matched directional coupler is given by

$$[S] = \begin{pmatrix} 0 & S_{12} & 0 & S_{14} \\ S_{12} & 0 & S_{23} & 0 \\ 0 & S_{23} & 0 & S_{34} \\ S_{14} & 0 & S_{34} & 0 \end{pmatrix}$$

Since the coupler is matched, $S_{ii} = 0$. Because of reciprocity,

$$\begin{aligned} S_{12} &= S_{21}, S_{14} = S_{41}, S_{23} \\ &= S_{32} \text{ and } S_{34} = S_{43} \end{aligned} \tag{7.18}$$

Since the ports 1 and 3, 2 and 4, 3 and 1 and 4 and 2 are decoupled,

$$S_{13} = S_{24} = S_{31} = S_{42} = 0 \tag{7.19}$$

(i) For a loss-less network, the unitary property is

$$|S_{12}|^2 + |S_{14}|^2 = 1 \tag{7.20}$$

$$|S_{12}|^2 + |S_{23}|^2 = 1 \tag{7.21}$$

$$|S_{23}|^2 + |S_{34}|^2 = 1 \tag{7.22}$$

$$|S_{14}|^2 + |S_{34}|^2 = 1 \tag{7.23}$$

From Eqs (7.20) and (7.21), we get

$$|S_{14}| = |S_{23}| \tag{7.24}$$

From Eqs. (7.21) and (7.22),. We obtain

$$|S_{12}| = |S_{34}| \tag{7.25}$$

By proper selection of the reference planes of port 1 with respect to port 2, and port 3 with respect to port 4, we can make S-parameters real.

$$S_{12} = S_{34} = \alpha \qquad (7.26)$$

α is a positive real number.

(ii) By applying the null property, we get

$$S_{12}S_{23}^* + S_{14}S_{34}^* = 0 \qquad (7.27)$$

or $\quad \alpha\,(S_{23}^* + S_{14}) = 0 \qquad (7.28)$

Since α is not equal to zero,

$$S_{23}^* + S_{14} = 0 \qquad (7.29)$$

We can make S_{14} real by properly selecting the reference plane of port 4 with respect to port 1, so that

$$S_{14} = S_{23} = -S_{23}^* = \beta \qquad (7.30)$$

Therefore

$$[S] = \begin{pmatrix} 0 & \alpha & 0 & \beta \\ \alpha & 0 & \beta & 0 \\ 0 & \beta & 0 & \alpha \\ \beta & 0 & \alpha & 0 \end{pmatrix} \qquad (7.31)$$

$\alpha^2 + \beta^2 = 1$ for conservation of energy. α is known as the *transmission factor* and β is the *coupling factor*.

Multi-hole directional couplers are designed for a desired coupling and directivity for the type of distribution selected by keeping the reverse voltage magnitude $|C_R|$ under a specified value C_m over the frequency band between the edges f_1 and f_2 as shown in Figs 7.14 and 7.15. The two important types of couplers are:

(i) Binomial couplers
(ii) Tchebychev couplers.

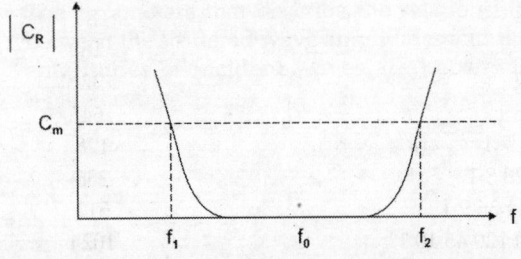

Fig. 7.14: Binomial distribution (maximally flat response)

7.13 BINOMIAL COUPLER

The binomial coupler has a flat response characteristic as shown in Fig. 7.14. For n-hole binomial couplers, the coupling coefficient C_k at the hole k is proportional to the corresponding binomial coefficient of $(a + b)^{n-1}$. Thus

$$C_k \propto a_k = a_k C_1 \qquad (7.32a)$$

$$a_k = {}^{n-1}C_{k-1}$$

$$= (n-1)!/[(k-1)!/(n-k)!] \qquad (7.32b)$$

For purpose of symmetry, the coupling coefficients are chosen as under:

$$C_1 = C_n,\ C_2 = C_{n-1} \text{ and so on.} \qquad (7.32c)$$

The reverse voltage C_R in the frequency band $(f_2 - f_1)$ is given by

For n is even:

$$|C_R| = 2C_1 \sum_{k=1}^{n/2} \left|{}^{n-1}C_{k-1} \cos[n-(2k-1)]\theta\right| \le C_m$$

$$(7.33a)$$

For n is odd:

$$|C_R| = 2C_1 \sum_{k=1}^{(n-1)/2} \left|{}^{n-1}C_{k-1} \cos[n-(2k-1)]\theta\right|$$

$$+ {}^{n-1}C_{(n-1)2} \le C_m \qquad (7.33b)$$

At frequency $f = f_o$, the derivatives of the reverse-coupled voltage C_R up to $(n-2)$ terms are zero and increase slowly on either side of f_o. Hence, the response is a maximally flat response without any ripple. The maximum value of C_k at the edges is C_m. The band edge frequency ratio r is given by

$$r = \lambda_{g_1}/\lambda_{g_2} = \theta_2/\theta_1 \qquad (7.34)$$

$$d = \lambda_{g_0}/4 \qquad (7.35)$$

$$\theta_1 = \pi/(1+r) = \pi/(1+\lambda_{g_1}/\lambda_{g_2})$$

$$= \pi\,\lambda_{g_2}/(\lambda_{g_1} + \lambda_{g_2})$$

$$= \pi\,\lambda_{g_0}/2\lambda_{g_1}$$

since $\ \lambda_{go} = 2\lambda_{g_1}\,\lambda_{g_2}/(\lambda_{g_1} + \lambda_{g_2})$

$$= 2\pi d/\lambda_{g_1}$$

since $\lambda_{g_0} = 4d$ (7.36)

$$\theta_2 = \pi r/(1+r)$$
$$= \pi \lambda_{g_1}/[\lambda_{g_2}(1+\lambda_{g_1}/\lambda_{g_2})]$$
$$= \pi \lambda_{g_1}/(\lambda_{g_1}+\lambda_{g_2})$$
$$= \frac{1}{2}\pi \lambda_{g_0}/\lambda_{g_2}$$

since $\lambda_{go} = 2\lambda_{g_1}\lambda_{g_2}/(\lambda_{g_1}+\lambda_{g_2})$

$$= 2\pi d/\lambda_{g_2}$$
$$= \pi - \theta_1 \qquad (7.37)$$

Here θ_1 and θ_2 are phase angles at f_1 and f_2 respectively.

The binomial coupling coefficients for a specified number of holes are given in Table 7.1

C_1 is obtained from the desired coupling C for a given number of holes.

$$C = 20 \log C/C_R \qquad (7.38)$$
$$C_m \geq C_1 2^{n-1} \cos^{n-1}\theta_1 \qquad (7.39)$$

A practical disadvantage of binomial couplers is the wide variation between the coupling coefficients for different holes, especially when n is large.

7.13.1 General Design Procedure

The design steps for binomial couplers are:

1. Obtain C from the given coupling, $C = 10^{-C(\text{dB})/20}$
2. Obtain C_m from the given coupling and directivity. $C_m = 10^{-(D+C)\text{dB}/20}$

3. Select the number of holes n.
4. Compute C_1 from $C = 2^{n-1}C_1$.
5. Test $\Sigma C_k \leq C_m$ for the selected n.
6. If the above condition is not satisfied, repeat steps 3 to 5.
7. Obtain the other values of C_k using Table 7.1 or Eq. (7.32)
8. From the designed values of C_k's, the hole dimensions are computed from the empirical formula
$$C = -20 \log(4\beta r_o^3/3ab) + [\cos\theta + (\lambda_g^2/2\lambda_o^2)]\,\text{dB}$$

7.13.2 Design Procedure when $r = 2$

If the frequency band ratio $r = 2$, then $C = 2^{n-1}C_1$. Within the band, $C_1 \leq C_m$. Hence, $C \leq 2^{n-1}C_m$. The simplified design procedure is given below:

1. Obtain C from the given coupling.
2. Obtain C_m from the given coupling and directivity. $C_m = 10^{-(D+C)\text{dB}/20}$
3. The number of holes is selected from $C/C_m \leq 2^{n-1}$.
4. Compute C_1 from $C = 2^{n-1}C_1$
5. Obtain the other values of C_k using Table 7.1 or Eq. (7.32).

From the designed values of C_k's, the hole dimensions are computed from the empirical formula

$$C = -20 \log(4\beta r_o^3/3ab)\,[\cos\theta + (\lambda_g^2/2\lambda_o^2)]\,\text{dB}$$

n	Binomial coefficients	Sum of coef. $= 2^n$
	Table 7.1: Pascal's triangle	
2	1 2 1	4
3	1 3 3 1	8
4	1 4 6 4 1	16
5	1 5 10 10 5 1	32
6	1 6 15 20 15 6 1	64
7	1 7 21 35 35 21 7 1	128
8	1 8 28 56 70 56 28 8 1	256
9	1 9 36 84 126 126 84 36 9 1	512
10	1 10 45 120 210 252 210 120 45 10 1	1024
11	1 11 55 165 330 462 462 330 165 55 11 1	2048
12	1 12 66 220 495 792 924 924 792 495 220 12 1	4056

7.14 TCHEBYSHEV COUPLER

The response of a Tchebyshev coupler is an equi-ripple characteristic as shown in Fig. 7.15. The reverse-coupling voltage C_R for n-hole coupler is proportional to the Tchebyshev polynomial of order $(n-1)$. The polynomial is given by

$$\Gamma_p(x) = \cos\{p\cos^{-1}(x)\}; -1 \le x \le +1 \quad (7.40a)$$
$$= \cosh\{p\cosh^{-1}(x)\}; x < -1; x > +1 \quad (7.40b)$$
$$p = n-1$$
$$x = \cos\theta/\cos\theta_1 = \cos\theta/|\cos\theta_2| \quad (7.41)$$

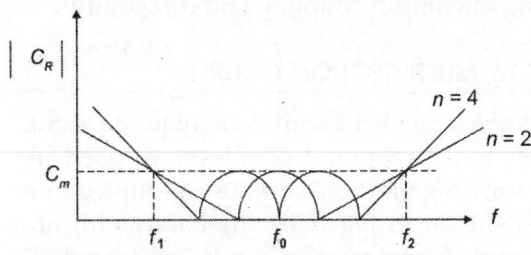

Fig. 7.15: Equiripple response (Tchebyshev distribution)

The properties of Tchebyshev polynomials are:

(a) As shown in Fig. 7.16, all polynomials pass through the point $(1, 1)$.

(b) For $-1 \le x \le +1$, $-1 \le \Gamma_p(x) \le +1$

(c) All roots lie within $-1 < x < 1$.

(d) All maxima have values of $+1$.

(e) All minima have values of -1.

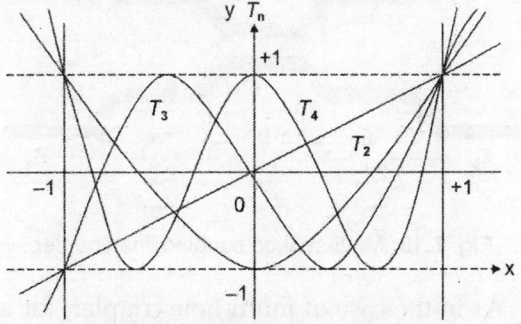

Fig. 7.16: Tchebyshev polynomial

The reverse-coupled voltage within the band is given by

For n is even:

$$C_R = 2\sum_{k=1}^{n/2} C_k \cos[n-(2k-1)\theta] \quad (7.42a)$$

For n is odd:

$$C_R = 2\sum_{k=1}^{(n-1)/2} C_k \cos[n-(2k-1)\theta] + {}^{n-1}C_{(n+1)/2}; \quad (7.43a)$$
$$= C_m \Gamma_{n-1}(x) \quad (7.43b)$$

For a specified C_m and n, Tchebyshev couplers give the largest bandwidth. In other words, it gives the lowest ripple C_m for a given bandwidth.

7.14.1 General Design Procedure

The design steps for Tchebyshev couplers are:

1. Obtain C from the given coupling. $C = 10^{-C(\text{dB})/20}$

2. Obtain C_m from the given coupling and directivity. $C_m = 10^{-(D+C)\text{dB}/20}$

3. Select the number of holes n.

4. Compute C_R in terms of powers of $\cos\theta$.

5. Substitute $\cos\theta = x\cos\theta_1$ and simplify.

6. Equate the similar coefficients with $C_m T_{n-1}(x)$.

7. Compute θ_1 from $C_p(\sec\theta_1) = 10^{-D(\text{dB})/20}$; $p = n/2$ for n even and $(n+1)/2$ for n odd.

8. ΣC_k is computed from C_i for the given coupling C for the selected number of holes n.

9. Test $|C_R| \le C_m$ for the selected n

10. If the above condition is not satisfied over the band, repeat the steps 3 to 9.

11. From the designed values of C_R's, the hole dimensions are determined from the empirical formula
$$C = -20\log(4\beta r_0^3/3ab) \times [\cos\theta + (\lambda_g^2/2\lambda_0^2)] \text{ dB} \quad (7.44)$$

7.14.2 Design Procedure When r = 2

1. Obtain **C** from the given coupling
$$C = 10^{-C(dB)/20}$$

2. Obtain C_m from the given Coupling and directivity.
$$C_m = 10^{-(D+C)dB/20}$$

3. Select the number of holes n.

4. Compute C_k using Table 7.2. $C_k = T_{n-1}C_m$.

5. From the designed values of C_R's, the hole dimensions are determined from the empirical formula
$$C = -20 \log (4\beta r_o^3/3ab) \times$$
$$[\cos \theta + (\lambda_g^2/2\lambda_o^2)] \text{ dB} \quad (7.45)$$

The coefficients of Tchebyshev polynomial are given in Table 7.2.

Table 7.2: Tchebyshev polynomial coefficients

$$[T_n(x) = 2x \, T_{n-1}(x) - T_{n-2}(x)]$$

n	Coefficients T				
1			1		
2			1	1	
3		2	5	2	
4		4	9	9	4
5	8	24	22	24	8

7.15 COUPLED TRANSMISSION LINE COUPLER

Figure 7.17 shows a coaxial line coupler. A narrow longitudinal slot cut on the common outer conductor joint couples the electromagnetic field from one coaxial line to another adjacent line. The transmission line that is excited is known as *primary line* and that in which the electromagnetic field is coupled is known as *secondary line*. An equal

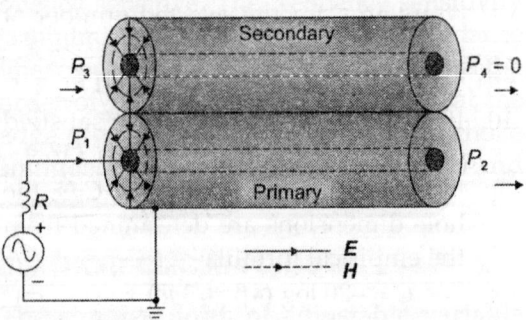

Fig. 7.17: Coupled coaxial line

and opposite charge is induced by the electric field in the primary line on the center conductor of the two lines. The resulting electric field in the secondary line is oppositely directed to that in the primary line. However, the magnetic field in both the lines is in the same direction. Hence, the power flow in the two guides is in opposite direction. When the power flow in the primary line is in the forward direction, the flow in the secondary line is in the backward direction. Hence, this coupler is known as *backward coupler* with port 4 being the *isolated port*. The coupling slot is $\lambda_g/4$ in length for achieving maximum coupling and directivity.

7.16 MULTI-SECTION COUPLER

When larger bandwidths are required, multi-section directional couplers are used. By cascading multiple sections of coupled lines as shown in Fig. 7.18, the bandwidth of a coupled-line coupler can be increased. To achieve perfect matching and improved directivity, the *even* and *odd* mode impedances of various sections are chosen such that

$$\sqrt{Z_{oe1}Z_{oo1}} = \sqrt{Z_{oe2}Z_{oo2}} = \cdots = \sqrt{Z_{oen}Z_{oon}}$$
$$= Z_0 \quad (7.46)$$

The mid-band coupling coefficient C_{ok} of the k-th section is
$$C_{ok} = (Z^2_{oek} - 1)/(Z^2_{ook} + 1) \quad (7.47)$$

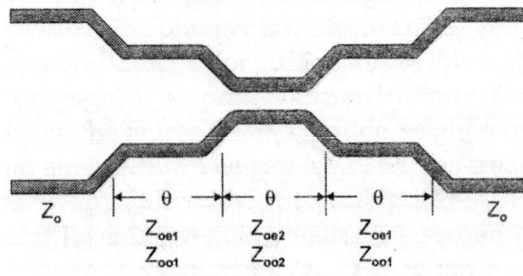

Fig. 7.18: Multi-section coupled line coupler

As in the case of multi-hole coupler, for a given coupling, the coupling coefficients can be determined from the binomial or Tchebyshev distribution.

7.17 BRANCH LINE COUPLER

Figure 7.19 shows a branch line coupler. It is a direct-coupled transmission structure. The main line is directly coupled to the secondary line by means of two shunt branches. This type of coupler handles high power and provides tight coupling. The length and spacing of the branches are quarter wavelength long at the mid-band frequency f_0. For a symmetrical coupler, the characteristic admittances of the series and shunt branches are Y_A and Y_B respectively. All input and output lines have the same characteristic admittance Y_0.

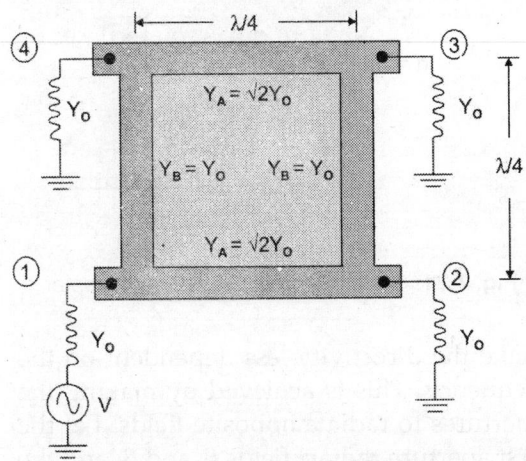

Fig. 7.19: Branch line coupler

The voltages at the ports are:

$$V_1 = V/2; \quad V_2 = -jV/2\sqrt{2};$$
$$V_3 = -V/2\sqrt{2} \text{ and } V_4 = 0 \quad (7.48)$$

The coupling, directivity and the transmission loss are given by

$$C = V_3/V_1 = -1/\sqrt{2} = 3\,\text{dB} \quad (7.49)$$
$$D = V_4/V_1 = 0 \quad (7.50)$$
$$T = V_2/V_1 = -j1/\sqrt{2} = 3\,\text{dB} \quad (7.51)$$

Hence, a branch coupler with single section is a 3 dB *forward coupler*.

7.18 HYBRID RING OR RAT-RACE COUPLER

Figure 7.20 shows a hybrid ring or rat race coupler. A wave incident at any one port can take the two available paths. Assuming that the other ports are match-terminated, the wave divides equally between the two paths. When the two waves arrive at a port, they combine. The phase difference between the two waves is determined by the difference in their path lengths. Thus, a wave incident in port 1 splits equally into two waves. They travel around the ring circuit in opposite directions. The two waves arrive at port 2 ($5\lambda/4 - \lambda/4 = \lambda = 0°$) and at port 4 ($3\lambda/4 - 3\lambda/4 = 0°$) in phase and at port 3 ($\lambda - \lambda/2 = \lambda/2 = 180°$) out of phase. Thus port 1 and 3 are uncoupled. Hence, port 3 is the *isolated* port. Similarly, the wave incident in port 2, splits equally into two waves. They travel around the ring circuit in opposite directions. The two waves arrive at port 1 and 3 in phase and at port 4 out of phase because the two coupling paths differ in length by $\lambda/2$. Thus port 2 and 4 are uncoupled. Hence, port 4 is the *isolated* port. The difference in path lengths and the corresponding phase difference are given in Table 7.3.

The characteristic impedance of each input line of the hybrid ring is Z_0. The ring has a characteristic impedance of Z_1. Let θ_1 be the electrical length of the ring between ports 1

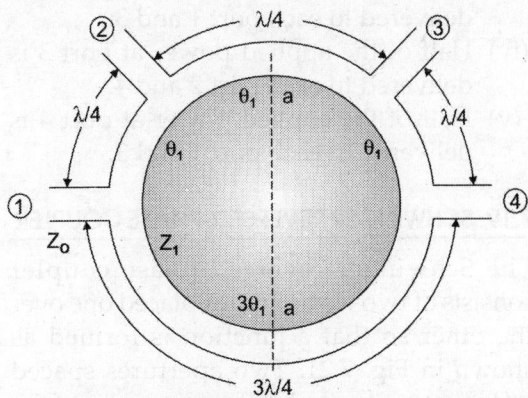

Fig. 7.20: Hybrid ring or rat-race coupler

Table 7.3: Differential path lengths and phase in hybrid ring

Input port	Output ports			
	1	2	3	4
1	—	$\lambda\,(0°)$	$\lambda/2\,(180°)$	0
2	$\lambda\,(0°)$	—	$\lambda\,(0°)$	$\lambda/2\,(180°)$
3	$\lambda/2\,(180°)$	$\lambda\,(0°)$	—	$l(0°)$
4	0	$\lambda/2\,(180°)$	$\lambda\,(0°)$	—

and 2, 2 and 3, 3 and 4, and $\theta_2 = 3\theta_1$. θ_2 represents the electrical length of the ring between ports 1 and 4. Excitations are chosen such that the symmetry plane aa is either an electric wall or magnetic wall. Thus, a two-port junction with ports 1 and 2 or ports 3 and 4 is formed. This enables us to describe one-half of the structure in terms of scattering matrix from the symmetry property[3]. The complete 4-port S-matrix can be found.

The 4-port S-matrix is given by

$$[S] = (-j/\sqrt{2})\begin{pmatrix} 0 & 1 & 0 & -1 \\ 1 & 0 & 1 & 0 \\ 0 & 1 & 0 & 1 \\ -1 & 0 & 1 & 0 \end{pmatrix} \quad (7.52)$$

The hybrid ring has the following properties:
  (i) Prot 1 and 3 are decoupled and so are ports 2 and 4.
  (ii) Half of the applied power at port 1 is delivered to each port 2 and 4.
  (iii) Half of the applied power at port 2 is delivered to each port 1 and 3.
  (iv) Half of the applied power at port 3 is delivered to each port 2 and 4.
  (v) Half of the applied power at port 4 is delivered to each port 1 and 3.

7.19 SCHWINGER REVERSED-PHASE COUPLER

The Schwinger reversed-phase coupler consists of two wave-guides placed one over the other so that a junction is formed as shown in Fig. 7.21. Two apertures spaced $\lambda/4$ apart are located at the center part of the junction. The coupler is designed so as to

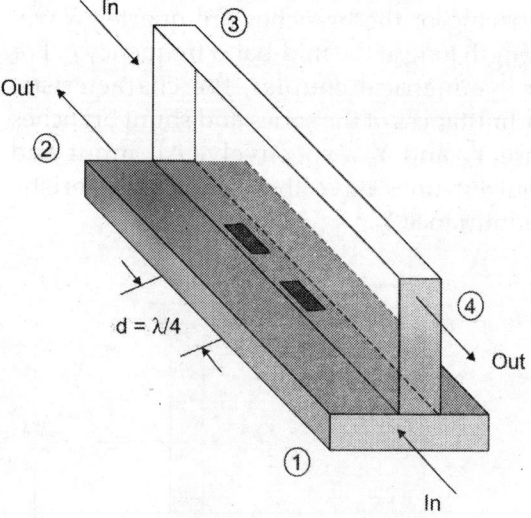

Fig. 7.21: Schwinger reversed phase coupler

make the directivity less dependent on the frequency. This is achieved by making the apertures to radiate opposite fields. Let the first aperture radiate fields B_f and B_b and the second one $-B_f$ and $-B_b$. At plane bb in the upper guide, the net field is $B_f - B_b = 0$ under all conditions. Thus, port 3 is not coupled to port 1. At the plane aa in the lower guide, the total field is

$$B_f - B_b\,e^{-2j\beta d} = e^{-j\beta d}\,B_b\,(e^{j\beta d} - e^{-j\beta d})$$
$$= e^{-j\beta d}\,B_b \times$$
$$[(\cos \beta d + j \sin \beta d) - (\cos \beta d - j \sin \beta d)]$$
$$= e^{-j\beta d}\,B_b\,2j\sin \beta d \quad (7.53)$$

Thus, the coupling between ports 1 and 4 is

$$C = -20 \log 2\,|B_b \sin \beta d| \quad (7.54)$$

It is maximum at $d = \lambda_g/4$ since $\beta = \lambda_g/2$. The directivity of this coupler is theoretically infinite and independent of frequency. However C is quite frequency-sensitive.

7.20 LONG SLOT COUPLER

The long slot coupler is shown in Fig. 7.22. In this, a single long slot is used instead of multiple holes. Each point in the plane of the slot acts like a coupling hole. The ends of the slot are properly tapered to prevent reflections from the ends of the slot. Therefore, perfect directivity is obtained even with a slot that is relatively short and wide. There is an optimum slot length for which all the power entering the main guide is transferred to the auxiliary guide. If the coupling is small, then coupled power is proportional to the square of slot length and to the sixth power of the slot width. This type of coupler has high directivity and high coupling. The coupling is markedly frequency sensitive.

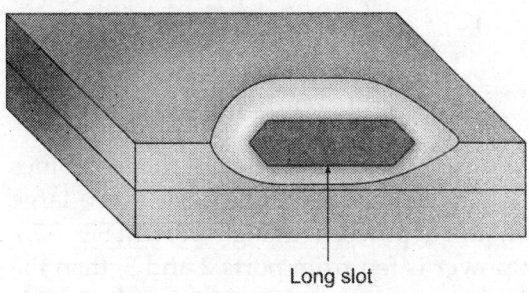

Fig. 7.22: Long slot coupler

7.21 LANGE DIRECTIONAL COUPLER

The Lange directional coupler consists of several coupled lines as shown in Fig. 7.23. In this, the coupling is larger than that in the coupled line coupler. The design of the coupler is such that wire connections are needed between some of the lines as shown in Fig. 7.23. This is the major disadvantage of Lange coupler.

The outstanding features are (i) its compact size and (ii) very broadband characteristics. This coupler is often used as an input coupler in balanced MW amplifiers. For this purpose, it is designed as 3 dB coupler and

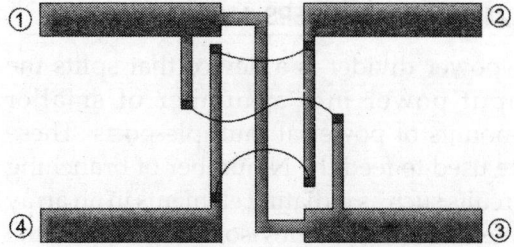

Fig. 7.23: Lange coupler

the output signals are in phase-quadrature so that it is a 90°-hybrid junction.

7.22 CAPACITANCE LOOP COUPLER

Another type of coupler is the capacitance loop coupler shown in Fig. 7.24. The loop is short with respect to a quarter wavelength. The **E**-field is equal in magnitude and direction in the two coaxial lines. However, the magnetic coupling is equal in magnitude but opposite in phase. For the EM wave moving to the right, the magnetic and electric couplings produce additive currents I_h and I_e respectively in cable A but subtractive currents in **B**. The currents in **B** can be made exactly equal in magnitude and opposite in phase by (i) varying the area or shape of the loop, (ii) the width of the conductor of the cable and (iii) by adding capacitance from the loop to the wall. At frequencies remote from the cut-off frequency of the guide, this coupler is independent of frequency.

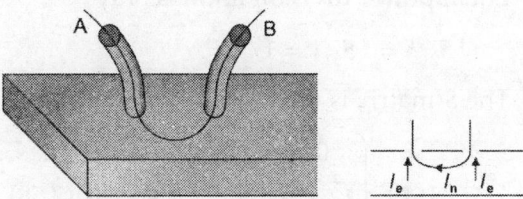

Fig. 7.24: Capacitance loop coupler

7.23 APPLICATIONS OF DIRECTIONAL COUPLERS

Directional couplers are used
 i. To measure transmitted power.
 ii. To measure power in reflectometers in both directions.
 iii. To measure VSWR.

7.24 POWER DIVIDERS AND COMBINERS

A power divider is a device that splits the input power into a number of smaller amounts of power at multiple ports. These are used to feed the N number of branching circuits such as radiating elements in an array antenna. This provides isolation between the output ports. Figure 7.25 shows a two-way equal (3 dB) power divider. It is a loss-less 3-port junction. The input port 1 is matched and the incident power is equally divided into two output ports 2 and 3. Therefore, the scattering matrix elements are given by

$S_{11} = 0$ (since port 1 is matched). (7.55)

$S_{21} = 1/\sqrt{2}$ (since one-half power goes into port 2) (7.56)

$S_{31} = 1/\sqrt{2}$ (since other-half power goes into port 3) (7.57)

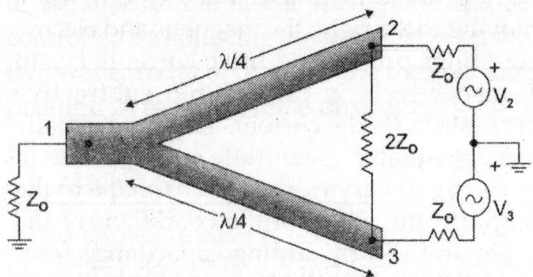

Fig. 7.25: Two-way equal power divider

Equal power division implies only

$$|S_{21}| = |S_{31}| = 1/\sqrt{2}.$$

The S-matrix is therefore

$$[S] = \begin{pmatrix} 0 & 1/\sqrt{2} & 1/\sqrt{2} \\ 1/\sqrt{2} & S_{22} & S_{23} \\ 1/\sqrt{2} & S_{32} & S_{33} \end{pmatrix} \quad (7.58)$$

Using the unitary property for loss-less network, we get

$$\frac{1}{2} + S_{22}S_{22}^* + S_{23}S_{23}^* = 1 \qquad 7.59)$$

$$\frac{1}{2} + S_{23}S_{23}^* + S_{33}S_{33}^* = 1 \qquad (7.60)$$

From the above two equations, we get

$$|S_{22}|^2 = |S_{33}|^2 \qquad (7.61)$$

Using the null property, we obtain

$$(1/\sqrt{2})S_{22}^* + (1/\sqrt{2})S_{23}^* = 0 \qquad (7.62)$$

This equation yields

$$S_{22} = -S_{23} \qquad (7.63)$$

Substituting this equation in Eq. (7.59), we have

$$\frac{1}{2} + S_{22}S_{22}^* + S_{22}S_{22}^* = 1$$

$$|S_{22}|^2 = \frac{1}{4} \qquad (7.64)$$

or, $\quad |S_{22}| = |S_{23}| = |S_{33}| = \frac{1}{2} \qquad (7.65)$

The last equation indicates that ports 2 and 3 are not matched. The voltage reflection coefficients at these ports are 1/2. Therefore, S-matrix of a 3-dB power divider is given by

$$[S] = \begin{pmatrix} 0 & 1/\sqrt{2} & 1/\sqrt{2} \\ 1/\sqrt{2} & 1/2 & -1/2 \\ 1/\sqrt{2} & -1/2 & 1/2 \end{pmatrix} \quad (7.66)$$

Power combiner is a device that combines the powers from multiple ports into a large amount of power at a single port. In Fig. 7.25, if power is fed from ports 2 and 3, then the two powers are combined at port 1 and it is the sum of these two powers.

Example 7.1: Calculate the input SWR and output ratio of a power divider under the following conditions: (a) Impedances are as shown in Fig. 7.25. (b) $Z_2 = Z_0$ and $Z_3 = 2Z_0$

Solution: (a) The two arm impedances are equal. Therefore, the input power divides equally. Hence,

$$P_2 = P_3 = 0.5\,P_{in}$$

or **3 dB** below the input power.

(b) Since the impedances are different, the power ratio is given by

$$P_2 : P_3 = Z_3 : Z_2 = 2 : 1$$

Therefore, $\quad P_2 = 2/3\,P_{in} = \mathbf{0.67}\,P_{in}$

$$P_3 = 1/3\,P_{in} = \mathbf{0.33}\,P_{in}$$

Thus, P_2 is **1.76** dB below P_{in} and P_3 is **4.77 dB** below P_{in}.

7.26 ADDITIONAL EXAMPLES

Example 7.2: Find the S-matrix of an isolator with 1 dB insertion loss and 25 dB isolation loss.

Solution: Insertion loss $= 1 = -20 \log |S_{21}|$

$\therefore \qquad S_{21} = 10^{-1/20} = 10^{-0.050} = 0.8913$

Isolation loss $= 25$ dB $= -20 \log |S_{12}|$

$\therefore \qquad S_{12} = 10^{-35/20} = 10^{-1.25} = 0.0562$

Since there is no reflection,

$$S_{11} = S_{22} = 0$$

Hence the S-matrix is given by

$$[S] = \begin{pmatrix} 0 & 0.0562 \\ 0.891 & 0 \end{pmatrix}$$

Example 7.3: Prove that a loss-less reciprocal three-port network cannot be matched at all the three ports.

Solution: The S-matrix of a matched 3-port junction is given by

$$[S] = \begin{pmatrix} 0 & S_{12} & S_{13} \\ S_{12} & 0 & S_{23} \\ S_{13} & S_{23} & 0 \end{pmatrix}$$

Since it is lossless, applying unitary property we get

$|S_{12}|^2 + |S_{13}|^2 = 1 \qquad \qquad$ (i)

$|S_{12}|^2 + |S_{23}|^2 = 1 \qquad \qquad$ (ii)

$|S_{13}|^2 + |S_{23}|^2 = 1 \qquad \qquad$ (iii)

The null property gives

$S_{13}S_{23}{}^* = S_{12}S_{23}{}^* = S_{12}S_{13}{}^* = 0 \qquad$ (iv)

Assume $S_{12} \neq 0$. Then from the last equation,

$$S_{13} = S_{23} = 0$$

This does not satisfy the Eq. (iii). Therefore it is not possible to construct a perfectly matched loss-less reciprocal 3-port network.

Example 7.4: Find the S-matrix of a 3-port circulator having an insertion loss of 0.5 dB, isolation loss of 30 dB and VSWR of 1.5.

Solution: $IL = 0.5 = 20 \log |S_{12}|$

$|S_{12}| = 10^{-0.5/20} = \mathbf{0.944}$

Since the IL between ports 1 and 2, 2 and 3 and 3 and $\perp$ are all same, we have

$|S_{21}| = |S_{32}| = |S_{13}| = \mathbf{0.944}$

Isolation loss $= 30$ dB $= -20 \log |S_{13}|$

$|S_{13}| = 10^{-30/20} = \mathbf{0.032}$

$= |S_{23}| = |S_{12}|$

The reflection coefficient is

$\Gamma = (S - 1)/(S + 1)$

$= (1.5 - 1)/(1.5 + 1) = 0.2$

$= |S_{11}| = |S_{22}| = |S_{33}|$

Hence, $\quad [S] = \begin{pmatrix} 0.200 & 0.032 & 0.944 \\ 0.944 & 0.200 & 0.032 \\ 0.032 & 0.944 & 0.200 \end{pmatrix}$

Example 7.5: Show that the S-matrix of an ideal loss-less N-port circulator is given by

$$[S] = \begin{pmatrix} 0 & 0 & 0 & \cdots & 1 \\ 1 & 0 & 0 & \cdots & 0 \\ \cdots & \cdots & \cdots & \cdots & \cdots \\ 0 & 0 & 1 & 10 & 0 \\ 0 & 0 & 1 & 01 & 0 \end{pmatrix}$$

by proper terminal plane locations.

Solution: The sequence followed by an ideal loss-less N-port circulator after the selection of proper terminal plane locations is $1 \to 2 \to 3 \to 4,\ldots N \to 1$.

Therefore, $S_{ij} = 1$ for $i = 1, 2, 3,\ldots n$ and $j = n, 1, 2,\ldots, (n - I)$.

All other s-parameters are zero. Hence proved.

Example 7.6: A rectangular waveguide with $a = 2b = 2.4$ cm is operating at 10 GHz. Design a maximally flat 20 dB directional coupler so that $D \geq 60$ dB in the band ratio of 2.

Solution: (i) To find coupling coefficients

$$C = 20 \text{ dB} = -20 \log C;$$
$$C = 10^{-20/20} = 0.1$$
$$D + |C| = -20 \log C_R = -20 \log C_m = 80$$

Therefore,

$$C_m = 10^{-80/20} = 10^{-4}$$
$$C/C_m = 1000 \le 2^{n-1}$$
$$\therefore \quad n-1 = 10 \text{ or } n = 11$$
$$C_1 = C_8 = C/2^{10} = 0.1/1024$$
$$= 9.766 \times 10^{-5}$$

From Table 7.1,

$$C_2 = C_7 = 7C_1 = 7 \times 9.766 \times 10^{-4}$$
$$= 6.84 \times 10^{-3}$$
$$C_3 = C_6 = 21C_1 = 21 \times 9.766 \times 10^{-4}$$
$$= 0.0205$$
$$C_4 = C_5 = 35C_1 = 35 \times 9.766 \times 10^{-4}$$
$$= 0.0342$$

(ii) To find r_o

$$C = (4/3) \, (\beta_{10} \, r_o^3/ab) \, (\lambda_{go}/\lambda_o)^2$$
$$\lambda_o = c/f = 3 \times 10^{10}/10 \times 10^9 = 3 \text{ cm}$$
$$k_o = 2\pi/\lambda_o = 6.28/3 = 2.093$$

$$\beta_{10} = \sqrt{k_o^2 - (\pi/a)^2}$$

$$= \sqrt{(2.093)^2 - (3.14/2.4)^2} = 1.634 \text{ rad.}$$

$$\lambda_{go} = 4d = \lambda_0\sqrt{1 - (\lambda_0/2a)^2}$$

$$= 3/\sqrt{1 - (3/4.8)^2} = 3.845 \text{ cm}$$

$$d = \lambda_{go}/4 = 3.845/4 = 0.961 \text{ cm}$$
$$C = (4/3) \, (\beta_{10} \, r_o^3/ab) \, (\lambda_{go}/\lambda_o)^2$$
$$= (4/3)(1.634 \, r_o^3/2.4 \times 1.2) \, (3.845/3)^2$$
$$= 1.241 \, r_o^3$$
$$r_o^3 = (C/1.241)^{1/3}$$
$$r_{01} = r_{08} = (C_1/1.241)^{1/3}$$
$$= (9.766 \times 10^{-5}/1.241)^{1/3} = 0.0197 \text{ cm}$$
$$r_{02} = r_{07} = (C_2/1.241)^{1/3}$$
$$= (7 \times C_1/1.241)^{1/3} = 0.0377 \text{ cm}$$
$$r_{03} = r_{06} = (C_3/1.241)^{1/3}$$
$$= (21 \times C_1/1.241)^{1/3} = 0.0543 \text{ cm}$$
$$r_{04} = r_{05} = (C_4/1.241)^{1/3}$$
$$= (35 \times C_1/1.241)^{1/3} = 0.1233 \text{ cm}$$

Example 7.7: Design a 3-hole center-hole Tchebyshev coupler with $C = 20 \text{ dB}$ and $D = 60 \text{ dB}$ at $f = 10 \text{ GHz}$. The waveguide dimensions are $a = 2b = 2.4 \text{ cm}$. Find the frequency band.

Solution: $C = 10^{-20}/20 = 0.1$

$$D + C = 80 = -20 \log C_m; \; C_m = 10^{-4}$$
$$0.1 = C = C_1 + C_2 + C_3 = 2C_1 + C_2 \text{ (i)}$$
$$C_R = 2C_1 \cos(n-1)\theta + C_2$$
$$= 2 \, [C_1 \cos 2\theta] + C_2$$
$$= 2C_1 \, (2\cos^2\theta - 1) + C_2$$

Let $\cos \theta = x \cos \theta_1$

$$C_R = 2C_1 \, (2x^2 \cos^2 \theta_1 - 1) + C_2$$
$$= 4C_1 \, x^2 \cos^2 \theta_1 - 2C_1 + C_2 \quad \text{(ii)}$$
$$= C_m T_2(x) = (2x^2 - 1) \quad \text{(iii)}$$

Equating the coefficients of (ii) and (iii), with $C_m T_2(x)$

$$4C_1 \cos^2 \theta_1 = 2C_m = 2 * 10^{-4}$$
$$C_2 - 2C_1 = -C_m = -10^{-4} \quad \text{(iv)}$$
$$D = 60 \text{ dB} = 20 \log |C_2 (\sec \theta_1)|$$
$$C_2 (\sec \theta_1) = 1000 = 2 \sec^2 \theta_1 - 1$$
$$\sec^2 \theta_1 = 999/2$$

$$\cos \theta_1 = \sqrt{2/999} = 0.0447$$

$$\theta_1 = 87.43°$$
$$4C_1 \cos^2 \theta_1 = 4C_1 \times 0.002 = 2 * 10^{-4}$$
$$C_1 = = 2 * 10^{-4}/4 \times 0.02$$
$$= 0.0025$$
$$C_2 - 2C_1 = -C_m = -10^{-4}$$
$$C_2 = 2C_1 - C_m$$
$$= 2 \times 0.025 - 0.0001 = 0.0249$$

At 10 GHz,

$$\lambda_o = 30/10 = 3 \text{ cm}$$
$$k_o = 2\pi/\lambda_o = 6.28/3 = 2.0933$$
$$\lambda_{go} = 4d = \lambda_o/\sqrt{1 - (\lambda_o/2a)^2}$$
$$= 3.87 \text{ cm}$$
$$d = 0.97 \text{ cm}$$

The electrical distance at one end of the band θ_1 is

$$\beta_1 d = \theta_1$$

$$\theta_1 = 87.43° = 2\pi d/\lambda_{g_1}$$

$$= 360 \times 0.97/\lambda_{g_1}$$

$$\lambda_{g_1} = 360 \times 0.97/87.43° = \textbf{3.994 cm}$$

$$= \lambda_1/\sqrt{1-(\lambda_1/2a)^2}$$

Here λ_1 is the wavelength at f_1.

$$1-(\lambda_1/4.8)^2 = (\lambda_1/\lambda_{g_1})^2;$$

$$(\lambda_1/\lambda_{g_1})^2 + (\lambda_1/4.8)^2 = 1;$$

$$\lambda_1^2 = \textbf{9.43}$$

$$\lambda_1 = \textbf{3.07 cm}$$

$$f_1 = c/\lambda_1 = 30/3.07 = \textbf{9.772 GHz}$$

$$f_o = \textbf{10 GHz}$$

$$\theta_2 = \pi - \theta_1 = 180° - 87.43° = 92.57°$$

$$\beta_2 d = \theta_2$$

$$\lambda_{g_2} = 2\pi d/\theta_2 = 360 \times 0.97/92.57$$

$$= \textbf{3.772 cm}$$

$$\lambda_2^2[(1/2a)^2 +(1/\lambda_{g_2})^2] = 1; 0.1231\,\lambda_2^2 = 1$$

$$\lambda_2 = \textbf{2.966 cm}$$

$$f_2 = c/\lambda_2 = 30/2.966 = \textbf{10.115 GHz}$$

Hence the bandwidth is given by

$$\Delta f = f_2 - f_1$$

$$= 10.115 - 9.772 = \textbf{0.343 GHz}$$

To find r_o: The phase constant β_{10} for TE_{10} is

$$\beta_{10} = \sqrt{k_0^2 -(\pi/a)^2} = \textbf{1.6348}$$

$$C = (4/3)\,(\beta_{10}\,r_o^3/ab)\,[1 + 1/2\,(\lambda_{go}/\lambda_o)^2]$$

$$= (4/3)\,(1.6348\,r_o^3)\,[1 + 1/2\,(3.87/3)^2]$$

$$= \textbf{3.993}\,r_o^3$$

$$r_o = (C/3.993)^{1/3}$$

The radii of the holes are

$$r_{o1} = r_{o3} = (C_1/3.993\}^{1/3}$$

$$= (0.025/3.993)^{1/3} = \textbf{0.185 cm}$$

$$r_{o2} = (C_2/3.993\}^{1/3} = (0.049/3.993)^{1/3}$$

$$= \textbf{0.23 cm}$$

Hole spacing $d = \lambda_{go}/4 = \textbf{0.97 cm}$

Example 7.8: Design a 4-hole 30 dB directional coupler with Tchebychev distribution for $r = 2$.

Solution: $C = 10^{-30/20} = 10^{-1.5}$

$$= \textbf{0.03162} = 26\,C_m$$

from Table 7.2.

$$C_m = 0.03162/26 = \textbf{1.22} \times 10^{-3}$$

$$C_1 = C_5 = 4C_m = \textbf{4.88} \times 10^{-3}$$

$$C_2 = C_4 = 9C_m = \textbf{10.98} \times 10^{-3}$$

$$D = -C + 20 \log 1/C_m$$

$$= -30 + 58.27 = \textbf{28.27 dB}$$

Example 7.9: For the rat-race hybrid coupler, (a) calculate the input admittance at port 1 when all the other ports are matched, (b) when input is fed at port 1, find signal distribution in all other ports, (c) if input is fed to port 3 and all other ports are matched, find power distribution in all other ports.

Solution: (a) The admittance matrix with all ports matched is given by

$$\begin{pmatrix} I_1 \\ I_2 \\ I_3 \\ I_4 \end{pmatrix} = \frac{j}{\sqrt{2}} \begin{pmatrix} 0 & 0 & 1 & 1 \\ 0 & 0 & 1 & -1 \\ 1 & 1 & 0 & 0 \\ 1 & -1 & 0 & 0 \end{pmatrix} \begin{pmatrix} V_1 \\ V_2 \\ V_3 \\ V_4 \end{pmatrix} \quad \text{(i)}$$

When all ports except port 1 are match-terminated by normalized impedance $z_0 = 1$, we get

$$V_2 = -I_2 z_0 = -I_2$$

$$V_3 = -I_3 z_0 = -I_3$$

$$V_4 = -I_4 z_0 = -I_4$$

Hence, substituting for V_2, V_3, V_4 in Eq. (i)

$$\begin{pmatrix} I_1 \\ I_2 \\ I_3 \\ I_4 \end{pmatrix} = \frac{j}{\sqrt{2}} \begin{pmatrix} 0 & 0 & 1 & 1 \\ 0 & 0 & 1 & -1 \\ 1 & 1 & 0 & 0 \\ 1 & -1 & 0 & 0 \end{pmatrix} \begin{pmatrix} V_1 \\ -I_2 \\ -I_3 \\ -I_4 \end{pmatrix} \quad \text{(ii)}$$

From Eq. (ii), we obtain

$$I_1 = -j/\sqrt{2}\,(I_3 + I_4) \quad \text{(iii)}$$

$$I_2 = -j/\sqrt{2}\,(I_3 - I_4) \quad \text{(iv)}$$

$$I_3 = -j/\sqrt{2}\,(-V_1 + I_2) \tag{v}$$

$$I_4 = -j/\sqrt{2}\,(-V_1 - I_2) \tag{vi}$$

Adding Eqs (v) and (vi), we get

$$I_3 + I_4 = -j/\sqrt{2}\,(-2V_1) = (j/\sqrt{2})\,V_1 \tag{vii}$$

Substituting Eq. (vii) in Eq. (iii), we get

$$I_1 = (-j/\sqrt{2})\,(j/\sqrt{2})\,(2V_1) = V_1$$

$$I_1/V_1 = Y_1 = 1 = \text{(normalized admittance at port 1}$$

Thus, port 1 is also matched if all other ports are matched.

(b) **Input to port 1:** The S-matrix is given by

$$\begin{pmatrix} b_1 \\ b_2 \\ b_3 \\ b_4 \end{pmatrix} = \frac{-j}{\sqrt{2}} \begin{pmatrix} 0 & 0 & 1 & 1 \\ 0 & 0 & 1 & -1 \\ 1 & 1 & 0 & 0 \\ 1 & -1 & 0 & 0 \end{pmatrix} \begin{pmatrix} a_1 \\ 0 \\ 0 \\ 0 \end{pmatrix}$$

$$\therefore \quad b_1 = b_2 = 0;$$
$$P_1 = P_2 = 0$$

$$b_3 = -ja_1/\sqrt{2}\,;$$
$$P_3 = |b_3|^2 = |a_1|^2/2$$

$$b_4 = -ja_1/\sqrt{2}\,;$$
$$P_4 = |b_4|^2 = |a_1|^2/2$$

Thus input power at port 1 equally splits into port 3 and port 4. No power is reflected to port 1 and no output at 4.

(c) **Input to port 3:** The S-matrix is

$$\begin{pmatrix} b_1 \\ b_2 \\ b_3 \\ b_4 \end{pmatrix} = \frac{-j}{\sqrt{2}} \begin{pmatrix} 0 & 0 & 1 & 1 \\ 0 & 0 & 1 & -1 \\ 1 & 1 & 0 & 0 \\ 1 & -1 & 0 & 0 \end{pmatrix} \begin{pmatrix} 0 \\ 0 \\ a_3 \\ 0 \end{pmatrix}$$

$$b_1 = (-j/\sqrt{2})a_3$$

$$P_1 = |b_1|^2 = |a_3|^2/2$$

$$b_2 = (-j/\sqrt{2})\,a_3$$

$$P_2 = |b_2|^2 a_3 = |a_3|^2/2a$$

$$b_3 = b_4 = 0$$

$$\therefore \quad P_3 = P_4 = 0$$

The input power at port 3 equally splits into ports 1 and 2. No power is reflected to port 3 and no output in port 4.

KEY POINTS

- Microwave passive devices are microwave isolators, circulators, directional couplers and power dividers
- An isolator is a two-port non-reciprocal microwave transmission device used to isolate one component from loading the other component.
- An ideal isolator completely absorbs the power propagated in one direction and transmits the signal power without any attenuation in the opposite direction. Therefore the isolator is also known as uniline.
- A microwave circulator is a multi-port device in which the wave can flow from the i-th port to $(i+1)$th port in one direction.
- The most common types of microwave circulators are 4-port and 3-port circulators.
- A directional coupler is a four-port waveguide junction used for coupling a known part of the microwave power to a port in the secondary waveguide, called a coupled port, while free transmission of power takes place from the input port to the output port in the primary line. No power reaches the fourth port, called isolated port. All ports of the directional couplers are matched.
- If the power flows in a forward direction in the secondary waveguide, then these directional couplers are known as forward directional couplers.
- In a backward directional coupler, power flows in the reverse or backward direction in the secondary wave-guide.
- Directional couplers are used (i) to measure transmitted power, (ii) in reflectometers to measure power in both directions and (iii) to measure VSWR.
- A power divider is a device that splits the input power into a number of smaller amounts of power at multiple N-ports.
- A power combiner is a device that combines the powers from multiple ports into a large amount of power at a single port.

FURTHER READING

1. Altman JL (1962). *Microwave Circuits*, Van Nostrand, NJ.

2. Chodorov M and Susskind C (1964). *Fundamentals of Microwave Electronics*, McGraw-Hill, NY.

3. Das A and Das SK (2004). *Microwave Engineering*, TMH, New Delhi.

4. Harvey AF. *Microwave Engineering*, Acad Press, NY, 1963

5. Liao SY (2000). *Microwave Devices and Circuits*, PHI, New Delhi.

REVIEW QUESTIONS

7.1 What is an isolator? Give its use.

7.2 What is a uniline? Why is it so called?

7.3 Mention the two types of isolators.

7.4 Give the S-matrix of an ideal loss-less matched isolator.

7.5 What is a circulator? Give its use.

7.6 Give the S-matrix of a matched loss-less and nonreciprocal 4-port circulator.

7.7 Distinguish between 4-port and 3-port circulators.

7.8 Give the S-matrix of a matched loss-less non reciprocal 3-port circulator.

7.9 What is a direction coupler?

7.10 Mention four important types of directional couplers.

7.11 Mention the characteristic of an ideal directional coupler.

7.12 Distinguish between forward and backward direction couplers. Give an example of each.

7.13 What are the important parameters of directional couplers?

7.14 Define mainline VSWR of a directional coupler.

7.15 Define the auxiliary line VSWR of a directional coupler.

7.16 Define the coupling coefficient of a directional coupler.

7.17 Define the mainline insertion loss of a directional coupler.

7.18 Define the directivity of a directional coupler.

7.19 What is a Bethe-hole directional coupler? Mention the two types.

7.20 What is a two-hole directional coupler?

7.21 What is a multi-hole coupler? How is it superior to two-hole coupler?

7.22 What is a binomial coupler?

7.23 What is a Tchebyshev coupler?

7.24 Mention the various steps in the design of multi-hole couplers.

7.25 Mention the use of coupled line coupler.

7.26 What is a multi-section coupler? What are its advantages?

7.27 What is the advantage of branch line coupler?

7.28 What is a hybrid ring or rat race coupler?

7.29 How many ports are there in hybrid ring? Give the spacing between them.

7.30 Give the S-matrix of a hybrid ring.

7.31 What is the merit of a Schwinger reversed phase coupler?

7.32 What is a long slot coupler?

7.33 What is a Lange coupler?

7.34 What is a capacitance loop coupler?

7.35 Give the S-matrix of a directional coupler.

7.36 Mention the applications of directional couplers.

7.37 What is a 3 dB coupler?

7.38 What is the value of transmission loss in a 3 dB coupler?

7.39 What is a power divider and power combiner?

7.40 What is a 3 dB power divider?

7.41 Write down the S-matrix of a 3 dB power divider.

DESCRIPTIVE QUESTIONS

7.1 What is Faraday rotation? Explain, with the help of appropriate diagram, the working of Faraday rotation isolator.

7.2 What is a resonance isolator? Explain, with the help of appropriate diagram, the working of a resonance isolator.

7.3 Derive the S-matrix of an ideal loss-less N-port circulator.

7.4 Explain, with a neat sketch, the construction and operation of the 4-port circulator using magic tees.

7.5 Explain the construction and operation of a 4-port circulator using directional coupler.

7.6 Explain the construction and operation of a 3-port circulator. Mention its uses.

7.7 Define and explain the important parameters of directional couplers.

7.8 Define coupling factor and directivity of a directional coupler. Give the significance of these terms.

7.9 Mention the various types of directional couplers. Describe any two in detail.

7.10 Explain the coupling mechanism in a Bethe-hole directional coupler and two-hole directional coupler.

7.11 Give the general design procedure of binomial directional coupler and the design procedure for $r = 2$.

7.12 Give the general design procedure of Tchebychev directional coupler and the design procedure for $r = 2$.

7.13 Prove that a loss-less reciprocal three-port network cannot be matched at all the three ports.

7.14 Explain a 3 dB power divider.

7.15 Derive the S-matrix of a 3 dB power divider.

PRACTICE PROBLEMS

7.1 Show that the S-matrix of an ideal isolator without loss in the direction from arm 1 to arm 2 is given by
$$[S] = \begin{pmatrix} 0 & 0 \\ 1 & 0 \end{pmatrix}$$

7.2 Show that the S-matrix of an ideal Y-circulator is given by
$$[S] = \begin{pmatrix} 0 & 0 & 1 \\ 1 & 0 & 0 \\ 0 & 1 & 0 \end{pmatrix}$$

7.3 Find the S-matrix of an isolator with 0.5 dB insertion loss and 25 dB isolation.
(**Ans:** $S_{11} = S_{22} = 0$; $S_{12} = 0.0562$; $S_{21} = 0.944$)

7.4 Find the S-matrix of a 3-port circulator having an insertion loss of 1 dB, isolation loss of 30 dB and VSWR of 1.5.
(**Ans:** $S_{11} = S_{22} = S_{33} = 0.2$; $S_{12} = S_{23} = S_{31} = 0.032$; $S_{13} = S_{21} = S_{32} = 0.89$)

7.5 A matched isolator has insertion loss of 0.5 dB and isolation loss of 25 dB. Find its S-matrix.
(**Ans:** $S_{11} = S_{22} = 0$, $S_{12} = 10^{-1.2}$, $S_{21} = 10^{-0.025}$)

7.6 A rectangular wave-guide with $a = 2b = 2.4$ cm is operating at 10 GHz. Design a maximally flat 20 dB directional coupler so that $D \geq 40$ dB in the band ratio of 2.
(**Ans:** $d = 0.961$ cm; $r_o^1 = r_o^8 = 0.0803$ cm; $r_o^2 = r_o^7 = 0.1588$ cm; $r_o^3 = r_o^6 = 0.2290$ cm; $r_o^4 = r_o^5 = 0.2715$ cm)

7.7 Design a 3-hole center-hole Tchebyshev coupler with $C = 20$ dB and $D = 40$ dB at $f = 10$ GHz. The wave-guide dimensions are $a = 2b = 2.4$ cm. Find the frequency band.
(**Ans:** d = 0.96 cm; $r_o^1 = r_o^3 = 0.263$ cm; $r_o^2 = 0.329$ cm; $r = 1.104$ GHz)

7.8 Design a 5-hole 30 dB directional coupler with Tchebychev distribution for $r = 2$.
(**Ans:** $C_1 = C_5 = 2.608 \times 10^{-3}$; $C_2 = C_4 = 7.824 \times 10^{-3}$; $C_5 = 1.0758 \times 10^{-2}$; $D = 39.74$ dB)

7.9 The specifications for a directional coupler give the directivity as 40 dB, the coupling as 10 dB and the transmission loss as 1 dB. For a power input of 5 mW at port 1, determine the power delivered at each of the other ports.
(**Ans:** $P_2 = 4.5$ mW, $P_3 = 0.5$ mW, $P_4 = 0.5$ mW)

7.10 The specifications for a directional coupler give the directivity as 40 dB, the coupling as 20 dB and the transmission loss as 0.4 dB. For a power input of 1 mW at port 1, determine the power delivered at each of the other ports. Also determine the power dissipated in the primary arm in dB relative to the input power.
(**Ans:** $P_2 = 0.912$ mW, $P_3 = 0.1$ mW, $P_4 = 10$ mW; −10.6 dBm)

7.11 A rectangular waveguide binomial coupler has 5 circular holes in the common side/narrow wall to produce 30 dB coupling at 10 GHZ. The guide width $a = 2.5$ cm and height $b = 1.2$ cm. The dominant input mode of unit amplitude radiates a field of amplitude $(4/3)$ $(r_o^3/ab\beta)$ $(\pi/a)^2$ in both directions in the other guide. Determine the required hole radii and the frequency ratio for which the directivity is greater than 50 dB.
(**Ans:** $r_{01} = 0.1677$ cm, $r_{02} = 0.26625$ cm, $r_{03} = 0.3047$ cm, $r = 1.074$)

REFERENCE

1. Liao SY (1985). *Microwave Solid State Devices*, PH. N.J.

2. Atwater HA (1962). *Introduction to Microwave Theory*, McGraw Hill, NY.

3. Collins RE (1996). *Foundations of Microwave Engineering*, McGraw Hill, NY.

4. Gandhi OP (1981). *Microwave Engineering and Applications*, Pergamon, NY.

5. Ghose RN (1963). *Microwave Circuit Theory and Analysis*, McGraw Hill, NY.

6. Lebedev I (1973). *Microwave Engineering*, MIR Publications, Moscow.

7. Montogomery CG et al (1948). *Principles of Microwave Circuits*, McGraw Hill, NY.

8. Pozar DM (1990). *Microwave Engineering*, Addison-Wesley, Mass.

9. Reich HJ et al (1953). *Microwave Theory and Techniques*, Van Nostrand, NJ.

10. Roddy D (1999). *Microwave Technology*, PH, NJ.

11. Roy SK and Mitra M (2003). *Microwave Semiconductor Devices*, PHI, New Delhi.

12. Seeger JA (1988). *Microwave Theory Components and Devices*, PH, NJ.

13. Veley VF (1987). *Modern Microwave Technology*, PH., N.J.

14. Wheeler GJ (1963). *Introduction to Microwave*, Englewood Cliffs, NJ.

15. Wolff EA and Kaul R (1988). *Microwave Engineering and Systems*, John Wiley, NY.

16. Terman FE (1955). *Electronic and Radio Engineering*, McGraw Hill Intl.

17. Reich HJ (1978). *Microwave Principles*, East-West, New Delhi.

18. Rizzi PA. *Microwave Engineering:* Passive Circuits, PH, NJ.

19. Soohoo RF (1971). *Microwave Electronics*, Addison-Wesley, Mass.

■ Microwave Resonators

Objectives

- Know the resonator types and parameters.
- Classify the various cavity resonator types.
- Understand the various quality factors associated with cavity resonators.
- Familiarize the applications of cavity resonators.

8.1 INTRODUCTION

Resonators are tuned circuits used at microwave frequencies. At low frequencies, less than 300 MHz, lumped inductances and capacitances are used to construct the tuned circuits. However, at higher frequencies beyond 300 MHz, lumped inductances and capacitances cannot be used because:

(i) Inductance and capacitance values are too small to use.

(ii) Losses due to skin effect increase.

To overcome these difficulties, coaxial and transmission line sections, rectangular and circular waveguides are employed as resonators. These are closed metallic cavities.

Any space enclosed by conducting walls possesses a resonant frequency for each particular type of field that can exist in the space. Resonators of this type are known as *cavity resonators*. Thus, a cavity resonator is a metallic enclosure that confines the electromagnetic energy. Electric and magnetic energies are stored in the cavity resonators. The stored electric energy inside the cavity determines the equivalent capacitance and the stored magnetic energy inside the cavity determines the equivalent inductance. The energy dissipated by the finite conductivity of the cavity walls determines the equivalent resistance. Thus, an LCR resonant circuit is formed. At resonance, the average energy stored in the electric field or the capacitor is maximum and is equal to W_e and the average energy stored in the magnetic field or the inductor is maximum and is equal to W_m and both the energies are equal. The mode having the lowest resonant frequency is known as *dominant mode*.

8.2 RESONATOR PARAMETERS

The important parameters of resonators are:
(i) Resonant frequency, (ii) Input impedance, (iii) Quality factor

(i) **Resonant frequency:** The resonant frequency of a resonator is that frequency at which the total energy stored in the cavity is maximum and is equal to $2W_e$ or $2W_m$. W_e is the the electric energy and W_m is the magnetic energy.

The circuit impedance of a resonator is then purely resistive.

(ii) *Input impedance*: The input impedance of the resonator corresponds to the parallel resonant impedance of a tuned circuit. At resonant frequency, the circuit impedance is purely resistive.

(iii) *Quality factor Q*: The quality factor Q of a resonator is the capacity of the resonant circuit for storing the electromagnetic energy. It is proportional to the ratio of maximum energy stored to the energy dissipated per cycle. It is given by

$Q = 2\pi$ (*maximum energy stored*)/*energy dissipated per cycle*

It is also a measure of frequency selectivity of the cavity. The *selectivity* is defined as the ratio of the resonant frequency to the bandwidth. Thus,

Selectivity = Resonant frequency/Bandwidth

$$= f_r/(f_1 - f_2) = f_r/\Delta_f = Q$$

since $(f_1 - f_2) = f_r/Q$ \hfill (8.1)

Thus, the quality factor Q is directly proportional to the selectivity at the resonant frequency $f_r \cdot \Delta_f = (f_1 - f_2)$ is the 3 dB bandwidth. In order to obtain high Q, the resonant circuit is made highly reactive. Values of Q as high as 10,000 can be achieved with microwave resonators.

8.2.1 Advantages of MW Resonators

The advantages of microwave resonators are:
 (i) Reasonable dimensions
 (ii) Simplicity
 (iii) Remarkably high Q
 (iv) Very high shunt impedance.

8.3 RESONATOR TYPES

A cavity resonator can be formed by an enclosed surface, irrespective of irregular outline. Therefore, it can take many forms. The important types of cavity resonators are:

 (i) Coaxial cavity resonators
 (ii) Rectangular cavity resonators
 (iii) Circular cavity resonators
 (iv) Semi-circular cavity resonators
 (v) Reentrant cavity resonators
 (vi) Hole-and-slot cavity resonators

A spherical cavity is also of interest from a theoretical point of view but not very useful in practice.

8.4 COAXIAL CAVITY RESONATOR

The coaxial cavity resonators are sections of coaxial lines with either open or short circuited at the ends. The three types of coaxial cavity resonators are:

 (i) Quarter-wave coaxial cavity resonator with one end short circuited and the other end open
 (ii) Half-wave coaxial cavity resonator with both ends shorted
 (iii) Capacitive end coaxial cavity resonator

Figure 8.1 shows these cavities with their field configurations and equivalent circuits.

We shall discuss the method of obtaining the length l for coaxial resonators for the three types.

 (i) *Quarter-wave coaxial cavity resonator*: This type of resonator has one end shorted and the other end open. As this resonator behaves like a parallel resonant circuit, the current at resonance is zero. Thus,

$$I = V/jZ_0 \tan \beta l = 0$$

Since the characteristic impedance is finite, the only possibility is that $\tan \beta l = \infty$.

or, $\qquad \beta l$ = odd multiples of $\pi/2$

$$= (2n - 1)\pi/2, n = 1, 2, 3, \ldots$$

Since $\beta = 2\pi/\lambda$,

$$l = (\lambda/2\pi)(2n - 1)\,\pi/2$$

$$= (2n - 1)\lambda/4$$

for $\qquad n = 1, 2, 3$ \hfill (8.2)

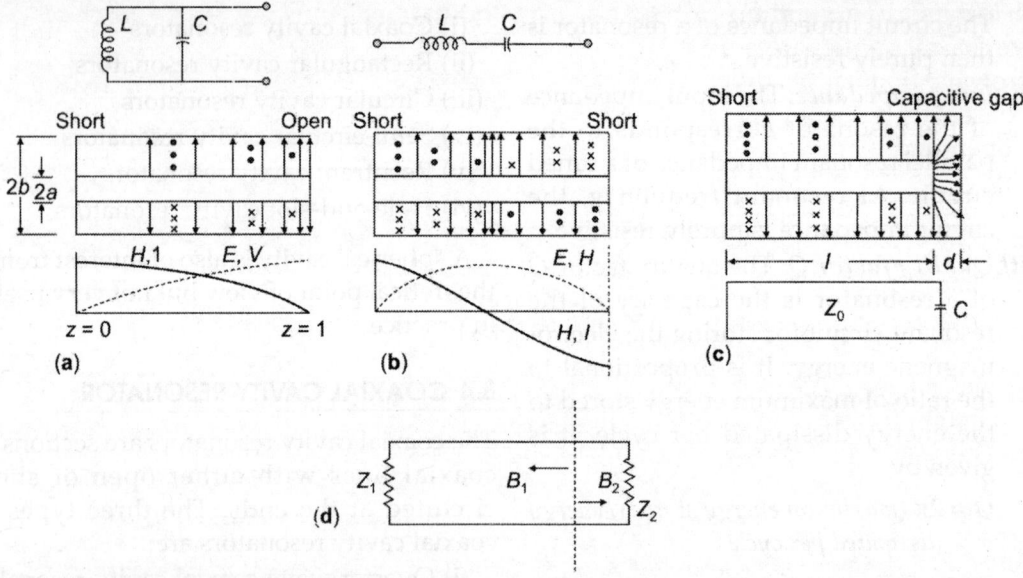

Fig. 8.1: Coaxial cavities (a) Quarter-wave (b) Half-wave (c) Capacitive end cavity (d) Equivalent circuit

Thus, the quarter-wave coaxial cavity is equivalent to parallel resonant circuit shown in Fig. 8.1(a) and the resonance occurs at frequencies at which the length of the cavity is an odd multiple of $\lambda/4$.

(ii) *Half-wave coaxial cavity resonator*: This type of resonator is shorted at both ends. As this resonator behaves like a series resonant circuit, the current at resonance is infinity. Thus,

$$I = V/jZ_0 \tan \beta l = \infty$$

Since the characteristic impedance is finite, the only possibility is that $\tan \beta l = 0$.

or, βl = odd multiples of π

$$= (2n-1)\pi , \, n = 1, 2, 3, ...$$

Since $\beta = 2\pi/\lambda$,

$$l = (\lambda/2\pi)(2n-1)\pi$$

$$= (2n-1)\lambda/2 \text{ for } n = 1,2,3 \quad (8.3)$$

Thus, the half-wave coaxial cavity is equivalent to series resonant circuit shown in Fig. 8.1(b) and the resonance occurs at frequencies at which the length of the cavity is an odd multiple of $\lambda/2$.

(iii) *Capacitive end coaxial cavity resonator*: This type of resonator has one end shorted and a capacitive gap at the other end. Parallel resonance occurs at frequencies at which the total circuit susceptance is zero. Thus, at resonance,

$$\omega_1 C = 1/(Z_0 \tan \beta l$$

or, $\beta l = \tan^{-1}(1/Z_0 w_r C)$

Since $\beta = 2\pi/\lambda$,

$$l = (\lambda/2\pi) \tan^{-1}(1/Z_0 \omega_r C) \quad (8.4)$$

Z_0 is the characteristic impedance of the coaxial cable and C is the gap capacitance between the center conductor and the open end as shown in Fig. 8.1(c). The electric field in the gap will be very large if d is made very small. This results in strong interaction between the electron beam passing through the gap and the MW field. This type of resonators find extensive use in MW amplifiers and oscillators. The higher order modes in all the coaxial cavities in **TEM** modes are avoided by restricting the dimensions a and b of the cavities to $\pi (a + b) < \lambda$.

The power loss in the coaxial cavity depends on the diameters of the coaxial cavities. Hence, the quality factor Q varies with b/a and is a maximum at $b/a = 3.6$. Half-wave coaxial cavities are preferred for use at microwave frequencies to the quarter-wave coaxial cavity because of radiation loss from the open end of the quarter-wave coaxial cavity.

The capacitive end coaxial cavity is tuned by

(i) Changing the gap length d with a capacitive ridge at a fixed cavity length l. This is known as *capacitive tuning*.

(ii) Varying the length l by a variable short-circuit plunger at a fixed gap length d. This is known as *inductive tuning*.

8.5 WAVEGUIDE CAVITY RESONATORS

Figure 8.2 shows the different types of cavity resonators. The simplest waveguide cavity resonator consists of a section of rectangular or circular waveguide short-circuited at both ends to form a rectangular or circular prism respectively. From the wave equations that satisfy the boundary conditions, the field components within the cavity are computed. Modes in a cavity are classified as transverse electric (**TE**) or transverse magnetic (**TM**)

modes, analogous to waveguide modes. The particular mode of such a class is then commonly designated by *three subscripts*. Thus, the field configuration, shown in Fig. 8.2(b), is the **TM**$_{010}$ mode. **TM** denotes that the magnetic field lies in a plane transverse to the axis of the cylinder, the first and third subscripts denote that the variation of the magnetic field is zero with radial direction and with position along the axis, and the second subscript indicates that there is one-half cycle of variation in the field along the radial line passing from one edge of the cylinder to the other edge. The field configuration shown in Fig. 8.2(c) is the **TE**$_{101}$ mode in that the electric field is transverse to an axis in the l-direction and that the variation of the electric field is one-half cycle, zero and one-half cycle in the a-, b- and l-directions respectively. Various **TE**$_{mnp}$ and **TM**$_{mnp}$ modes exist inside the cavity. Very high Q factors can be obtained with these resonators accompanied by narrow bandwidth.

8.5.1 Rectangular Cavity Resonators

The rectangular cavity resonator is a rectangular waveguide with two ends closed by

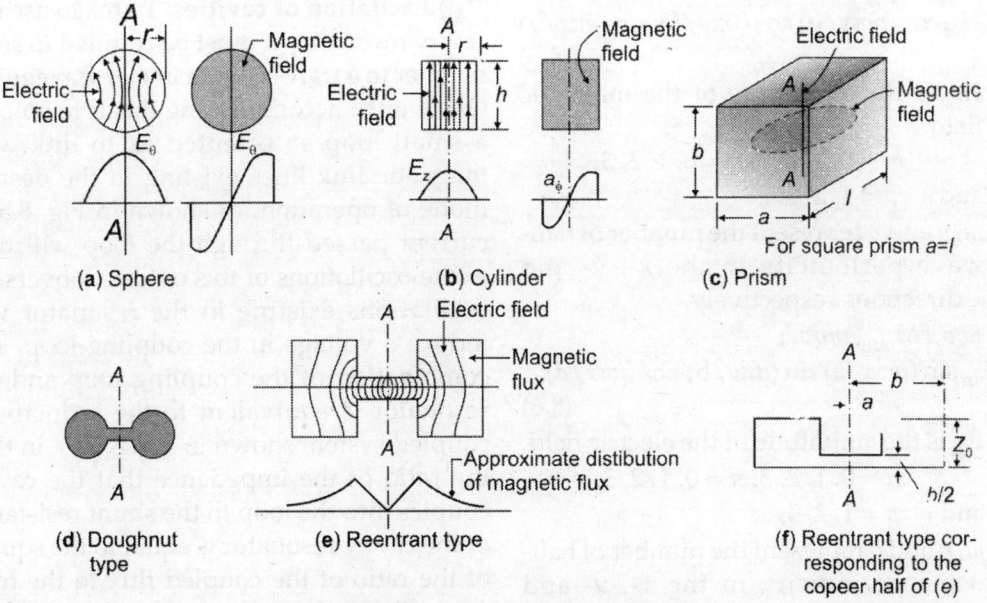

Fig. 8.2: Types of cavity resonators

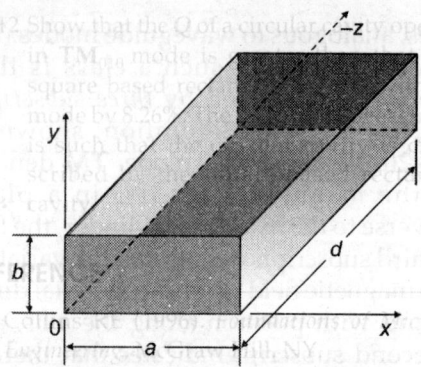

Fig. 8.3: Rectangular cavity resonator

a metal wall as shown in Fig. 8.3. The field inside the rectangular cavity should satisfy the Maxwell's equations with the following boundary conditions:

(i) The electric field tangential to the metal walls is zero

(ii) The magnetic field normal to the metal walls is also zero.

Since the boundary condition is zero tangential E at the four walls, the harmonic functions in z-direction is so chosen as to satisfy this condition at the remaining two end walls. Hence,

(i) *For TE_{mnp} mode:*

$$H_z = H_{0z} \cos(m\pi x/\alpha) \cos(n\pi y/b) \cdot \sin(p\pi z/d)$$
$$(8.5)$$

H_{0z} is the amplitude of the magnetic field.

$$m = 0, 1, 2, 3; n = 0, 1, 2, 3,$$
and $\quad p = 1, 2, 3, \ldots$

m, n and p represent the number of half-wave periodicity in the x-, y- and z-directions respectively.

(ii) *For TM_{mnp} mode:*

$$E_z = E_{0z} \sin(m\pi x/a) \sin(n\pi y/b) \cdot \cos(p\pi z/d)$$
$$(8.6)$$

E_{0z} is the amplitude of the electric field.

$$m = 0, 1, 2, 3; n = 0, 1, 2, 3,$$
and $\quad p = 1, 2, 3, \ldots$

m, n and p represent the number of half-wave periodicity in the x-, y- and z-directions respectively.

For both TE_{mnp} and TM_{mnp} modes, the separation equation is given by

$$k^2 = (m\pi/a)^2 + (n\pi/b)^2 + (p\pi/d)^2$$
$$(8.7)$$

$k_c^2 = \omega^2 \mu\varepsilon$ *for a lossless dielectric.* Therefore, the resonant frequency for both the TE_{mnp} and TM_{mnp} modes is given by

$$f_r = \frac{1}{2\sqrt{\mu\varepsilon}} \sqrt{\left(\frac{m}{a}\right)^2 + \left(\frac{n}{b}\right)^2 + \left(\frac{p}{d}\right)^2} \quad (8.8)$$

The dimensions of the resonant cavity determine the dominant mode. For $a > b < d$, the *dominant mode* is TE_{101} mode. Figure 8.4 shows the field configurations of the dominant mode.

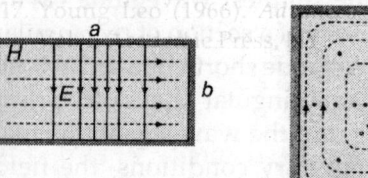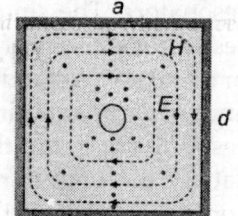

Fig. 8.4: Dominant mode (TE_{101})field configuration of a rectangular cavity

(i) **Excitation of cavities:** To make use of a cavity resonator, it must be coupled in some manner to a transmission line or waveguide. One way of accomplishing this is to employ a small loop so oriented as to link with magnetic flux lines existing in the desired mode of operation, as shown in Fig. 8.5. A current passed through the loop will then excite oscillations of this mode. Conversely, oscillations existing in the resonator will induce a voltage in the coupling loop. The combination of the coupling loop and the resonator is equivalent to the inductively coupled system shown in Fig. 8.5(b). In this, the ratio of the impedance that the cavity couples into the loop to the shunt resistance of the cavity resonator is equal to the square of the ratio of the coupled flux to the total magnetic flux lying to one side of the cylinder

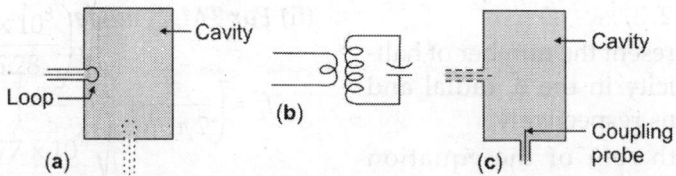

Fig. 8.5: Loop and probe coupling to cavity resonators

axis. The magnitude of the magnetic coupling can be readily controlled by the orientation of the loop and its location with respect
to the magnetic field. Thus, the coupling can
be reduced to zero when the plane of the loop
is rotated so that it is parallel to the magnetic
flux. The coupling will be low if the loop is
placed at a point of low magnetic flux
density. Thus, a loop near the vertical axis
as shown dotted in Fig. 8.5(a) will have zero
coupling to the dominant mode.

Coupling to the cavity can also be achieved
by means of a probe as shown in Fig. 8.5(c).
A voltage applied to the probe produces
electric fields inside the cavity that excite the
desired mode of oscillations. Thus, this is a
form of capacitive coupling. The magnitude
of the coupling is determined by (i) the
surface that the probe exposes to the electric
field of oscillations of the desired mode and
(ii) the intensity of the electric field at the
position of the probe. Thus, maximum coupling is obtained in a cylindrical cavity operating in the **TM$_{010}$** when the probe is located
on the axis as shown. The coupling to this
mode will be zero if the probe projects into
the cavity from the side wall as shown by
dotted lines.

(ii) **Tuning of cavities:** The cavity resonators are tuned mechanically
  (i) by moving a short-circuit plunger
      parallel to the axis. This changes the
      length of the cavity and hence the
      resonant frequency is changed.
  (ii) by inserting a metallic screw into the
       curved wall of the cavity. This increases
       the resonant frequency
  (iii) by placing a small plate at the center of
        the cavity and varying its position.

Hence the resonant frequency is changed.

8.5.2 Circular Cavity Resonators

Figure 8.6 shows a circular cavity resonator.
It consists of a circular waveguide with two
ends closed by a metal wall. The electromagnetic field inside the cavity should
satisfy the Maxwell's equations with the
following boundary conditions:
  (i) The electric field tangential to the metal
      walls is zero
  (ii) The magnetic field normal to the metal
       walls is also zero.

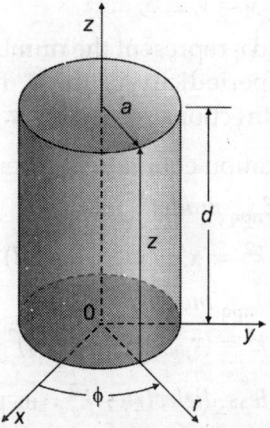

Fig. 8.6: Circular resonator

Since the boundary condition is zero
tangential E at four walls, the harmonic
functions in z is so chosen as to satisfy this
condition at the remaining two end walls.
Hence,

(i) *For TE$_{npq}$ mode:*
$$H_z = H_{0z} J_n (x'_{np} r / a) \cos (n\phi) \sin (q\pi z / d)$$
$$(8.9)$$

H_{0z} is the amplitude of the magnetic
field

J_n is the Bessel function of the first kind.

$n = 0, 1, 2, 3; p = 0, 1, 2, 3,$

and $q = 1, 2, 3, ...$

n, p and q represent the number of half-wave periodicity in the ϕ, radial and axial directions respectively.

x'_{np} is the p-th root of the equation $J_n(x'_{np}) = 0$. Some of the roots for various modes are given below:

TE_{01x} modes: $x'_{01} = 3.832$

TE_{11x} modes: $x'_{11} = 1.841$

TE_{12x} modes: $x'_{12} = 5.331$

TE_{21x} modes: $x'_{21} = 3.054$.

(ii) *For TM$_{npq}$ mode:*

$$E_z = E_{0z} J_n(x_{np}r/a) \cos(n\phi) \cos(q\pi z/d)$$
(8.10)

E_{0z} is the amplitude of the electric field.

J_n is the Bessell function of the first kind.

$$n = 0, 1, 2, 3; p = 0, 1, 2, 3,$$

and $q = 1, 2, 3, ...$

n, p and q represent the number of half-wave periodicity in the ϕ, radial and axial directions respectively.

The separation equation is given by

(i) *For TE$_{npq}$ mode:*

$$k^2 = (x'_{np}/a)^2 + (q\pi/d)^2$$
(8.11)

(ii) *For TM$_{npq}$ mode:*

$$k^2 = (x_{np}/a)^2 + (q\pi/d)^2$$
(8.12)

For a lossless dielectric, $k_c^2 = \omega^2 \mu \varepsilon$. Therefore, the resonant frequency is given by

(i) *For TE$_{npq}$ mode:*

$$f_r = \left(\frac{1}{2\pi\sqrt{\mu\varepsilon}}\right) \sqrt{\left(\frac{x'_{np}}{a}\right)^2 + \left(\frac{q\pi}{d}\right)^2} \text{ Hz}$$
(8.13)

(ii) *For TM$_{npq}$ mode:*

$$f_r = \left(\frac{1}{2\pi\sqrt{\mu\varepsilon}}\right) \sqrt{\left(\frac{x_{np}}{a}\right)^2 + \left(\frac{q\pi}{d}\right)^2} \text{ Hz}$$
(8.14)

x_{np} is the p-th root of the equation $J_n(x_{np}) = 0$. Some of the roots for various modes are given below:

TM_{01x} modes: $x_{01} = 2.405$

TM_{11x} modes: $x_{11} = 3.832$

TM_{12x} modes: $x_{12} = 5.520$

TM_{21x} modes: $x_{21} = 5.135$.

Table 8.1 shows the variation of frequency ratio $(f_r)_{npq} / (f_r)_{dominant}$ with $d/2a$ for different modes

From Table 8.1, it can be seen that, if $d/2a < 1$, the dominant mode is TM_{010} mode and, if $d/2a > 1$, the dominant mode is TE_{0111} mode.

8.5.3 Semicircular Cavity Resonator

In Fig. 8.7, a semicircular cavity resonator is shown. In the semicircular cavity resonator, the wave function is given by

(i) *For TE$_{npq}$ mode:*

$$H_z = H_{0z} J_n(x'_{np}r/a) \cos(n\phi) \sin(qpz/d)$$
(8.15)

H_{0z} is the amplitude of the magnetic field

J_n is the Bessell function of the first kind.

$$n = 0, 1, 2, 3; p = 0, 1, 2, 3,$$

and $q = 1, 2, 3, ...$

n, p and q represent the number of half-wave periodicity in the ϕ, radial and axial directions respectively.

Table 8.1: Variation of $(f_r)_{npq}/(f_r)_{dominant}$ with $d/2a$ for various modes of circular resonator

$d/2a$	TM_{010}	TE_{111}	TM_{110}	TM_{011}	TE_{211}	TM_{111}, TE_{011}
0.5	1.0	1.5	1.59	1.63	1.80	2.05
1.0	1.0	1.0	1.59	1.19	1.42	1.72
1.5	1.13	1.0	1.80	1.24	1.52	1.87

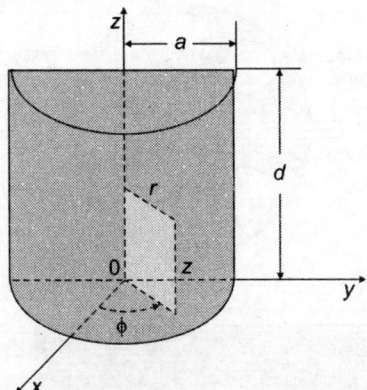

Fig. 8.7: Semicircular resonator

a = radius of the semicircular cavity resonator

d = length of the resonator

(ii) *For TM$_{npq}$ mode:*

$$E_z = E_{0z} J_n(x_{np}r/a) \sin(n\phi) \cos(qpz/d)$$
$$(8.16)$$

E_{0z} is the amplitude of the electric field.

J_n is the Bessell function of the first kind.

$$n = 0, 1, 2, 3; p = 0, 1, 2, 3$$
and $\quad q = 1, 2, 3, ...$

n, p and q represent the number of half-wave periodicity in the ϕ, radial and axial directions respectively.

The separation equation is given by

(i) *For TE$_{npq}$ mode:*

$$k^2 = (x'_{np}r/a)^2 + (q\pi/d)^2 \quad (8.17)$$

(ii) *For TM$_{npq}$ mode:*

$$k^2 = (x_{np}/a)^2 + (q\pi/d)^2 \quad (8.18)$$

For a lossless dielectric, $k^2 = \omega^2\mu\varepsilon$. Therefore, the resonant frequency is given by

(i) *For TE$_{npq}$ mode:*

$$f_r = \left(\frac{1}{2\pi a\sqrt{\mu\varepsilon}}\right)\sqrt{(x'_{np})^2 + \left(\frac{q\pi a}{d}\right)^2} \text{ Hz}$$
$$(8.19)$$

(ii) *For TM$_{npq}$ mode:*

$$f_r = \left(\frac{1}{2\pi a\sqrt{\mu\varepsilon}}\right)\sqrt{(x_{np})^2 + \left(\frac{q\pi a}{d}\right)^2} \text{ Hz}$$
$$(8.20)$$

The values n, p, and q for a semicircular cavity resonator differ from that of the circular cavity resonator. If $d > a$, TE_{111} mode is the dominant mode. If $d < a$, TE_{110} mode is the dominant mode.

8.5.4 Reentrant Cavity Resonator

A reentrant cavity resonator is that in which the opposite sides are brought closer together to form a reentrant structure. Several types of reentrant cavities are shown in Fig. 8.8. The most commonly used reentrant cavity is shown in Fig. 8.9 with field configurations. The electric field is concentrated in the small gap g. The cavity is tuned by means of short-circuit plungers. The reentrant cavity of length d and gap width $g \ll d$, may be considered as a coaxial line with radii of the inner and outer conductors as a and b. The characteristic impedance of the coaxial line is given by

$$Z_0 = \left(\frac{1}{2\pi}\right)\sqrt{\frac{\mu}{\varepsilon}} \ln(b/a)$$

$$= 60 \ln(b/a) \text{ for air dielectric} \quad (8.21)$$

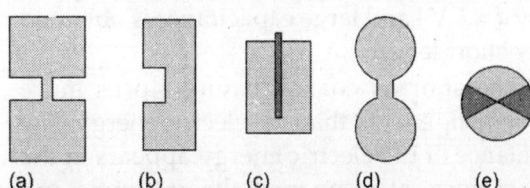

(a)   (b)   (c)   (d)   (e)

Fig. 8.8: Resonant cavity types (a) Coaxial (b) Radial (c) Tunable (d) Toroidal (e) Butterfly

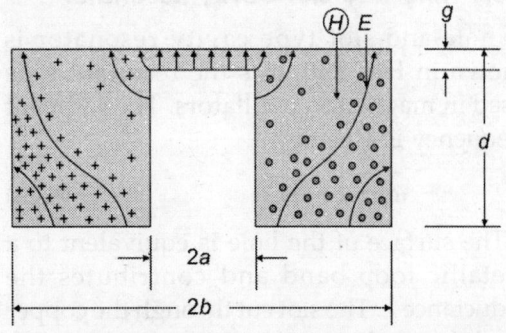

Fig. 8.9: Reentrant cavity with field configuration

The input impedance to each shorted coaxial line is given by

$$Z_{in} = jZ_0 \tan (2\pi d/\lambda_g) \qquad (8.22)$$

Substituting for Z_0 in the above equation, we obtain

$$Z_{in} = j\left(\frac{1}{2\pi}\right)\sqrt{\frac{\mu}{\varepsilon}} \ln\left(\frac{b}{a}\right) \tan\left(\frac{2\pi a}{\lambda_g}\right) \qquad (8.23)$$

The inductance of the cavity is given by

$$L = \frac{2X_{in}}{\omega} = \left(\frac{1}{\pi\omega}\right)\sqrt{\frac{\mu}{\varepsilon}} \ln\left(\frac{b}{a}\right) \tan\left(\frac{2\pi d}{\lambda_g}\right) \qquad (8.24)$$

The capacitance of the gap is given by

$$C = \varepsilon a^2 \pi/g \qquad (8.25)$$

At resonance, the gap capacitance C and the coaxial line below the gap provide equal and opposite reactance. Hence,

$$1/\omega_r C = Z_0 \tan (2\pi a/\lambda_g) \qquad (8.26)$$

The length d of the reentrant cavity resonator is

$$d = (\lambda_g/2\pi) \tan^{-1}(1/Z_0\omega_r C) \qquad (8.27)$$

For low capacitance, the length d is given by $d = \lambda_g/4$ and large capacitance is obtained by short length.

The shorted coaxial cavity stores more magnetic energy than the electric energy. The balance of the electric energy appears in the gap since, at resonance, the magnetic and electric energies are equal.

8.5.5 Hole-and-Slot Cavity Resonator

A hole-and-slot type cavity resonator is shown in Fig. 8.10. It is the reentrant type used in magnetron oscillators. The resonant frequency is given by

$$\omega_r = 1/\sqrt{LC} \qquad (8.28)$$

The surface of the hole is equivalent to a metallic loop band and contributes the inductance L. The slot cut through the copper block forms the capacitance gap.

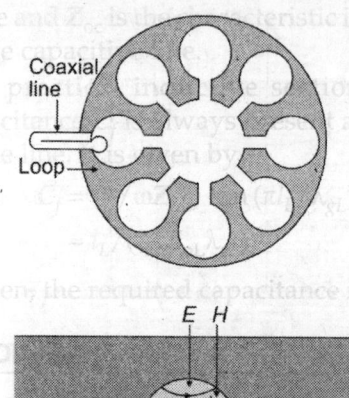

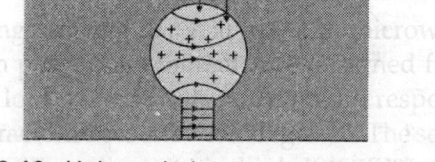

Fig. 8.10: Hole-and-slot type cavity with field configuration

8.6 QUALITY FACTOR OF CAVITIES

The *quality factor* Q of a cavity has the same significance as for conventional resonant circuit. It is defined as the ratio of maximum energy stored to the energy dissipated per cycle. It is also a measure of frequency selectivity of the cavity. It is, thus, given by

$$Q = 2\pi \,(maximum\ energy\ stored)/energy$$
$$dissipated\ per\ cycle$$
$$= \omega W/P$$
$$= f_r/\Delta f \qquad (8.29)$$

W is the maximum energy stored, P is the average power dissipated or loss, f_r is the resonant frequency and Δf is the 3 dB bandwidth. In order to obtain high Q, the circuit is made highly reactive. The energy stored is proportional to the square of the magnetic flux density integrated throughout the volume of the resonator while the energy lost per cycle in the walls is proportional to the skin depth and to the square of the magnetic flux density integrated over the surface of the cavity. Thus, to obtain high Q, the resonator should have a large volume to surface ratio since it is the volume that stores the energy and it is the surface area that dissipates the energy. As a result of this, resonators such as spheres, cylinders and prisms have higher Q's than reentrant resonators.

8.6.1 Unloaded Q-factor (Q_o)

The quality factor of a cavity, when it is not connected to any external circuit or load, is known as *unloaded Q-factor* (Q_o). At resonant frequency, the electric and magnetic energies are equal and in time quadrature. When the electric energy is at its maximum, the magnetic energy is at its minimum and *vice versa*. The total energy stored in the resonator is given by

$$W_e = \int_v (\varepsilon/2)\,|E|^2 dv$$
$$= W_m = \int_v (\mu/2)\,|H|^2 dv = W \quad (8.30)$$

$|E|$ and $|H|$ are the peak values of the electric and magnetic field intensities and v is the volume of the cavity.

The average power loss in the resonator is evaluated by integrating the power density over the inner surface of the resonator. Thus,

$$P = (R_s/2)\int_s |H_t|^2\,da \quad (8.31)$$

H_t is the peak value of the tangential magnetic intensity and R_s is the surface resistance of the resonator. Hence, Q_o is given by

$$Q_o = W/P$$
$$= \omega_r \mu \int_v |H|^2\,dv / (R_s \int_s |H_t|^2\,ds)$$
$$\quad (8.32)$$

The peak value of the magnetic intensity is related to its tangential and normal components and is given by

$$|H|^2 = |H_t|^2 + |H_n|^2$$

H_t is the tangential component and H_n is the normal component of the magnetic intensity. The value of the $|H_t|^2$ at the resonator walls is approximately twice the value of $|H|^2$ averaged over the volume. Hence Q is given by

$$Q = w_r \mu / 2R_s \quad (8.33)$$
$$= volume / surface\ area$$

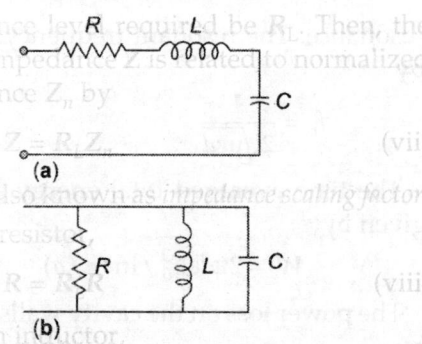

(a)

(b)

Fig. 8.11: Unloaded cavity equivalent circuit (a) Series (b) Parallel

As shown in Fig. 8.11, an unloaded cavity resonator can be represented by an equivalent series or parallel resonant circuit. The resonant frequency of the cavity resonator is

$$f_r = \frac{1}{2\pi\sqrt{LC}} \quad (8.34)$$

The unloaded Q_o is given by

$$Q_o^{'} = \omega_r L/R \quad (8.35)$$

In practical cavity resonators, there may be power loss due to

(i) Conductors, P_c

(ii) Dielectric fills, P_d

(iii) Radiation from the openings, P_r

Therefore, the unloaded Q_o is given by

$$Q_o = \omega_r W/P$$
$$= \omega_r W/(P_c + P_d + P_r) \quad (8.36)$$

Equation (8.36) may be written as

$$1/Q_o = P_c/\omega_r W + P_d/\omega_r W + P_r/\omega_r W$$
$$= 1/Q_c + 1/Q_d + 1/Q_r \quad (8.37)$$

where

$$Q_c = \omega_r W/P_c \quad (8.38)$$
$$Q_d = \omega_r W/P_d \quad (8.39)$$
$$Q_r = \omega_r W/P_r \quad (8.40)$$

(i) Coaxial cavity resonators: Short-circuiting the two ends of an air-filled coaxial line of length d forms a coaxial cavity resonator. The radii of the conductors, a and b, are such that only **TEM** mode exists at resonance. The resonant frequency is given by

$$f_r = \frac{1}{2\sqrt{\mu\varepsilon d}} \qquad (8.41)$$

The time averaged total energy stored is given by

$$W = 2\pi d\varepsilon E_0^2 / \ln(b/a) \qquad (8.42)$$

The power loss on the cavity walls is given by

$$P = \left(\frac{\pi R_s}{2}\right) \left[\frac{2E_o}{\eta \ln \dfrac{b}{a}}\right]^2 \left[\frac{d}{a} + \frac{d}{b} + 4\ln\frac{b}{a}\right] \qquad (8.43)$$

Hence,

$$Q_{\text{oTEM}} = \frac{\pi\eta \ln\left(\dfrac{b}{a}\right)}{\left[R_s\left(\dfrac{d}{a} + \dfrac{d}{b} + 4\ln\dfrac{b}{a}\right)\right]} \qquad (8.44)$$

(ii) **Rectangular cavity resonators:** The dominant mode in a rectangular cavity resonator of dimensions $a \times b \times d$ with $d > b > a$, is **TE$_{101}$** mode. The unloaded quality factor is given by

$$Q_{\text{oTE}_{101}} = \left(\frac{\pi\eta}{4R_s}\right) \frac{2b(a^2 + d^2)^{3/2}}{ad(a^2 + d^2) + 2b(a^3 + d^3)}$$
$$(8.45)$$

For a *square base cavity resonator*, $a = d$. Hence Q_o is maximum and is given by

$$Q_{\text{omax}} = 1.11 \frac{\sqrt{\mu/\varepsilon}}{[R_s(1 + a/2b)]} \qquad (8.46)$$

For an *air-filled cubic cavity resonator*, $a = b = d$. Hence Q_o is given by

$$Q_o = 0.74\eta/R_s = 279/R_s \qquad (8.47)$$

Example 8.1 A cube shaped cavity is required to resonate at 7.5 GHz in the **TE$_{101}$** mode. Determine its unloaded Q if the cavity is air-filled.

Solution: Given:

f_r =7.5 GHz in the **TE$_{101}$** mode.

(i) $f_r = c/a\sqrt{2\varepsilon_r}$

$a = c/f_r\sqrt{2\varepsilon_r}$

$= 3 \times 10^{10}/(7.5 \times 10^9 \times 1.414 \times 1)$

since air-filled.

$= \mathbf{2.828}$ cm

(ii) The unloaded Q is

$Q_U = 0.74\eta/R_s$

$= 0.74 \times 377/R_s$

$= 279/R_s$

$= 279/0.023$ (since $R_s = 0.023$ ohm per square)

$= \mathbf{12{,}130}$

The general expressions for Q_o for **TE$_{nmp}$** and **TM$_{mnp}$** is given by

(i) **For TE$_{mnp}$:**

$$Q_o = \frac{\eta\, abd\, k_c^2\, k^3}{4R_s[bd(k_c^2 + k_y^2 + k_z^2) + ad(k_c^2 + k_y^2 + k_z^2) + abk_c^2 k_z^2]} \qquad (8.48)$$

(ii) **For TM$_{mnp}$:**

$$Q_o = \frac{\eta\, abd\, k_c^2\, k}{4R_s[b(a + d)k_x^2 + a(b + d)k_y^2]} \qquad (8.49)$$

$k_x = m\pi/a,\ k_y = n\pi/b,\ k_x = p\pi/d,$

$k^2 = (k_x^2 + k_y^2 + k_z^2),\ k_c^2 = k_x^2 + k_y^2 \qquad (8.50)$

(iii) **Circular cavity resonators:** The three important modes of circular cavity resonator are **TM$_{010}$, TE$_{011}$** and **TE$_{111}$** modes. Consider a circular cavity resonator of radius a and length d, For $d/2a < 1$, the dominant mode is. **TM$_{010}$.** For $d/2a \geq 1$, the dominant mode is **TE$_{111}$. TE$_{011}$** mode is the ϕ-symmetric mode. Its Q is *two* to *three times* that of dominant modes and there is no axial current; i.e. $H_\phi = 0$.

(a) *Q for dominant TM$_{010}$ mode:* For this mode, $d < 2a$ and $n = 0, m = 1$ and $p = 0$. Hence, the resonant frequency from Eq. (8.14) is given by

$$f_r = x_{o1}/[2\pi a\sqrt{\varepsilon_o\mu_o}] \qquad (8.51)$$

The average stored energy is given by

$$W = (\varepsilon_o E_o^2/4)\pi da^2 J_1^2(x_{o1}) \qquad (8.52)$$

The total power loss is given by

$$P = (R_s E_o^2 / \eta^2) \, \pi a J_1^2(x_{01}) \, (a + d) \tag{8.53}$$

Hence, Q_o is given by

$$Q_o = x_{01} \eta / [2R_s (1 + a/d)] \tag{8.54}$$

For $p = 0$, $x_{01} = 2.405$. Therefore

$$Q_{TM_{010}} = 1.202 \, \eta / [R_s(1 + a/d)] \tag{8.55}$$

(b) Q for dominant TE$_{111}$ mode: For this mode, $d \geq 2a$ and $n = 1$, $m = 1$ and $p = 1$. The Q_o for this mode is given by

$$Q_{oTE_{111}} = \left(\frac{\lambda_o}{2\pi\delta_s}\right) \frac{[1 - (1/x_{11}')^2][(x_{11}')^2 + (\pi a/d)^2]^{3/2}}{\left[(x_{11}')^2 + 2\frac{a}{d}\left(\frac{\pi a}{d}\right)^2 + \left(1 - 2\frac{a}{d}\right)\left(\frac{\pi a}{x_{11}'d}\right)^2\right]} \tag{8.56}$$

Q_o varies inversely proportional to $\sqrt{f}$.

(c) Q for dominant TE$_{011}$ mode: The field distribution is ϕ independent and $n = 0$, $m = 1$ and $p = 1$. The Q_o for this mode is given by

$$Q_{oTE_{011}} = \left(\frac{\eta}{2R_s}\right) \frac{\left[\left(\frac{x_{01}'}{a}\right)^2 + \left(\frac{\pi}{d}\right)^2\right]^{3/2}}{\frac{1}{a}\left(\frac{x_{01}'}{a}\right)^2 + \left(\frac{2}{d}\right)\left(\frac{\pi}{d}\right)^2} \tag{8.57}$$

$$\eta = \sqrt{\mu / \varepsilon} \text{ and } R_s = \sqrt{\omega\mu / 2\sigma}$$

The variation of normalized value of $Q_o \delta_s / \lambda_o$ with $2a/d$ for several modes is shown in Fig. 8.12 for circular cavity resonators. Q_o varies inversely proportional to $\sqrt{f}$. From Fig. 8.12, it is seen that **TE$_{011}$** mode has higher Q_o compared to the dominant mode **TM$_{010}$** (for $2a/d > 1$) or **TE$_{111}$** (for $2a/d \leq 1$).

8.6.2 Advantages of TE$_{011}$ Mode

The advantages of **TE$_{011}$** mode are:

(i) The unloaded Q_o is *two* to *three times* that of **TE$_{111}$** mode.

(ii) There is no axial current on the walls since $H_\varphi = 0$.

(iii) For tuning purposes, a short-circuit plunger at one end can be moved freely without intersecting the current path.

(iv) There is no leakage of signal through the gap between the circular walls and the plunger plate.

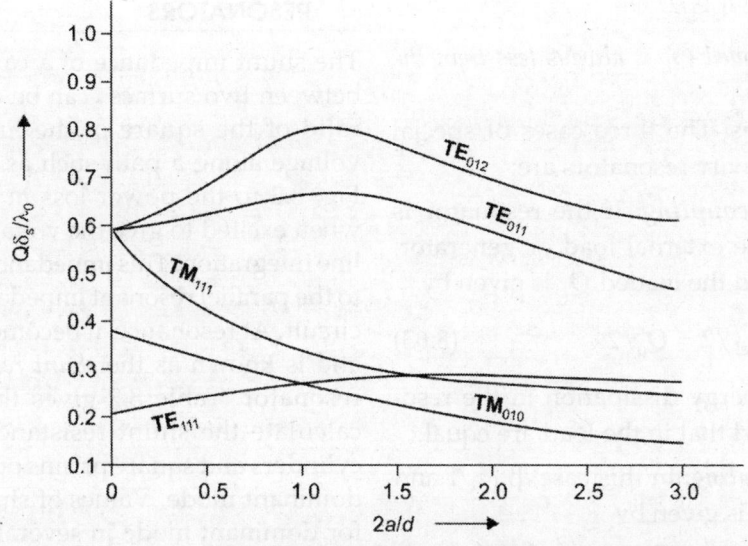

Fig. 8.12: Q_o of circular cavity

8.6.3 Loaded and External Q

Generally a cavity resonator is coupled to a generator and load by means of a slot in the common wall of the waveguide or coaxial line probe. Hence, the energy loss is calculated taking into account the loss due to external load or circuit. If the energy loss in the cavity per cycle is P_c and that due to external load is P_{el}, then the loaded quality factor Q_L is given by

$$Q_L = 2\pi \text{ (maximum energy stored)/}$$
$$\text{(Total energy loss)} \quad (8.58)$$

$$= \omega_r W/(P_c + P_{el})$$
$$= (P_c/\omega_r W) + (P_{el}/\omega_r W) \quad (8.59)$$

Eq.(8.59) may be written as

$$1/Q_L = 1/Q_o + 1/Q_{el} \quad (8.60)$$
$$1/Q_o = \omega_r W/P_c \quad (8.61)$$
$$1/Q_{el} = \omega_r W/P_{el} \quad (8.62)$$

Q_o is the unloaded Q and Q_{el} is the external load.

The load-coupling coefficient is given by

$$\beta_{el} = P_{el}/P_c$$
$$\therefore \quad Q_L = [\omega_r W/P_c]/(1 + \beta_{el})$$
$$= Q_o/(1 + \beta_{el})$$

Thus, *the loaded* Q_L *is always less than the unloaded* Q_o.

Special cases: The three cases of special interests for cavity resonators are:

(i) *Critical coupling*: If the resonator is matched to the external load or generator, then $\beta_{el} = 1$ and the loaded Q_L is given by

$$Q_L = Q_{el}/2 = Q_o/2 \quad (8.63)$$

Thus, the energy dissipation in the resonant cavity and that in the load are equal.

(ii) *Overcoupling*: In this case, $\beta_{el} > 1$ and the loaded Q_L is given by

$$Q_L = Q_o/(1 + \beta_{el}) < Q_o \quad (8.64)$$

The energy loss in the cavity walls is less than that in the load.

(iii) *Undercoupling*: In this case, $\beta_{el} < 1$ and the loaded Q_L is given by

$$Q_L = Q_o/(1 + \beta_{el}) < Q_o \quad (8.65)$$

The energy loss in the cavity walls is greater than that in the load.

When the resonator is matched with the generator, the SWR $S = \beta_{el} = 1$. When it is overcoupled, $S = \beta_{el}$ while it is undercoupled, $S = 1/\beta_{el}$. The variation of S with β_{el} is shown in Fig. 8.13.

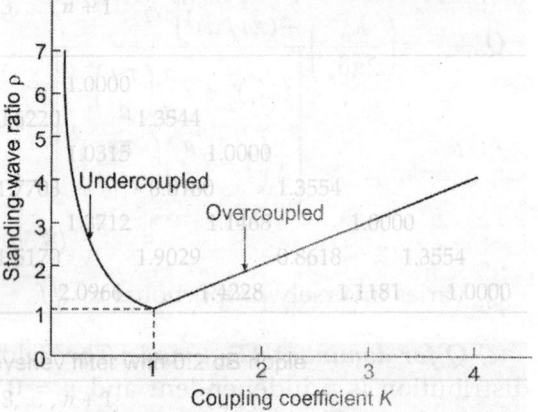

Fig. 8.13: Variation of SWR with coupling coefficient

8.7 SHUNT IMPEDANCE OF CAVITY RESONATORS

The shunt impedance of a cavity resonator between two surfaces can be defined as the ratio of the square of the line integral of voltage along a path such as *AA* shown in Fig. 8.2 to the power loss in the resonator when excited to give the voltage used in the line integration. This impedance corresponds to the parallel resonant impedance of a tuned circuit. At resonance, it becomes a resistance and is known as the *shunt resistance* of the resonator. Table 8.2 gives the formula to calculate the shunt resistance of spheres, cylinders and square prisms operating in the dominant mode. Values of shunt resistance for dominant mode in several typical cases are given in Table 8.3. It can be seen that it is

Table 8.2: Formulae for properties of cavity resonators for dominant mode

Cavity type	Wavelength λ_o	Q	R_s
Sphere	228 r	$0.318\lambda_o/\delta$	$104.4\lambda_o/\delta$
Cylinder	2.61 r	$0.383(\lambda_o/\delta)/[1+(r/h)]$	$72(h/r)(\lambda_o/\delta)/[1+(r/h)]$
Square prism	1.414 a	$0.353(\lambda_o/\delta)/[1+(a/2b)]$	$120(b/a)(\lambda_o/\delta)/[1+(a/2b)]$

(All dimensions are in cm, λ_o is the wavelength at resonance, d is the skin depth $=0.62/\sqrt{f}$)

Table 8.3: Properties of cavity resonators for dominant mode

Resonator type	Dimensions (cm)	Wavelength λ_o (cm)	Q (copper walls)	R_s MΩ (Cu walls)
Sphere	r = 5	11.4	28,000	9.7
Cylinder	r = h/2 = 5	13.0	24,000	9.1
Square prism	a = b = d = 10	14.1	23,000	7.8
Reentrant	a = 0.81, b = 1.69, d = 0.40	12.8	4,000	0.17

very large compared with shunt resistance obtainable with lumped resonant circuits. Although the shunt resistance of the reentrant cavity is much less than that of the other cavities, this shunt resistance is developed across such a short gap that the shunt resistance per unit length is of the same order of magnitude as the maximum value obtainable with other cavities.

8.8 NUMERICAL EXAMPLES

Example 8.1: Calculate the resonant frequency for TE_{101} mode of a rectangular cavity formed by shorting the ends with $a = 2$ cm, $b = 1$ cm and $d = 5$ cm.

Solution: Given: $a = 2$ cm, $b = 1$ cm, $d = 5$ cm, TE_{101} mode, $m = 1$, $n = 0$, $p = 1$

The resonant frequency for rectangular resonator is given by

$$f_r = \frac{\sqrt{(m/a)^2+(n/b)^2+(p/d)^2}}{(2\sqrt{\mu\varepsilon})}$$

$$= \left(\frac{3\times10^8}{2}\right)\sqrt{\left(\frac{1}{0.02}\right)^2+\left(\frac{1}{0.05}\right)^2}$$

$$= 1.5\times10^8\times\sqrt{2500+400}$$

$$= 1.5\times10^8\times53.85$$

$$= \textbf{8.08 GHz}$$

Example 8.2: A rectangular waveguide resonator of dimensions 2 cm $\times 1$ cm is filled with air. What should be the length of the resonator for TE_{101} mode resonance at 10 GHz?

Solution: Given: $a = 2$ cm, $b = 1$ cm, TE_{101} mode, $m = 1$, $n = 0$, $p = 1$, $f_r = 10\times10^9$.

The resonant frequency for rectangular resonator is given by

$$f_r = \frac{\sqrt{(m/a)^2+(n/b)^2+(p/d)^2}}{(2\sqrt{\mu\varepsilon})}$$

$$10\times10^9 = \left(\frac{3\times10^8}{2}\right)\sqrt{\left(\frac{1}{0.02}\right)^2+\left(\frac{1}{d}\right)^2}$$

$$\frac{10\times10^9}{1.5\times10^8} = \left(\frac{200}{3}\right) = \sqrt{2500+(1/d)^2}$$

$$(1/d)^2 = (200/3)^2 - 2500 = 1944.4$$

$$d^2 = 1/1944.4 = 5.14\times10^{-4}$$

$$d = 2.267\times10^{-2}\,\text{m} = \textbf{2.267 cm}$$

Example 8.3: Design a rectangular cavity resonator to have a resonant frequency of 10 GHz having dimensions of $a = d$ and $b = a/2$.

Solution: Given: $a = d$, $b = a/2$, $f_r = 10$ GHz.

The resonant frequency for rectangular resonator is given by

$$f_r = \frac{\sqrt{(m/a)^2 + (n/b)^2 + (p/d)^2}}{(2\sqrt{\mu\varepsilon})}$$

$$10 \times 10^9 = \left(\frac{3 \times 10^8}{2}\right)\sqrt{\left(\frac{1}{a}\right)^2 + \left(\frac{2}{a}\right)^2 + \left(\frac{1}{a}\right)^2}$$

$$\left(\frac{200}{3}\right) = \sqrt{6/a^2}$$

$$6/a^2 = (200/3)^2$$

$$a = \textbf{3.675 cm}$$

Example 8.4: A rectangular cavity resonator has dimensions of 5 cm × 2 cm × 15 cm. Determine the resonant frequency of the dominant mode.

Solution: Given:

$$a = 5 \text{ cm}, b = 2 \text{ cm } d = 15 \text{ cm}.$$

Since $a > b < d$, the dominant mode is $\textbf{TE}_{101}$.

The resonant frequency for rectangular resonator is given by

$$f_r = \frac{\sqrt{(m/a)^2 + (n/b)^2 + (p/d)^2}}{(2\sqrt{\mu\varepsilon})}$$

$$= \left(\frac{3 \times 10^8}{2}\right)\sqrt{\left(\frac{1}{0.05}\right)^2 + \left(\frac{0}{0.02}\right)^2 + \left(\frac{1}{0.15}\right)^2}$$

$$= 1.5 \times 10^9 \times \sqrt{400 + 44.5}$$

$$= \textbf{3.164 GHz}$$

Example 8.5: An air-filled cylindrical cavity resonates at 3 GHz in $\textbf{TM}_{010}$ mode. The resonator is now filled with a loss-less material of dielectric constant 2.56. Calculate the new resonant frequency.

Solution: Given: $f_r = 3$ GHz, dielectric constant = 2.56, $\textbf{TM}_{010}$ mode

$$f_r \propto 1/\sqrt{\varepsilon}$$

The new resonant frequency $f_{r(\text{new})}$ is given by

$$f_{r(\text{new})} = f_r / \sqrt{\varepsilon_r} = 3/\sqrt{2.56}$$

$$= 3/1.6 = \textbf{1.875 GHz}$$

Example 8.6: An air-filled circular has a radius of 3 cm and is used as a resonator for $\textbf{TE}_{011}$ mode at 10 GHz by placing two perfectly conducting plates at its two ends. Determine the minimum distance between the two plates.

Solution: Given: $r = 3$ cm, $f_r = 10$ GHz, $\textbf{TE}_{011}$ mode

$$x'_{np} \text{ for } \textbf{TE}_{011} \text{ mode is } x'_{01} = 3.832.$$

For $\textbf{TE}_{npq}$ mode

$$f_r = \frac{\sqrt{\left(\frac{x'_{np}}{a}\right)^2 + \left(\frac{q\pi}{d}\right)^2}}{(2\pi\sqrt{\mu\varepsilon})} \text{ Hz}$$

$$10 \times 10^9 = \left(\frac{3 \times 10^8}{2 \times 3.14}\right)\sqrt{\left(\frac{3.832}{0.03}\right)^2 + \left(\frac{3.14}{d}\right)^2}$$

$$(209.33) = \sqrt{16315.8 + (1/d)^2}$$

$$(1/d)^2 = (209.33)^2 - 16315.8 = 27503.25$$

$$d^2 = 1/27503.25 = 3.64 \times 10^{-5}$$

$$d = 1.91 \times 10^{-2} \text{ m} = \textbf{1.91 cm}$$

Example 8.7: The resonant frequency of a cavity is 8 GHz. It is critically coupled to an external circuit. The bandwidth with loading is 4 MHz. Calculate the loaded and unloaded **Q**.

Solution: Given: $f_r = 8$ GHz, $\Delta f = 4$ MHz, $Q_L = f_r / \Delta f = 8 \text{ GHz}/4 \text{ MHz} = 2000$

For critical coupling, $Q_L = Q_o/2$. Therefore, Q_o is given by

$$Q_o = 2Q_L = \textbf{4000}$$

Example 8.8: Find the resonant frequencies for the first five lowest modes of an air-filled cylindrical cavity of radius 2 cm and length 3 cm.

Solution: Given: $a = 2$ cm, $d = 3$ cm

For $\textbf{TE}_{npq}$ mode:

$$f_r = \frac{\sqrt{\left(\frac{x'_{np}}{a}\right)^2 + \left(\frac{q\pi}{d}\right)^2}}{(2\pi\sqrt{\mu\varepsilon})} \text{ Hz}$$

$$= \left(\frac{3 \times 10^8}{6.28}\right)\sqrt{\left(\frac{x'_{np}}{a}\right)^2 + \left(\frac{q\pi}{d}\right)^2}$$

$$= 4.777 \times 10^7 \sqrt{\left(\frac{x'_{np}}{a}\right)^2 + \left(\frac{q\pi}{d}\right)^2}$$

TE$_{011}$ mode:

$n = 0, p = 1, q = 1, x'_{01} = 3.832,$
$f_r = 10.43$ GHz

TE$_{111}$ mode:

$n = 1, p = 1, q = 1, x'_{11} = 1.841,$
$f_r = 6.66$ GHz

TE$_{211}$ mode:

$n = 2, p = 1, q = 1, x'_{21} = 3.0534,$
$f_r = 8.84$ GHz

For TM$_{npq}$ mode:

$$f_r = \frac{\sqrt{\left(\frac{x_{np}}{a}\right)^2 + \left(\frac{q\pi}{d}\right)^2}}{(2\pi\sqrt{\mu\varepsilon})} \text{ Hz}$$

$$= \left(\frac{3 \times 10^8}{6.28}\right)\sqrt{\left(\frac{x'_{np}}{a}\right)^2 + \left(\frac{q\pi}{d}\right)^2}$$

$$= 4.777 \times 10^7 \sqrt{\left(\frac{x'_{np}}{a}\right)^2 + \left(\frac{q\pi}{d}\right)^2}$$

TM$_{010}$ mode:

$n = 0, p = 1, q = 0, x_{01} = 2.405,$
$f_r = 5.74$ GHz

TM$_{011}$ mode:

$n = 0, p = 1, q = 1, x_{01} = 2.405,$
$f_r = 7.60$ GHz

TM$_{111}$ mode:

$n = 1, p = 1, q = 1, x_{11} = 3.832,$
$f_r = 10.43$ GHz

Therefore the lowest five modes and frequencies are:

TM$_{010}$ mode: $f_r = 5.74$ GHz;
TE$_{111}$ mode: $f_r = 6.66$ GHz;
TM$_{011}$ mode: $f_r = 7.60$ GHz;
TE$_{211}$ mode: $f_r = 8.84$ GHz;
TM$_{111}$ and TE$_{011}$ modes: $f_r = 10.43$ GHz;

Example 8.9: A circular air-filled cavity with radius 4 cm and length 12 cm is excited in TE$_{111}$ mode. The 3 dB bandwidth is 3 MHz. Calculate the resonant frequency and Q.

Solution: Given: $a = 4$ cm, $d = 12$ cm, TE_{111} mode, $\Delta f = 3$ MHz

$$f_r = \frac{\sqrt{\left(\frac{x'_{np}}{a}\right)^2 + \left(\frac{\pi}{d}\right)^2}}{(2\sqrt{\pi\varepsilon})} \text{ Hz}$$

$$= \left(\frac{3 \times 10^8}{2}\right)\sqrt{\left(\frac{1.841}{0.04}\right)^2 + \left(\frac{3.14}{0.12}\right)^2}$$

$$= 1.5 \times 10^8 \sqrt{2118.3 + 684.7}$$

$$= 1.5 \times 10^8 \sqrt{2803}$$

$$= 7.94 \text{ GHz}$$

$$Q_o = f_r / \Delta f = 7.94 \times 10^9 / 3 \times 10^6 = \mathbf{2647}$$

Example 8.10: A circular air-filled copper cavity is excited in the TM$_{010}$ mode at 10 GHz. The cavity has length : radius as 2. Find the Q.

Solution: Given:

$f_r = 10$ GHz, $d/a = 2, a/d = 1/2$

$Q = 1.202 \times 377 / [R_s(1 + a/d)]$

$$R_s = \sqrt{\frac{\omega\mu}{2\sigma}}$$

$$= \sqrt{\frac{6.28 \times 10 \times 10^9 \times 4 \times 3.14 \times 10^{-7}}{(2 \times 5.8 \times 10^7)}}$$

$$= 2.5 \times 10^{-2}$$

$$Q = 1.202 \times 377 / [2.5 \times 10^{-2}(1 + 0.5)]$$

$$= \mathbf{12084.1}$$

KEY POINTS

- A cavity resonator is a metallic enclosure that stores electric and magnetic energies.
- The important parameters of resonators are (i) Resonant frequency, (ii) Quality factor Q and (iii) Input impedance.

- The advantages of microwave resonators are (i) Reasonable dimensions, (ii) Simplicity, (iii) Remarkably high Q and (iv) Very high shunt impedance.
- The important types of cavity resonators are (i) Coaxial cavity resonators, (ii) Rectangular cavity resonators, (iii) Circular cavity resonators, (iv) Semi-circular cavity resonators, (v) Reentrant cavity resonators and (vi) Hole-and-Slot cavity resonators.
- The three types of coaxial cavity resonators are (i) quarter-wave coaxial cavity, (ii) half-wave coaxial cavity and (iii) capacitive end coaxial cavity resonators.
- The simplest waveguide cavity resonator is a length of rectangular or circular wave-guide short-circuited at both ends to form a rectangular or circular prism respectively.
- The resonant frequency of rectangular resonator for both the **TE**$_{mnp}$ and **TM**$_{mnp}$ modes is given by

$$f_r = \frac{\sqrt{\left(\frac{m}{a}\right)^2 + \left(\frac{n}{b}\right)^2 + \left(\frac{p}{d}\right)^2}}{(2\sqrt{\mu\varepsilon})} \text{ Hz}$$

- For $a > b < d$, the dominant mode is **TE**$_{101}$ mode.
- The resonant frequency of circular resonator is given by
  (i) For **TE**$_{npq}$ mode:

$$f_r = \frac{\sqrt{\left(\frac{x'_{np}}{a}\right)^2 + \left(\frac{q\pi}{d}\right)^2}}{(2\pi\sqrt{\mu\varepsilon})} \text{ Hz}$$

  (ii) For **TM**$_{npq}$ mode:

$$f_r = \frac{\sqrt{\left(\frac{x_{np}}{a}\right)^2 + \left(\frac{q\pi}{d}\right)^2}}{(2\pi\sqrt{\mu\varepsilon})} \text{ Hz}$$

- The resonant frequency of a semi-circular resonator is given by
  (i) For **TE**$_{npq}$ mode

$$f_r = \frac{\sqrt{\left(x'_{np}\right)^2 + (q\pi a/d)^2}}{(2\pi a\sqrt{\mu\varepsilon})} \text{ Hz}$$

  (i) For **TM**$_{npq}$ mode

$$f_r = \frac{\sqrt{\left(x_{np}\right)^2 + (q\pi a/d)^2}}{(2\pi a\sqrt{\mu\varepsilon})} \text{ Hz}$$

- A reentrant cavity resonator is one in which the opposite sides are brought closer together to form a reentrant structure. It is used in klystron and magnetron tubes.
- The quality factor **Q** of a cavity is defined as the ratio of maximum energy stored to the energy dissipated per cycle. It is also a measure of frequency selectivity of the cavity. It is, thus, given by

$$Q = 2\pi \times \text{(maximum energy stored)}/\text{energy dissipated per cycle}$$
$$= \omega_r W/P = f_r/\Delta f$$

- The quality factor of a cavity, when it is not connected to any external circuit or load, is known as unloaded Q-factor **Q**$_o$.
- Generally a cavity resonator is always connected to a load or external circuit such as a generator. If the energy loss in the cavity per cycle is P_c and that due to external load is P_{el}, then the quality factor is given by

$$Q_L = \omega_r W/(P_c + P_l)$$

For critical coupling,

$$Q_L = Q_e/2 = Q_o/2, \text{ since } P_c = P_e.$$

FURTHER READING

1. Argence E and Hahan T (1967). Theory of Waveguides and Cavity Resonators, Blackie & Sons, London.
2. Collins RE (1996). Foundations of Microwave Engineering, McGraw Hill. NY.
3. Davis WA (1984). Microwave Semiconductor Circuit Design, Van Nostrand, NY.
4. Kaifez D and Guilon P (1986). Electron Resonators, Artech., Mass.
5. Terman FE (1934). Resonant Lines in Radio Circuits, *Elec. Engg.*, Vol. 53, p 1046.
6. Das A and Das SK (2004). Microwave Engineering, TMH, New Delhi.

REVIEW QUESTIONS

8.1 Define a cavity resonator. Mention four configurations

8.2 What are the important parameters of resonators?

8.3 What are the advantages of MW resonators?

8.4 Mention the various types of MW resonators.

8.5 Write down expression for lengths of three types of coaxial resonators.

8.6 Write down expression for resonant frequency of a rectangular resonator.

8.7 How is the cavity resonator excited?

8.8 Mention the methods of tuning a resonant cavity resonator.

8.9 Write down expression for resonant frequency of a circular resonator in TE_{mnp} mode.

8.10 Write down expression for resonant frequency of a circular resonator in TM_{mnp} mode.

8.11 Write down expression for resonant frequency of a semi-circular resonator in TE_{npq} mode.

8.12 Write down expression for resonant frequency of a semi-circular resonator in TM_{npq} mode.

8.13 Define unloaded Q of a resonator.

8.14 What are the losses that occur in a practical resonator?

8.15 How do the cavity losses affect the unloaded Q?

8.16 Write down the expression for Q of a cubic cavity resonator.

8.17 Define loaded and external Q.

8.18 What is a reentrant cavity? Where it is used?

8.19 What is a hole-and-slot cavity? Where it is used?

DESCRIPTIVE QUESTIONS

8.1 What is a cavity resonator? What are their configurations? What are the important parameters of a resonator?

8.2 Explain the excitation and tuning methods of a resonator.

8.3 Define unloaded Q of a resonator. What are the losses that occur in a practical resonator? How do they affect the unloaded Q?

8.4 Write down the expression for Q of a cubic cavity resonator. Define loaded and external Q.

8.5 Explain, with a neat sketch, the reentrant cavity resonator and hole-and-slot resonator.

PRACTICE PROBLEMS

8.1 Calculate the resonant frequency for TE_{101} mode of a rectangular cavity formed by shorting the ends with $a = 3$ cm, $b = 1.5$ cm and $d = 5$ cm.
(**Ans:** 5.183 GHz)

8.2 A rectangular wave-guide resonator of dimensions 3 cm × 1.5 cm is filled with air. What should be the length of the resonator for TE_{101} mode resonance at 10 GHz?
(**Ans:** 2 cm)

8.3 Design a rectangular cavity resonator to have a resonant frequency of 10 GHz having dimensions of $d = 2a$ and $b = a/2$.
(**Ans:** 2.7 cm)

8.4 A rectangular cavity resonator has dimensions of 4 cm × 2 cm × 10 cm. Determine the resonant frequency of the dominant mode.
(**Ans:** 3.88 GHz)

8.5 An air-filled cylindrical cavity resonates at 3 GHz in TM_{010} mode. The resonator is now filled with a loss-less material of dielectric constant 2.2. Calculate the new resonant frequency.
(**Ans:** 2.02 GHz)

8.6 An air-filled circular has a radius of 3 cm and is used as a resonator for TE_{011} mode at 9 GHz by placing two perfectly conducting plates at its two ends. Determine the minimum distance between the two plates.
(**Ans:** 1.72 cm)

8.7 The resonant frequency of a cavity is 10 GHz. It is critically coupled to an external circuit. The bandwidth with loading is 4 MHz. Calculate the loaded and unloaded Q.
(**Ans:** 2500, 5000)

8.8 Find the resonant frequencies for the first five lowest modes of an air-filled rectangular cavity of dimension 5 cm × 4 cm × 2.5 cm.
(**Ans:** TE_{mns} and TM_{mnp}: 110, 101, 011/210, 111 and 120)

8.9 Find the resonant frequencies for the first five lowest modes of an air-filled cylindrical cavity of radius 1.905 cm and length 2.54 cm.
(**Ans:** TM_{010}, 6.03 Ghz; TE_{111}, 7.49 GHz; TM_{011}, 8.44 GHz; TE_{211}, 9.67 GHz; TM_{111} and TE_{011}, 11.27 GHz)

8.10 A circular air-filled cavity with radius 3 cm and length 10 cm is excited in TE_{111} mode. The 3-dB bandwidth is 2.5 MHz. Calculate the resonant frequency and Q.
(**Ans:** 10.42 GHz, 4168)

8.11 A circular air-filled copper cavity is excited in the TM_{010} mode at 9.375 GHz. The cavity has length: radius as 1.5. Find the Q.
(**Ans:** 108764)

8.12 Show that the Q of a circular cavity operating in $\mathbf{TM}_{010}$ mode is greater than that of the square based rectangular cavity with $\mathbf{TE}_{101}$ mode by 8.26%. The dimension of each cavity is such that the circular cavity is circumscribed by the square based rectangular cavity.

REFERENCE

1. Collins RE (1996). *Foundations of Microwave Engineering*, McGraw Hill. NY.

2. Gandhi OP (1981), *Microwave Engineering and Applications*, Pergamon, NY.

3. Lance AL (1964). *Introduction to Microwave Theory and Measurements*, McGraw Hill, NY.

4. Lebedev I (1973). *Microwave Engineering*, MIR Publications, Moscow.

5. Liao SY (2000). *Microwave Devices and Circuits*, PHI, New Delhi.

6. Montogomery CG et al (1948). *Principles of Microwave Circuits*, McGraw Hill, NY.

7. Reich HJ et al (1953). *Microwave Theory and Techniques*, Van Nostrand, NJ.

8. Rizzi PA. *Microwave Engineering: Passive Circuits*, PH, NJ.

9. Roddy D (1999). *Microwave Technology*, PH, N.J.

10. Slater JC (1950). *Microwave Electronics*, Van Nostrand, NJ.

11. Soohoo RF (1971). *Microwave Electronics*, Addison-Wesley, Mass.

12. Terman FE (1955). *Electronic and Radio Engineering*, McGraw Hill, NY.

13. Veley VF (1987). *Modern Microwave Technology*, PH., NJ.

14. Wolff EA and Kaul R (1988). *Microwave Engineering and Systems*, John Wiley, NY.

15. Wilkinson EJ (1960). An N-way hybrid power divider, IEEE, Trans. MTT-8, No.1, p 116–118.

16. Wheeler GJ (1963). *Introduction to Microwave*, Englewood Cliffs, NJ.

17. Young Leo (1966). *Advances in Microwaves*, Vol. I, Academic Press, NY.

Microwave Filters

Objectives

- Identify the various MW filter parameters and mismatch loss.
- Design prototype low pass MW filter.
- Compare the Binomial and Tchebyshev filter response.
- Understand the need for frequency transformation.
- Design Low pass, high pass, band pass and band stop MW filters.

9.1 INTRODUCTION

A filter is a frequency selective device. It is a passive, reciprocal, linear two port network formed with inductive and capacitive elements. It is designed to transmit without attenuation a specified band of frequencies known as the *pass band* while attenuating heavily all frequencies outside this band, known as the *stop band*. Such ideal filters are not practicable and hence, they are designed within an acceptable tolerance. However, the practical filters do have a very low attenuation in the pass band and a small output signal in the stop band due to the presence of resistance in the reactive elements.

9.2 CLASSIFICATION OF FILTERS

Filters are classified based on the frequency band it passes or stops as:
- (i) Low-pass filters
- (ii) High-pass filters
- (iii) Band-pass filters
- (iv) Band rejection or band stop filters.

9.2.1 Low-Pass Filters

Low-pass filters (LPF) transmit all frequencies from zero to some upper frequency f_c known as *cut-off frequency* and attenuate all frequencies above cut-off frequency. Thus, it passes low frequencies below the cut-off frequency and stops higher frequencies beyond the cut-off frequency. An ideal low pass filter provides constant gain from zero to the cut-off frequency f_c. Fig. 9.1(a) shows the characteristic of the ideal and practical low pass filter with pass band and stop band. The *pass band* is the range of frequencies from 0 to f_c and is also known as the *bandwidth* of the low pass filter. The *stop band* is the frequency range beyond f_c. Due to presence of resistance in the inductive elements, the response of practical low pass filters in the pass band decreases as the frequency is increased and the gain drops by 3 dB at the cut-off frequency. Thereafter, the response decreases further and is small at the end of the *transition band*.

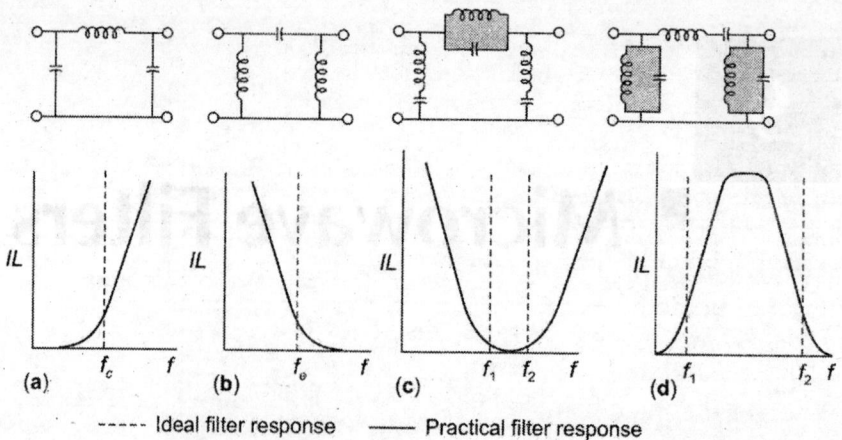

----- Ideal filter response   —— Practical filter response

Fig 9.1: Characteristics of ideal and practical filters

9.2.2 High-Pass Filters

High-pass filters (HPF) transmit all frequencies above a lower frequency f_c known as *cut-off frequency* and attenuate all frequencies below the cut-off frequency. Thus, it passes high frequencies above the cut-off frequency and stops lower frequencies below the cut-off frequency. An ideal high pass filter provides constant gain from the cut-off frequency f_c to infinity. Figure 9.1(b) shows the characteristic of the ideal and practical high pass filter with pass band and stop band. The *pass band* is the range of frequencies from f_c to infinity and is also known as the *bandwidth* of the high pass filter. The *stop band* is the frequency range from 0 to f_c. Due to presence of resistance in the inductive elements, the response of practical high pass filters in the pass band decreases as the frequency is decreased and the gain drops by 3 dB at the cut-off frequency. Thereafter, the response decreases as the frequency is further decreased and is small at the end of the *transition band*.

9.2.3 Band-Pass Filters

Band-pass filters (BPF) transmit all frequencies in the range f_1 to f_2 and attenuate all frequencies outside this range. Thus, it passes a frequency band f_1 to f_2. The frequency f_1 is known as *lower cut-off frequency* and f_2 is

known as *upper cut-off frequency*. An ideal band pass filter provides constant gain from f_1 to f_2. Figure 9.1(c) shows the characteristic of the ideal and practical band pass filter with pass band and stop band. The *pass band* is the range of frequencies from f_1 to f_2 and is also known as the *bandwidth* of the band pass filter. It has two stop bands, one from zero to f_1 and the other from f_2 to infinity. Due to presence of resistance in the inductive elements, the response of practical band pass filters in the pass band decreases on either side as the frequency is varied and the gain drops by 3 dB at the cut-off frequencies. Thereafter, the response decreases as the frequency is further varied and is small at the end of the *transition band*.

9.2.4 Band Rejection Filters

Band rejection filters (BRF) attenuate frequencies from f_1 to f_2 and transmit all frequencies outside this range. Thus, it attenuates a frequency band f_1 to f_2. The frequency f_1 is known as *lower cut-off frequency* and f_2 is known as *upper cut-off frequency*. An ideal band rejection filter provides infinite attenuation from f_1 to f_2. Figure 9.1(d) shows the characteristic of the ideal and practical band rejection filter with pass band and stop band. The *stop band* is the range of frequencies from f_1 to f_2. It has two pass bands, one from zero to f_1 and the other from f_2 to infinity. Due to presence of resistance in the inductive elements, the response of practical band rejection filters in the stop band decreases on either side as the frequency is varied and the gain drops by 3 dB at the cut-off frequencies. Thereafter, the response decreases as the frequency is further varied and is small at the end of the *transition band*.

For designing microwave filters, first a low-frequency low-pass prototype filter is designed and then the microwave filter is realized by replacing all inductors and capacitors by suitable microwave circuit elements. In most microwave systems, a microwave filter is designed to operate between a resistive source of 50 ohm and a resistive load of 50 ohm. In this chapter, we shall discuss mainly the design of reflective type filters.

9.3 FILTER PARAMETERS

The various parameters used in the design of microwave filters are:

  (i) Pass band

 (ii) Stop band attenuation

(iii) Input and output impedances

(iv) Insertion loss

 (v) Return loss

(vi) Group delay

Of these parameters, the *amplitude response* of the microwave filter is the *important* parameter. It is expressed in terms of insertion loss as a function of frequency .

A microwave filter connected to a generator and a load is shown in Fig. 9.2. Let the *incident power, reflected power* and *the power delivered to the load* be P_i, P_r and P_L respectively. Then, the insertion loss (*IL*) of the microwave filter is given by

$$IL_{dB} = 10 \log (P_i/P_L)$$
$$= 10 \log P_i/(P_i - P_r) \qquad (9.1)$$
$$= 10 \log 1/[1 - (P_i/P_r)]$$
$$= 10 \log 1/(1 - |\Gamma|^2) \qquad (9.2)$$

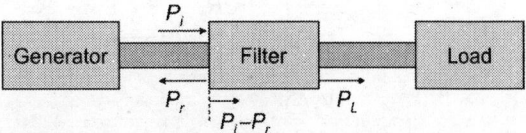

Fig. 9.2: Microwave filter with source and load

P_L is the power delivered to the load if the filter is lossless and is equal to $P_i - P_r \cdot |\Gamma|$ is the magnitude of the voltage reflection coefficient and is equal to $|\Gamma| = (P_i/P_r)^{1/2}$.

The return loss of the microwave filter is given by

$$RL_{dB} = 10 \log (P_i/P_r)$$
$$= 10 \log 1/|\Gamma|^2 \qquad (9.3)$$

The amount of impedance matching at the input port of the microwave filter is measured by the return loss.

The group delay of a microwave filter is given by

$$t_d = \frac{\frac{1}{2} d\phi}{df} \qquad (9.4)$$

ϕ_t is the *transmission phase angle*. When multi-frequency or pulsed signals are passed through the microwave filter, the group delay is an important parameter. It is used to determine the *frequency dispersion or deviation* from constant group delay over a given frequency band.

9.4 INSERTION LOSS DUE TO MISMATCH

When a microwave filter with characteristic resistive impedance R_o is terminated at both ends with this impedance, then it is matched. Hence, it has no reflection at either port. If the filter is not match terminated, then a mismatch occurs and the insertion loss will be present. *The insertion loss is defined as the ratio of the power delivered to the load when it is directly connected to the generator to the power delivered to the load due to the insertion of the filter.*

Figure 9.3 shows a loss-less microwave filter coupling a generator with a load. Let

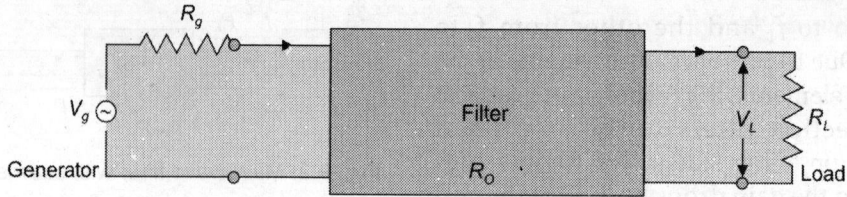

Fig. 9.3: Microwave filter with mismatch terminations

the characteristic resistive impedance be R_o, the generator voltage at the input port be V_g and the generator resistive impedance be R_g. The filter is terminated with a resistive load R_L at the output port.

In the absence of the filter, the power delivered to the load is $[V_g/(R_g + R_L)]^2 \cdot R_L$. If $R_g = R_L$, the maximum power P_1 delivered to the load is given by

$$P_1 = [V_g/(2R_g)]^2$$
$$= V_g^2/4R_g \qquad (9.5)$$

When the filter is inserted, the power P_2 delivered to the load is given by

$$P_2 = |V_L|^2/R_L \qquad (9.6)$$

The insertion loss (IL) of the filter is given by

$$IL_{dB} = 10 \log P_1/P_2$$
$$= 10 \log [V_g/2V_L]^2 (R_L/R_g)$$
$$= 20 \log [\tfrac{1}{2}(V_g/V_L)] + 10 \log(R_L/R_g)$$
$$= \alpha \qquad (9.7)$$

If $R_L = R_g$, then it is image impedance matched. In this case, the insertion loss (**IL**) of the filter is given by

$$IL_{dB} = 20 \log [\tfrac{1}{2} | V_g/V_L | = \alpha_o \qquad (9.8)$$

When α_o is inserted in Eq. (9.7), we get

$$IL_{dB} = \alpha_o + 10 \log (R_L/R_g) \qquad (9.9)$$

If the microwave filter is matched to the generator and the load, then $R_g = R_o = R_L$ and $\alpha = \alpha_0$. Then the voltage across the load is given by $V_L = \tfrac{1}{2}V_g$ and the insertion loss is given by

$$IL_{dB} = 20 \log [\tfrac{1}{2} | V_g/V_L |]$$
$$= 20 \log 1 = 0 \qquad (9.10)$$

From Eq. (9.9), it is seen that the insertion loss is a function of R_L and R_g. If $R_L > R_g$, then $\alpha > \alpha_0$, and if $R_L < R_g$, $\alpha < \alpha_0$, and $R_L = R_g$, $\alpha = \alpha_0$. Thus the insertion loss is less than the image impedance matched insertion loss. This implies that the output signal level is higher than the input signal level in the pass band.

9.5 MICROWAVE FILTER ELEMENTS

Series and shunt elements of microwave filters are realized with sections of coaxial lines, wave-guides, strip or microstrip lines, cavity resonators or resonant irises. Fig. 9.4 shows MW filter elements. A short circuit stub of length less than $\lambda/4$, formed in the narrow walls of a rectangular wave-guide simulates a series inductance as shown in Fig. 9.4(a). Similarly, a short circuit stub of length greater than $\lambda/4$ but less than $\lambda/2$, formed in the narrow wall of a rectangular wave-guide simulates a series capacitance. It can also be realized by a coaxial line gap formed by choke of length l less than $\lambda/4$ as shown in Fig. 9.4(b). A short circuit stub of length less than $l/4$ in the plane parallel to the broad wall of a rectangular wave-guide or an inductive iris simulates a shunt inductance as shown in Fig. 9.4(c). A capacitive iris simulates a shunt capacitance as shown in Fig. 9.4(d).

9.6 MICROWAVE FILTER DESIGN TECHNIQUES

Two commonly used MW filter design techniques are (i) *image parameter* and (ii) *insertion loss* method. However, only the insertion loss method results in complete specifications of

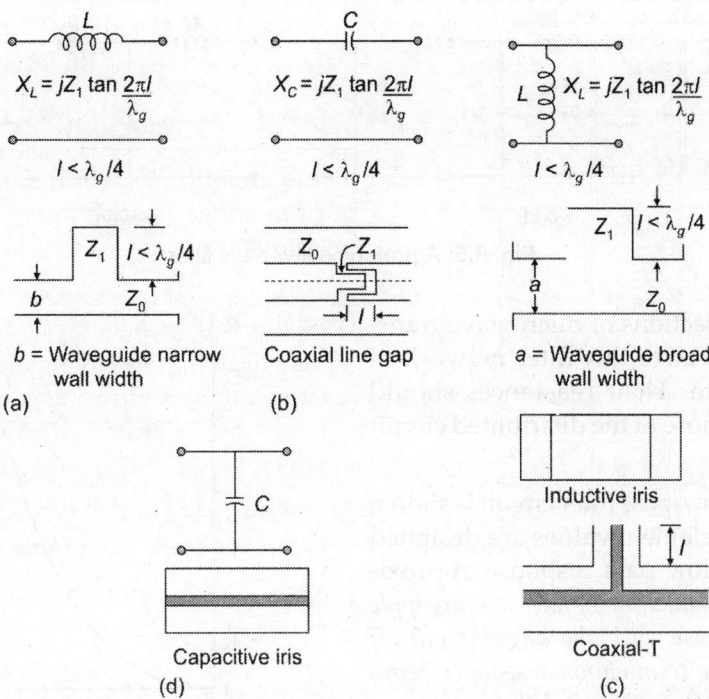

Fig.9.4: Microwave filter elements (a) Series *L* (b) Series *C* (c) Shunt *L* (d) Shunt *C*

a physically realizable frequency characteristic over the entire pass band and the stop band. Hence, insertion loss method is preferred for the design of microwave filters.

Figure 9.1 shows the equivalent circuits of the most commonly used microwave filters: *low-pass, high-pass, band pass* and *band stop* filters and their typical response characteristics. The equivalent lumped element values of microwave filter components are functions of frequency. In general, MW have an infinite number of poles and zeros. *According to Foster's reactance theorem, a physically realizable filter should have a finite number of poles and zeros.* Therefore, microwave filters are designed only for a narrow frequency band. *The magnitude of the reflection coefficient* $|\Gamma(\omega)|$ *should be less than or equal to unity for physical realization of passive microwave filters.* The reflection coefficient is expressed as a ratio of two even polynomials so that the insertion loss may be expressed as

$$IL = 1 + [M\,(\omega^2)/N\,(\omega^2)] \qquad (9.11)$$

In the design of microwave filters, the polynomials *M* and *N* are chosen such that the desired response characteristics is obtained.

9.6.1 Prototype Low-pass Filter Design

In the microwave filter design by insertion loss method, the general procedure is first to design a low-pass prototype filter and then frequency transform this design to the required type such as low-pass, high pass, band pass or band stop filter with specified center and band-edge frequencies. The steps involved in the design are:

Step **1:** With the specified pass band characteristics, design a low-pass prototype filter.

Step **2:** This prototype filter is frequency transformed to the required type such as low-pass, high pass, band pass or band stop filter with the specified center and band-edge frequencies.

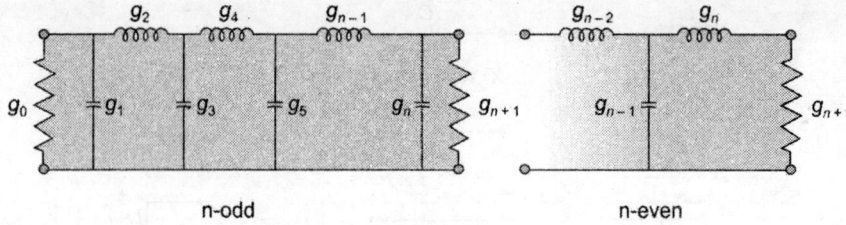

n-odd   n-even

Fig. 9.5: A prototype low-pass filter

Step 3: With sections of microwave transmission lines, realize this filter network in microwave form. Their reactances should correspond to those of the distributed circuit elements.

A prototype low-pass filter circuit is shown in Fig. 9.5. The element values are designed from standard low-pass response approximations such as *maximally flat* or *equi-ripple pass band response with the angular cut-off frequency and the termination resistance being both normalized to unity.*

(i) Maximally Flat Response Filter

The *maximally flat response* is also known as *Butterworth response* or *binomial response*. It exhibits approximately a flat response characteristic in the pass band and monotonically increasing attenuation in the stop band. The insertion loss for a prototype low-pass Butterworth filter is given by

$$IL = 1 + a_m^2 \omega_n^{2n} \qquad (9.12)$$

The normalized angular frequency $\omega_n = \omega/\omega_c$. The pass band is from $\omega = 0$ to $\omega = \omega_c$. For $a_m^2 = 1$, the maximum insertion loss in the pass band is 3 dB at the cut-off frequency ω_c. The rate of increase in insertion loss beyond ω_c depends on the exponent $2n$, where n is the number of reactive elements used in the filter network. IL_x represents the insertion loss at a given frequency $\omega_{nx} = \omega_x/\omega_c$ in the stop band. The Butterworth insertion loss response is shown in Fig. 9.6. The element values of low-pass ladder network derived from Butterworth response for normalized values of $\omega_{nc} = 1$ and norma-

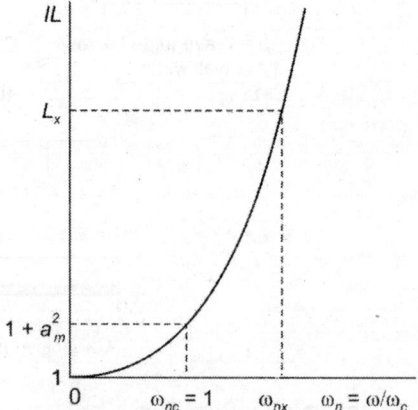

Fig. 9.6: Butterworth response

lized load resistance $r = 1$ are calculated from the following equations (refer to Fig. 9.5).

$$g_o = 1$$
$$g_k = 2 \sin \left[(2k - 1)\pi/2n\right],$$
$$k = 1, 2, 3, \ldots, n$$
$$g_{n+1} = 1, \text{ for all } n. \qquad (9.13)$$

Table 9.1 gives the values of g_k for 3 dB insertion loss at $w_n = 1$.

(ii) Equiripple Response Filter

The *equiripple response* is also known as *Tchebyshev response*. It exhibits equiripple response in the pass band and monotonically increasing attenuation in the stop band. The insertion loss for a prototype low-pass Tchebyshev filter is given by

$$IL = 1 + a_m^2 \Gamma_n^2(\omega_n) \qquad (9.14)$$

a_m is the ripple factor and n is the number of reactive elements or the degree of approximation. The normalized angular frequency $\omega_n = \omega/\omega_c$. The pass band is from $\omega = 0$ to

n	g_k $k = 1, 2, 3, ..., n$						
1				2.0			
2			1.414		1.414	1.0	
3			1.0	2.0	1.0	1.0	
4		0.7654	1.8480	1.8480	0.7654	1.0	
5		0.618	1.618	2.0	1.618	0.618	
6	0.5176	1.414	1.9320	1.9320	1.4140	0.5176	1.0
7	0.445	1.247	1.802	2.000	1.802	1.247	0.445

Table 9.1: Values of g_k for Butterworth filter with 3 dB insertion loss at $w_n = 1$

$\omega = \omega_c$. $\Gamma_n(\omega_n)$ is the Tchebyshev cosine polynomial of degree n and is given by

$$\Gamma_n = \cos(n \cos^{-1}\omega_n) \quad \text{for } \omega_n \leq 1$$
$$= \cosh(n \cosh^{-1}\omega_n) \quad \text{for } \omega_n > 1 \tag{9.15}$$

For $n = 0$,

$$\Gamma_0(\omega_n) = \cos(0 \cdot \cos^{-1}\omega_n) = \cos(0) = 1$$

For $n = 1$,

$$\Gamma_1(\omega_n) = \cos(1 \cdot \cos^{-1}\omega_n) = \omega_n$$

For $n \geq 2$, the Tchebyshev cosine polynomials are obtained by the recursive formula

$$\Gamma_n(\omega_n) = 2\omega_n\Gamma_{n-1}(\omega_n) - \Gamma_{n-2}(\omega_n) \tag{9.16}$$

For $n = 2$,

$$\Gamma_2(\omega_n) = 2\omega_n\Gamma_{2-1}(\omega_n) - \Gamma_{2-2}(\omega_n)$$
$$= 2\omega_n\Gamma_1(\omega_n) - \Gamma_0(\omega_n)$$
$$= 2\omega_n\omega_n - 1$$
$$= 2\omega_n^2 - 1;$$

Similarly,

$$\Gamma_3(\omega_n) = 4\omega_n^3 - 3\omega_n$$

$$\Gamma_4(\omega_n) = 8\omega_n^4 - 8\omega_n^2 + 1.$$

Table 9.2 shows the Tchebyshev cosine polynomials for various values of n.

The insertion loss response characteristic oscillates between 1 and $1 + a_m^2$ in the pass band, equals to $1 + a_m^2$ at the cut-off frequency w_c, and monotonically increases beyond cut-off frequency in the stop band. The rate of increase is much faster compared to the Butterworth filter. IL_x represents the inser-

n	Tchebyshev cosine polynomials
0	1
1	ω_n
2	$2\omega_n^2 - 1$
3	$4\omega_n^4 - 3\omega$
4	$8\omega_n^4 - 8\omega_n^2 + 1$
5	$16\omega_n^5 - 20\omega_n^3 + 5\omega$
6	$32\omega_n^6 - 48\omega_n^4 + 18\omega_n^2 - 1$
7	$64\omega_n^7 - 112\omega_n^5 + 56\omega_n^3 - 7\omega$
8	$128\omega_n^8 - 256\omega_n^6 + 160\omega_n^4 - 32\omega_n^2 - 1$
9	$256\omega_n^9 - 576\omega_n^7 + 432\omega_n^5 - 120\omega_n^3 + 9\omega$
10	$512\omega_n^{10} - 1280\omega_n^8 + 1120\omega_n^6 - 400\omega_n^4 + 50\omega_n^3 - 1$

Table 9.2: Tchebyshev cosine polynomials $C_n = \cos(n \cdot \cos^{-1}\omega_n)$

tion loss at a given frequency $\omega_{nx} = \dfrac{\omega_x}{\omega_c}$ in the stop band. The Tchebyshev insertion loss response is shown in Fig. 9.7. The element

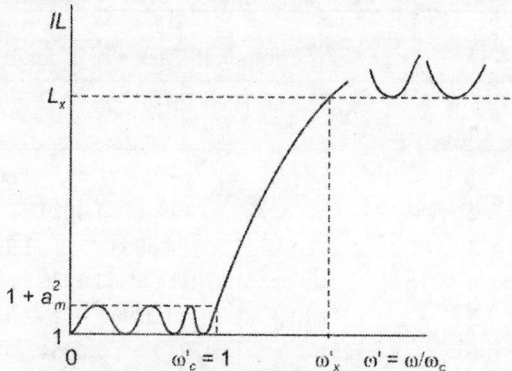

Fig. 9.7: Tchebyshev response

values of low-pass ladder network derived from Tchebyshev response for normalized values of $\omega_{nc} = 1$ and normalized load resistance $r = 1$ are calculated from the following equations (refer to Fig. 9.5):

$$g_0 = 1$$

$$g_1 = 2 \sin (\pi/2n)/\sinh (\beta/2n)$$

$$g_k = 4 p_{k-1} p_k/(q_{k-1} g_{k-1}):$$

$$k = 2, 3, \ldots, n$$

$$g_{n+1} = \tanh^2 (\beta/4) \text{ for even } n.$$
$$= 1, \text{ for odd } n \quad (9.17)$$
$$p_k = \sin [(2k-1)\pi/2n];$$
$$k = 1, 2, 3, \ldots, n$$
$$q_k = \sinh^2 (\beta/2n) + \sin h^2 (k\pi/n);$$
$$k = 1, 2, 3, \ldots, n$$
$$\beta = \ln(\coth a_m^2/17.37) \quad (9.18)$$

Tables 9.3 to 9.5 give the values of g_k for 0.1 dB ripple, 0.2 dB ripple and 0.5 dB ripple of Tchebyshev filter respectively.

Table 9.3: Values of g_k for Tchebyshev filter with 0.1 dB ripple

n	$g_k \quad k = 1, 2, 3, \ldots, n+1$							
1				0.3052	1.0000			
2			0.8430	0.6220	1.3544			
3		1.0315	1.1474	1.0315	1.0000			
4	1.1088	1.3061	1.7703	0.8180	1.3554			
5	1.1468	1.3712	1.9750	1.3712	1.1468	1.0000		
6	1.1681	1.4039	2.0562	1.5170	1.9029	0.8618	1.3554	
7	1.1181	1.4228	2.0966	1.5733	2.0966	1.4228	1.1181	1.0000

Table 9.4: Values of g_k for Tchebyshev filter with 0.2 dB ripple

n	$g_k \quad k = 1, 2, 3, \ldots, n+1$							
1				0.4342	1.0000			
2			1.0378	0.6745	1.5386			
3		1.2275	1.1525	1.2275	1.000			
4	1.3028	1.2844	1.9761	0.8468	1.5386			
5	1.3394	1.3370	2.1660	1.3370	1.3394	1.0000		
6	1.3598	1.3632	2.2934	1.4555	2.0974	0.8838	1.5386	
7	1.3722	1.3781	2.2756	1.5001	2.2756	1.3781	1.3722	1.0000

Table 9.4: Values of g_k for Tchebyshev filter with 0.5 dB ripple

n	$g_k \quad k = 1, 2, 3, \ldots, n+1$							
1				0.6986	1.0000			
2			1.4029	0.7071	1.9841			
3		1.5963	1.0969	1.5963	1.0000			
4	1.6703	1.1926	2.3661	0.8419	1.9841			
5	1.7058	1.2296	2.5408	1.2296	1.7058	1.0000		
6	1.7254	1.2479	2.6064	1.3137	2.4758	0.8696	1.9841	
7	1.7372	1.2583	2.6381	1.3444	2.6381	1.2583	1.7372	1.0000

9.7 TRANSFORMATION OF PROTOTYPE FILTER

In the previous section, we discussed the design of prototype low pass filter with normalized cut-off frequency of $\omega_{nc} = 1$ and normalized source and load resistance of 1 ohm. *Frequency* and *impedance normalization* or *scaling* are used to obtain the parameters of the actual low pass filter with the arbitrary cut-off frequency and impedance requirements. This is described below.

9.7.1 Low-pass Filter Elements

The parameters of prototype low-pass filter are frequency and impedance scaled to satisfy the specified cut-off frequency w_c and the impedance levels.

(i) *Frequency scaling*: Let the normalized cut-off frequency be ω_n, the normalized element value be g_k and the actual cut-off frequency be ω_c. The relationship between actual and the normalized frequency is given by

$$\omega_n = \omega/\omega_c \qquad \text{(i)}$$
$$\text{or,} \qquad \omega = \omega_n\omega_c \qquad \text{(ii)}$$

The actual cut-off frequency be ω_c is also known as *frequency scaling factor*. We obtain the actual element values by equating normalized value to the actual value.

For an inductor,
$$\omega_n g_k = \omega L = \omega_n \omega_c L \qquad \text{(iii)}$$
$$\therefore \qquad L = g_k/\omega_c \qquad \text{(iv)}$$

For a capacitor,
$$1/\omega_n g_k = 1/\omega C = 1/\omega_n \omega_c C \qquad \text{(v)}$$
$$C = g_k/\omega_c \qquad \text{(vi)}$$

As the resistances are independent of frequency, they remain unaffected in the frequency scaling. Thus, *the frequency scaling is achieved by dividing all inductances and capacitances by ω_c without altering the resistances.*

(ii) *Impedance scaling*: The normalized filters are terminated in 1 ohm. Let the actual impedance level required be R_L. Then, the actual impedance Z is related to normalized impedance Z_n by

$$Z = R_L Z_n \qquad \text{(vii)}$$

R_L is also known as *impedance scaling factor*. For a resistor,

$$R = R_L R \qquad \text{(viii)}$$

For an inductor,
$$L_k = R_L L_p \qquad \text{(ix)}$$

For a capacitor,
$$C_k = C/R_L \qquad \text{(x)}$$

The impedance scaling is accomplished by multiplying all resistances and inductances by R_L and dividing all capacitors by R_L.

Since both the transformations are to be performed simultaneously, the actual low-pass filter elements are:

(i) *Series arm inductance*:
$$L_k = g_k R_L/\omega_c = R_L L_p \text{ henry} \qquad (9.19)$$

(ii) *Shunt arm capacitances*:
$$C_k = g_k/(\omega_c R_L) = C_p R_L \text{ farad} \qquad (9.20)$$

9.7.2 Low Pass Filter to High Pass Filter Transformation

Let the normalized cut-off frequency be ω_n, the normalized element value be g_k and the actual cut-off frequency be ω_c. The equation to transform low pass filter to high pass filter is given by

$$\omega = \omega_c/\omega_n \qquad (9.21)$$

For capacitor, the transformation is given by
$$1/\omega_n g_k = \omega/\omega_c, \; g_k = \omega L_{hp}$$
$$\text{or,} \qquad L_{hp} = 1/\omega_c g_k$$

For the inductor, the transformation is given by
$$\omega_n g_k = g_k \omega_c/\omega = 1/\omega C_{hp}$$
$$\text{or,} \qquad C_{hp} = 1/g_k \omega_c$$

After applying the impedance transformation, the inductance and capacitance element values of actual high-pass filter are:

(i) *Series arm capacitance:*

$$C_k = 1/(g_k \omega_c R_L) \quad \text{farad} \qquad (9.22)$$

(ii) *Shunt arm inductances:*

$$L_k = R_L/(g_k \omega_c) \quad \text{henry} \qquad (9.23)$$

Thus, *the series inductance of prototype low-pass filter is transformed into series capacitance and shunt capacitance of prototype low-pass filter into shunt inductances in the high-pass filter.*

9.7.3 Low Pass Filter to Band Pass Filter Transformation

Let the normalized cut-off frequency be ω_n and the normalized element value be g_k. Let lower and upper cut-off frequencies of the band pass filter be ω_{c1} and ω_{c2}. Then, the equation to transform low pass filter to band pass filter is given by

$$\omega_n = (\omega_o/\text{BW}) \, [(\omega/\omega_o) - \omega_o/\omega)] \qquad (9.24)$$

The bandwidth BW of the band pass filter is given by

$$\text{BW} = \omega_{c2} - \omega_{c1}$$

The center frequency ω_o is the geometric mean of the two cut-off frequencies, ω_{c2} and ω_{c1}. Thus,

$$\omega_o^2 = \omega_{c1}\omega_{c2}$$

For the inductor, the transformation is given by

$$\omega_n g_k = g_k \omega/\text{BW} + \omega_o^2 g_k/(\omega\,\text{BW})$$
$$= \omega\,L_{bp1} + 1/(\omega C_{bp1})$$

For the capacitor, the transformation is given by

$$\omega_n g_k = g_k \omega/\text{BW} + \omega_o^2 g_k/(\omega\,\text{BW})$$
$$= \omega C_{bp2} + 1/(\omega L_{bp2})$$

Application of impedance transformation results into:

(i) *Series-tuned series arm elements:*

$$L_{k1} = g_k R_L/\,\text{BW} \qquad \text{henry} \qquad (9.25)$$

$$C_{k1} = \text{BW}/(g_k R_L \,\omega_o^2) \quad \text{farad} \qquad (9.26)$$

(ii) *Shunt-tuned shunt arm elements:*

$$L_{k2} = \text{BW}\, R_L/(g_k \omega_o^2) \quad \text{henry} \qquad (9.27)$$

$$C_{k2} = g_k/(\text{BW}\, R_L) \quad \text{farad} \qquad (9.28)$$

9.7.4 Low Pass Filter to Band Stop or Rejection Filter Transformation

Let the normalized cut-off frequency be ω_n and the normalized element value be g_k. Let lower and upper cut-off frequencies of the band stop filter be ω_{c1} and ω_{c2}. Then, the equation to transform low pass filter to band stop filter is given by

$$\omega_n = \text{BW}/[\omega_o(\omega/\omega_o) + \omega_o(\omega_o/\omega)] \quad (9.29)$$

The bandwidth BW of the band atop filter is given by

$$\text{BW} = \omega_{c2} - \omega_{c1}.$$

The center frequency ω_o is the geometric mean of the two cut-off frequencies, ω_{c2} and ω_{c1} Thus,

$$\omega_o^2 = \omega_{c1}\omega_{c2}$$

For the inductor, the transformation is given by

$$\omega_n g_k = 1/[(\omega/\text{BW}\, g_k) + \omega_o^2 \omega/(\text{BW}\, g_k)]$$
$$= 1/[\omega C_{bs1} + 1/(\omega L_{bs1})$$

For the capacitor, the transformation is given by

$$\omega_n g_k = (g_k\,\text{BW})/(\omega + \omega_o^2/\omega)$$
$$= 1/[\omega/(\text{BW}\, g_k) + (\omega_o^2/\text{BW}\, g_k)]$$
$$= \omega L_{bs2} + 1/(\omega C_{bs2})$$

Application of impedance transformation results into:

(i) *Series-tuned series arm elements:*

$$L_{k1} = g_k\,\text{BW}\, R_L/\omega_o^2 \quad \text{henry} \qquad (9.30)$$

$$C_{k1} = 1/(g_k R_L\,\text{BW}) \quad \text{farad} \qquad (9.31)$$

(ii) *Shunt-tuned shunt arm elements:*

$$L_{k2} = R_L/(g_k\,\text{BW}) \quad \text{henry} \qquad (9.32)$$

$$C_{k2} = g_k\,\text{BW}/(R_L\,\omega_o^2) \quad \text{farad} \qquad (9.33)$$

The above results are summarized in Table 9.6.

Table 9.6: Summary of filter element values

Prototype element	Low-pass filter element	High-pass filter element	Band pass filter element	Band stop filter element
Series arm g_k	$L = g_k R_L / \omega_c$	$C_k = 1/(g_k \omega_c R_L)$	$L_k = g_k R_L / BW$ $C_k = BW/(g_k R_L \omega_0^2)$	$L_k = g_k\, BW\, R_L / \omega_0^2$ $C_k = 1/(g_k R_L\, BW)$
Shunt arm g_k	$C = g_k/(\omega_c R_L)$	$L_k = R_L / g_k \omega_c$	$L_k = BW\, R_L/(g_k \omega_0^2)$ $C_k = g_k/(BW\, R_L)$	$L_k = R_L/(g_k\, BW)$ $C_k = g_k\, BW/(R_L \omega_0^2)$

9.8 DESIGN OF MW LOW-PASS FILTER

Microwave low-pass filters with waveguide sections cannot be realized since waveguides are basically high-pass lines. Hence, low-pass filters are constructed with coaxial lines, strip lines or microstrip lines. Reactive elements are realized using sections of coaxial lines, strip lines or microstrip lines having appropriate impedances.

The series inductive elements in low-pass filters are realized with short sections of coaxial strip line with length $l < \lambda_g/4$ and having relatively high characteristic impedance. The shunt capacitive elements are realized with very short sections of coaxial strip line with length $l \ll \lambda_g/4$ and having relatively low characteristic impe-dance. Figure 9.8 shows the realization of some filter elements. The length of the inductive and capacitive sections is obtained from the input reactance and susceptance formulae of filter sections. The response characteristic of a microwave low-pass filter is shown in Fig. 9.9.

9.8.1 Length of Inductive Line

A short length l_L of a loss-less line offers inductive reactance X_L when terminated with short-circuit. It is given by

$$\omega_c L = Z_{oL} \tan \beta l_L \qquad (9.34)$$

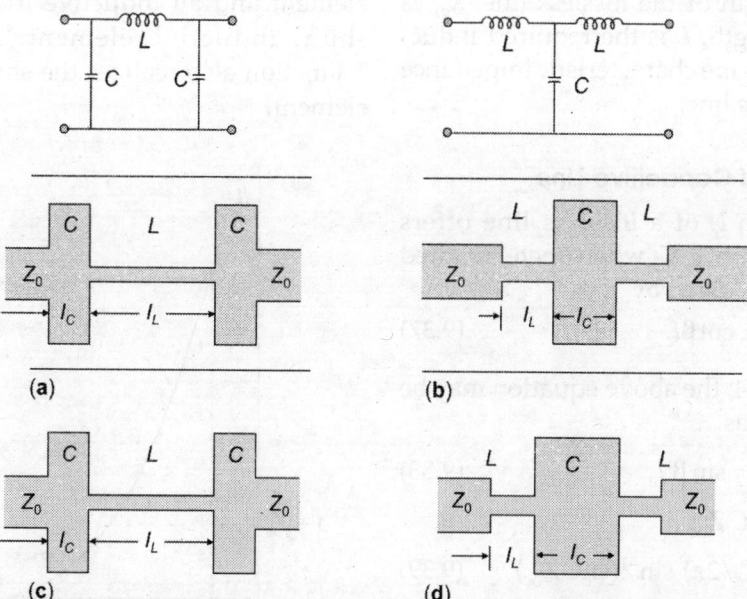

Fig. 9.8: Microwave low-pass filters (a) Coaxial Pi-section (b) Microstrip Pi-section (c) Coaxial T-section (d) Microstrip T-section

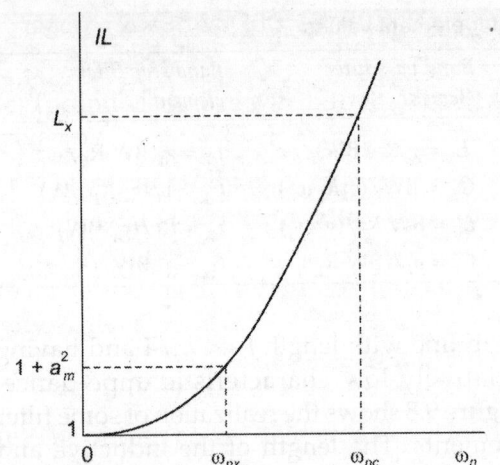

Fig 9.9: Low pass Butterworth filter response

For $\beta l_L << \lambda_{gL}/4$, Eq. (9.34) may be approximated as

$$\omega_c L \approx (Z_{oL} \sin \beta l_L) \qquad (9.35)$$

$$\sin \beta l_L = \omega_c L/Z_{oL}$$

or, $\qquad l_L = (1/\beta) \sin^{-1}(\omega_c L/Z_{oL})$

Substituting $\beta = 2\pi/\lambda_{gL}$, we get

$$l_L = (\lambda_{gL}/2\pi) \sin^{-1}(\omega_c L/Z_{oL}) \qquad (9.36)$$

l_L is the length of the lossless line, λ_{gL} is guide wavelength, L is the required inductance and Z_{oL} is the characteristic impedance of the inductive line.

9.8.2 Length of Capacitive Line

A short length l_c of a lossless line offers capacitive reactance X_C when open-circuited at one end. It is given by

$$1/\omega_c C = Z_{oc} \cot \beta l_c \qquad (9.37)$$

For $l_c << \lambda_{gc}/4$, the above equation may be approximated as

$$1/w_c C \approx Z_{oc}/\sin \beta \, l_c \qquad (9.38)$$

or, $\sin \beta l_C = \omega_c C Z_{oc}$

$\therefore \qquad l_c = (\lambda_{gc}/2\pi) \sin^{-1}(\omega_c C Z_{oc}) \qquad (9.39)$

l_c is the length of the lossless line, λ_{gc} is guide wavelength, C is the required capaci-

tance and Z_{oc} is the characteristic impedance of the capacitive line.

In practical inductive sections, fringe capacitance C_f is always present at the ends of the line. It is given by

$$C_f = (1/\omega Z_{oL}) \tan (\pi l_L/\lambda_{gL})$$
$$\approx l_L/(2f Z_{oL} \lambda_{gL}) \qquad (9.40)$$

Then, the required capacitance is $(C + C_f)$.

9.9 DESIGN OF MW HIGH-PASS FILTER

Using scaled Eqs (9.20 to 9.22), microwave high pass filter elements are designed from the low-pass prototype filter. Its response characteristic is shown in Fig. 9.10. The series capacitive elements in high-pass filters are realized with very small gaps in the coaxial and strip line of gap length $l << \lambda_g/4$, as shown in Fig. 9.11. The shunt inductive elements are realized with short sections of the coaxial and strip line of length $l < \lambda_g/4$ and having relatively low characteristic impedance and tee-connected to the main line. In the waveguide configuration, a capacitive iris realizes the series capacitive element and an inductive iris realizes the shunt inductive element. An *H*-plane *T*-junction also realizes the shunt inductive element.

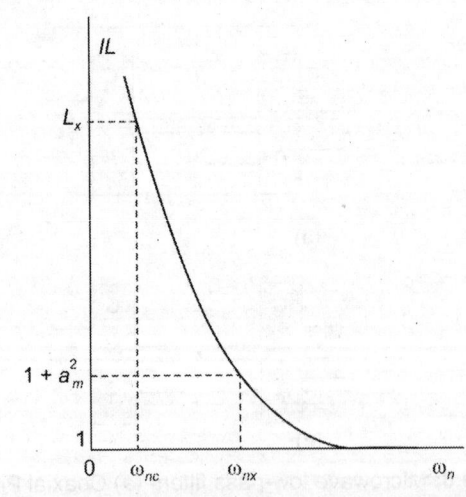

Fig. 9.10: High-pass Butterworth filter response

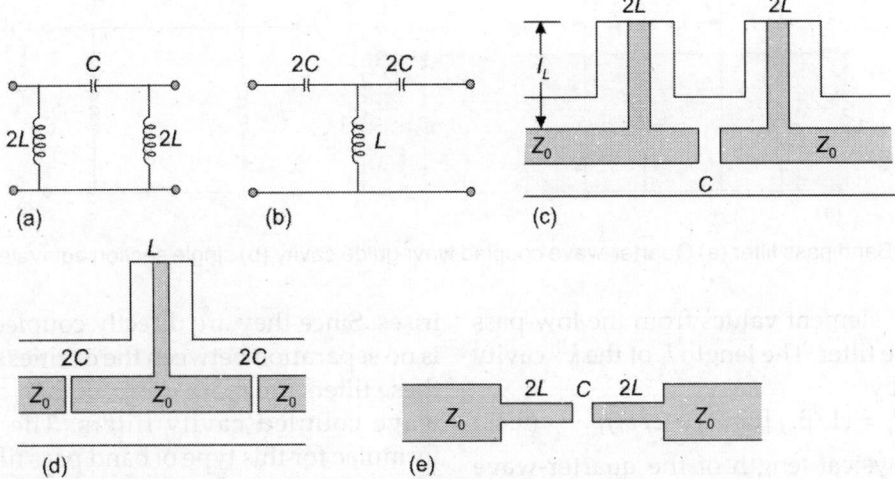

Fig 9.11: Microwave high-pass filters (a) Pi-section (b) T-section (c) Coaxial line Pi-section (d) Coaxial T-section (e) Microstrip Pi-section

9.10 DESIGN OF MW BAND-PASS FILTER

Figure 9.12(a) shows the circuit of a microwave band pass filter. These filters are narrow band filters. They are designed from the low pass prototype filter by using scaled Eqs (9.23) to (9.26). Its response characteristic is shown in Fig. 9.12. The resonator circuits of these filters are realized by coaxial lines, cascaded strip lines or cavity resonators of suitable configurations. They are described in the following sections.

9.10.1 Quarter Wave Coupled Cavity Band Pass Filter

Figure 9.13(a) shows a band pass circuit derived from the prototype low-pass filter. The MW band pass filters are realized with waveguide cavities that are coupled through the irises. Figure 9.13(b) shows the equivalent circuit of any k^{th} section loaded with two identical inductive irises with normalized susceptance $-jb_k$. The kth cavity is formed by a pair of irises separated by a distance l_k. The design formulae for this type of band pass filters are given below.

The susceptance b_k of the kth cavity resonator is given by

$$b_k = 2\sqrt{Q_k^2 - 1} \qquad (9.41)$$

The quality factor Q_k of the kth cavity resonator is given by

$$Q_k = (g_k/2)[\beta_0/(\beta_2 - \beta_1)] \qquad (9.42)$$

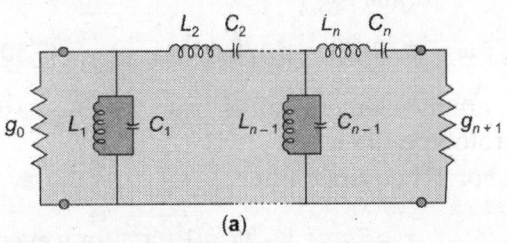

(a)

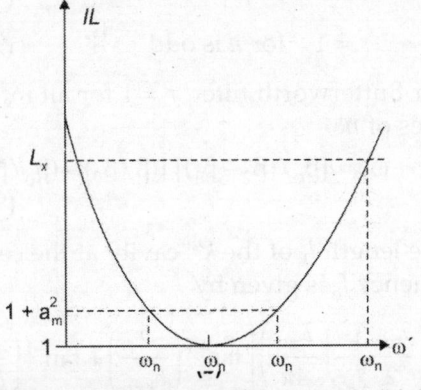

Fig. 9.12: (a) Band pass filter circuit (b) Filter response

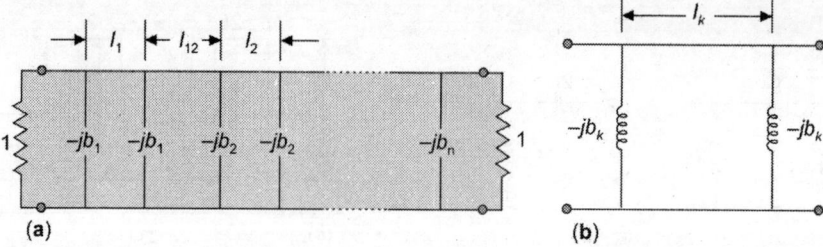

Fig. 9.13: Band pass filter (a) Quarter-wave coupled waveguide cavity (b) single section equivalent circuit

g_k's are element values from the low-pass prototype filter. The length l_k of the kth cavity is given by

$$l_k = (1/\beta_o) \left[\tan^{-1}(-2/b_k)\right] \qquad (9.43)$$

The physical length of the quarter-wave coupling line between the adjacent cavities is given by

$$l_{k,k+1} = \left[(l_k + l_{k+1})/2\right] - \lambda_{go}/4 \qquad (9.44)$$

The required iris dimensions can be calculated.

The insertion loss of the Tchebyshev band pass filter is

$$IL = 1 + a_m^2 \Gamma_n^2 \left[\frac{\beta_0}{(\beta_2 - \beta_1)}\right] \left[\left(\frac{\beta}{\beta_0}\right) - \left(\frac{\beta_0}{\beta}\right)\right] \qquad (9.45)$$

$$\beta_o = \sqrt{\beta_1 \beta_2} \qquad (9.46)$$

β_1 and β_2 are the coupling coefficients and β_o *is the geometric mean of the* coupling coefficients.

9.10.2 Direct Coupled Cavity Band Pass Filter

Figure 9.14 shows a direct-coupled cavity band pass filter. It has a number of cavity resonators directly coupled by inductive

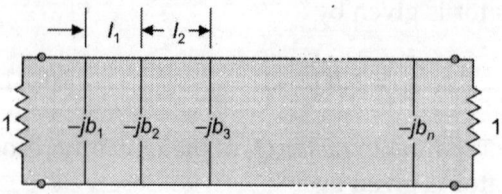

Fig. 9.14: Direct coupled cavity band pass filter

irises. Since they are directly coupled, there is no separation between the cavities. Hence, these filters are more compact than quarter-wave coupled cavity filters. The design formulae for this type of band pass filters are given below.

The normalized susceptance of the irises are given by

$$b_1 = (1 - \omega/g_1)/\sqrt{(\omega/g_1)} \qquad (9.47)$$

$$b_k = \left(\frac{1}{\omega}\right) \left[1 - \frac{\omega^2}{(g_k g_{k-1})}\right] \sqrt{(g_k g_{k-1})} \qquad (9.48)$$

$$b_n = \frac{(1 - \omega r/g_n)}{\sqrt{(\omega r/g_n)}} \qquad (9.49)$$

$$\omega = (\pi/2)\left[(\beta_2 - \beta_1)/\beta_0\right] \qquad (9.50)$$

g_k are the element values from the low-pass prototype filter.

For Tchebyshev filter,

$$r = 2a_m^2 + 1 - 2a_m\sqrt{1 + a_m^2} \quad \text{for } n \text{ even} \qquad (9.51)$$

$$r = 1 \quad \text{for } n \text{ is odd} \qquad (9.52)$$

For Butterworth filter, $r = 1$ for all integer values of n.

$$\omega_n = \left[\beta_o/(\beta_2 - \beta_1)\right] \left[(\beta/\beta_0) - (\beta_0/\beta)\right] \qquad (9.53)$$

The length l_k of the kth cavity at the center frequency f_o is given by

$$l_k = \left(\frac{\lambda_{go}}{2}\right) - \left(\frac{\lambda_{go}}{4\pi}\right) \left[\tan^{-1}\left(\frac{2}{b_{k+1}}\right) + \tan^{-1}\left(\frac{2}{b_k}\right)\right] \qquad (9.54)$$

9.11 MICROWAVE BAND STOP FILTER DESIGN

Microwave band stop filters are narrow band filters. They are obtained from the low-pass prototype filter by using frequency transformation given by

$$\frac{1}{\omega_n} = \left[\frac{\omega_0}{\omega_2 - \omega_1}\right]\left(\frac{\omega}{\omega_0} - \frac{\omega_0}{\omega}\right); \omega_0 = \sqrt{\omega_2\omega_1}$$
(9.55)

The low-pass prototype filter circuit, the band stop filter circuit and their equiripple response characteristics are shown in Fig. 9.15. w_x represents a frequency in the stop band at which the attenuation is high.

9.11.1 Quarter Wave Coupled Band Stop Filter

When a band stop filter is to be realized with transmission lines, it is convenient to use either resonant series or shunt branches only that are linked by quarter-wave sections of the transmission line. Thus, a quarter-wave coupling network shown in Fig. 9.16 can replace the ladder filter network shown in Fig. 9.15. The characteristic impedance of the quarter-wave coupling sections is Z_0 for n odd and Z' for n even where n is the number of resonators. Hence,

For n = odd: $Z'/Z_0 = 1$
For n = even:

$$Z'/Z_0 = \frac{1}{\sqrt{g_0 g_{n+1}}}$$
(9.56)

The design formulae for this type of band stop filters are given below:

$$x_1/Z_0 = \omega_0/[g_0 g_1(\omega_2 - \omega_1)]$$
(9.57)
$$x_k/Z_0 = (Z'/Z_0)^2 [g_0\omega_0/ g_k(\omega_2 - \omega_1)];$$
$$k = \text{even}$$
(9.58)

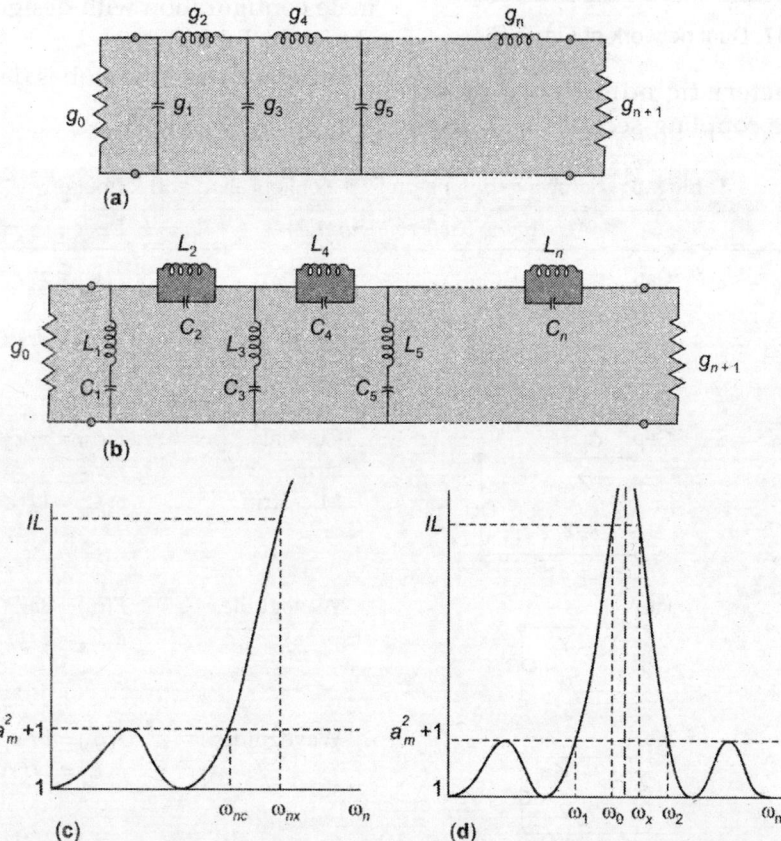

Fig. 9.15: (a) Prototype filter (b) Equivalent stop-band circuit (c) Prototype low-pass response (d) Band-stop response

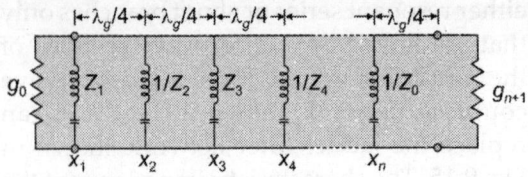

Fig. 9.16: Microwave equivalent circuit of a ladder band stop filter

$$x_k/Z_o = \omega_o/[g_o\, g_k(\omega_2 - \omega_1)]; \quad k = \text{odd} \neq 1 \tag{9.59}$$

where x_k are reactance slope parameters.

The dual realization of the circuit shown in Fig. 9.16 is shown in Fig. 9.17. The parallel resonant circuits are cascaded in series by quarter-wave coupled network.

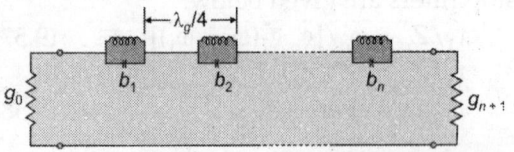

Fig. 9.17: Dual network of Fig. 9.16

The characteristic admittance of the quarter-wave coupling sections is Y_o for n odd and Y' for n even, where n is the number of resonators. Hence,

$$Y'/Y_o = \frac{1}{\sqrt{g_o g_{n+1}}} \tag{9.60}$$

The design formulae for this type of band stop filters are given below:

$$b_1/Y_o = \omega_o/[g_o\, g_1(\omega_2 - \omega_1)] \tag{9.61}$$

$$b_k/Y_o = (Y'/Y_o)^2\, [g_o\omega_o/g_k(\omega_2 - \omega_1)]; \quad k = \text{even} \tag{9.62}$$

$$b_k/Y_o = \omega_o/[g_o\, g_k(\omega_2 - \omega_1)]; \quad k = \text{odd} \neq 1 \tag{9.63}$$

The series and parallel resonant circuits in Figs 9.16 and 9.17 are realized by short-circuited or open-circuited resonant stubs with a series gap capacitance in coaxial lines, strip and microstrip lines, and with shunt inductive irises in waveguides. The approximate configuration with design formulae is shown in Table 9.6.

The length l_k of the stub is determined by

$$l_k = \lambda_g\, \phi_o/2\pi \tag{9.64}$$

Table 9.6: Microwave band stop filter configuration and formulae			
Resonator	*Approximate configuration*		*Design formulae*
Gap C_g — Z_1 — SC, $\lambda_g/4$ (x)		Coaxial strip Microtrip	$F(\phi_0) = 2x/Z_1$ $\omega_0 C_g = 1/(Z_1 \tan\phi_0)$
Gap C_g — Z_1 — OC, $\lambda_g/2$ (x)		Coaxial strip Microtrip	$F(\phi_0) = x/Z_1$ $\omega_0 C_g = 1/(Z_1 \tan\phi_0)$
Iris L_g Y_1 — OC, $\lambda_g/4$ (b)		Waveguide	$F(\phi_0) = 2b/Y_1$ $\omega_0 C_g = 1/(Y_1 \tan\phi_0)$
Iris L_g Y_1 — SC, $\lambda_g/2$ (b)		Waveguide	$F(\phi_0) = b/Y_1$ $\omega_0 L_g = 1/(Y_1 \tan\phi_0)$
			$F(\phi_0) = \phi_0 \sec^2\phi_0 + \tan\phi_0$

Table 9.7: Values of $F(\phi_0)$ for various values of ϕ_0 in degrees

ϕ	$F(\phi)$	ϕ	$F(\phi)$	ϕ	$F(\phi)$	ϕ	$F(\phi)$	ϕ	$F(\phi)$	ϕ	$F(\phi)$	ϕ	$F(\phi)$
20.00	0.76	68.00	10.96	75.50	24.99	80.55	58.56	83.30	116.58	86.00	328.42	88.70	3226.52
21.00	0.80	68.50	11.47	75.60	25.34	80.60	59.18	83.35	118.24	86.05	426.85	88.76	2497.78
22.00	0.85	69.00	12.01	75.70	25.69	80.65	59.81	93.40	120.40	86.10	345.61	88.80	3804.74
23.00	0.90	69.50	12.60	75.80	26.80	80.70	60.46	83.45	121.89	86.15	354.72	88.85	4153.96
24.00	0.95	70.00	13.23	75.90	26.42	80.75	61.11	83.50	123.77	86.20	364.20	88.90	4553.58
25.00	1.00	70.50	13.91	76.00	26.79	80.80	61.78	83.55	125.70	86.25	374.06	88.95	5013.77
26.00	1.06	70.60	14.06	76.10	27.17	80.86	62.45	83.60	127.68	86.30	384.33	89.00	5547.42
27.00	1.10	70.70	14.19	76.20	27.57	80.90	63.14	83.65	129.70	86.25	395.02	89.05	6171.05
28.00	1.16	70.80	14.34	76.30	27.97	80.95	63.84	83.70	131.77	86.40	406.17	89.10	6906.09
29.00	1.22	70.90	14.49	76.40	28.38	81.00	64.55	83.75	133.90	86.45	417.80	89.15	7780.72
30.00	1.28	71.00	14.64	76.50	28.80	81.05	65.27	83.80	136.07	86.50	429.93	89.20	8832.70
31.00	1.34	71.10	14.79	76.60	29.22	81.10	66.00	83.85	138.00	86.55	442.61	89.25	10113.40
32.00	1.40	71.20	14.95	76.70	29.66	81.15	66.75	83.90	140.58	86.60	455.85	89.30	11694.29
33.00	1.47	71.30	15.11	76.80	30.11	81.20	67.51	83.95	142.92	86.65	469.69	89.35	13677.07
34.00	1.54	71.40	15.27	76.90	30.57	81.25	68.28	84.00	145.32	86.70	484.18	89.40	16210.46
35.00	1.61	71.50	15.43	77.00	31.04	81.30	69.07	84.05	147.78	86.75	499.35	89.45	19518.95
36.00	1.69	71.60	15.60	77.10	31.52	81.35	69.87	84.10	150.31	86.80	515.24	89.50	23954.27
37.00	1.77	71.70	15.77	77.20	32.01	81.40	70.68	84.15	152.90	86.85	531.91	89.55	30092.89
38.00	1.85	71.80	15.94	77.30	32.51	81.45	71.51	84.20	155.55	96.90	549.39	89.60	38933.26
39.00	1.94	71.80	16.11	77.40	33.02	81.50	72.35	84.25	158.28	86.95	576.76	89.65	52329.04
40.00	2.03	72.00	16.29	77.50	33.55	81.55	73.21	84.30	161.08	87.00	587.06	89.70	74046.28
41.00	2.13	72.10	16.47	77.60	34.09	81.60	74.08	84.35	163.95	87.05	607.36	89.75	112731.26
42.00	2.23	72.20	16.65	77.70	36.64	81.65	74.97	84.40	166.91	87.10	628.74	89.80	192063.13
43.00	2.34	72.30	16.84	77.80	35.21	81.70	75.88	84.45	169.94	87.15	651.27	89.85	397933.81
44.00	2.45	72.40	17.03	77.90	35.79	81.75	76.80	84.50	173.06	87.20	675.03	89.90	1266238.98
45.00	2.57	72.50	17.22	78.00	36.39	81.80	77.74	84.55	176.26	87.25	700.11	89.95	27096342.23
46.00	2.70	72.60	17.42	78.10	37.00	81.85	78.70	84.60	179.55	87.30	726.63		
47.00	2.84	72.70	17.62	78.20	37.62	81.90	79.67	84.65	182.94	87.35	754.67		
48.00	2.98	72.80	17.82	78.30	38.27	81.95	80.66	84.70	186.42	87.40	784.38		
49.00	3.14	72.90	18.03	78.40	38.92	82.00	81.67	84.75	190.01	87.45	815.87		
50.00	3.31	73.00	18.24	78.50	39.60	82.05	82.70	84.80	193.70	87.50	849.30		
51.00	3.49	73.10	18.45	78.60	40.29	82.10	83.75	84.85	197.49	87.55	884.83		
52.00	3.68	73.20	18.67	78.70	41.01	82.15	84.82	84.90	201.40	87.60	922.64		
53.00	3.89	73.30	18.80	78.80	41.74	82.20	85.92	84.95	205.43	87.65	962.92		
54.00	4.11	73.40	19.12	78.90	42.49	82.25	87.03	85.00	209.58	87.70	1005.91		
55.00	4.35	73.50	19.35	79.00	43.26	82.30	88.16	85.05	213.86	87.75	1051.84		
56.00	4.61	73.60	19.58	79.10	44.06	82.35	89.32	85.10	218.27	87.80	1100.00		
57.00	4.90	73.70	19.82	79.20	44.87	82.40	90.50	85.15	222.82	87.55	1153.67		
58.00	5.21	73.80	20.06	79.30	45.71	82.45	91.70	85.20	227.51	87.90	1210.22		
59.00	5.55	73.90	20.31	79.40	46.58	82.50	92.93	85.25	232.36	97.95	1271.04		
60.00	5.93	74.00	20.56	79.50	47.46	82.55	94.18	85.30	237.36	88.00	1336.56		
61.00	6.34	74.10	20.82	79.60	48.38	82.60	95.46	85.35	242.52	88.05	1407.28		
61.50	6.57	74.20	21.08	79.70	49.32	82.65	96.76	85.40	247.85	88.10	1483.78		
62.00	6.80	74.30	21.35	79.80	50.29	82.70	98.09	85.45	253.36	88.15	1566.68		
62.50	7.05	74.40	21.62	79.90	51.28	82.75	99.45	85.50	259.06	88.20	1656.74		

(Contd...)

Table 9.7: Values of $F(\phi_0)$ for various values of ϕ_0 in degrees (Contd.)

ϕ	$F(\phi)$	ϕ	$F(\phi)$	ϕ	$F(\phi)$	ϕ	$F(\phi)$	ϕ	$F(\phi)$	ϕ	$F(\phi)$	ϕ	$F(\phi)$
63.00	7.31	74.50	21.90	80.00	52.31	82.80	100.84	85.55	264.95	88.25	1754.79		
63.50	7.59	74.60	22.18	80.10	53.37	82.85	102.26	85.60	271.05	88.30	1861.81		
64.00	7.88	74.70	22.47	80.15	53.91	82.90	103.70	85.65	277.36	88.35	1978.94		
64.50	8.19	74.80	22.76	80.20	54.46	82.95	105.18	85.70	283.89	88.40	2107.48		
65.00	8.51	74.90	23.06	80.25	55.02	83.00	106.69	85.75	290.66	88.45	2248.96		
65.50	8.86	75.00	23.37	80.30	55.59	83.05	108.24	85.80	297.67	88.50	2405.19		
66.00	9.23	75.10	23.68	80.35	56.16	83.10	109.81	85.85	304.94	88.55	2578.29		
66.50	9.62	75.20	24.00	80.40	56.75	83.15	111.42	85.90	312.48	88.60	2770.77		
67.00	10.04	75.30	24.32	80.45	57.34	83.20	113.07	85.95	320.30	88.65	2985.64		
67.50	10.48	75.40	24.65	80.50	57.94	83.25	114.76						

The line width is determined from the characteristic impedance. The gap length d_k for the capacitance C_g is approximately given by

$$d_k = \lambda_g/4; \text{ short-circuit condition} \quad (9.65)$$

$$= (\lambda_g/2) - l_k; \text{ open-circuit condition} \quad (9.66)$$

The inductive iris is obtained by calculating the value of the inductance L_g from Table 9.6. Table 9.7 gives the values of $F(\phi_0)$ for various values of ϕ_0.

The design procedure for band stop filter involves the following steps:

Step 1: Determine the number of resonators n from the maximum attenuation at band edge frequencies and the value of given attenuation at a given frequency w_x in the stop band using frequency transformation.

Step 2: Determine the prototype element values from the band edge attenuation and the number of resonators n determined in step 1.

Step 3: Determine the parameters for a selected realizable configuration.

Step 4: Select the stub impedances and determine gap capacitances or iris inductances and electrical length of the stubs at resonant frequency.

Step 5: Determine the stub lengths and dimensions of the capacitance gaps or irises.

Figure 9.18 shows some forms of microwave band stop filters.

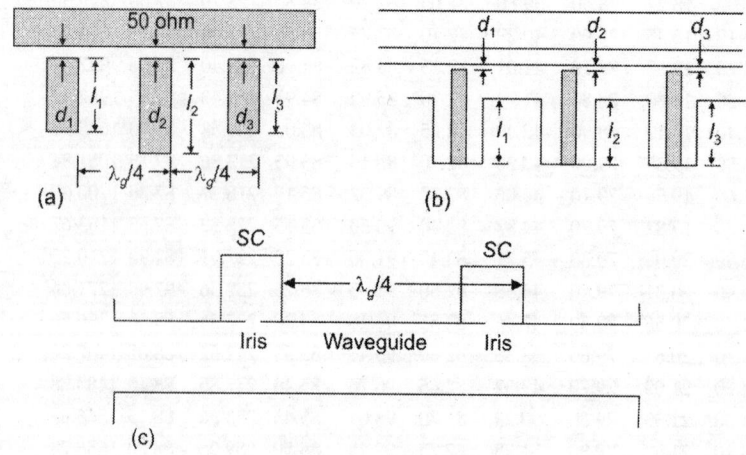

Fig. 9.18: Microwave band-stop filters (a) Strip line (b) Coaxial line (c) Waveguide

9.12 NUMERICAL EXAMPLES

Example 9.1 Design a low-pass microwave filter with cut-off frequency of 1 GHz, 30dB attenuation at 1.75 GHz with 0.2 dB ripple. Use alumina substrate of thickness 0.63 mm.

Solution: Given: f_c = 1 GHz, f_x = 1.75 GHz, IL = 30 dB and ripple = 0.2 dB

(i) *Low-pass prototype design:*

$$IL = 1 + a_m^2 \Gamma_n^2(\omega_n); \quad \omega_n = \omega/\omega_c$$

For 0.2 dB ripple, we have

$$10 \log(1 + a_m^2) = 0.2$$

$$a_m^2 = 10^{0.2/10} - 1$$

$$= 1.047 - 1 = 0.047$$

At stop band frequency f_{nx},

$$10 \log(1 + a_m^2 \cosh^2(n \cosh^{-1}\omega_{nx}) = 30 \text{ dB}$$

$$\omega_{nx} = \frac{\omega_x}{\omega_c} = \frac{1.75}{1} = 1.75$$

$$\therefore 1 + a_m^2 \cosh^2[n \cosh^{-1}(1.75)] = 10^{30/10}$$

$$= 1000$$

$$\cosh^2[n \cosh^{-1}(1.75)] = \frac{(1000 - 1)}{0.047}$$

$$\therefore n \approx 5$$

Hence, *a five section low-pass filter is to be designed.*

The prototype elements for $n = 5$ and 0.2 dB ripple (from Table 9.3) are:

$$g_0 = g_6 = 1, g_1 = g_5 = 1.3394,$$

$$g_2 = g_4 = 1.337 \text{ and } g_3 = 2.166$$

(ii) *Microwave filter lumped element values:* With -50-ohm termination, R_L = 50 ohm. The lumped element values for cascaded Pi-section are given by

$$C_k = g_k / R_L w_c$$

and $\quad L_k = g_k R_L / w_c$

$$\therefore C_1 = C_5 = 1.3394/(50 \times 6.28 \times 2 \times 10^9)$$

$$= \textbf{2.132 pF}$$

$$C_3 = 2.166/(50 \times 6.28 \times 2 \times 10^9)$$

$$= \textbf{3.447 pF}$$

$$L_2 = L_4 = (1.337 \times 50)/(6.28 \times 2 \times 10^9)$$

$$= \textbf{5.32 nH}$$

Example 9.2 Design a quarter-wave coupled three-cavity filter having maximum pass band ripple of 0.1 dB. The pass band extends from 10 GHz to 10.4 GHz. Use waveguides of dimensions $a = 2.5$ cm and $b = 1.2$ cm and inductive diaphragm with circular holes.

Solution: Given: Ripple = 0.1 dB, f_1 = 10 GHz, f_2 = 10.4 GHz, a = 2.5 cm, b =1.2 cm

(i) *At center frequency,*

$$\beta_o = 2p/\lambda_{gp}$$

$$\tan \beta_o l_k = -2/b_k$$

The distance between cavity k and $k + 1$ is given by

$$l_{k, k+1} = [(l_k + l_{k+1})/2] - \lambda_{go}/4$$

For 0.1 dB ripple, we have

$$10 \log(1 + a_m^2) = 0.1$$

$$a_m^2 = 10^{0.1/10} - 1 = 1.0233 - 1$$

$$= 0.0233$$

The prototype elements for $n = 3$ and 0.1 dB ripple (from Table 9.2) are:

$$g_1 = g_3 = 1.0315 \text{ and } g_2 = 1.1474$$

The propagation constants k_o in free space at the band edges and b in a rectangular waveguide in dominant TE_{10} mode are given by

$$k_{ok} = w/c$$

$$\therefore k_{o1} = 6.28 \times 10^{10}/(3 \times 10^{10}) = 2.0944$$

$$k_{o2} = 6.28 \times 10.4 \times 10^9/(3 \times 10^{10})$$

$$= 2.1782$$

$$\beta_k = [k_{ok}^2 - (\pi/a)^2]^{1/2}$$

$$\beta_1 = [k_{o1}^2 - (\pi/a)^2]^{1/2} = 1.5805$$

$$\beta_2 = [k_{o2}^2 - (\pi/a)^2]^{1/2} = 1.6899$$

Center of the frequency band occurs at

$$\beta_o = \sqrt{\beta_1 \beta_2} = 1.6343$$

$$f_o = \sqrt{f_1 f_2} = 10.198 \text{ GHz}$$

$$\lambda_o = 30/f_o = 2.942 \text{ cm}$$
$$\lambda_{go} = 2\pi/\beta_o = 6.28/1.6343$$
$$= 3.845 \text{ cm}$$
$$\beta_o/(\beta_2 - \beta_1) = 1.707/(1.7796 - 1.6373)$$
$$= 11.996$$

(ii) *For narrow band and large susceptance values of the irises:*

$$Q_k = (g_k/2)[\beta_o/(\beta_2 - \beta_1)]$$
$$b_k = 2(Q_k^2 - 1)^{1/2}$$
$$\therefore \quad Q_1 = (11.996/2) \times 1.0315 = 6.1869$$
$$Q_2 = (11.996/2) \times 1.1474 = 6.8821$$
$$Q_3 = (11.996/2) \times 1.0315 = 6.1869$$
$$b_1 = 2 \times (6.1869^2 - 1)^{1/2} = 12.21$$
$$b_2 = 2 \times (6.8821^2 - 1)^{1/2} = 13.24$$
$$b_3 = b_1 = 12.21$$

(iii) *Calculation of cavity length l_k:*
$$\tan \beta_o l_k = -2/b_k$$
$$\tan (1.707 \times 180°/3.1415) l_k = -2/b_k$$
$$\tan 97.81 \ l_k = -2/b_k$$

(a) *For k = 1,*
$$\tan 97.81 \ l_1 = -2/b_1 = -2/12.21$$
$$= -0.1638$$
$$= -\tan 9.3°$$
$$= \tan (180° - 9.3°)$$
$$= \tan 170.7°$$
$$\therefore \quad l_1 = 170.7/97.81 = 1.745 \text{ cm}$$

(b) *For k = 2,*
$$\tan 97.81 \ l_2 = -2/b_2 = -2/13.24$$
$$= -0.11511$$
$$= -\tan 8.6°$$
$$= \tan (180° - 8.6°)$$
$$= \tan 171.4$$
$$\therefore \quad l_2 = 171.4/97.81 = 1.752 \text{ cm}$$
$$l_3 = l_1 = 1.745 \text{ cm}$$

(c) *Distance between the cavities:*
$$l_{k,\ k+1} = [(l_k + l_{k+1})/2] - \lambda_{go}/4$$
$$= [(l_k + l_{k+1})/2] - (3.679/4)$$
$$= [(l_k + l_{k+1})/2] - 0.9198$$
$$\therefore \ l_{1,2} = [(l_1 + l_2)/2] - 0.9198$$
$$= (1.745 + 1.752)/2 - 0.9189$$

$$= 0.8287 \text{ cm}$$
$$l_{2,3} = [(l_2 + l_3)/2] - 0.9189$$
$$= (1.745 + 1.752)/2 - 0.9189$$
$$= 0.8287 \text{ cm}$$

(d) *Radii of diaphragm holes:* For $\mathbf{TE_{10}}$ mode, radius of the *k-th* hole is given by

$$r_k^3 = 3ab/8\beta_o b_k$$

$$\therefore \ r_1 = \left(\frac{3 \times 2.5 \times 1.2}{8 \times 1.707 \times 12.21}\right)^{1/3}$$
$$= 0.3783 \text{ cm}$$

$$\therefore \ r_2 = \left(\frac{3 \times 2.5 \times 1.2}{8 \times 1.707 \times 13.24}\right)^{1/3}$$
$$= 0.3684 \text{ cm}$$
$$r_3 = r_1 = 0.3783 \text{ cm}$$

Example 9.3 Design a symmetrical three section maximally flat band pass quarter-wave coupled filter with center frequency in pass band and bandwidth are 9 GHz and 90 MHz respectively. Assume 3 dB insertion loss.

Solution: Given: $f_2 - f_1 = 90$ MHz, $f_o = 9$ GHz, $n = 3$

Fractional bandwidth of the filter
$$= \text{bandwidth/center frequency}$$
$$= 90/9,000 = 1/100 = 1\%$$

(a) The elements of low-pass prototype filter for maximally flat response with $n = 3$ and insertion loss of 3 dB at band edges, (from Table 9.1) are given by
$$g_o = 1,$$
$$g_1 = g_3 = 1,$$
$$g_2 = 2.$$

$$f_o = 9 \text{ GHz} = \sqrt{f_1 f_2} = 9 \times 10^3 \text{ Hz}$$
$$f_2 - f_1 = 90 \text{ MHz}$$
$$\therefore f_1 = 9.045 \text{ GHz}$$
$$f_2 = 8.955 \text{ GHz}$$

(b) *X-band waveguide dimensions:*
$$a = 2.286 \text{ cm}$$
$$b = 1.016 \text{ cm}$$

$\beta_o = 2\pi[(f_o/c)^2 - (1/2a)^2]^{1/2}$

$\quad = 6.28[(9/30)^2 - (1/2 \times 2.286)^2]^{1/2}$

$\quad = 1.851 \text{ rad/cm}$

$\quad = 106.6°$

$\lambda_{go} = 2\pi/\beta_o = 6.28/1.851 = 3.393 \text{ cm}$

$\beta_1 = 2\pi[(f_1/c)^2 - (1/2a)^2]^{1/2}$

$\quad = 6.28\left[\left(\dfrac{8.955}{30}\right)^2 - \left(\dfrac{1}{2 \times 2.286}\right)^2\right]^{1/2}$

$\quad = 1.28 \text{ rad/cm}$

$\beta_2 = 2\beta\pi\,[(f_2/c)^2 - (1/2a)^2]^{1/2}$

$\quad = 6.28\left[\left(\dfrac{9.045}{30}\right)^2 - \left(\dfrac{1}{2 \times 2.286}\right)^2\right]^{1/2}$

$\quad = 1.31 \text{ rad/cm}$

$\dfrac{\beta_o}{\beta_2 - \beta_1} = 1.851/(1.31 - 1.28) = 61.7$

(c) *Loaded Q of the section:*

$\quad Q_k = (g_k/2)[\beta_o/(\beta_2 - \beta_1)]$

$\therefore \quad Q_1 = (1/2) \times 61.7 = 30.85$

$\quad Q_2 = (2/2) \times 61.7 = 61.7$

$\quad Q_3 = (1/2) \times 61.7 = 30.85$

(d) The hole susceptance are given by

$\quad b_k = 2(Q_k^2 - 1)^{1/2}$

$\therefore \quad b_1 = 2(Q_1^2 - 1)^{1/2} = 61.6$

$\quad b_2 = 2(Q_2^2 - 1)^{1/2} = 123.32$

$\quad b_3 = 2(Q_3^2 - 1)^{1/2} = 61.6$

(e) *Computation of l_k at f_o:*

$$\tan \beta_o l_k = -2/b_k$$

$$\tan (1.851 \times 180°/3.1415)l_k = -2/b_k$$

$$\tan 106.06\, l_k = -2/b_k$$

(i) *For k = 1,*

$\tan 106.06\, l_1 = -2/b_1 = -2/61.66$

$\quad = -0.0324$

$\quad = -\tan 1.61$

$\quad = \tan (180° - 1.6°)$

$\quad = \tan 178.4$

$\therefore \quad l_1 = 178.4/106.06 = 1.82 \text{ cm}$

(ii) *For k = 2,*

$\tan 106.06\, l_2 = -2/b_2 = -2/123.32$

$\quad = -0.0162$

$\quad = -\tan 0.6$

$\quad = \tan (180° - 0.6°)$

$\quad = \tan 179.4$

$\therefore \quad l_2 = 179.4/106.06$

$\quad = 1.691 \text{ cm}$

$\quad l_3 = l_1 = 1.682 \text{ cm}$

(f) *Distance between the sections:*

$\quad l_{k,\,k+1} = [(l_k + l_{k+1})/2] - \lambda_{go}/4$

$\quad = [(l_k + l_{k+1})/2] - (3.393/4)$

$\quad = [(l_k + l_{k+1})/2] - 0.8483$

$\therefore \quad l_{1,2} = [(l_1 + l_2)/2] - 0.8483$

$\quad = (1.682 + 1.691)/2 - 0.8483$

$\quad = 0.84 \text{ cm}$

$\quad l_{2,3} = [(l_2 + l_3)/2] - 0.8483$

$\quad = (1.687 + 1.677)/2 - 0.8483$

$\quad = 0.84 \text{ cm}$

(g) *Radii of diaphragm holes:* For **TE$_{10}$** mode, radius of the *k-th* hole is given by

$$r_k^3 = 3ab/8\beta_o b_k$$

$\therefore \quad r_1 = \left(\dfrac{3 \times 2.286 \times 1.016}{8 \times 1.851 \times 66.66}\right)^{1/3}$

$\quad = 0.1916 \text{ cm}$

$\therefore \quad r_2 = \left(\dfrac{3 \times 2.286 \times 1.016}{8 \times 1.851 \times 123.32}\right)^{1/3}$

$\quad = 0.1563 \text{ cm}$

$\quad r_3 = r_1 = 0.1916 \text{ cm}$

Example 9.4 Design a strip line Tchebyshev narrow band-stop filter having frequency of infinite attenuation at 4 GHz, fractional bandwidth of 0.05, pass band ripple of 0.5 dB and 26 dB minimum attenuation at 2% of the center frequency. Use dielectric substrate of $\varepsilon_r = 2.25$ and $h = 0.125''$. Nominal characteristic impedance of the filter is 50 ohm. Assume resonator line impedances $Z_{b1} = Z_{b2} = Z_{b3} = 60$ ohm and $W_o/h = 0.80$ and $W_1/h = 0.62$

Solution: Given: At 4 GHz, attenuation = Γ, $\Delta f/f_o = 0.05$, ripple = 0.5 dB, 26 dB at 2% of the center frequency

(a) To find number of resonators n: 2% of the center frequency = $0.02 \times 4 = 80$ MHz

The frequency f_x at which attenuation is 26 dB is given by

$$f_x = 4 \text{ GHz} + 80 \text{ MHz}/2 = 4.04 \text{ GHz}$$

$$\therefore \quad f_x/f_o = 4.04/4 = 1.01$$

$$\Delta f/f_o = 0.05$$

(b) From frequency transformation at 26 dB attenuation point, we get

$$1/\omega_{nx} = (f_o/\Delta f) [(f_x/f_o) - (f_o/f_x)]$$
$$= (1/0.05)(1.01 - 0.99) = 2/5$$
$$\omega_{nx} = 2.5$$

(c) Ripple = 0.5 dB

$$10 \log (1 + a_m^2) = 0.5 \text{ dB}$$

$$1 + a_m^2 = 10^{0.5/10} = 1.122$$

$$\therefore \qquad a_m^2 = 0.122$$

(d) At 26 dB attenuation point,

$$w_{nx} = 2.5, \quad a_m^2 = 0.122$$

$$10 \log (1 + a_m^2 \cosh^2(n \cosh^{-1} w_{nx})) = 26 \text{ dB}$$

$$\therefore \quad 1 + a_m^2 \cosh^2 [n \cosh^{-1} (2.5)] = 10^{26/10}$$
$$= 398.11$$

$$\cosh^2 [n \cosh^{-1}(2.5)] = \frac{(3.98 - 1)}{0.122}$$

$$\cosh [n \cosh^{-1}(2.5)] = 57.1$$
$$= \cosh 4.74°$$

$$\therefore \qquad n = \frac{4.74}{\cosh^{-1}(2.5)}$$
$$= 3$$

(e) *Element values of low-pass prototype filter:* For $n = 3$, ripple = 0.5 dB, the element values from Table 9.2 are:

$$g_0 = g_4 = 1.0$$
$$g_1 = g_5 = 1.5963$$
$$g_2 = 1.0969$$
$$\omega_{nc} = 1$$

(f) *Microwave realization:* $n = 3$ (odd), the impedance of the quarter wavelength coupling lines are $Z' = Z_o$. The parameters of series resonators are:

$$x_1/R_o = x_3/R_o = \omega_o/[g_0 g_1(\omega_o - \omega_1)]$$
$$= 1/(1.5963 \times 0.05) = 12.53$$

$$x_2/R_o = (Z_1/R_o)^2 (\omega_o g_o)/[g_2(\omega_2 - \omega_1)]$$
$$= 1/(1.0969 \times 0.05) = 18.23$$

$$\therefore \quad x_1 = x_3 = 12.53 \times 50 = 626.5 \text{ ohm}$$
$$x_2 = 18.23 \times 50 = 911.6 \text{ ohm}$$

The gap capacitive reactance at resonant frequency is given by

$$\omega_o C_{gk} = 1/(Z_k \tan \varphi_o)$$
$$F(\varphi_o) = \varphi_o \sec^2\varphi_o + \tan \varphi_o = x_k/Z_k$$

(g) *To find guide wavelength:*

$$h = 0.125'' = 0.3175 \text{ cm}$$

$$\varepsilon_r = 2.25$$

$$\lambda_{go} = \frac{\lambda_o}{\sqrt{\varepsilon_r}} = \frac{(30/4)}{\sqrt{2.25}} = 5.0 \text{ cm}$$

$$\lambda_{go}/4 = 1.25 \text{cm}$$

(h) *To find line widths*: Resonator line impedances

$$Z_{b1} = Z_{b2} = Z_{b3} = 60 \text{ ohm}$$

$$W_o/h = 0.80, \quad W_1/h = 0.62.$$

• For $Z_o = 50$ ohm line:

$$Z_o\sqrt{\varepsilon_r} = 50 \times \sqrt{2.25} = 75 \text{ ohm}.$$

$$W_o = 0.80 \times 0.3175 = 2.5 \text{ mm}$$

• For $Z_o = 60$ ohm line:

$$Z_o\sqrt{\varepsilon_r} = 60 \times \sqrt{2.56} = 90 \text{ ohm}.$$

$$W_1 = 0.62 \times 0.3175 = 1.97 \text{ mm}$$

$$W_2 = W_3 = 2.5 \text{ mm}$$

(i) *Stub length:*

$$F(\varphi_{o1}) = F(\varphi_{o3}) = \varphi_{o1} \sec^2\varphi_{o1} + \tan \varphi_{o1}$$
$$= x_1/Z_{b1}$$
$$= 626.5/60 = 10.442$$

$$F(\varphi_{o2}) = 911.6/60 = 15.19$$

From Table 9.5, we find

$$\varphi_{o1} = \varphi_{o3} = 67.5° = 1.1781 \text{ rad.}$$
$$\varphi_{o2} = 71.35° = 1.2453 \text{ rad.}$$

$\therefore \qquad l_1 = l_3 = \lambda_{go}\varphi_{o1}/2\pi$
$\qquad \qquad = (5 \times 1.1781)/6.28 = 0.938 \text{ cm}$
$\qquad l_2 = \lambda_{go}\varphi_{o2}/2\pi$
$\qquad \qquad = (5 \times 1.2453)/6.28 = 0.9915 \text{ cm}$

(j) *Capacitance gap diameter:*

$\qquad d_k = (\lambda_{go}/4) - l_k$
$\qquad d_1 = d_3 = 1.25 - 0.938 = 0.312 \text{ cm}$
$\qquad d_3 = 1.25 - 0.9915 = 0.2585 \text{ cm}$

KEY POINTS

- An ideal filter is a passive, reciprocal, linear two-port device that provides perfect transmission for all frequencies in the pass band and infinite attenuation in the stop-band.

- Filters are classified as (i) low-pass, (ii) high-pass, (iii) band pass and (iv) band rejection filters.

- Low-pass filters transmit all signal frequencies from zero to f_c known as cut-off frequency and attenuate all frequencies above the cut-off frequency.

- High-pass filters transmit all signal frequencies above a low cut-off frequency f_c and reject all frequencies below the cut-off frequency.

- Band pass filters transmit all signal frequencies in a range f_1 (lower cut-off frequency) to f_2 (upper cut-off frequency) and attenuate all frequencies outside this range.

- Band rejection filters attenuate all signal frequencies in a range f_1 to f_2 and transmit all frequencies outside this range.

- Practical filters have a very low attenuation in the pass band and a small output signal in the stop band due to the presence of resistance in the reactive elements.

- Microwave filter elements are realized by means of sections of coaxial lines, waveguides, strip or microstrip lines, cavity resonators and resonant irises.

- A series inductance is realized by a short circuit stub of length less than $\lambda/4$.

- A series capacitance is realized by a short circuit stub of length greater than $\lambda/4$ but less than $\lambda/2$.

- A shunt inductance is realized by a short circuit stub of length less than $\lambda/4$ in the plane parallel to the broad wall of a rectangular waveguide or by means of inductive iris.

- A shunt capacitance is realized by means of capacitive iris.

- According to Foster's reactance theorem, a physically realizable filter should have a finite number of poles and zeros.

- In the microwave filter design by insertion loss method, the general procedure is first to design a low-pass prototype filter and then frequency transform this design to the required type with specified center and band-edge frequencies.

- The Butterworth response or maximally flat response or binomial response exhibits a flat response in the pass band and monotonically increasing attenuation in the stop band.

- The Tchebyshev response or equiripple response exhibits equi-ripple response in the pass band and monotonically increasing attenuation in the stop band.

- Microwave low pass filters with wave-guide sections cannot be realized since wave-guides are basically high-pass lines. Hence, low-pass filters are designed with coaxial lines, strip lines or microstrip lines.

FURTHER READING

1. Collins RE (1996). Foundations of Microwave Engineering, McGraw Hill, NY.
2. Soohoo RF (1971). Microwave Electronics, Addison-Wesley, Mass.
3. Fox AG (1941). Wave Guide Filters and Transformers, BST, Rep. MM-41, pp. 160–250..
4. Liao SY (2000). Microwave Devices and Circuits, PHI, New Delhi.
5. Malherbe JAG (1979). Microwave Transmission Line Filters, Aptech, Dedham, Mass.

REVIEW QUESTIONS

9.1 Define an ideal filter.

9.2 How does a practical filter differ from the ideal one? Mention the reasons.

9.3 Define a low-pass filter and draw the ideal and practical response of the filter.

9.4 Define a high-pass filter and draw the ideal and practical response of the filter.

9.5 Define a band pass filter and draw the ideal and practical response of the filter.

9.6 Define a band stop filter and draw the ideal and practical response of the filter.

9.7 Mention four important parameters of a filter.

9.8 Define group delay.

9.9 Define insertion loss.

9.10 Mention the components used in MW filters.

9.11 State the Foster's reactance theorem.

9.12 Explain the reason for using insertion loss method to design a filter.

9.13 Explain the concept of designing a microwave filter.

9.14 What is meant by flat response of a filter?

9.15 What is meant by equiripple response of a filter?

9.16 Explain frequency and impedance transformation.

9.17 Draw the Butterworth response characteristic of low pass filter.

9.18 Draw the Tchebyshev response characteristic of low pass filter.

DESCRIPTIVE QUESTIONS

9.1 What are the parameters of the filters? Explain insertion loss, return loss and group delay.

9.2 Derive an expression for the insertion loss of a filter with mismatch terminations.

9.3 Explain clearly the method of designing a prototype low pass filter by insertion loss method.

9.4 Explain the transformations required to transform low pass prototype filter into low-pass microwave filter.

9.5 Explain the transformations required to transform low pass prototype filter into high-pass microwave filter.

9.6 Explain the transformations required to transform low pass prototype filter into band pass microwave filter.

9.7 Explain the transformations required to transform low pass prototype filter into band pass microwave filter.

PRACTICE PROBLEMS

9.1 Design a low pass microwave filter with cut-off frequency of 2 GHz, 30 dB attenuation at 3.5 GHz with 0.2 dB ripple. Use alumina substrate of thickness 0.63 mm. Assume $\varepsilon_r = 9.9$, $Z_{oc} = 20\ \Omega$, $Z_{oL} = 100\ \Omega$.

(**Ans:** $C_1 = C_5 = 2.132$ pF, $C_3 = 3.447$ pF, $L_2 = L_4 = 5.32$ nH, $l_{c1} = l_{c5} = 4.605$ mm, $l_{c3} = 7.445$ mm, $l_{L2} = l_{L4} = 6.501$ cm)

9.2 Design a quarter-wave coupled three-cavity filter having maximum pass band ripple of 0.1 dB. The pass band extends from 10 GHz to 10.4 GHz. Use wave-guides of dimensions $a = 2.286$ cm and $b = 1.016$ cm and inductive diaphragm with circular holes.

(**Ans:** $l_1 = l_3 = 1.843$ cm, $l_2 = 1.851$ cm, $l_{1,2} = l_{1,3} = 0.885$ cm, $r_1 = 0.3538$ cm, $r_2 = 0.3267$ cm)

9.3 Design a symmetrical three-section maximally flat band pass quarter-wave coupled filter with center frequency in pass band and band-width are 10 GHz and 100 MHz respectively. Assume 3 dB insertion loss.

(**Ans:** $l_1 = l_3 = 1.965$ cm, $l_2 = 1.977$ cm, $l_{1,2} = l_{2,3} = 0.9772$, $r_1 = 0.2136$ cm, $r_2 = 0.1693$ cm)

9.4 Design a strip line Tchebyshev narrow band-stop filter having frequency of infinite attenuation at 4 GHz, fractional bandwidth of 0.05, pass band ripple of 0.5 dB and 26 dB minimum attenuation at 2% of the center frequency. Use dielectric substrate of $\varepsilon_r = 2.56$ and $h = 0.125"$. Nominal characteristic impedance of the filter is 50 ohm. Assume resonator line impedances $Z_{b1} = Z_{b2} = Z_{b3} = 60$ ohm and $W_o/h = 0.74$ and $W_1/h = 0.55$.

(**Ans:** $l_1 = l_3 = 0.8779$ cm, $l_2 = 0.9280$ cm, $d_1 = d_3 = 0.2921$ cm, $d_2 = 0.242$ cm)

REFERENCE

1. Matthaei GL et al (1964). *Microwave Filters, Impedance Matching Networks and Coupling Structures*, McGraw Hill, NY.

2. Rizzi PA. *Microwave Engineering: Passive Circuits*, PH, NJ.

3. Das A and Das SK (2004). *Microwave Engineering*, TMH, New Delhi.

4. Ghose RN (1963). *Microwave Circuit Theory and Analysis*, McGraw Hill, NY.

5. Harvey AF (1963). *Microwave Engineering*, Acad. Press, NY.

6. Montogomery CG et al (1948). *Principles of Microwave Circuits*, McGraw Hill, NY.

7. Pozar DM (1990). *Microwave Engineering*, Addison-Wesley, Mass.

8. Reich HJ et al (1953). *Microwave Theory and Techniques*, Van Nostrand, NJ.

9. Slater JC (1950). *Microwave Electronics*, Van Nostrand, NJ.

10. Atwater HA (1962). *Introduction to Microwave Theory*, McGraw Hill, NY.

11. Altman JL (1962). *Microwave Circuits*, Van Nostrand, NJ.

12. Gandhi OP (1981). *Microwave Engineering and Applications*, Pergamon, NY.

13. Veley VF (1987). *Modern Microwave Technology*, PH, NJ.

Klystron Amplifier

Objectives

- Understand the HF limitations of LF electron tubes.
- Know the constructional details of klystron tube.
- Appreciate the velocity modulation and the bunching process.
- Evaluate the effect of beam loading on the klystron amplifier.
- Derive expressions for output power and voltage gain.
- Identify the advantages of multicavity klystron tubes.

10.1 INTRODUCTION

The conventional vacuum tubes such as triodes and pentodes, cannot be used at microwave frequencies because of the following limitations:

i. Transit time effects

ii. Lead reactance and interelectrode capacitances

iii. Cathode emission and plate heat dissipation

iv. Power loss due to skin effect

v. Constant gain-bandwidth product.

Because of these, the design and the principle of operation of microwave tubes differ from those of conventional vacuum tubes. The commonly used microwave vacuum tubes are klystron, reflex klystron, travelling wave tube (TWT) and magnetron. In this chapter, we shall discuss the constructional details, mechanism of operation and applications of klystron tubes.

10.2 LIMITATIONS OF CONVENTIONAL VACUUM TUBES

In this section, we shall study in detail the effect of the above limitations on conventional vacuum tubes.

10.2.1 Transit Time Effect

Transit time is the time duration for an electron to travel from cathode to anode. The transit time is given by

$$t = d/v \qquad (10.1)$$

Here d is the distance between the cathode and the anode, v is the velocity of the electrons. At frequencies below the microwave frequencies, the transit time is negligible compared to the period of the signal. However, at microwave frequencies, the transit time is comparable to the period of the microwave signal. The potential between the grid and the cathode may alternate several times during the electron transit. The grid potential during the negative half cycle

223

removes energy that was given to the electron during the positive half cycle. Consequently, the electrons may oscillate back and forth between the cathode-grid space or return to the cathode. The overall effect is to reduce the operating efficiency. The degeneration becomes more serious when frequencies are well above 1 GHz. Once the electrons pass the grid, they are quickly accelerated to the anode by the high plate voltage. At MW frequencies, since the transit time is not negligible, the transconductance becomes a complex number with a relatively small magnitude and hence, the output power is decreased.

The transit time may be minimized by first accelerating the electron beam with a very high dc voltage and then velocity modulating it. This principle is used in microwave tubes such as klystrons and magnetrons.

10.2.2 Lead Reactance and Interelectrode Capacitance Effects

The lead reactance at low frequencies is negligible and the interelectrode capacitive reactance is very large; hence they may be neglected. However, at microwave frequencies, the lead reactances are large enough that they cannot be neglected. The interelectrode capacitive reactances reduce to reasonable values so that they have to be taken into account while analyzing microwave circuits. The effect of these is to load the input circuit so as to reduce the operating efficiency.

These effects are better understood by considering the triode circuit shown in Fig. 10.1. Figure 10.1(a) shows the triode circuit at high frequencies and Fig. 10(b) shows its equivalent circuit. The grid-plate capacitance is C_{gp} and L_k is the cathode inductance.

Since $C_{gp} \ll C_{gk}$ and $\omega L_k \ll 1\lambda(\omega C_{gh})$, the input voltage V_{in} is given by

$$V_{in} = V_g + V_k = V_g + j\omega L_k g_m V_g \quad (10.2a)$$

and the input current I_{in} is given by

$$I_{in} = j\omega C_{gk} V_g \quad (10.2b)$$

From the above equations, we obtain

$$V_{in} = \frac{I_{in}(1 + j\omega L_k g_m)}{j\omega C_{gk}} \quad (10.3)$$

The input admittance is approximately

$$Y_{in} = \frac{I_{in}}{V_{in}}$$

$$= \frac{j\omega C_{gk}}{1 + j\omega L_k g_m}$$

$$= \omega^2 L_k C_{gk} g_m + j\omega C_{gk} \quad (10.4)$$

in which $(\omega L_k g_m) \ll 1$ has been dropped. Since the cathode lead is usually short and quite large in diameter, the transconductance is much less than 1/millimho.

The input impedance Z_{in} at very high frequencies is given by

$$Z_{in} = \frac{1}{\omega^2 L_k C_{gk} g_m} - \frac{jl}{\omega^3 L_k^2 C_{gk} g_m^2} \quad (10.5)$$

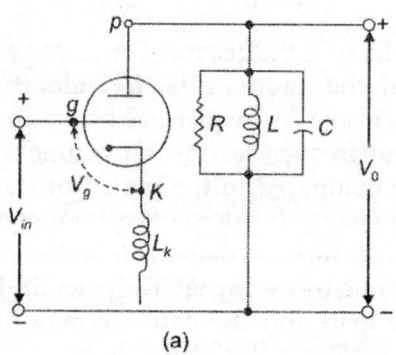

(a)

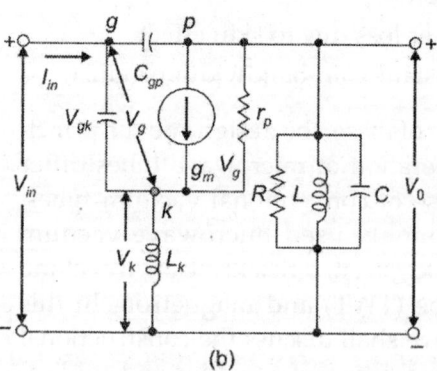

(b)

Fig. 10.1: (a) Triode circuit (b) Equivalent circuit

The real part of Z_{in} is inversely proportional to f^2 and the imaginary part is inversely proportional to f^3. When the frequency is above 1 GHz, the real part becomes small enough to nearly short the signal source. Hence, the output power P_o is decreased rapidly.

Reduction in the lead length and electrode area minimizes this effect. However, this limits the power-handling capacity of the devices.

10.2.3 Cathode Emission and Plate Heat Dissipation Limitation

Microwave sources should generate high power for transmission. The conventional vacuum tubes are low power devices. To increase the power, the cathode emission should be copious. For this, the cathode area should be very large. This, in turn, will increase the heat on the anode as well as the inter-electrode capacitance problem. To dissipate the heat produced, the anode area has to be large. Klystron and reflex klystron tubes utilize an electron beam on which space-charge waves and cyclotron waves can be excited. The space charge waves are primarily longitudinal oscillations of the electron and interact with electromagnetic fields in cavities and slow wave structures to cause amplification.

10.2.4 Power Loss due to Skin Effect

At higher frequencies, the current has the tendency to flow through the outer surface of the conductors. This gives raise to higher resistance and hence higher losses.

10.2.5 Gain-Bandwidth Product

The gain-bandwidth product for an amplifier is a constant quantity. To obtain higher gain, we have to sacrifice bandwidth. At microwave frequencies, higher gain over a broad bandwidth is required for transmission purposes. This is achieved with re-entrant cavities and slow-wave structures in microwave tubes.

10.3 CLASSIFICATION OF MICROWAVE VACUUM TUBES

To overcome the limitations of the conventional vacuum tubes at microwave frequencies, the microwave tubes utilize the transit time for microwave amplification and oscillations. Microwave tubes consist of an electron gun that produces electron beam. The microwave tubes are classified based on the device used for transfer of amplified energy as

(i) Cavity structures

(ii) Slow-wave structures

The klystron, reflex klystron and magnetron belong to the cavity type (tubes) and the traveling wave tube is a slow-wave structure. They may also be classified based on the direction of electric and magnetic fields within the structure as

(i) Linear-beam or "O" type tubes

(ii) Cross field or "M" type tubes.

In the linear-beam tubes, the accelerating electric field is in the same direction as that of the static magnetic field used to focus the electron beam. In the cross-field type tubes, the accelerating electric field is perpendicular to the static magnetic field. The klystron, reflex klystron and the traveling wave tubes are linear-beam tubes and the magnetron is the cross-field device.

10.4 TWO CAVITY KLYSTRON AMPLIFIER

A widely used microwave amplifier is the two-cavity klystron amplifier. It operates on the principle of velocity and current modulation. Figure 10.2 shows a two-cavity klystron amplifier tube. It consists of an electron gun, a buncher cavity, a catcher cavity and the collector. The space between the two cavities is known as *drift space*. A high velocity electron beam from the electron gun passes through the two cavities and drift space. Then, the collector that is at a very high dc potential with respect to the cathode

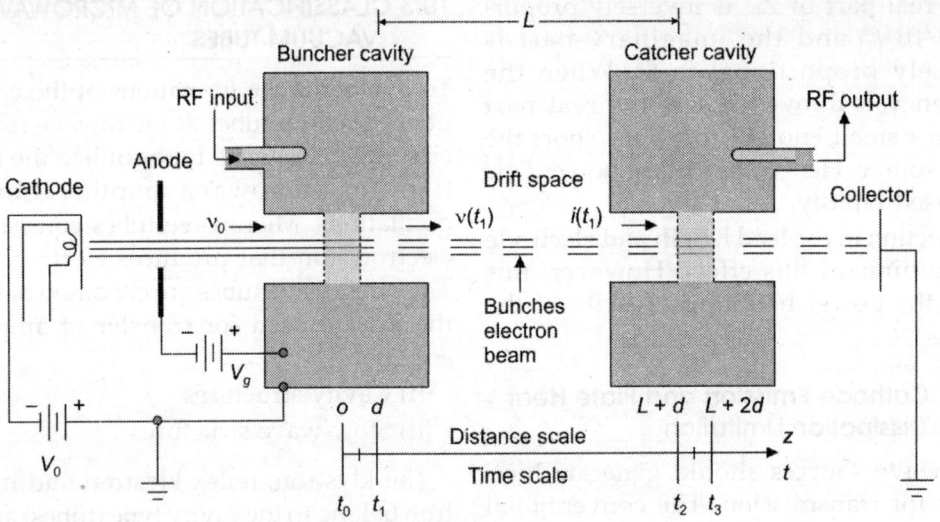

Fig. 10.2: Two-cavity Klystron amplifier

collects the electrons. The input RF signal to be amplified is used to excite the input cavity through a coupling loop. The output RF signal is collected at the catcher or the output cavity through another coupling loop. An axial magnetic field is applied so that the electron beam does not spread during transit. The anode voltage V_0 and the cavity gap width d are such that the transit time through each gap is less than one-fourth of the period of the RF signal.

10.5 MECHANISM OF OPERATION

All electrons emitted from the electron gun arrive at the buncher or input cavity with uniform velocity. Those electrons passing the first cavity gap when the input RF signal is zero, pass through it without change in the velocity. Those passing through the positive half cycle of the input RF signal get accelerated and pass faster. Those electrons that pass through the negative half cycle of the input RF signal get decelerated and pass slowly. As a result of these actions, the electrons gradually bunch together as they travel down the drift space L. Thus the electrons form bunches. This variation in electron velocity is known as *velocity modula-*

tion. The density of electrons in the second cavity gap varies cyclically in time. The electron beam contains an ac component and is said to be *density* or *current modulated*. Thus, the effect of drift space is to convert velocity modulation into current modulation. While this beam passing through the catcher or output cavity induces RF current in the cavity and thereby excites RF field in the output cavity. The phase of the induced voltage in the output cavity is opposite to that of the input cavity. Hence, the output-gap voltage retards the bunched electrons. The maximum bunching should occur approximately midway between the catcher cavity grids during its retarding phase. The kinetic energy of electrons during the retardation process is transferred to the output cavity. The electrons come out of the output cavity with reduced velocity and are collected by the collector. The signal amplitude at the output cavity attains a large steady value when the kinetic energy compensates the output cavity circuit losses. The amplified signal is coupled to the output circuit from the catcher cavity through a current loop. The output signal is rich in harmonics. Hence the cavity can be tuned to fundamental or any harmonic frequency.

10.6 ANALYSIS OF TWO CAVITY KLYSTRON AMPLIFIER

On the basis of the following assumptions, the quantitative analysis of the two cavity klystron amplifier is carried out:

1. The electrons leave the cathode with zero velocity.
2. The electron beam has a uniform density in the cross-section of the beam.
3. Compared to the periodic time of the input RF signal, transit time in the cavity gap is small.
4. Input RF signal amplitude is very small compared to the accelerating anode potential.
5. The anode, cathode, collector and the cavity grids are all parallel.
6. Cavity grids do not intercept any electron while passing through it.
7. No de-bunching takes place at the bunching point.
8. The drift space is free of RF field.

10.6.1 Reentrant Cavity Resonator

A reentrant cavity resonator is a cavity resonator in which the opposite sides are brought closer together to form a reentrant structure. Several types of reentrant cavities are shown in Fig. 10.3. The most commonly used reentrant cavity is shown in Fig. 10.4 with field configurations. The electric field is concentrated in the small gap g. The tuning of the cavity is accomplished by means of short-circuit plungers. The reentrant cavity of length d and gap width $g << d$ may be considered as a coaxial line with radii of the

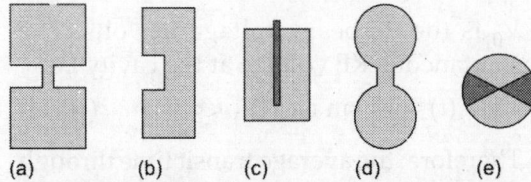

(a)   (b)   (c)   (d)   (e)

Fig. 10.3: Several types of reentrant cavities (a) Coaxial (b) Radial (c) Tunable (d) Tovoidal (e) Butterfly

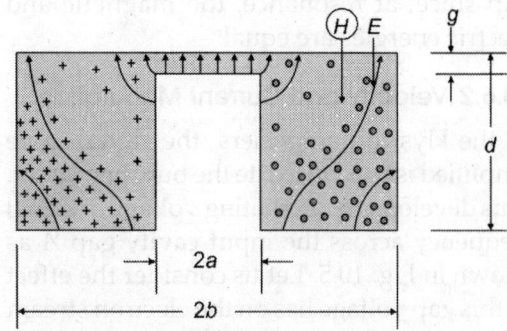

Fig. 10.4: Commonly used reentrant cavity

inner and outer conductors as a and b. The characteristic impedance of the coaxial line is given by

$$Z_0 = \left(\frac{1}{2\pi}\right)\sqrt{\frac{\mu}{\varepsilon}}\ln\left(\frac{b}{a}\right) \qquad (10.6)$$

The input impedance to each shorted co-axial line is given by

$$Z_{in} = jZ_0 \tan\left(2\pi d/\lambda_g\right) \qquad (10.7)$$

Substituting for Z_0 in the above equation, we obtain

$$Z_{in} = j\left(\frac{1}{2\pi}\right)\sqrt{\frac{\mu}{\varepsilon}}\ln\left(\frac{b}{a}\right)\tan\left(\frac{2\pi d}{\lambda_g}\right) \qquad (10.8)$$

The inductance of the cavity is given by

$$L = \frac{2X_{in}}{\omega} = \left(\frac{1}{\pi\omega}\right)\sqrt{\frac{\mu}{\varepsilon}}\ln\left(\frac{b}{a}\right)\tan\left(\frac{2\pi d}{\lambda_g}\right) \qquad (10.9)$$

The capacitance of the gap is given by

$$C_g = \varepsilon a^2\pi/d \qquad (10.11)$$

The gap capacitance C_g and the coaxial line below the gap provide, at resonance, equal and opposite reactance at the plane of the capacitance. Hence,

$$1/\omega_r C = Z_0 \tan\left(2\pi d/\lambda_g\right) \qquad (10.11)$$

or, $\quad d = (\lambda_g/2\pi)\tan^{-1}(1/Z_0\omega_r C) \quad (10.12)$

The shorted coaxial cavity stores more magnetic energy than the electric energy. The balance of the electric energy appears in the gap since, at resonance, the magnetic and electric energies are equal.

10.6.2 Velocity and Current Modulation

In the klystron amplifiers, the signal to be amplified is used to excite the buncher cavity. This develops an alternating voltage of signal frequency across the input cavity gap A as shown in Fig. 10.5. Let us consider the effect of this gap voltage has on the electron stream passing the gap A when the RF signal is zero while going positive. The electron passing through the gap A travels towards the gap C without any change in velocity. Let this electron be designated as *reference electron*. However, an electron passing through the gap A slightly later than this reference electron is accelerated by the positive RF field at the input gap. Hence, it travels from A to C with increased velocity. This electron therefore tends to overtake the reference electron. Similarly, the electron that passes through A slightly before the reference electron encounters a negative RF filed at the gap and therefore slowed down. This earlier electron tends to drop back and overtaken by the reference electron. As a result of these, the electrons gradually *bunch* together as they travel along the drift space ABC as illustrated in Fig. 10.5. Thus, a pulsating stream of electrons passes through the output cavity gap C and excites oscillations in the output cavity. The voltage developed across C is the alternating component of the bunched beam flowing through the shunt impedance that the output cavity develops across the gap C. When the amplifier system is properly designed and adjusted, the power delivered to the output cavity is much greater than the power in the input cavity. Thus, signal amplification is achieved.

Electrons that pass the buncher cavity gap A at uniform time intervals have their velocities varied in accordance with the gap voltage at that moment. As a result of this, after the electrons have traveled the distance

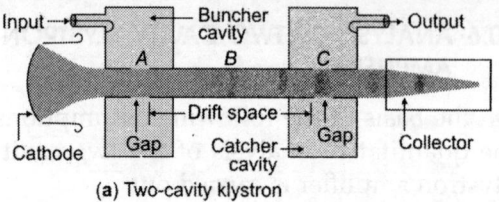

(a) Two-cavity klystron

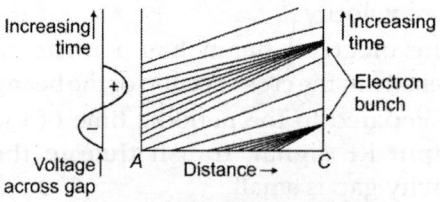

(b) Distance-time diagrgam showing bunching of electron stream

Fig. 10.5: Two cavity klystron amplifier

AC, they tend to be bunched together about the reference electron. The electrons pass the input gap A at a uniform rate but they emerge from the gap with velocities that are a function of time. Such an electron beam is said to be *velocity modulated*. However, after the electrons traveled sufficient distance down the drift space, bunching occurs and the density of the electrons in the stream varies cyclically in time. Under these conditions, as the electron beam contains an ac component, it is said to be *current modulated*.

10.6.3 Transit Time and Angle

The velocity of electrons accelerated by high dc voltage V_o before entering the buncher grids is given by

$$v_0 = \sqrt{2\left(\frac{e}{m}\right)V_o} = 5.93 \times 10^5 \sqrt{V_o} \text{ m/s}$$

(10.13)

V_0 is the dc beam voltage in volts. The instantaneous RF voltage at the cavity is

$$v_s(t) = V_1 \sin \omega t \quad (V_1 \ll V_0) \qquad (10.14)$$

Therefore, the average transit time through cavity gap d is given by

$$t_g = d/v_0 = (t_1 - t_0) \qquad (10.15)$$

The average transit angle is

$$\theta_g = \omega t_g = \omega d/v_o = \omega(t_1 - t_0) \quad (10.16)$$

10.6.4 Beam Coupling Coefficient

The average microwave voltage in the cavity gap shown in Fig. 10.6 is given by

$$V_{av} = \left(\frac{1}{t_g}\right)\int_{t_0}^{t_1} V_1 \sin \omega t \, dt$$

$$= -(V_1/\omega t_g)\,[\cos \omega t_1 - \cos \omega t_0]$$

$$= (V_1/\omega t_g)\,[\cos \omega t_0 - \cos (\omega t_0 + \omega d/u_o)]$$

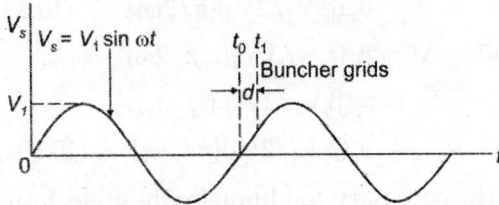

Fig. 10.6: Signal voltage in the input gap

Let $A = (\omega t_o + \omega d/2v_o) = (\omega t_o + \theta_g/2)$ and $B = \omega d/2v_o = \theta_g/2$. Using the trigonometric identity $\cos(A-B) - \cos(A+B) = 2\sin A \sin B$, we get

$$V_{av} = V_1 \frac{\sin(\omega d/2v_o)\cdot\sin(\omega t_o + \omega d/2v_o)}{(\omega d/2v_o)}$$

$$= V_1 \frac{\sin(\theta_g/2)\cdot\sin(\omega t_o + \theta_g/2)}{(\theta_g/2)}$$

$$= V_1 \beta_i \sin(\omega t_o + \omega d/2v_o)$$

$$= V_1 \beta_i \sin(\theta_g/2)/(\theta_g/2) \quad (10.17)$$

$$\beta_i = \sin(\omega d/2v_o)/(\omega d/2v_o)$$

$$= \sin(\theta_g/2)/(\theta_g/2) \quad (10.18)$$

β_i is known as *beam coupling coefficient* of the input buncher cavity gap. Thus, the coupling between the electron beam and the input cavity varies with gap d in the form of $(\sin\theta)/\theta$. As the gap d tends to zero, the beam-coupling coefficient also tends to zero.

10.6.5 Depth of Velocity Modulation

As the gap transit angle θ_g increases, the coupling coefficient between the electron beam and the buncher cavity decreases as shown in Fig. 10.7. Thus, the velocity modulation of the beam decreases for a given microwave signal. Immediately after the velocity modulation, the exit velocity of the electron beam from the buncher gap is given by

$$v(t_1) = \sqrt{2\left(\frac{e}{m}\right)(V_o + V_{av})} \quad (10.19)$$

$$= v_o\sqrt{1 + \left(\frac{V_1\beta_i}{V_o}\right)\sin\left(\omega_o + \frac{\theta_g}{2}\right)} \quad (10.20)$$

$$= v_o\sqrt{1 + d\sin\left(\omega t_o + \frac{\theta_g}{2}\right)} \quad (10.21)$$

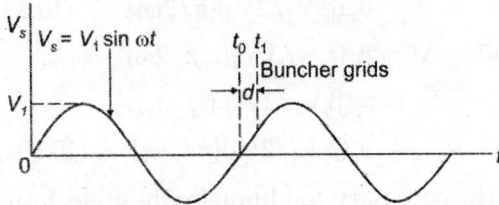

Fig. 10.7: Input beam coupling coefficient vs gap transit angle

The term $d = (V_1\beta_i/V_0)$ is known as *depth of velocity modulation*. If the modulation depth $m \ll 1$, then Eq. (10.21) for velocity modulation becomes

$$v(t_1) = v_o\left[1 + \frac{1}{2}d\sin\left(\omega t_0 + \frac{\theta_g}{2}\right)\right] \quad (10.22)$$

Alternatively, the velocity modulation equation may also be expressed as

$$v(t_1) = v_o\left[1 + \frac{1}{2}d\sin\left(\omega t_0 - \frac{\theta_g}{2}\right)\right] \quad (10.23)$$

since $\omega t_0 = \omega t_1 - \theta_g$

10.6.6 Bunching Process

The electrons leave the buncher gap with a velocity given by Eq. (10.22) or (10.23). They drift with this velocity in the field-free drift space between the two cavities. The effect of the velocity modulation is to produce bunching of the electron beam or *current modulation*. The electrons with velocity v_o that pass the buncher cavity gap at $V_s = 0$ travel through it with unchanged velocity v_o. These are the reference electrons and become the bunching center. Those electrons that pass the buncher cavity gap during the positive half cycle of the microwave input voltage V_s travel faster than the reference electrons. Those electrons that pass the buncher cavity gap during the negative half cycle of the microwave input voltage V_s travel slower than the reference electrons. At a distance ΔL along the beam from the input cavity, the electrons in beam have drifted into dense clusters. Fig. 10.8 shows the trajectories of minimum, zero and maximum electron acceleration.

Let us consider the electron that leaves the buncher at time t_0 and reaches the launching centre at t_d the distance ΔL is given by

$$\Delta L = v_o (t_d - t_b) \qquad (10.24)$$

Similarly, the distances for electrons at t_a and t_c are

$$\Delta L = v_{min} (t_d - t_a)$$
$$= v_{min} (t_d - t_b + \pi/2\omega) \qquad (10.25)$$
$$\Delta L = v_{max} (t_d - t_c)$$
$$= v_{min} (t_d - t_b - \pi/2\omega) \qquad (10.26)$$

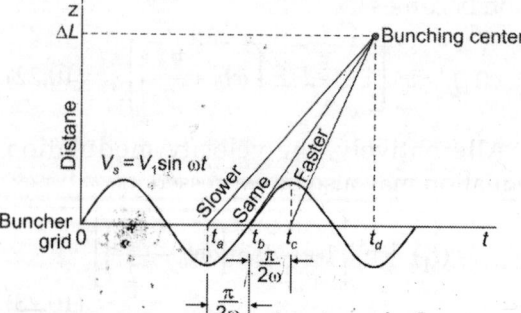

Fig. 10.8: Electron bunching distance

since $\quad t_a = t_b - (\pi/2\omega)$
and $\quad t_c = t_b + (\pi/2\omega)$

The maximum and minimum velocities obtained from Eqs (10.22) and (10.23) are

$$v_{min} = v_o(1 - V_1\beta_i/2V_0) \qquad (10.27)$$
$$v_{max} = v_o(1 + V_1\beta_i/2V_0) \qquad (10.28)$$

Substituting these values in Eqs (10.25) and (10.26), we get

$$\Delta L = v_o (t_d - t_b) + [(v_o\pi/2\omega) - v_o (\beta_iV_1/2V_0) (t_d - t_b) - v_o (\beta_iV_1/2V_0)(\pi/2\omega)] \qquad (10.29)$$

and $\quad \Delta L = v_o (t_d - t_b) - [(v_o\pi/2\omega) - v_o(\beta_iV_1/2V_0) (t_d - t_b) - v_o(\beta_iV_1/2V_0)(\pi/2\omega)] \qquad (10.30a)$

The necessary condition for these electrons to meet at the same distance ΔL is

$$\left(\frac{v_o\pi}{2\omega}\right) - v_o\left(\frac{\beta_iV_1}{2V_0}\right)(t_d - t_b) - v_o\left(\frac{\beta_iV_1}{2V_0}\right)\left(\frac{\pi}{2\omega}\right) = 0$$

$$(10.30b)$$

and

$$-\left(\frac{v_o\pi}{2\omega}\right) + v_o\left(\frac{\beta_1v_1}{2v_o}\right)(t_d - t_b) + v_o\frac{\beta_1v_1}{2v_o}\cdot\frac{\pi}{2\omega} = 0$$

$$(10.31)$$

Assuming $(\beta_iV_1/2V_o)$ is negligible, we obtain

$$(t_d - t_b) = \pi V_o/\omega\beta_iV_1 \qquad (10.32)$$
and $\quad \Delta L = v_o\pi V_o/\omega\beta_iV_1 \qquad (10.33)$

In deriving the above, the effect of space charge in the drift space is neglected. The distance-time plot of the electron trajectories is shown in Fig. 10.9 and it is known as *applegate diagram*.

10.6.7 Applegate Diagram

This diagram illustrates the launching action in a klystron amplifier. Each line in the Applegate diagram represents the distance-time history of an individual electron. The slope of each line is inversely proportional to the velocity of the electron it represents.

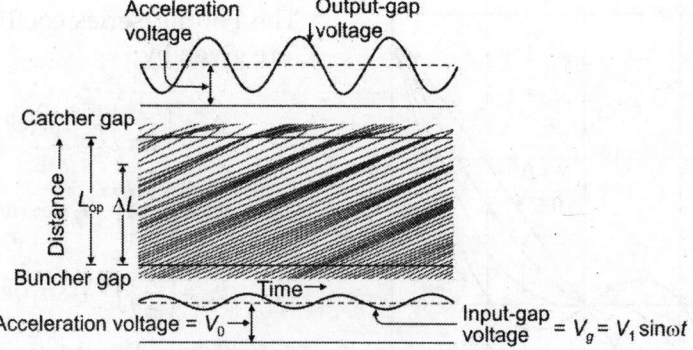

Fig. 10.9: Applegate diagram

10.6.8 Drift Space Transit Time

The drift space is assumed to be field free. The T transit time drift for an electron to travel a drift space distance L as shown in Fig. 10.2 is given by

$$T = (t_2 - t_1) = L/v(t_1)$$
$$= L/v_o\ [1 + (\beta_i V_1/2V_0) \sin (\omega t_o + \theta_g/2)]$$
$$= (L/v_o)\ [1 - (\beta_i V_1/2V_0) \sin (\omega t_1 - \theta_g/2)] \tag{10.34}$$
$$= T_o\ [1 - (\beta_i V_1/2V_0) \sin (\omega t_1 - \theta_g/2)] \tag{10.35}$$

$T_o = (L/v_o)$ is the dc transit time. Equation (10.30) is obtained assuming that $(\beta_i V_1/2V_0) \ll 1$ and using the binomial expansion $(1 + x)^{-1} = 1 - x$ for $x \ll 1$.

The drift transit angle is given by

$$\theta = \omega T = (\omega L/v_o)\ [1 - (\beta_i V_1/2V_o).$$
$$\sin (\omega t_1 - \theta_g/2)] \tag{10.36}$$
$$= \theta_o - X \sin (\omega t_1 - \theta_g/2) \tag{10.37}$$
$$\theta_o = \omega L/v_o = 2\pi N \tag{10.38}$$

θ_o is the dc transit angle, N is the number of electron transit cycles in the drift space and

$$X = (\beta_i V_1/2V_0)\theta_o \tag{10.39}$$

is the *bunching parameter* of a klystron.

10.6.9 Catcher Cavity Current

During a time interval dt_o, a charge dQ_o passing through the buncher gap is given by

$$dQ_o = I_o\ dt_o \tag{10.40}$$

I_o is the dc beam current. The same charge also passes through the catcher at a later time dt_2. Therefore,

$$I_o\ |dt_o| = i_2 |dt_o| \tag{10.41}$$

Current i_2 is the current at the catcher gap. From Fig. 10.2, we obtain

$$t_2 = t_o + t_g + T_o\ [1 - (\beta_i V_1/2V_o).$$
$$\sin (\omega t_o + \theta_g/2)] \tag{10.42}$$

Multiplying by ω we obtain

$$\omega t_2 = \omega t_o + \omega t_g + \omega T_o\ [1 - (\beta_i V_1/2V_0).$$
$$\sin (\omega t_o + \theta_g/2)] \tag{10.43}$$

After rearranging we get

$$\omega t_2 - (\theta_o + \theta_g/2) = (\omega t_o + \theta_g/2) -$$
$$X \sin (\omega t_o + \theta_g/2)] \tag{10.44}$$

$(\omega t_o + \theta_g/2)$ is the buncher cavity departure angle and $\omega t_2 - (\theta_o + \theta_g/2)$ is the catcher cavity arrival angle. Fig. 10.10 shows the catcher cavity arrival angle curves as a function of buncher departure angle for various bunching parameter values.

Differentiating Eq. (10.42) with respect to t_o, we obtain

$$dt_2 = dt_o\ [1 - X \cos (\omega t_o + \theta_g/2)] \tag{10.45}$$

The current arriving at the catcher cavity is then given by

$$i_2 (t_o) = I_o/[1 - X \cos (\omega t_o + \theta_g/2)] \tag{10.46}$$

Since, $\omega t_2 = \omega t_o + \theta_g + \theta_o$, the catcher current in terms of t_2 is given by

$$i_2(t_2) = I_o/[1 - X \cos (\omega t_2 - \theta_o - \theta_g/2)] \tag{10.47}$$

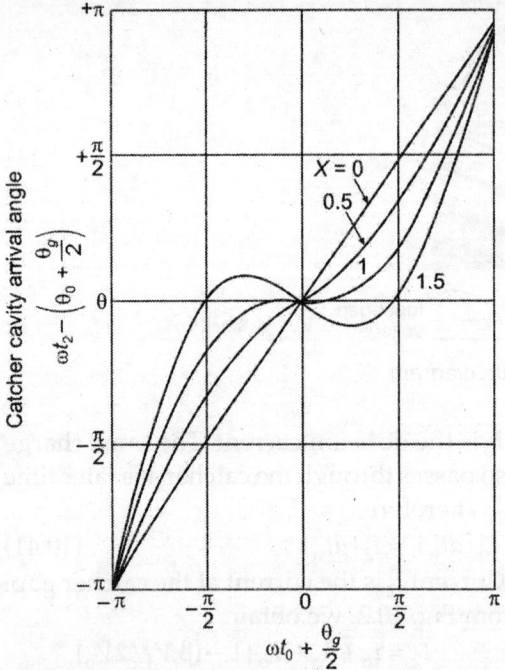

Fig. 10.10: Catcher cavity arrival angle versus buncher departure angle

Fig. 10.11 shows the curves of beam current $i_2(t_2)$ as a function of catcher arrival angle for various values of bunching parameter.

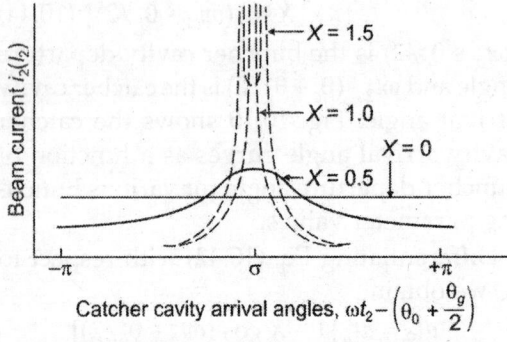

Fig. 10.11: Beam current $i_2(t_2)$ as a function of catcher arrival angle

The beam current at the catcher cavity is a periodic waveform of period $2\pi/\omega$ about dc current. Hence, the catcher current i_2 can be expanded in a Fourier series as

$$i_2 = a_o + \sum_{n=1}^{\infty} [a_n \cos(n\omega t_2) + b_n \sin(n\omega t_2)]$$

$$\text{(10.48)}$$

The Fourier series coefficients a_o, a_n, and b_n are given by

$$a_o = \left(\frac{1}{2\pi}\right) \int_{-\pi}^{\pi} i_2 d(\omega t_2) \qquad \text{(10.49)}$$

$$a_n = \left(\frac{1}{\pi}\right) \int_{-\pi}^{\pi} i_2 \cos(n\omega t_2) \, d(\omega t_2) \quad \text{(10.50)}$$

$$b_n = \left(\frac{1}{\pi}\right) \int_{-\pi}^{\pi} i_2 \sin(n\omega t_2) \, d(\omega t_2) \quad \text{(10.51)}$$

Substituting Eq. (10.41) in Eq. (10.49) and integrating, we get

$$a_o = \left(\frac{1}{2}\pi\right) \int_{-\pi}^{\pi} I_o d(\omega t_2) = I_o \qquad \text{(10.52)}$$

Substituting Eq. (10.41) and (10.44) in Eqs (10.50) and (10.51) yields

$$a_n = \frac{1}{\pi} \int_{-\pi}^{\pi} I_o \cos \left[(n\omega t_o + n\theta_g + n\theta_o) + nX \sin(\omega t_o + \theta_{g/2})\right] d(\omega t_o) \qquad \text{(10.53)}$$

$$b_n = \left(\frac{1}{\pi}\right) \int_{-\pi}^{\pi} I_o \sin \left[n\omega t_o + n\theta_g + n\theta_o) + nX \sin \left(\omega t_o + \frac{\theta}{2} \right) \right] d(\omega t_o) \qquad \text{(10.54)}$$

substituting the trigonometric identities

$$\cos(A \pm B) = \cos A \cos B \pm \sin A \sin B$$
$$\sin(A \pm B) = \sin A \cos B \pm \cos A \sin B$$

The two integrals in Eqs (10.53) and (10.54) involve cosine and sine functions.

Each term in the integrand has an infinite number of terms of *Bessel functions*. These are

$$\left[\cos\left[nX \sin\left(\omega t_o + \frac{\theta_g}{2}\right)\right] = 2 J_0(nX) + 2 [J_2(nX) \cos 2(\omega t_o + \theta_g/2)] + 2 [J_4(nX) \cos 4(\omega t_o + \theta_g/2)] + \dots \right. \qquad \text{(10.55)}$$

and

$$\left[\sin\left[nX \sin\left(\omega t_o + \frac{\theta_g}{2}\right)\right] = 2[J_1(nX) \sin(\omega t_o + \theta_g/2)] + 2 [J_3(nX) \sin 3(\omega t_o + \theta_g/2)] + \dots \right. \qquad \text{(10.56)}$$

Substituting the above series into the integrands of Eqs (10.53) and (10.54) respectively, the integrals are readily evaluated term by term. Then, the Fourier series coefficients are

$$a_n = 2I_o J_n(nX) \cos(n\theta_g + n\theta_o) \quad (10.57)$$
$$b_n = 2I_o J_n(nX) \sin(n\theta_g + n\theta_o) \quad (10.58)$$

$J_n(nX)$ is the n-th order *Bessel function of the first kind*. It is shown in Fig. 10.12 for $n = 1$ to 5.

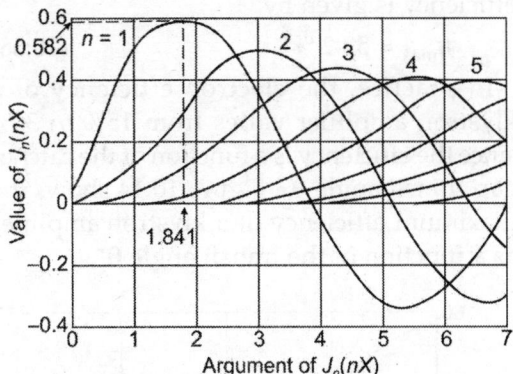

Fig. 10.12: Bessel functions of the first kind

Substitution of Eqs (10.49), (10.57) and (10.58) in Eq. (10.48) gives the beam current as

$$i_2 = I_o + \sum_{n=1}^{\infty} 2I_o J_n(nX) \cos[n\omega(t_2 - \tau_g - T_o)]$$
$$(10.59)$$

The fundamental component I_f of the beam current at the catcher cavity has a magnitude

$$I_f = 2I_0 J_1(nX) \quad (10.60)$$

This current has its maximum amplitude at

$$X = 1.841 \quad (10.61)$$

10.6.9 Optimum Distance *L*

The optimum distance L at which the maximum fundamental component of the current occurs is obtained from Eqs. (10.38), (10.39) and (10.57). It is given by

$$L_{opt} = 3.682 \, v_o V_0 / \omega\beta_i V_1 \quad (10.62)$$

The distance given by Eq. (10.33) is approximately 15% less than that of Eq. (10.62). This is due to approximations made in deriving Eq. (10.33) and the fact that the maximum fundamental component of the current will not coincide with the maximum electron density along the beam because of the presence of harmonics.

10.7 BEAM LOADING

When the buncher cavity gap is negligibly small, the average energy of the electron beam leaving the cavity over a cycle is nearly equal to the energy with which they enter the cavity. However, if the buncher cavity gap is large, the average energy of the electrons leaving buncher gap is larger than that when they entered the gap. This is because the electrons interact with the RF field for a longer duration while passing the gap. This excess energy has to be supplied by the buncher cavity to the electron beam for bunching. Thus the electron beam is loaded by the excess cavity energy. This phenomenon is known as *beam loading*.

10.8 OUTPUT POWER

For efficient operation of the klystron amplifier, the maximum bunching should occur approximately midway between the catcher cavity grids. The phase of the catcher cavity gap voltage must be such that the bunched electrons encounter a retarding phase while passing through the catcher cavity grids. During this retarding phase, its kinetic energy is transferred to the field of the catcher cavity. Hence, the electrons emerging from the catcher grids, have reduced velocity and are finally collected at the collector.

10.8.1 Induced Current in Catcher Cavity

The current induced in the walls of the catcher cavity by the electron beam is directly proportional to the amplitude of the microwave input voltage V_1. From Fig. 10.13, the fundamental component of the induced microwave current in the catcher cavity is given by

$$i_{2\,\text{ind}} = 2\beta_o I_0 J_1(X) \cos [\omega(t_2 - t_g - T_0)]$$
(10.63)

β_o is the output beam coupling coefficient of the catcher gap. If the buncher and catcher cavities are identical, then $\beta_i = \beta_o$ and the magnitude of fundamental component of the induced microwave current in the catcher cavity is given by

$$I_{2\,\text{ind}} = \beta_o I_2 = 2\beta_o I_0 J_1(X)$$
(10.64)

10.8.2 Output Equivalent Circuit

An equivalent circuit of the output cavity is shown in Fig. 10.13. In this circuit, R_{sho} represents the output shunt resistance of the output cavity walls. R_B is the beam loading resistance and R_L is the external load resistance.

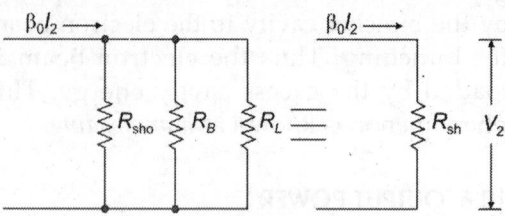

Fig. 10.13: Equivalent circuit

10.8.3 Output Power

The output power delivered to the catcher cavity and the load is given by

$$P_o = \frac{1}{2}(\beta_o I_2)^2 R_{\text{sh}} = \frac{\beta_o I_2 V_2}{2}$$
(10.65)

Here β_o is the output beam-coupling coefficient of the catcher gap, R_{sh} is the effective shunt resistance due to parallel combination of R_{sho}, R_B and R_L. V_2 and I_2 are the fundamental components of the catcher gap voltage and current respectively.

10.8.4 Electronic Efficiency

The electronic efficiency of the two-cavity klystron amplifier is defined as the ratio of

the output power to the input dc power. Thus

$$\text{Efficiency } \eta = \left(\frac{P_o}{P_i}\right) = \left(\frac{\beta_o I_2 V_2}{2 I_0 V_0}\right)$$
(10.66)

The power loss due to beam loading and cavity walls are included.

If the coupling is perfect, then $\beta_o = 1$. The maximum output current is

$$I_{2\,\text{max}} = 2I_0 \times 0.582 = 1.164\,I_0$$
(10.67)

In addition, if $V_2 = V_0$, then the maximum efficiency is given by

$$\eta_{\text{max}} = 58.2\,\%$$
(10.68)

In practice, the electron efficiency of a klystron amplifier varies from 15% to 30% since the efficiency is a function of the catcher gap transit angle θ_g. Figure 10.14 shows the maximum efficiency of a klystron amplifier as a function of the transit angle θ_g.

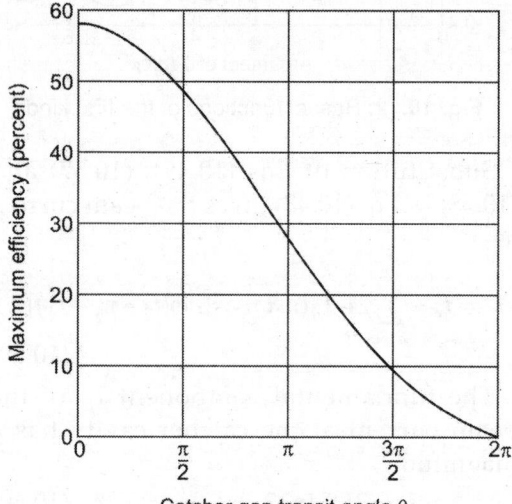

Fig. 10.14: Maximum efficiency of a klystron amplifier versus the transit angle θ_g

10.9 TYPICAL CHARACTERISTICS

Typical characteristics of a klystron amplifier are:

1. Efficiency is about 30%
2. Average output power P_o is up to 500 kW
3. Pulse output power P_0 is up to 30 MW

4. Fundamental frequency is 10 GHz

5. Power gain is 30 dB

10.10 MUTUAL CONDUCTANCE

The equivalent mutual conductance of a klystron amplifier is defined as the ratio of the induced current to the input voltage. Thus,

$$|G_m| = i_{2\text{ind}}/V_1 = 2\beta_o I_0 J_1(X)/V_1 \quad (10.69)$$

The input voltage V_1 in Eq. (10.35) can be expressed in terms of the bunching parameter X assuming $\beta_o = \beta_i$ as

$$V_1 = (2V_0/\beta_o\theta_o)\, X \quad (10.70)$$

Substituting the above equation in Eq. (10.65), we obtain

$$|G_m| = \beta_o^2\theta_o I_0 J_1(X)/XV_0 \quad (10.71)$$

or, $\quad \dfrac{|G_m|}{G_o} = \beta_o^2\theta_o J_1(X)/X \quad (10.72)$

$G_o = I_0/V_0$ is the dc beam conductance and $|G_m|/G_o$ is the normalized mutual conductance. The mutual conductance is inversely proportional to the bunching parameter X and decreases with increase in X as shown in Fig. 10.15.

From Fig. 10.15, it is seen that the normalized mutual conductance is maximum for $X = 1.841$, for $J_1(X)/X = 0.361$. Hence, the maximum value of the normalized mutual conduc-tance is given by

$$\dfrac{|G_m|}{G_o} = 0.316\beta_o^2\theta_o \quad (10.73)$$

10.11 VOLTAGE GAIN

The voltage gain of a klystron amplifier is defined as the ratio of the output voltage V_2 to the input voltage V_1. Thus

$$A_v = |V_2|/|V_1|$$

$$V_2 = \beta_2 I_2 R_{\text{sh}} = 2\beta_2 I_0 J_1(X)R_{\text{sh}}$$

$$V_1 = XV_0/\pi N\beta_1 = 2V_0/\beta_1\theta_0$$

$$A_v = |V_2|/|V_1|$$

$$= (\beta_o^2\theta_o I_0 J_1(X)R_{\text{sh}}/XR_o$$

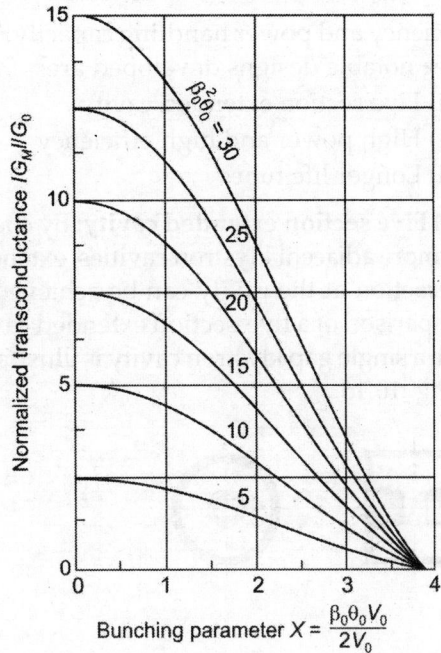

Fig. 10.15: Normalized mutual conductance versus bunching parameter

$$= (\beta_o^2\theta_o/R_o)\,[J_1(X)/X]R_{\text{sh}} \quad (10.74)$$

$$= G_m R_{\text{sh}} \quad (10.75)$$

Here θ_o is the transit angle given by $\theta_o = \omega t_o$ at the output cavity, $R_o = V_0/I_0$ is the dc beam resistance, $\beta_i = \beta_o$ for identical cavities, $J_1(X)$ is the Bessel function of first order and X is the bunching parameter and is given by

$$X = \beta_0 V_1\theta_0/2V_0 \quad (10.76)$$

10.12 APPLICATIONS OF TWO-CAVITY KLYSTRON AMPLIFIER

The two-cavity klystron amplifiers are used in

 (i) Troposcatter transmitters

(ii) Satellite communication ground stations

(iii) UHF TV transmitter power amplifiers

(iv) Pulsed radars

10.13 MODERN KLYSTRON TUBES

As far back as 1960s, efforts were undertaken to develop klystron tubes to improve efficiency and power handling capacity. The three notable designs developed are:

(i) Five section extended cavity

(ii) High power and high efficiency

(iii) Longer life tubes

(i) **Five section extended cavity:** By coupling more adjacent klystron cavities, extended interaction at the cavity can be achieved. A comparison of a five-section extended cavity with a single gap klystron cavity is illustrated in Fig. 10.16.

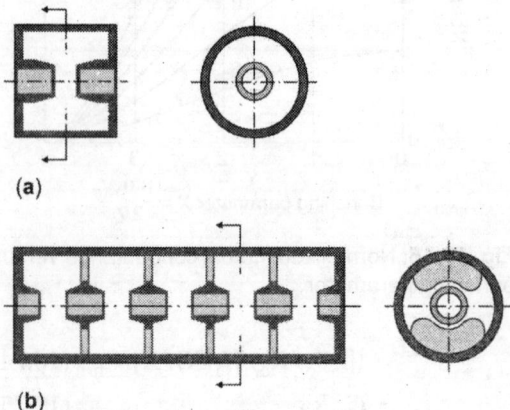

(a)

(b)

Fig. 10.16: (a) Single-gap cavity (b) five-gap extended interaction cavity

(ii) **High power and high efficiency:** In 1960s, effects were undertaken to improve the efficiency of klystron amplifiers. As a result, high power and high efficiency klystron tubes such as VA-884D, Stanford high power klystron and VKC8269A were developed. A 50 kW experimental klystron tube in the industrial heating frequency band with 75 % efficiency has been demonstrated. The operating characteristics of the VA-884D

Table 10.1: Operating characteristics of VA-884D

Beam voltage	16.5 kV
Beam current	2.4 A
Power output	14 kW
Gain	52 dB
Efficiency	36%
Frequency	10.9 to 6.45 GHz
Electronic 1 dB BW	75 MHz

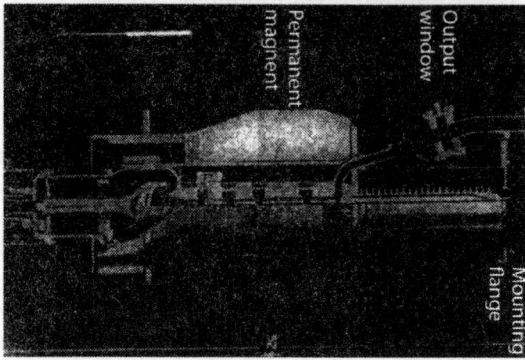

Fig. 10.17: Cut-away view of 24-MW klystron

klystron amplifier with five-cavity is listed in Table 10.1.

Fig. 10.17 shows a cut-away view of 24-MW S-band high peak power permanent-magnet-focused klystron tube developed for use in 2-mile Standford Linear Accelerator. The operating characteristics of this klystron tube are given in Table 10.2.

Table 10.2: Operating characteristics of 24-MW klystron

Beam voltage	250 kV
Beam current	250 A
Pulse repetition rate	60 to 360 pps
RF pulse width	2.5 µs
Peak power output	24 MW
Gain	50 to 55 dB
Efficiency	36% (approx.)
Frequency	2.856 GHz
Electronic 1 dB BW	20 MHz
Weight of focussing PM	363 kg

The Varian continuous superpower klystron amplifier VKC-8269A is shown in Fig. 10.18. Its operating characteristics are tabulated in Table 10.3.

Table 10.3: Operating characteristics of 24-MW klystron

Beam voltage	62 kV
Beam current	16.5 A
Peak power output	500 kW
Gain	56 dB
Efficiency	50%
Frequency	2.114 GHz

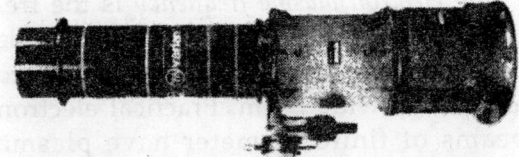

Fig. 10.18: Varian VKC-8269C CW superpower klystron

(iii) **Long-life tubes:** The Electron Dynamics Division of the Hughs Aircraft Company has developed long-life klystron tube that has a life of more than ten years. This long-life was possible because of the development of the reduction in the operating temperature of the cathode. This was achieved by unique construction of the cathode. The cathode is constructed with porous tungsten impregnated with calcium, aluminium and barium oxides. It is coated with a layer of osmium ruthenium alloy. This lowers its work function and hence emission takes place at reduced temperature. This temperature reduction slows down evaporation of barium *ten-fold* and extends the life of the cathode to several years.

10.14 MULTI CAVITY KLYSTRON

A two cavity klystron amplifier has a power gain of about 30 dB. To achieve higher power gain, several two cavity tubes are connected in cascade. The output of each tube feeds the input of the following tube. Besides this, a multi cavity klystron is also designed to give higher gain. Figure 10.19 shows a four-cavity klystron amplifier. In this, intermediate cavities are used. The intermediate cavities are placed at a distance of the bunching parameter X of 1.841 away from the previous cavity. Each intermediate cavity acts as a buncher cavity with the passing electron beam and induces a more enhanced RF voltage than the previous cavity. This, in turn, causes an *increased velocity modulation*. This increases considerably, the voltage amplification the power output and the efficiency. Higher bandwidth can be obtained by using stagger-tuned multiple cavities but with decreased gain.

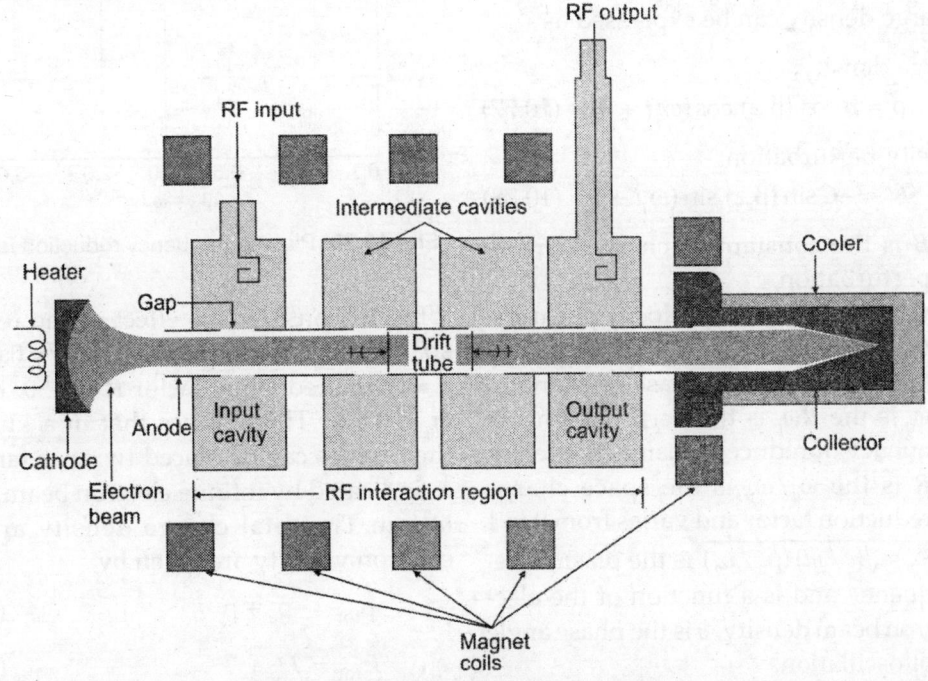

Fig. 10.19: Four-cavity klystron amplifier

10.14.1 Beam Current Density

In the low-power klystron amplifiers, the electron density in the beam is small. Hence, the effect of space charge was neglected. In high power tubes, the electron density is large and the electrons undergo mutual repulsion in the drift space. Therefore, the space charge effect cannot be neglected. In a high power klystron tube, the electron density has a dc part and an RF perturbation caused by the electron bunches. The space-charge-forces within the electron bunches vary with the size and shape of the electron beam. In an infinitely wide beam, the electric fields are constrained to act only in the axial direction. In a finite size electron beam, the electric fields are radial as well as axial. As a result of this, the axial component is reduced in comparison with the infinite beam. With the reduced space-charge force, the axial plasma frequency is reduced and hence the plasma wavelength is increased.

Let us assume that the charge density and velocity perturbation are simple sinusoidal variations in both time and position. Then, the charge density can be expressed as

Charge density:
$$\rho = B \cos (\beta_e z) \cos (\omega_q t + \theta) \quad (10.77)$$

Velocity perturbation:
$$\mathcal{V} = -C \sin (\beta_e z) \sin (\omega_q t + \theta) \quad (10.78)$$

Here B is the constant of charge density perturbation,

C is the constant of velocity perturbation,

$\beta_e = \omega/\mathcal{V}$ is the dc phase constant,

ω_q is the $R\omega_p$ is the perturbation frequency or reduced plasma frequency,

R is the ω_q/ω_p is the space charge reduction factor and varies from 0 to 1

$\omega_p = \sqrt{(e/m)(\rho_0/\varepsilon_0)}$ is the plasma frequency and is a function of the electron beam density, θ is the phase angle of oscillation.

The *electron plasma frequency* is the frequency at which the electrons oscillate in the beam. This plasma frequency applies only to an infinite wide beam. Practical electron beams of finite diameter have plasma frequency less than ω_p. This lower plasma frequency is known as *reduced plasma frequency* and is denoted by ω_q. The *space charge reduction factor R* is a function of the electron beam radius r and the ratio n of the beam-tunnel radius to the beam radius as shown in Fig. 10.20.

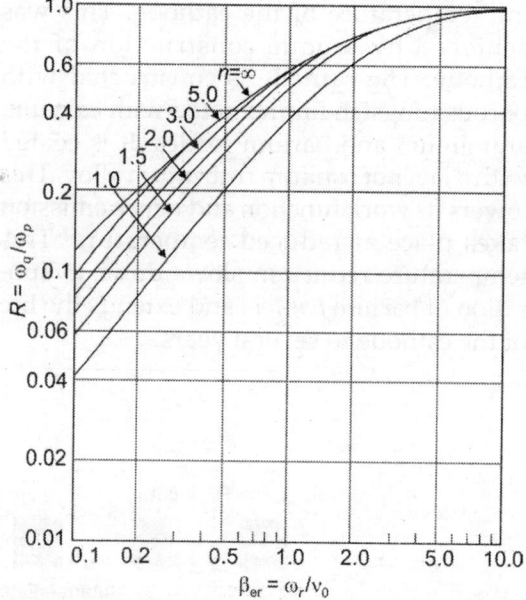

Fig. 10.20: Plasma frequency reduction factor **R**

Let us consider the effect of the reduced space charge forces. If $\beta_e r = \omega r / \mathcal{V} = 0.85$ and $n = 2$, the reduction factor $R = 0.50$. Hence, $\omega_q = 0.5\omega_p$. This implies that in a klystron, the cavities can be placed twice as far apart as indicated by infinite electron beam calculation. The total charge density and the electron velocity are given by

$$\rho_{tot} = -\rho_0 + \rho \quad (10.79)$$

$$\mathcal{V}_{tot} = \mathcal{V}_0 + \mathcal{V} \quad (10.80)$$

Here, ρ_o is the dc electron charge density,

ρ is the instantaneous RF charge density,

$\mathcal{V}_o$ is the dc electron velocity,

$\mathcal{V}$ is the instantaneous electron velocity perturbation.

In practical microwave tubes, ω_p/ω is much smaller than unity. Hence, the current density can be shown to be

$$J = \mathcal{V}_o B \cos(\beta_e z - \omega t) \cos(\omega_q t + \theta) \tag{10.81}$$

The electrons leaving the input buncher cavity gap of a klystron amplifier have a velocity at the exit grid given by

$$\mathcal{V}(t_1) = \mathcal{V}_o[1 + (\beta_i V_1/2V_0)\sin(\omega t_g)] \tag{10.82}$$

The electrons under the influence of space charge effect exhibit simple harmonic motion, the velocity at a later tome is given by

$$\mathcal{V}_{tol} = \mathcal{V}[1+(\beta_i V_1/2V_0)\sin(\omega t_g) \\ \cos(\omega_p t - \omega_p t_g)] \tag{10.83}$$

Hence, the current density equation is given by

$$J = -\frac{1}{2}\left(\frac{J_0 \omega}{V_0 \omega_q}\right)\beta_i V_1 \sin(\beta_q z) \cos(\beta_e z - \omega t) \tag{10.84}$$

$\beta_q = \omega_q/\mathcal{V}_o$ is the plasma phase constant.

10.14.2 Advantages

The advantages of multi-cavity klystron amplifiers are

(a) High gain-bandwidth product

(b) High efficiency

(c) High power output

10.14.3 Typical Characteristics

Typical characteristics of a multi-cavity klystron amplifier are

(a) Efficiency is 35 to 50 %.

(b) Power output is 30 dB at UHF and 60 dB in X-band.

(c) Bandwidth is 8 to 60 MHz.

10.14.4 Applications

The applications of multi-cavity klystron amplifiers are

(a) As high power microwave amplifiers

(b) In UHF TV transmitters

10.15 SPACE-CHARGE EFFECTS IN TWO CAVITY KLYSTRON

In this section, we shall discuss the effect of space charge on the performance of a two-cavity klystron amplifier.

10.15.1 Output Current and Voltage with Space Charge Effect

Assuming identical cavities in a two-cavity klystron amplifier are placed at the point where the RF current is maximum, the magnitude of RF current at the output cavity is given by

$$|i_2| = \frac{1}{2}\left(\frac{I_o \omega}{V_o \omega_q}\right)\beta_i |V_1| \tag{10.85}$$

V_1 is the magnitude of the input signal voltage. Then, the magnitudes of the induced current and voltage in the output cavity are given by

$$|I_2| = \beta_o|i_2| = \frac{1}{2}\left(\frac{I_o \omega}{V_o \omega_q}\right)\beta_o^2 |V_1| \tag{10.86}$$

$$|V_2| = |I_2| R_{shl}| = \frac{1}{2}\left(\frac{I_o \omega}{V_o \omega_q}\right)\beta_o^2 |V_1| R_{shl}^{\cdot} \tag{10.87}$$

$\beta_o = \beta_i$ is the beam coupling coefficient, R_{shl} = total shunt resistance of the output cavity including the external load.

10.15.2 Output Power with Space Charge Effect

The output power delivered to the load in a two-cavity klystron amplifier is given by

$$P_{out} = |I_2|^2 R_{shl}$$

$$= \frac{1}{4} \left(\frac{I_0 \omega}{V_0 \omega_q} \right)^2 \beta_o^4 \, |V_1|^2 \, R_{shl} \quad (10.88)$$

The power gain of the two-cavity klystron amplifier is given by

$$\text{Power gain} = \frac{P_{out}}{P_{in}} = \frac{P_{out}}{(|V_1|^2 R_{sh})}$$

$$= \frac{1}{4} \left(\frac{I_0 w}{V_0 \omega_q} \right)^2 \beta_o^4 R_{shl} \cdot R_{sh}$$

$$(10.89)$$

R_{sh} is the total shunt resistance at the input cavity.

10.15.3 Electronic Efficiency with Space Charge Effect

The electronic efficiency of the two-cavity klystron amplifier is given by

$$\eta = P_{out}/P_{in} = P_{out}/(I_0 V_0)$$

$$= \frac{1}{4} \left(\frac{|V_1| \omega}{V_0 \omega_q} \right)^2 \beta_o^4 \, R_{shl} \quad (10.90)$$

10.16 NUMERICAL EXAMPLES

Example 10.1 A two-cavity klystron amplifier is tuned at 2 GHz. The drift space is 2 cm. The beam current is 50 mA. The catcher voltage is 0.3 times the beam voltage. Assume $\beta = 1$. Calculate beam voltage, input voltage, output voltage, power and efficiency for maximum output for $N = 3\frac{1}{4}$.

Solution: Given: $f = 2 \times 10^9$, $L = 2 \times 10^{-2}$, $I_o = 50 \times 10^3$, $V_2 = 0.3 \, V_0$, $\beta = 1$.

Beam voltage

$$V_0 = (m/2e)(Lf/N)^2$$

$$= \left(\frac{9.1 \times 10^{-31}}{2 \times 1.6 \times 10^{-19}} \right) \left(2 \times 10^{-2} \times 2 \times \frac{10^9}{3\frac{1}{4}} \right)^2$$

$$= 430.8 \text{ V}$$

For maximum power output, the bunching parameter $X = 1.841 = \pi N V_1/V_0$ where V_1 is

the buncher voltage and V_0 is the beam voltage. Therefore V_1 is given by

$$V_1 = X V_0/\pi N$$

$$= (1.841 \times 430.8)/(8.1415 \times 3\frac{1}{4})$$

$$= \textbf{77.67 V}$$

Catcher voltage

$$V_2 = 0.3 V_0 = 0.3 \times 430.8$$

$$= \textbf{129.24 V}$$

Output power

$$P_0 = \beta I_0 V_2 J_1(X) \cos\phi$$

$$P_{0\,max} = I_0 V_2 J_1(X) \ (\text{since } \beta = 1 \text{ and } \phi = 0)$$

$$= 0.582 \times 50 \times 10^{-3} \times 129.24$$

$$= \textbf{3.761 W}$$

DC input power

$$P_{dc} = V_0 I_0 = 430.8 \times 50 \times 10^{-3}$$

$$= \textbf{21.54 W}$$

The maximum efficiency

$$\eta_{max} = 0.582 \, V_2/V_0$$

$$= 0.582 \times 129.24/430.8$$

$$= \textbf{17.46 \%}$$

Example 10.2 A two-cavity klystron operates at 10 GHz with $I_0 = 40$ mA and $V_0 = 1600$V. The drift space length is 2 cm. The output cavity total shunt resistance is 40 k-ohms. The beam-coupling coefficient is 0.92. Compute the maximum voltage gain.

Solution: Given: $f = 10 \times 10^9$, $I_0 = 40 \times 10^{-3}$, $N_0 = 1600$, $L = 2 \times 10^{-2}$, $R_{sh} = 40 \times 10^3$, $\beta = 0.92$.

Max. voltage gain

$$A_{V\,max} = \beta^2 \theta_o I_0 J_1(X)_{max} R_{sh}/X \, V_0.$$

The transit angle θ_o in the drift space is

$$\theta_o = \omega L/v_0.$$

The beam velocity V_o is given by

$$v_0 = 5.93 \times 10^5 \sqrt{V_o}$$

$$= 5.93 \times 10^5 \sqrt{1600}$$

$$= 2.37 \times 10^7 \text{ m/s}.$$

$$\therefore \ \theta_o = \omega L/v_o$$

$$= 2 \times 3.1415 \times 10 \times 10^9 \times 2 \times 10^{-2}/$$

$$2.37 \times 10^7$$

$$= 53 \text{ rad}.$$

$A_{v\max} = -\beta^2\theta_o I_0 J_1(X)_{\max} R_{sh}/X V_0$

$= (0.92)^2 \times 253 \times 40 \times 10^{-3} \times 0.582 \times$

$40 \times 10^3/(1.841 \times 1600)$

$= -14.2$

Example 10.3 A two-cavity klystron amplifier has $V_0 = 1$ kV, $I_0 = 25$ mA, $f = 3$ GHz, $d = 1$ mm, $L = 4$ cm, $R_0 = 40$ kΩ and $R_{sh} = 30$ kΩ. Find (a) input gap voltage for maximum voltage V_2, (b) voltage gain neglecting beam loading, (c) efficiency and (d) beam loading conductance.

Solution: Given: $V_0 = 1$ kV, $I_0 = 25$ mA, $f = 3$ GHz, $d = 1$ mm, $L = 4$ cm, $R_0 = 40$ kΩ and $R_{sh} = 30$ kΩ.

(a) For maximum V_2, $J_1(X)$ must be maximum. It is maximum at $X = 1.841$ and is equal to 0.582.

$v_o = 5.93 \times 10^5 \sqrt{V_0}$ m/s

$= 5.93 \times 10^5 \sqrt{1000}$ m/s

$= 1.88 \times 10^7$ m/s

The gap transit angle is

$\theta_g = \omega d/v_o$

$= 2 \times 3.14 \times 3 \times 10^9 \times 1 \times 10^{-3}/1.88 \times 10^7$

$= 1$ rad.

The beam-coupling coefficient is

$\beta_i = \beta_o = \sin(\theta_g/2)/(\theta_g/2)$

$= \sin(1/2)/(1/2) = 0.959$

The dc transit angle between the cavities is

$\theta_o = \omega T_0 = \omega L/v_o$

$= 2 \times 3.14 \times 3 \times 10^9 \times 4 \times 10^{-2}/1.88 \times 10^7$

$= 40$ rad.

The maximum input voltage $V_{1\max}$ is given by

$V_{1\max} = 2V_0 X/\beta_i\theta_o$

$= 2 \times 10^3 \times 1.841/(0.959 \times 40)$

$= 96.0$ V

(b) The voltage gain is given by

$A_v = -\left(\dfrac{\beta_o^2\theta_o}{R_o}\right)\left[\dfrac{J_1(X)}{X}\right]R_{sh}$

$= -\dfrac{(0.959)^2 \times 40 \times 0.582 \times 30 \times 10^3}{(4 \times 10^4 \times 1.841)}$

$= -7.2$

(c) Efficiency is given by

$\eta = (\beta_o I_2 V_2)/(2I_0 V_0)$

$I_2 = 2I_0 J_1(nX) = 2 \times 25 \times 10^{-3} \times 0.582$

$= 29.1 \times 10^{-3}$

$V_2 = \beta_o I_2 R_{sh}$

$= 0.959 \times 29.1 \times 10^{-3} \times 30 \times 10^3$

$= 837$ V

$\eta = \dfrac{0.959 \times 29.1 \times 10^3 \times 837}{(2 \times 25 \times 10^{-3} \times 1000)}$

$= 46.7\%$

(d) The beam-loading conductance is given by

$$G_B = \left(\frac{G_o}{2}\right)\left(\frac{\beta_o^2 - \beta_o \cos\theta_g}{2}\right)$$

$= 1/(40 \times 10^3 \times 2)[(0.959)^2 -$

$(0.959 \times \cos 28.6°)]$

$= 9.7 \times 10^{-7}$ mho

Example 10.4 A two-cavity klystron amplifier has $V_0 = 20$ kV, $I_0 = 2$ A, $f = 10$ GHz, $V_1 = 10$ V rms, $\beta_i = \beta_o = 1$, dc electron beam current density $\rho_o = 10^{-6}$ C/m³, $R_{sh} = 10$ kΩ and $R_{shl} = 30$ kΩ. Find (a) plasma frequency, (b) reduced plasma frequency for $R = 0.5$, (c) induced current in the output cavity, (d) induced voltage in the output cavity, (e) output power delivered to the load, (f) power gain and (g) electronic efficiency.

Solution: Given: $V_0 = 20$ kV, $I_0 = 2$ A, $f = 10$ GHz, $\beta_i = \beta_o = 1$, $\rho_o = 10^{-6}$ C/m³, $R_{sh} = 10$ kΩ and $R_{shl} = 30$ kΩ.

(a) The plasma frequency is given by

$\omega_p = \sqrt{(e/m)(\rho_o/\varepsilon_o)}$

$= [1.759 \times 10^{11} \times 10^{-6}/(8.854 \times 10^{-12})]^{1/2}$

$= 1.41 \times 10^8$ rad/s

(b) The reduced plasma frequency is given by

$\omega_q = R\omega_p = 0.5 \times 1.41 \times 10^8$

$= 0.705 \times 10^8$ rad/s

$\omega/\omega_q = 2 \times 3.14 \times 10 \times 10^9/(0.705 \times 10^8)$

$\qquad = 891$

(c) The induced current in the output cavity is given by

$|I_2| = \frac{1}{2}(I_0\omega/V_0\omega_q)\, \beta_o^2\, |V_1|$

$\qquad = \frac{1}{2}(2 \times 891 \times 1^2 \times |10|/(20 \times 10^3)$

$\qquad = \mathbf{0.4455\ A}$

(d) The induced voltage in the output cavity is given by

$|V_2| = |I_2|\, R_{shl} = 0.4455 \times 30 \times 10^3$

$\qquad = \mathbf{13.37\ kV}$

(e) The output power delivered to the load is given by

$P_o = |I_2|^2 R_{shl} = 0.4455^2 \times 30 \times 10^3$

$\qquad = \mathbf{5.95\ kW}$

(f) Power gain is given by

Power gain

$\quad = \frac{1}{4}(I_0\omega/V_0\omega_q)^2\, \beta_o^4\, |V_1|^2\, R_{shl}$

$\quad = (0.25 \times [2 \times 891]/(20 \times 10^3))^2 \times$

$\qquad 1^4 \times 30 \times 10^3 \times 10 \times 10^3 = 5.98 \times 10^5$

$\quad = \mathbf{77.67\ dB}$

(g) The electronic efficiency is given by

$\eta = (P_o/P_i) = (\beta_o I_2 V_2)/(2 I_0 V_0)$

$\quad = 5.95 \times 10^3/(2 \times 2 \times 20 \times 10^3)$

$\quad = \mathbf{7.48\%}$

Example 10.5 A four-cavity klystron amplifier has $V_0 = 14.5$ kV, $I_0 = 1.4$ A, $f = 8$ GHz, dc electron beam current density $\rho_o = 10^{-6}$ C/m^3, RF charge density $\rho = 10^{-8}$ C/m^3, velocity perturbation $\mathscr{V} = 10^5$ m/s. Find (a) dc electron velocity, (b) dc phase constant, (c) plasma frequency, (d) reduced plasma frequency, for $R = 0.4$, (e) dc beam current density and (f) instantaneous beam current density.

Solution: Given: $V_0 = 14.5$ kV, $I_0 = 1.4$ A, $f = 8$ GHz, $\rho_o = 10^{-6}$ C/m^3, $\rho = 10^{-8}$ C/m^3, $\mathscr{V} = 10^5$ m/s, $R = 0.4$.

(a) The dc electron velocity is given by

$\mathscr{V}_o = 5.93 \times 10^5\sqrt{V_0}$

$\qquad = 5.93 \times 10^5\sqrt{14500}$

$\qquad = \mathbf{7.14 \times 10^7\ m/s.}$

(b) The dc phase constant is given by

$\beta_e = \omega/\mathscr{V}_o$

$\qquad = 6.28 \times 8 \times 10^9/(7.14 \times 10^7)$

$\qquad = \mathbf{7.04 \times 10^2\ rad/m}$

(c) The plasma frequency is given by

$\omega_p = \sqrt{(e/m)(\rho_o/\varepsilon_o)}$

$\qquad = \left[\dfrac{1.759 \times 10^{11} \times 10^{-6}}{8.854 \times 10^{-12}}\right]^{1/2}$

$\qquad = \mathbf{1.41 \times 10^8\ rad/s}$

(d) The reduced plasma frequency for $R = 0.4$ is given by

$\omega_q = R\omega_p = 0.4 \times 1.41 \times 10^8$

$\qquad = \mathbf{0.564 \times 10^8\ rad/s}$

(e) The dc beam current density is given by

$J_o = \rho_o\mathscr{V}_o = 10^{-6} \times 7.14 \times 10^7$

$\qquad = \mathbf{71.4\ A/m^2}$

(f) The instantaneous beam current density is given by

$J = \rho\mathscr{V}_0 - \rho_o\mathscr{V}_o$

$\qquad = 10^{-8} \times 7.14 \times 10^7 - 10^{-6} \times 10^5$

$\qquad = \mathbf{0.614\ A/m^2}$

Example 10.6 A four-cavity klystron amplifier has $V_0 = 18$ kV, $I_0 = 2.25$ A, $f = 8$ GHz, $d = 1$ cm, signal voltage $V_1 = 10$ V rms, $\beta_i = \beta_o = 1$, and dc electron beam current density $\rho_o = 10^{-8}$ C/m^3. Find (a) dc electron velocity, (b) dc phase constant, (c) plasma frequency, (d) reduced plasma frequency, for $R = 0.5$, (e) reduced phase constant, (f) transit time across the input gap, (g) electron velocity leaving the input gap.

Solution: Given: $V_0 = 18$ kV, $I_0 = 2.25$A, $f = 8$ GHz, $d = 1$ cm, $\rho = 10^{-8}$ C/m^3, $\beta_i = \beta_o = 1$, $\mathscr{V} = 10^5$ m/s.

(a) The dc electron velocity is given by

$\mathscr{V}_o = 5.93 \times 10^5\sqrt{V_0}$

$\qquad = 5.93 \times 10^5\sqrt{18000}$

$\qquad = \mathbf{7.96 \times 10^7\ m/s.}$

(b) The dc phase constant is given by

$$\beta_e = \beta / \mathcal{V}_o$$
$$= 6.28 \times 8 \times 10^9 / (7.96 \times 10^7)$$
$$= \textbf{6.31} \times \textbf{10}^2 \,\textbf{rad/m}$$

(c) The plasma frequency is given by

$$\omega_p = \sqrt{(e/m)(\rho_o/\varepsilon_o)}$$
$$= \left[\frac{1.759 \times 10^{11} \times 10^{-8}}{(8.854 \times 10^{-12})} \right]^{1/2}$$
$$= \textbf{1.41} \times \textbf{10}^7 \,\textbf{rad/s}$$

(d) The reduced plasma frequency for $R = 0.5$ is given by

$$\omega_q = R\omega_p = 0.5 \times 1.41 \times 10^8$$
$$= \textbf{7.05} \times \textbf{10}^7 \,\textbf{rad/s}$$

(e) The reduced plasma phase constant is given by

$$\beta_e = \omega_q / \mathcal{V}_0 = 7.05 \times 10^7 / (7.96 \times 10^7)$$
$$= \textbf{0.886} \,\textbf{rad/m}$$

(f) The transit time across the gap is given by

$$t_g = d / \mathcal{V}_o = 1 \times 10^{-2} / (7.96 \times 10^7)$$
$$= \textbf{0.1256} \,\textbf{ns}$$

(g) The electron velocity leaving the gap is given by

$$\mathcal{V}(t_1) = \mathcal{V}_o [1 + (\beta_i V_1 / 2V_0) \sin(\omega t_g)]$$
$$= 7.96 \times 10^7 [1 + (1 \times 10)/(2 \times 18 \times 10^3) \sin(6.28 \times 0.1256 \times 10^{-9})$$
$$= \textbf{7.96} \times \textbf{10}^7 + \textbf{2.21} \times \textbf{10}^4 \,\textbf{ms}$$

Example 10.7 A four-cavity klystron amplifier has $V_0 = 10$ kV, $I_0 = 1$ A, $f = 4$ GHz, signal voltage $V_1 = 2$ V rms, $\beta_i = \beta_o = 1$, and dc electron beam current density $\rho_o = 5 \times 10^{-5}$ C/m^3, $R_{sh} = 10$ kΩ and $R_{shl} = 5$ kΩ. Find (a) plasma frequency, (b) reduced plasma frequency for $R = 0.6$, (c) induced current in the output cavity, (d) induced voltage in the output cavity, (e) output power delivered to the load.

Solution: Given: $V_0 = 10$ kV, $I_0 = 1$ A, $f = 4$ GHz, $\beta_i = \beta_o = 1$, $\rho_o = 5 \times 10^{-5}$ C/m^3, $V_1 = 2$ V, $R_{sh} = 10$ kΩ and $R_{shl} = 5$ kΩ.

(a) The plasma frequency is given by

$$\omega_p = \sqrt{(e/m)(\rho_o/\varepsilon_o)}$$
$$= \left[\frac{1.759 \times 10^{11} \times 5 \times 10^{-5}}{(8.854 \times 10^{-12})} \right]^{1/2}$$
$$= \textbf{0.997} \times \textbf{10}^8 \,\textbf{rad/s}$$

(b) The reduced plasma frequency is given by

$$\omega_q = R\omega_p = 0.6 \times 0.997 \times 10^8$$
$$= \textbf{0.598} \times \textbf{10}^9 \,\textbf{rad/s}$$
$$\omega/\omega_q = 2 \times 3.14 \times 4 \times 10^9 / (0.598 \times 10^8)$$
$$= \textbf{42.03}$$

(c) The induced current in the output cavity is given by

$$|I_4| = (1/8)(I_0 \omega / V_0 \omega_q)^3 \beta_o^6 |V_1| R_{sh}^2$$
$$= \left(\frac{1}{8}\right) \left(\frac{1 \times 42.03}{10^4}\right)^3 \times 1^6 \times |2| \times (10 \times 10^3)^2$$
$$= \textbf{1.856 A}$$

(d) The induced voltage in the output cavity is given by

$$|V_4| = |I_4| R_{shl} = 1.856 \times 5 \times 10^3$$
$$= \textbf{9.28 kV}$$

(e) The output power delivered to the load is given by

$$P_o = |I_4|^2 R_{shl} = 1.856^2 \times 5 \times 10^3$$
$$= \textbf{17.22 kW}$$

KEY POINTS

- The conventional vacuum tubes such as triodes and pentodes, cannot be used at microwave frequencies because of certain limitations. Their effects may be overcome by proper design.
- At microwave frequencies, reentrant cavities and slow-wave structures are used to obtain higher gain-bandwidth products.
- A reentrant cavity resonator is that in which the opposite sides are brought closer together to form a reentrant structure.
- Based on the device used for transfer of amplified energy, the microwave tubes are classified as (i) cavity structure and (ii) slow-wave structure tubes.

- The klystron, reflex klystron and magnetron belong to the cavity type tubes and the traveling wave tube is a slow-wave structure.
- Based on the direction of electric and magnetic fields within the structure, the MW tubes can also be classified as (i) linear-beam or "O" type tubes and (ii) cross-field or "M" type tubes.
- In the linear-beam tubes, the accelerating electric field is in the same direction as that of the static magnetic field used to focus the electron beam.
- In the cross-field type tubes, the accelerating electric field is perpendicular to the static magnetic field.
- The klystron, reflex klystron and the traveling wave tubes are linear-beam tubes and the magnetron is the cross-field device.
- A widely used microwave amplifier is the two-cavity klystron amplifier.
- Reference electron is the electron passing through the reentrant cavity when the RF signal is zero and going positive.
- Electrons passing through the input cavity gap later than the reference electron are accelerated by positive field and those that pass the input cavity before the reference electron are slowed down by negative field. As a result of these, the bunching process takes place and the electrons are velocity modulated.
- After the electrons are bunched in the drift space, the density of the electrons in the stream passing a given point varies cyclically in time. Under these conditions, the electron beam contains an ac component and is said to be current modulated.
- The distance-time plot of the electron trajectories in the drift space is known as Applegate diagram.
- Excess energy supplied by the buncher cavity to the electron beam is known as beam loading.
- The fundamental component of the beam current I_f at the catcher cavity has a magnitude $I_f = 2I_oJ_1(nX)$.
- Typical characteristics of a klystron amplifier are (i) efficiency is about 40% (ii) average output power P_o is up to 500 kW (iii) pulse output power P_o is up to 30 MW (iv) fundamental frequency is 10 GHz (v) power gain is 30 dB
- The two-cavity klystron amplifiers are used in (i) tropo-scatter transmitters, (ii) satellite communication ground stations, (iii) UHF TV transmitter power amplifiers and (iv) pulsed radars.
- The advantages of a multi-cavity klystron amplifier are (i) high gain-bandwidth product, (ii) high efficiency and (iii) high power output.
- The applications of a multi-cavity klystron amplifier are (i) as high power microwave amplifiers and (ii) in UHF TV transmitters.

FURTHER READING

1. Altman JL (1962). *Microwave Circuits*, Van Nostrand, NJ.
2. Chodorov M and Susskind C (1964). *Funda-mentals of Microwave Electronics*, McGraw Hill, NY.
3. Hamilton DR et al (1948). *Klystron and Microwave Triodes*, McGraw Hill, NY.
4. Harvey AF (1963). *Microwave Engineering*, Acad. Press, NY.
5. Howes MJ and Morgan DV (1976). *Microwave Devices*, John Wiely, NY.
6. Gilmour AS Jr (1986). Microwave Tubes, Artech., Massachusetts.

REVIEW QUESTIONS

10.1 Mention the limitations of conventional vacuum tubes at microwave frequencies.

10.2 Explain the effect of transit time? How can it be minimized?

10.3 Discuss the effects of lead inductance and interelectrode capacitance at microwave frequency? How are they minimized?

10.4 Mention four commonly used microwave tubes.

10.5 How are the microwave tubes classified?

10.6 Explain the velocity modulation in klystron amplifier.

10.7 Explain the bunching or current modulation in klystron amplifier.

10.8 What is an applegate diagram? Explain.

10.9 Mention the assumptions made while analyzing a klystron amplifier.

10.10 What is meant by beam loading?

10.11 Draw the equivalent circuit of the output cavity of a klystron amplifier.

10.12 Define the efficiency of a klystron amplifier.. What is the maximum efficiency?

10.13 Mention the typical characteristics of a klystron amplifier.

10.14 Define the voltage gain of a klystron amplifier.

10.15 What are the applications of a klystron amplifier?

10.16 What is a multi-cavity klystron amplifier? What are its advantages?

10.17 Mention the typical characteristics of a multi-cavity klystron amplifier.

10.18 Mention the applications of a multi-cavity klystron amplifier.

DESCRIPTIVE QUESTIONS

10.1 Discuss in detail, the limitations of conventional tubes at microwave frequencies.

10.2 Explain the velocity modulation. How is it achieved in two-cavity klystron?

10.3 Describe the construction and operation of the klystron amplifier.

10.4 Explain, in detail, the bunching process and derive an expression for the bunching parameter.

10.5 Describe the phenomenon of velocity modulation in a two-cavity klystron.

10.6 Explain how microwave power is amplified by the interaction of velocity-modulated beam with electromagnetic field in the two-cavity klystron amplifier.

10.7 Explain briefly (i) velocity modulation and electron bunching and (ii) condition for obtaining maximum power output in a klystron.

PRACTICE PROBLEMS

10.1 A two-cavity klystron amplifier is tuned at 3 GHz. The drift space is 2 cm. The beam current is 25 mA. The catcher voltage is 0.3 times the beam voltage. Assume $\beta = 1$. Calculate beam voltage, input voltage, output voltage, power and efficiency for maximum output for $N = 5 \frac{1}{4}$.
[**Ans:** 371.4 V, 41.43 V, 1.621 W and 17.46%]

10.2 A two-cavity klystron operates at 10 GHz with $I_0 = 36$ mA and $V_0 = 10$ kV. The drift space length is 2 cm. The output cavity total shunt conductance is 20 mmhos. The beam-coupling coefficient is 0.92. Compute the maximum voltage gain.
[**Ans:** 10.2]

10.3 A two-cavity klystron amplifier is operated with $V_0 = 3$ kV. The coupling coefficient is 0.9 and the magnitude of the signal voltage at the input gap is 100 V. Calculate the velocities of the electrons leaving the input gap.
[**Ans:** Max. velocity = 3.3×10^7, Min. velocity $= 3.2 \times 10^7$]

10.4 A two-cavity klystron amplifier has a beam current of 400 mA, an output cavity coupling coefficient of 0.95 and the magnitude of the voltage across the output cavity gap is 75 V. Calculate (a) the maximum magnitude of the fundamental induced current and (b) the maximum power output.
[**Ans:** (a) 4610.6 mA., (b) 14.81 W]

10.5 A two-cavity klystron is operated at 10 GHz with $V_0 = 1200$ V, $I_0 = 30$ mA, $d = 1$ mm, $L = 4$ cm and $R_{sg} = 40$ k-ohms. Calculate (a) the input RF voltage V_1 for maximum output, (b) voltage gain and (c) efficiency. Assume $\beta = 0.7810$. Neglect beam loading.
[**Ans:** 96.3 V; 21.12 dB and 12.52%]

10.6 An identical two-cavity klystron amplifier operates at 4 GHz with $V_0 = 1600$ V, $I_0 = 25$ mA, $d = 1$ mm and $L = 3$ cm. If DC conductance and catcher cavity total equivalent conductance are 0.25×10^4 and 0.3×10^4 mhos respectively. Calculate (a) beam coupling coefficient, (b) DC transit angle in the drift space, (c) magnitude of the input cavity voltage for maximum output voltage, (d) voltage gain and (e) efficiency. Neglect beam loading.
[**Ans:** (a) 0.954; (b) 1.0589 rad or 60.67°; (c) 158.34 V; (d) 3.277 and (e) 9.0%]

10.7 A two-cavity klystron amplifier has $V_0 = 20$ kV, $I_0 = 2$ A, $f = 10$ GHz, $\beta_i = \beta_o = 1$, dc electron beam current density $\rho_o = 10^{-6}$ C/m^3, $R_{sh} = 10$ kΩ and $R_{shl} = 30$ kΩ. Find (a) plasma fre-quency, (b) reduced plasma frequency, (c) induced current in the output cavity, (d) induced voltage in the output cavity, (e) output power delivered to the load, (f) power gain and (g) electronic efficiency.
(**Ans:** 1.41×10^8 rad/s, 0.705×10^8 rad/s, 0.3565 A, 10.71 kV, 3.82 kW, 58.21 dB, 4.8 %)

10.8 The modulation depth in a klystron amplifier is 0.08. Calculate the maximum and minimum electron velocities relative to the average velocity.
(**Ans:** $1.04v_0$, $0.96v_0$)

REFERENCE

1. IEEE Proc. Vol.61, No.3, Mar. (1973) Special Issue on High Power Microwave Tubes.

2. Das A and Das SK (2004). *Microwave Engineering*, TMH, New Delhi.

3. Hamilton DR et al (1948). *Klystron and Microwave Triodes*, McGraw Hill, NY.

4. IEEE Trans. Electron Devices (1973). Special Issue on Microwave Theory and Tech-niques, MTT-21, No.11.

5. IEEE Trans. Electron Devices (1976). Special Issue on Microwave Theory and Tech-niques, MTT-24, No.11.

6. IEEE Trans. Electron Devices (1979). Special Issue on Microwave Theory and Tech-niques, MTT-27, No. 5

7. IEEE Trans. Electron Devices (1980). Special Issue on Microwave Theory and Techniques, MTT-28, No. 12.

8. IEEE Trans. Electron Devices (1982). Special Issue on Microwave Theory and Techniques, MTT-30, No. 4.

9. IEEE Trans. Electron Devices (1982). Special Issue on Microwave Theory and Techniques, MTT-30, No. 10.

10. Lebedev I (1973). *Microwave Engineering*, MIR Publications, Moscow.

11. Liao SY (2000). *Microwave Devices and Circuits*, PHI, New Delhi

12. Liao SY (1988). *Microwave Electron Tubes*, PH, NJ.

13. Pulfrey DL and Tarr NG (1989). *Introduction to Microelectronic Devices*, PH. NJ.

14. Seeger JA (1988). Microwave Theory *Components and Devices*, PH., NJ.

15. Spangenberg KR (1948). *Vacuum Tubes*, McGraw Hill, NY.

Reflex Klystron Oscillator

Objectives

- Understand the velocity modulation in a reflex klystron oscillator.
- Know various modes of operation.
- Analyze and derive expressions for impedance parameters.
- Identify the applications of a reflex klystron oscillator.

11.1 INTRODUCTION

A two-cavity klystron tube can be used as a microwave oscillator to generate microwave power. If a fraction of the output power of a two-cavity klystron is fedback to the input cavity and if the loop gain has a magnitude of unity with a phase shift of multiple of 2π, it will oscillate. However, the difficulty with this is as the oscillation frequency is varied, the resonant frequency of each cavity and the feedback path phase shift must also be readjusted for positive feedback. To overcome this disadvantage, the reflex klystron with a single cavity is developed.

11.2 REFLEX KLYSTRON TUBE

A common source of microwave power is the reflex klystron oscillator. It uses a single resonant cavity. Its efficiency is low and hence, it is a low power device. It can operate from 4 GHz to 200 GHz. It is a microwave oscillator tube with a built-in feedback mechanism. It uses the same cavity for bunching and for the output.

Figure 11.1 shows a reflex klystron oscillator. It consists of an electron gun, a single reentrant cavity resonator that also serves as anode, output coupling and repeller electrode. The repeller voltage is negative with respect to the cathode. It repels the partially bunched electron beam back to the resonator

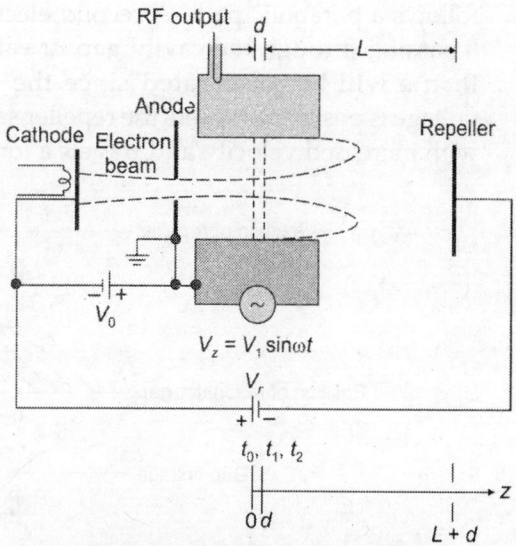

Fig. 11.1: Reflex klystron oscillator

cavity. This provides the necessary positive feedback to sustain the oscillations.

11.3 VELOCITY MODULATION

On application of dc voltage to the cavity, RF noise voltage is generated in the cavity. This electromagnetic noise field in the cavity is pronounced at cavity resonance frequency. This RF field acts on the electrons travelling towards the repeller electrode and causes the velocity of electrons emerging from the gap into the repeller space to vary with time in accordance with the RF voltage. Thus, the electron beam entering the repeller space is first velocity modulated by the RF cavity gap voltage. This causes the electrons to take different lengths of time to return to the gap. This results in the formation of electron bunches.

Figure 11.2 shows the trajectory of some typical electrons in the anode-repeller space. The electron a, passing through the cavity gap d at the instant when the gap voltage is zero and just going negative, enters the repeller space L with unchanged velocity, repelled back and return to the cavity resonator at a time t_0 later. In the distance-time coordinate system shown, this electron follows a parabolic path. A second electron b passing through the cavity gap Δt earlier than a will be accelerated since the gap voltage is positive. It enters the repeller space with increased velocity and travels a longer distance towards the repeller electrode and takes a longer time to return back to the cavity resonator. It thus tends to bunch with electron a. Similarly, an electron c passing through the cavity gap Δt after a, is decelerated and travel a shorter distance towards the repeller electrode and takes a shorter time to return back to the resonator. Thus, electron c catches with electron a and tend to bunch with it. This gives rise to a bunch around the electron a as shown in Fig. 11.2. This is known as applegate diagram. Thus the electrons *are velocity modulated* and form bunches that occur once per cycle centered on a reference electron such as a in Fig. 11.2. On their return journey, the bunched electrons pass through the cavity gap during the retardation phase of the gap voltage and give up their kinetic energy to the RF field in the cavity. A close examination of Fig. 11.2 shows that this condition occurs when the transit time N in the repeller space in cycles is

$$N = n + 3/4 \text{ cycles}; \quad n = 0, 1, 2, 3, \ldots$$
$$(11.1)$$

Thus, to generate and sustain the oscillations, the resonant system is tuned to the desired frequency and the negative repeller voltage is adjusted to give a transit time N that approximately satisfies Eq. (11.1). The more negative the repeller voltage, the more quickly the electrons passing into the repeller space are returned to the gap. Hence, the less will be the value of N of the transit time.

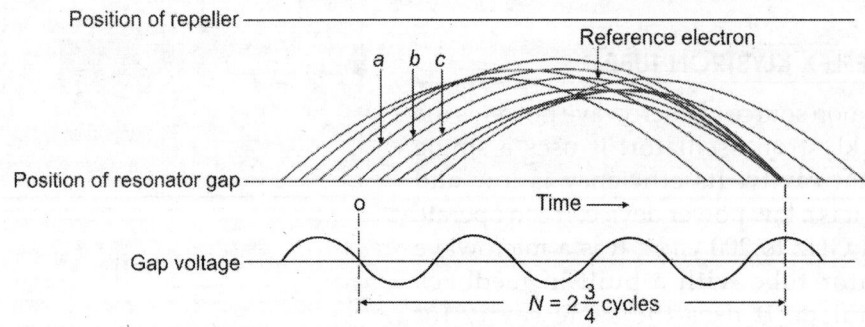

Fig. 11.2: Applegate diagram for reflex klystron

Klystron oscillator output energy is obtained from the cavity through a coupling loop. Finally the walls of the cavity collect the electrons.

11.4 OSCILLATION MODES

The electron bunches formed in a reflex klystron would deliver maximum power to the resonator if they pass the resonator gap at an instant when the RF field in the cavity corresponds to the positive peak of the RF cycle. From Fig. 11.2, it can be seen that this happens when $t_0 = 2\frac{3}{4}T$, where T is the periodic time of resonant frequency. In general, the above condition is satisfied for

$$t_0 = (n + \tfrac{3}{4})\, T = NT;\ n = 0, 1, 2, 3, \dots$$
$$(11.2)$$

The *mode number N* is given by $N = (n + \frac{3}{4})$. Thus, there are several values of N that satisfy the above oscillation condition. These values correspond to various modes of oscillation. A particular mode of operation is selected by choice of the repeller voltage. Various modes of the reflex klystron are presented in power output versus repeller voltage diagram shown in Fig. 11.3. The mode corresponding to $N = 1\frac{3}{4}$ occurs at maximum negative repeller voltage and the output power is also maximum. For $N = \frac{3}{4}$, the gain mechanism is usually not strong enough to overcome system losses. Higher modes ($N > \frac{3}{4}$) occur at lower repeller voltages with lower output power.

11.5 ANALYSIS OF REFLEX KLYSTRON OSCILLATOR

The output power of a reflex klystron oscillator attains the maximum value when the bunched electrons, on return, cross the cavity gap at the time the cavity gap velocity is positive and is maximum. The output power is a function of various parameters as explained below.

11.5.1 Assumptions

For calculation of RF power output, the following assumptions are made:
  (i) The gap RF voltage V_1 is small compared to the dc beam voltage V_0 ($V_1 << V_0$).
  (ii) Cathode, anode, cavity grids and the repeller electrode are all perfectly parallel.
  (iii) Cavity grids do not intercept any electron while passing through it.
  (iv) No debunching takes place in the repeller space.
  (v) The repeller space is free of RF field.

11.5.2 Transit Angle and Beam Coupling Coefficient

The analysis of a reflex klystron oscillator is similar to two-cavity klystron amplifier. The electron velocity v_0 at the cavity gap at $t = 0$ when it enters the gap is uniform and is given by

$$v_o = \sqrt{2\left(\frac{e}{m}\right)V_o} = 5.93 \times 10^5 \sqrt{V_0}\ \text{m/s} \quad (11.3)$$

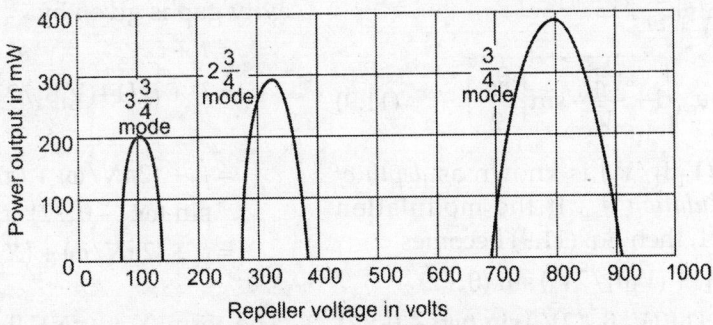

Fig. 11.3: Mode curves of reflex klystron

V_o is the dc beam voltage in volts. Let the RF voltage at the cavity be

$$v_1(t) = V_1 \sin \omega t \quad (V_1 << V_0) \quad (11.4)$$

The average transit time t_g through cavity gap d is given by

$$t_g = d/v_o \quad (11.5)$$

The average transit angle is

$$\theta_g = \omega t_g = \omega d/v_o \quad (11.6)$$

The average microwave voltage in the cavity gap is given by

$$V_{av} = (1/t_g) \int_0^{t_q} V_1 \sin \omega t \, dt$$

$$= V_1 [1 - \cos \omega t_g]/(\omega t_g)$$

Substituting $(1 - \cos 2\theta) = 2\sin^2\theta$ and $\omega t_g = \theta_g$ and rearranging, we get

$$V_{av} = V_1 \sin^2 (\theta_g/2)/(\theta_g/2)$$

$$= V_1\beta_1 \sin (\theta_g/2) \quad (11.7)$$

β_1 is known as *beam coupling coefficient* of the cavity gap and is given by

$$\beta_1 = \sin (\theta_g/2)/(\theta_g/2) \quad (11.8)$$

Thus, the coupling between the electron beam and the cavity varies with gap d in the form of $(\sin \theta)/\theta$. As the gap d tends to zero, the beam-coupling coefficient also tends to zero.

11.5.3 Modulation Depth

After the velocity modulation, the same electron leaves the cavity gap at time t_1. The exit velocity of the electron from the gap is given by

$$v(t_1) = \sqrt{2\left(\frac{e}{m}\right)(V_0 + V_{av})}$$

$$= v_o\sqrt{1 + \frac{V_1\beta_1}{V_0} \sin\left(\frac{\theta_g}{2}\right)} \quad (11.9)$$

The term $(V_1\beta_1/V_o)$ is known as *depth of velocity modulation* d_m. If the modulation depth $d_m << 1$, then Eq. (11.9) becomes

$$v(t_g) = v_o [1 + (V_1\beta_1/2V_0) \sin (\theta_g/2)$$

$$= v_o [1 + (V_1 \beta_1/2V_0) \sin (wt_g - \theta_g/2) \quad (11.10)$$

11.5.4 Transit Time

The electron beam traverses the cavity gap twice, once while crossing and again while returning. Hence, the round trip transit time is given by

$$t_r = 2v(t_g)/(\text{acceleration } a) \quad (11.11)$$

The acceleration is given by

$$a = eE/m$$

$$= (e/m) [V_o + V_R + V_1 \sin \omega t]/L$$

$$= (e/m) [V_o + V_R]/L \quad (11.12)$$

since $V_1 << V_0$.

Hence,

$$t_r = 2v(t_g)/a$$

$$= 2v_omL[1+(V_1\beta_1/2V_0)$$

$$\sin (\omega t_g - \theta_g/2)]/[e(V_o +V_R)] \quad (11.13)$$

The reference electron does not undergo any velocity modulation. Hence, its transit time in the repeller space is

$$t_o = 2v_o/a = 2v_omL]/[e(V_o +V_R)]$$

$$= NT \quad (11.14)$$

$$= 2\pi N/\omega \quad (11.15)$$

Combining Eqs (11.13) and (11.15), the round trip transit time is given by

$$t_r = t_o[1+(V_1\beta_1/2V_o) \sin (\omega t_g - \theta_g/2)] \quad (11.16)$$

11.5.5 Bunching Parameter

The time at which the electron arrives at the cavity gap is given by

$$t_b = t_g + t_r$$

$$= t_g + t_o [1+(V_1\beta_1/2V_o) \sin (\omega t_g - \theta_g/2)] \quad (11.17)$$

$$= t_g + (2\pi N/\omega) + (\pi N/\omega)(V_1\beta_1/V_o).$$

$$\sin (\omega t_g - \theta_g/2)$$

$$= t_g + (2\pi N/\omega) + (X/\omega) \sin (\omega t_g - \theta_g/2) \quad (11.18)$$

The term $X = (\pi NV_1\beta_1/V_o)$ is known as *bunching parameter of the reflex klystron.*

11.5.6 Fundamental RF Current

On return, the bunched electrons constitute the bunched beam current i_b. According to the theory of conservation of charges, the dc and RF charges are equal. Thus, we get

$$I_o \mid dt_g \mid = i_b \mid dt_b \mid \qquad (11.19)$$

Here I_o is the dc beam current and i_b is the RF current. The differentiation of Eq. (11.18) with respect to t_g gives

$$dt_b / dt_g = 1 + X \cos (\omega t_g - \theta_g/2) \qquad (11.20)$$

Therefore, the RF current i_b is given by

$$
\begin{aligned}
i_b &= I_o / (\mid dt_b \mid / \mid dt_g \mid) \\
&= I_o / [1 + X \cos (\omega t_g - \theta_g/2)]
\end{aligned}
$$
$$(11.21)$$

Since $V_1 \ll V_0$ and $X \ll 1$, we get from Eq. (11.18),

$$t_b = t_g + (2\pi N/w).$$

Hence,

$$i_b = I_o / [1 + X \cos (\omega t_b - 2\pi N - \theta_g/2)] \qquad (11.22)$$

By expanding the above equation in Fourier series, we obtain the beam current of reflex klystron oscillator as

$$
\begin{aligned}
i_b &= I_o + 2I_o \sum_{n=1}^{\infty} J_n (nX) \cdot \\
&\quad \cos n(\omega t_b - 2\pi N - \theta_g/2) \\
&= I_o + 2I_o J_1(X) \cos \omega(t_b - t_o - t_g/2) + \\
&\quad 2I_o \sum_{n=2}^{\infty} J_n (nX) \cos n(\omega t_b - \omega t_o - \theta_g/2)
\end{aligned}
$$
$$(11.23)$$

The fundamental component of the RF induced current in the cavity is given by

$$
\begin{aligned}
I_1 &= 2\beta_i I_o J_1(X) \cos \omega(t_b - t_o - t_g/2) \\
&= 2\beta_i I_o J_1(X) \cos \omega(t_b - 2\pi N)
\end{aligned}
$$
$$(11.24)$$

since $t_g/2 \ll 2\pi N$.

11.6 EQUIVALENT CIRCUIT

If the electron bunch returns to the cavity a little earlier then the time $t_o = (n + 3/4)$ T, the current lags behind the field and an inductive reactance is presented to the circuit. Similarly, if the electron bunch returns to the cavity a little later then the time $t_o = (n + 3/4)$ T, the current leads the field and a capacitive reactance is presented to the circuit. The equivalent circuit of a reflex klystron is shown in Fig. 11.4. Here $Y_e = G_e + jB_e$ is the electronic admittance. L, C and R represent the equivalent lumped circuit components of the microwave resonator cavity.

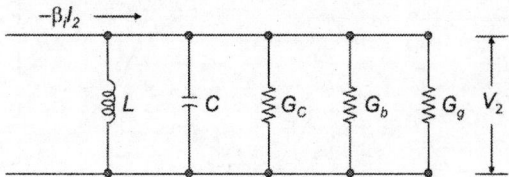

Fig.11.4: Equivalent circuit

The necessary conditions for sustained oscillations are G_e should be negative. Its magnitude should not be less than the total conductance of the cavity circuit. That is, $\mid -G_e \mid \geq G$ where $G = G_c + G_b + G_g$.

11.7 ELECTRONIC ADMITTANCE

The electronic admittance is given by

$$
\begin{aligned}
Y_e &= \frac{I_o}{V_o} \cdot \frac{\beta_i^2 \theta_o}{2} \cdot \frac{2J_1(X)}{X} \cdot e^{j\left(\frac{\pi}{2} - \theta_o\right)} \\
&= G_e + jB_e
\end{aligned}
$$
$$(11.25)$$

The amplitude of Y_e indicates that the electronic admittance is a function of the dc beam admittance (I_o/V_o), the dc transit angle $\theta_o = 2\pi N$ and the transit angle θ_o through the cavity gap.

Variations of G_e and B_e are shown in Fig. 11.5, the variations being a spiral. Infinite repeller voltage corresponds to the origin. As the repeller voltage is reduced, Y_e moves outwards along the spiral. Oscillations take place whenever $\mid G_e \mid$ is greater than G, the conductance of the external circuitry. That is when

$$t_o = (n + 3/4) T = NT, n = 0, 1, 2, ... \qquad (11.26)$$

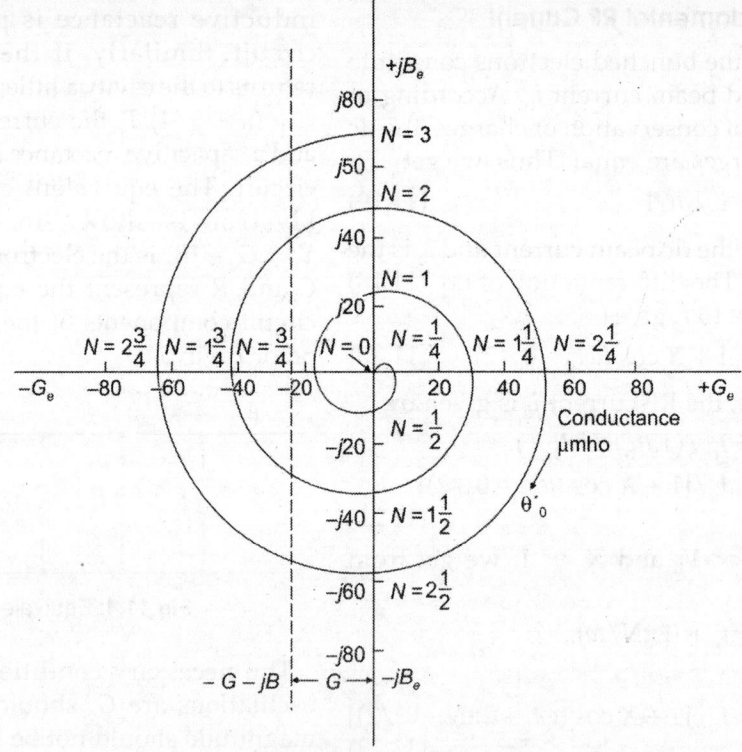

Fig. 11.5: Electronic admittance diagram

If jB_e is negative, oscillations take place at a frequency higher than the resonance frequency of the cavity. If it is positive, the oscillation frequency is lower than the resonant frequency of the cavity. This leads to frequency variations with the repeller voltage as shown in Fig. 11.6.

11.8 POWER OUTPUT

The RF power output delivered to the load is given by

$$P_0 = V_1 I_1/2 = V_1 \beta_i I_0 J_1(X) \qquad (11.27)$$

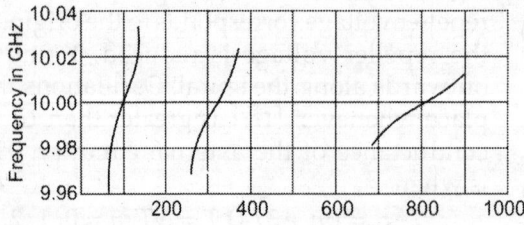

Fig. 11.6: Frequency variation with repeller voltage

Here V_1 is the amplitude of RF voltage, I_1 is the amplitude of RF current, β_i is the beam coupling coefficient, X is the bunching parameter, I_0 is the dc current and $J_1(X)$ is the Bessel function. The ratio of V_1 to V_0 is given by

$$V_1/V_0 = 2X/(2\beta_i \pi N) = X/(\beta_i \pi N) \qquad (11.28)$$

Substituting for V_1 from Eq. (11.28) into Eq. (11.27), we obtain

$$P_o = V_o I_o X J_1(X)/\pi N \qquad (11.29)$$

The factor $X J_1(X)$ reaches the maximum value of 1.25 at $X = 2.408$ and therefore, $J_1(X) = 0.52$. Hence the maximum RF power output is given by

$$P_{o\,max} = \frac{2.408 \times 0.52\, V_o I_o}{3.14\, N}$$

$$= 0.3986\, V_o I_o/N \qquad (11.30)$$

Figure 11.7 shows the variation of $X J_1(X)$ with X.

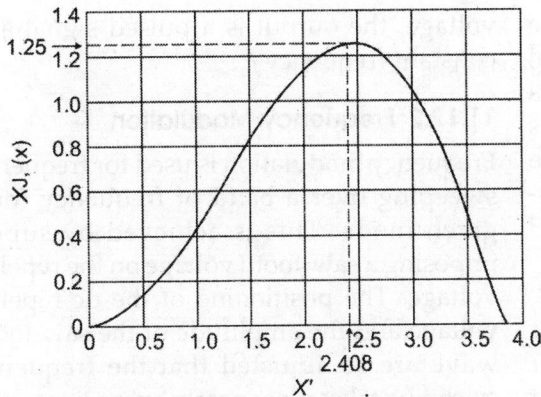

Fig.11.7: Variation of $X\,J_1(X)$ versus X'

11.9 EFFICIENCY

The electronic efficiency of a reflex klystron is defined as the ratio of the output power P_o to the input dc power P_i. They are given by

$$P_o = V_o I_o X J_1(X)/\pi N$$
$$P_i = V_o I_o$$

Hence,

$$\eta = P_o/P_i = V_o I_o X J_1(X)/ V_o I_o \pi N$$
$$= X J_1(X)/\pi N \qquad (11.31)$$

The maximum or the optimum efficiency is given by

$$\eta_{max} = P_{o\,max}/P_i = 0.3986/1.75$$
$$= 22.7\% \qquad (11.32)$$

The RF output is maximum when $n = 1$, i.e. $N = (n + 3/4) = 1.75$.

11.10 MODE CURVES

The output power and frequency can be electronically controlled by varying the repeller voltage of a reflex klystron. These parameters are expressed in terms of repeller voltage. The RF output power is given by

$$P_{rf} = \left[\frac{0.3986\,V_o I_o\,(V_o + V_R)}{2fL}\right]\sqrt{\frac{(e/m)}{2V_o}} \qquad (11.33)$$

The operating frequency of the reflex klystron oscillator is given by

$$f_{MHz} = (V_o + V_R)N/(0.0674 \times L_{cm}\sqrt{V_o}) \qquad (11.34)$$

The magnitude of repeller electrode voltage is given by

$$|V_R| = \sqrt{\left(\frac{8m}{e}\right)}\left(\frac{fL}{N}\right)\sqrt{V_o} - V_o \qquad (11.35)$$

$$= 6.74 \times 10^{-6}(fL/N)\sqrt{V_o} - V_o \qquad (11.36)$$

Here, f is in Hz and L is in meters. The variation of output power with repeller voltage is shown in Fig. 11.3. Figure 11.6 shows the variation of frequency with repeller voltage.

From Eq. (11.36), the change in repeller voltage with respect to frequency is given by

$$\frac{\Delta|V_R|}{\Delta f_{Hz}} = 6.74 \times 10^{-6} L \frac{\sqrt{V_o}}{N} \qquad (11.37)$$

To obtain maximum output power for a given mode N, the reflex klystron oscillator is tuned to the desired frequency f_o and then, the beam voltage V_o and the repeller voltage V_R are adjusted. The frequency f_o can be varied mechanically by using a short-circuit plunger and adjusting the beam voltage with klystron power supply.

11.11 TYPICAL CHARACTERISTICS

The typical characteristics of a reflex klystron oscillator are:

Frequency range:	4 to 200 GHz
Output RF power:	10 mW to 2.5 W
Max. efficiency:	22.7%

11.12 REFLEX KLYSTRON MODULATORS

Reflex Klystron oscillators are widely used as microwave sources in the laboratory to find the characteristics of a line or load. The most measurable parameters are VSWR and the position of the voltage minimum of the standing wave. These can be measured with microwave receivers or power meters but they are expensive. Hence reflex klystron oscillators are preferred. Microwave signals are low frequency modulated. This modulated signal is probed and detected by a crystal detector. The amplitude and phase variation information of the detected signal are measured using low frequency receivers to obtain the desired characteristics. For this purpose, amplitude modulation by square waves and frequency modulation by saw-tooth waves, as shown in Figs 11.8 and 11.9 are employed.

11.12.1 Amplitude Modulation

In the amplitude modulation, the repeller voltage is adjusted so that the operating point is at the left edge of the mode power curve. A low frequency (1 KHz) square wave is superimposed on the dc repeller voltage. The amplitude of the square pulse is adjusted to attain maximum power point and maintained throughout the measurements. Due to the square wave variation of the repeller

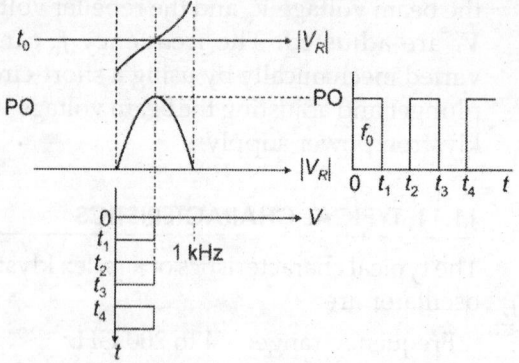

Fig. 11.8: Amplitude modulation with square wave

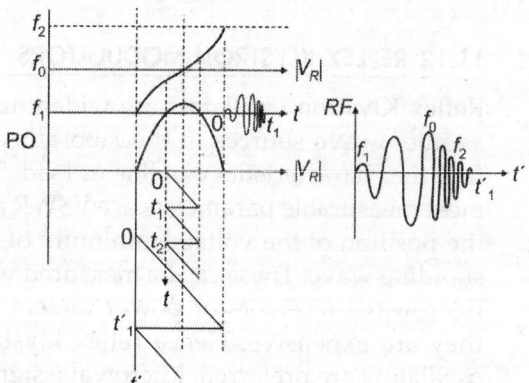

Fig. 11.9: Frequency modulation with sawtooth wave

voltage, the output is a pulsed signal at a constant frequency f_o.

11.12.2 Frequency Modulation

Frequency modulation is used for frequency sweeping over a band of frequency for a given mode. This is achieved by superimposing a saw-tooth voltage on the repeller voltage. The positioning of the dc repeller voltage and the amplitude of the saw-tooth wave are so adjusted that the frequency sweeping takes place nearly over a linear part of the frequency curve as shown in Fig.11.9 and at the same time over a small part of the power output curve so as to maintain almost constant power output and linear frequency sweeping. The response characteristic is displayed in the oscilloscope with the detected output fed to the y-plates and the modulating signal to the x-axis.

11.13 APPLICATIONS

The reflex klystron oscillators are used as
   (i) Microwave signal sources
  (ii) Local oscillator in microwave receivers
 (iii) FM oscillator in low power microwave links
 (iv) Parametric amplifiers

11.14 NUMERICAL EXAMPLES

Example 11.1 A reflex klystron is operated at 10 GHz with $V_o = 600$ V and $N = 1\frac{3}{4}$. The repeller space is 1 mm length and $I_o = 10$ mA. Assume $\beta_o = 1$. Compute the repeller voltage, maximum electronic efficiency and maximum output power.

Solution: Given: $f = 10 \times 10^9$, $V_o = 600$ V, $N = 1\frac{3}{4}$, $L = 1 \times 10^{-3}$, $I_o = 10 \times 10^{-3}$, $\beta = 1$.

The repeller voltage V_R is given by

$$|V_R| = (6.74 \times 10^{-6} \times fL/N)\sqrt{V_o - V_o}$$
$$= \left(\frac{6.64 \times 10^{-6} \times 10 \times 10^9 \times 1 \times 10^{-3}}{1.75}\right)\sqrt{600 - 600}$$
$$= 343.4 \text{ V}$$

The maximum efficiency

$$\eta_{max} = 0.3986/N = 0.3986/1.75$$
$$= 22.78\%$$

Maximum RF power

$$P_{o\,max} = 0.3986\,V_o I_o/N$$
$$= 0.3986 \times 600 \times 10 \times 10^{-3}/1.75$$
$$= 1.36 \text{ W}$$

Example 11.2 A reflex klystron is operated at 5 GHz with $V_o = 400$ V, repeller spacing of 0.5 cm and $N = 3\frac{3}{4}$. Calculate the bandwidth over $\Delta V_R = 1$ V.

Solution: Given: $f = 5 \times 10^9$, $V_o = 400$ V, $L = 5 \times 10^{-3}$, $N = 3\frac{3}{4}$, $\Delta V_R = 1$ V.

Bandwidth

$$B = \Delta f = \Delta V_R N/(6.74 \times 10^{-6} \times L \sqrt{V_o})$$
$$= 1 \times 3.75/(6.74 \times 10^{-6} \times 0.5 \times 10^{-2} \times \sqrt{400})$$
$$= 5.56 \text{ MHz}.$$

Example 11.3 A reflex klystron is operated at 9 GHz with $V_o = 600$ V, repeller spacing of 1 mm, $R_{sh} = 15$ kΩ and $N = 1\frac{3}{4}$. Calculate (a) the repeller voltage, (b) the dc current necessary to produce microwave gap voltage of 200 V and (c) the maximum efficiency. Assume $\beta_o = 1$.

Solution: Given: $f = 9 \times 10^9$, $V_o = 600$ V, $L = 1 \times 10^{-3}$, $R_{sh} = 15$ kΩ, $N = 1\frac{3}{4}$, $\beta_o = 1$.

(a) The repeller voltage V_R is given by

$$|V_R| = (6.74 \times 10^{-6} \times f \times L/N)\sqrt{V_o - V_o}$$
$$= \left(\frac{6.74 \times 10^{-6} \times 9 \times 10^9 \times 1 \times 10^{-3}}{1.75}\right)\sqrt{600 - 600}$$
$$= 249 \text{ V}$$

(b) The dc current I_o is given by

$$I_o = V_2/2J_1(X)\,R_{sh}$$
$$= 200/(2 \times 0.582 \times 15 \times 10^3)$$
$$= 11.45 \text{ mA}$$

(c) The maximum efficiency

$$\eta_{max} = 0.3986/N = 0.3986/1.75$$
$$= 22.78\%$$

KEY POINTS

- A common source of microwave power is the reflex klystron oscillator. It uses a single resonant

cavity. Its efficiency is low and hence, it is a low power device. It can operate from 1 GHz to 200 GHz. It is a microwave oscillator tube with a built-in feedback mechanism. It uses the same cavity for bunching and for the output.

- A reflex klystron oscillator consists of an electron gun, a single reentrant cavity resonator that also serves as anode, output coupling and repeller electrode. The repeller voltage is negative.
- The electrons are velocity modulated in the drift space and form bunches that occur once per cycle centered on a reference electron.
- The mode number N is given by $N = (n + \frac{3}{4})$.
- β_i is the beam coupling coefficient of the cavity gap and is given by $\beta_i = \sin(\theta_g/2)/(\theta_g/2)$.
- $d_m = V_1\beta_i/V_o$ is known as depth of velocity modulation.
- The round trip transit time is $t_r = t_o[1+(V_1\beta_1/2V_o)\sin(\omega t_1 - \theta_g/2)]$
- $X = (\beta NV_1\beta_1/V_o)$ is known as bunching parameter of the reflex klystron.
- The fundamental component of the RF induced current in the cavity is given by $I_1 = 2\beta_1 I_o\,J_1(X)\cos\omega(t_b - t_o - t_g/2) = 2\beta_1 I_o J_1(X)\cos\omega(t_b - 2\pi N)$
- The RF power output to the load is given by $P_o = V_1 I_1 X J_1(V)/\pi N$ and $P_{o\,max} = 0.3986\,V_o I_o/N$.
- The electronic efficiency of a reflex Klystron is defined as the ratio of the output power P_o to the input dc power P_i. Thus $\eta = P_o/P_i = XJ_1(X)/\pi N$ and $\eta_{max} = P_{o\,max}/P_i = 0.3986/N$.
- The reflex klystron oscillators are used as (i) Microwave signal sources, (ii) Local oscillators in microwave receivers, (iii) FM oscillators in low power microwave links and (iv) Parametric amplifiers.

FURTHER READING

1. Collins RE (1996). *Foundations of Microwave Engineering*, McGraw-Hill. NY.
2. Chodorov M and Susskind C (1964). *Fundamentals of Microwave Electronics*, MGH, NY.
3. Gewartowski JW and Watson HA (1965). *Principles of Electron Tubes*, Van Nostrand, NJ.
4. Gilmour AS Jr (1986). *Microwave Tubes*, Artech., Mass.
5. Liao SY (1988). *Microwave Electron Tubes*, PH, N.J.

REVIEW QUESTIONS

11.1 What is a reflex klystron?

11.2 What is meant by mode number of a reflex klystron oscillator? Which mode gives maximum output power?

11.3 Mention the assumptions made in the analysis of a reflex klystron oscillator.

11.4 Draw the equivalent circuit of a reflex klystron oscillator.

11.5 Give the expression for the output power of a reflex klystron oscillator.

11.6 When does the output power maximum and what is its value?

11.7 Define the efficiency of a reflex klystron oscillator. What is its value for $n = 1$?

11.8 Mention the typical characteristics of a reflex klystron oscillator.

11.9 What are the applications of a reflex klystron oscillator?

DESCRIPTIVE QUESTIONS

11.1 Describe the construction and working of a reflex klystron.

11.2 Describe, with necessary theory, the working of a reflex klystron. Explain how frequency stabilization is achieved.

11.3 Explain the working of a reflex klystron. Discuss its operating characteristics and applications.

11.4 Draw the electronic admittance diagram of a reflex klystron and explain the phenomenon of electronic tuning.

11.5 With mathematical substantiation, explain the velocity modulation and bunching process in a reflex klystron.

PRACTICE PROBLEMS

11.1 A reflex klystron is operated at 9 GHz with $V_o = 300$ V and $N = 1\frac{3}{4}$. The repeller space is 1mm length and $I_o = 10$ mA. Assume $\beta = 1$. Compute (a) the repeller voltage, (b) maximum electronic efficiency and (c) maximum output power.
   [**Ans:** (a) 249 V, (b) 22.74%, (c) 1.36 W]

11.2 A reflex klystron is operated at 5 GHz with $V_o = 350$ V, repeller spacing of 0.5 cm and $N = 3\frac{3}{4}$. Calculate the bandwidth over $\Delta V_R = 1$ V.
   [**Ans:** 5.948]

11.3 The reflector-to-cavity voltage for a reflex klystron is – 300 V. Calculate the magnitude of the deceleration produced given that the reflector is 0.8 cm from the nearest cavity grid.
   (**Ans:** 1.76×10^{16} m/s²)

REFERENCE

1. Atwater HA (1962). *Introduction to Microwave Theory*, McGraw-Hill, NY.
2. Das A and Das SK (2004). *Microwave Engineering*, TMH, New Delhi.
3. Gandhi OP (1981). *Microwave Engineering and Applications*, Pergamon, NY.
4. Ghose RN (1963) *Microwave Circuit Theory and Analysis*, McGraw Hill, NY,
5. Lance AL (1964). *Introduction to Microwave Theory and Measurements*, McGraw Hill, NY.
6. Lebedev I (1973). *Microwave Engineering*, MIR Publications, Moscow.
7. Liao SY (2000). *Microwave, Devices and Circuits,* PHI. New Delhi.
8. Pozar DM (1990). *Microwave Engineering*, Addison-Wesley, Massachutts.
9. Roddy D (1999). *Microwave Technology*, PH, NJ.
10. Sims GD and Stephen IM (1963). *Microwave Tubes and Semiconductor Devices*, Interscience Publication, NY.
11. Spangenberg KR (1948). *Vacuum Tubes*, McGraw Hill, N.Y,
12. Wolff EA and Kaul R (1988). *Microwave Engineering and Systems*, John Wiley, NY.
13. Terman FE (1955). *Electronic and Radio Engineering*, McGraw-Hill.
14. IEEE Proc. Vol.61, No.3, Mar. (1973) Special Issue on High Power Microwave Tubes.
15. IEEE Proc. Vol.70, No.1, Jan., 1962. Special Issue on Very Fast Solid State Technology.
16. IEEE Trans. Electron Devices (1973 Nov.). Special Issue on Microwave Theory and Techniques, MTT-21, No.11.
17. IEEE Trans. Electron Devices, (1976 Nov.) Special Issue on Microwave Theory and Techniques, MTT-24, No.11.
18. IEEE Trans. Electron Devices, (1979 May.) Special Issue on Microwave Theory and Techniques, MTT-27, No. 5.
19. IEEE Trans. Electron Devices, (1980 Dec.) Special Issue on Microwave Theory and Techniques, MTT-28, No.12.
20. IEEE Trans. Electron Devices, (1982 Apl.) Special Issue on Microwave Theory and Techniques, MTT-30, No. 4.
21. IEEE Trans. Electron Devices, (1982 Oct.) Special Issue on Microwave Theory and Techniques, MTT-30, No.10.

■ Travelling Wave Tube Amplifier

Objectives

- Understand the slow wave structure of the TWT.
- Explain the Brillouin diagram.
- Know the amplification process.
- Derive expressions for gain of the amplifier.
- Compare TWT amplifier with klystron amplifier.

12.1 INTRODUCTION

The traveling wave tube consists of a *long helix slow-wave non-resonant* microwave guiding structure. It makes use of a distributed interaction between an electron beam and a traveling wave. It is used for broadband microwave signal amplification. The electron beam from the cathode interacts continuously with an axial RF field over a long distance inside the helix structure where both velocity and density modulation take place.

12.2 TRAVELING WAVE TUBE (TWT)

The construction details of a TWT are shown in Fig. 12.1. It consists of an electron gun, a long helix slow-wave structure, a collector, input and output couplers and an external magnetic focusing structure. There is an attenuator near the input end. The electron gun produces a pencil-like beam of electrons having a velocity that typically corresponds to an accelerating potential of the order of

1500 V. This beam is shot through a long loosely wound helix and is collected by a collector. An axial magnetic focusing field is provided to prevent the beam from spreading and to guide it through the center of the helix. The signal to be amplified is applied to the input end of the helix. Under appropriate operating conditions, an amplified signal appears at the output end of the helix.

12.3 SLOW-WAVE STRUCTURE ANALYSIS

The gain-bandwidth product of a microwave amplifier is limited by the resonant circuit. Hence, the conventional resonators cannot produce large output. Therefore, several non-resonant periodic circuits are used to provide large gain over a wide bandwidth. Such structures are known as *slow-wave structures*. They are special circuits used in microwave tubes to reduce the wave velocity in certain direction so that the electron beam and the signal wave can interact. In waveguide, the phase velocity of a wave is greater than the velocity of light in vacuum. In the operation

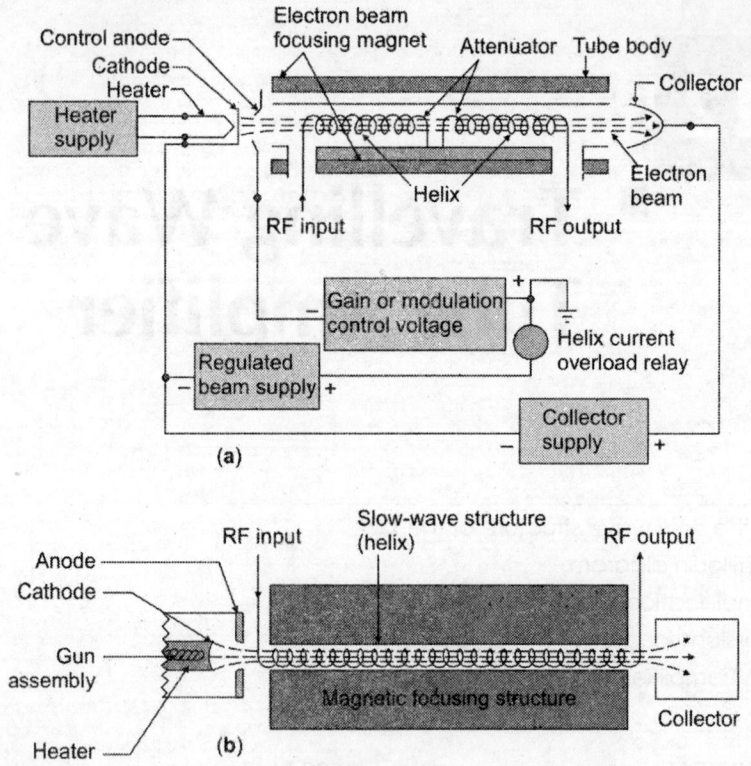

Fig. 12.1: TWT (a) Schematic diagram of helix TWT (b) Simplified diagram

of traveling-wave amplifier, the electron beam must be kept in step with the micro-wave signal. Hence, a slow-wave structure is used in the microwave devices so that the phase velocity of the microwave signal can keep pace with that of the electron beam for effective interaction. Fig. 12.2 shows several types of slow-wave structures.

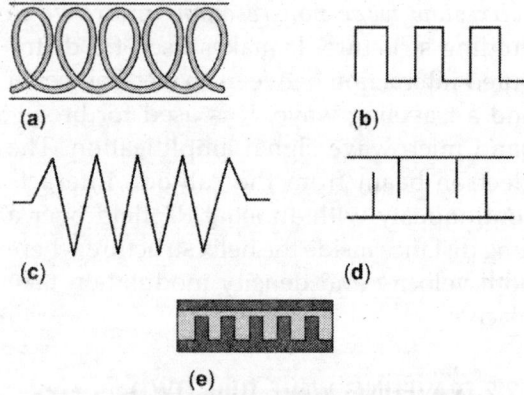

Fig. 12.2: Slow-wave structures (a) Helix (b) Folded line (c) Zigzag line (d) Inter-digital line and (e) Corrugated waveguide

12.4 BRILLOUIN DIAGRAM

The most commonly used slow-wave structure consists of a helical coil with concentric conducting cylinder shown in Fig. 12.3. The ratio of phase velocity v_p along the pitch to the phase velocity along the coil is given by

$$v_p/c = \frac{p}{\sqrt{p^2 + (\pi d)^2}} = \sin \psi \qquad (12.1)$$

Here, v_p is the phase velocity in the conducting medium in the coil

c is the velocity of light in free space
= 3×10^8 m/s

p is the pitch of the helix

d is the diameter of the helix

ψ is the pitch angle.

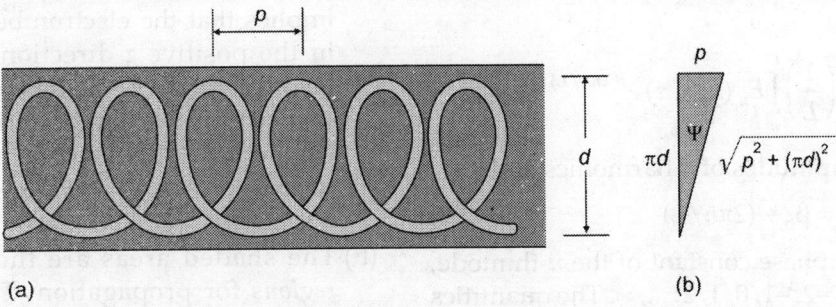

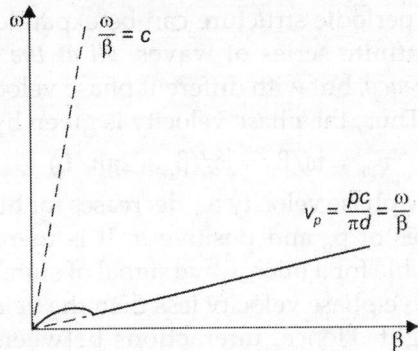

Fig. 12.3: Helical slow-wave structure (a) Helical coil (b) One turn of helix

Usually, the helical coil is inside a dielectric-filled cylinder. The phase velocity along the axial direction in the dielectric medium is given by

$$v_{pe} = p/\sqrt{\mu\varepsilon(p^2 + (\pi d)^2)} \qquad (12.2)$$

The slow-wave structure introduces considerable loss, if the dielectric constant is large. Hence, the efficiency is reduced. If the pitch angle, $p << \pi d$, the phase velocity along the coil in free space is approximately equal to

$$v_p \approx pc/(\pi d) = \omega/\beta \qquad (12.3)$$

The variation of ω with β for a helical slow-wave structure is shown in Fig. 12.4. This diagram is known as *Brillouin* diagram. The helix ω–β diagram is much useful in designing a helix slow-wave structure. Once β is found, v_p for a given helix dimension can be computed using Eq. (12.3). The group velocity is the slope of the ω–β curve and is given by

$$v_{gr} = \partial\omega/\partial p \qquad (12.4)$$

To be a slow-wave structure, the circuit must have the property of periodicity in the axial direction. In the helical slow-wave structure, a translation back and forth through a distance of one pitch length results in identically the same structure again. Thus, the period of the helical slow-wave structure is its pitch.

The field of a slow-wave structure must be distributed according to the Flouqet's

Fig. 12.4: ω–β or Brillouin diagram of a helical structure

theorem for periodic boundaries. The theorem states that *"the steady state solutions for the electromagnetic fields of a single propagating mode in a periodic structure have the property that the fields in adjacent cells are related by a complex constant."* The theorem is expressed mathematically as

$$E(x, y, z - L) = E(x, y, z)e^{j\beta_o L} \qquad (12.5)$$

Here, $E(x, y, z)$ is a periodic function of z with period L. β_o in the slow-wave structure is the phase constant of average electron velocity. The field distribution of $E(x, y, z)$ is expanded into a Fourier series of fundamental period L as

$$E(x, y, z) = \sum_{n=-\infty}^{\infty} E_n(x, y)e^{-j\left(\frac{2\pi n}{L}\right)z}e^{-j\beta_o z}$$

$$= \sum_{n=-\infty}^{\infty} E_n(x, y)e^{-j\beta_n z} \qquad (12.6)$$

Here,

$$E_n(x, y) = \left(\frac{1}{L}\right)\int_0^L E_n(x, y, z)\, e^{j(2\pi n/L)z}\,dz \quad (12.7)$$

are the amplitudes of n harmonics and

$$\beta_n = \beta_0 + (2\pi n/L) \quad (12.8)$$

β_n is the phase constant of the n-th mode, $n = -\infty, ..., -2, -1, 0, 1, 2, ..., \infty$. The quantities $E_n(x, y)\, e^{-j\beta_n z}$ are known as *spatial harmonics*.

From Eq. (12.6), it can be seen that the field in a periodic structure can be expanded as an infinite series of waves, *all at the same frequency*, but with different phase velocities v_{pn}. Thus, the phase velocity is given by

$$v_{pn} = \omega/\beta_n = \omega/(\beta_0 + 2\pi n/L) \quad (12.9)$$

The phase velocity v_{pn} decreases for higher values of β_0 and positive n. It is therefore possible for a microwave signal of suitable n to have phase velocity less than the velocity of light. Hence, interactions between the electron beam and the microwave signal are possible and thus, the microwave signal gets ampli-fied.

The group velocity

$$v_{gr} = \partial\omega/\partial\beta_0 \quad (12.10)$$

Thus, the group velocity is independent of n.

Figure 12.5 shows the ω–β or Brillouin diagram for a helix with several spatial harmonics. The properties of this diagram are:

(a) The second quadrant of the Brillouin diagram corresponds to negative n and hence the *negative* phase velocity. This

implies that the electron beam moves in the positive z-direction while the beam velocity coincides with phase velocity of the the negative spatial harmonics. This type of microwave tube is known as *backward-wave oscillator*.

(b) The shaded areas are the *forbidden regions* for propagation. This occurs because energy is radiated if the axial phase velocity of any spatial harmonic exceeds the velocity of light.

12.5 AMPLIFICATION PROCESS

The signal to be amplified is applied to the input end of the helix. It propagates around the turns of the helix and produces an electric field at the center of the helix along the helix axis. If the frequency is high, the velocity propagating signal along the helix approximates the velocity of light. The axial electric field signal advances with a velocity that is approximately the velocity of light multiplied by the ratio of helix pitch to helix circumference. When the velocity of the electrons in the helix approximates the rate of advance of the axial field, interaction takes place between this moving axial electric field and the moving electrons. On an average, the electrons deliver energy to the wave on the helix and the signal wave on the helix becomes larger at the output end of the helix. Thus the amplification of the signal is achieved.

12.5.1 Mechanism of Energy Transfer

The mechanism of energy conversion is illustrated in Fig. 12.6. Consider a group of electrons near the input end of the helix in the vicinity of A. Let the axial electric field be zero at this point and is negative towards the output end of the helix. An electron exactly located at A encounters zero axial electric field and hence is not affected by the signal on the helix. However, electron B, just to the left of A, encounters a positive axial

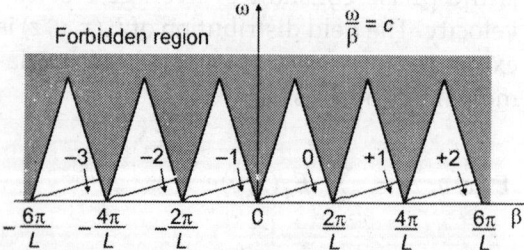

Fig. 12.5: Brillouin diagram of spatial harmonics for helical structure

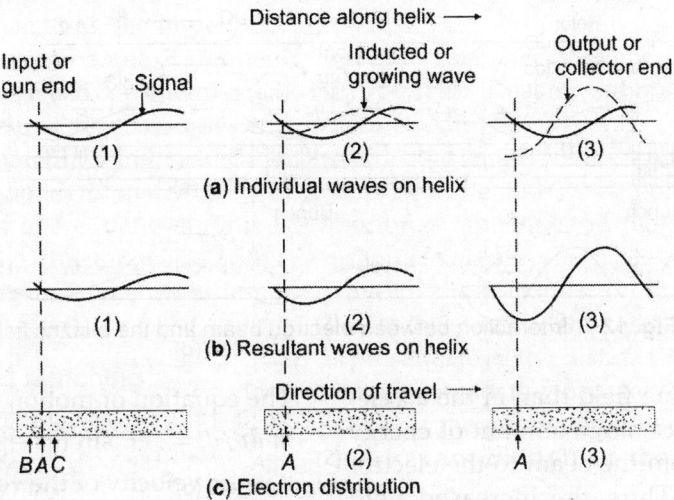

Fig.12.6: Mechanism of energy transfer

field and is accelerated, thus tend to catch up with electron A. Similarly, electron c, just to the right of A, encounters a negative axial field and is decelerated. It slows down and tends towards A. Thus, the electrons centered about A are velocity modulated. The velocity modulation takes place continuously as the electrons travel with the wave towards the collector. Thus bunching of electrons takes place.

These bunched electrons centered around A induce a second wave on helix and produces an axial electric field that lags behind by $\lambda/4$. Because of this action, the electrons encounter retarding field. As a result, they deliver energy to the wave on the helix. As the electrons travel further along the helix, the bunching is more and the induced wave grows in amplitude. A large and increasing amount of energy is thereby delivered by the electron bunch to the wave on the helix and the output is much larger than the original signal. Thus, power amplification, typically from 20 to 40 dB can be achieved in a single tube.

The slow-wave structure of the helix is characterized by the ω–β or Brillouin diagram shown in Fig. 12.6. The phase shift

of the fundamental wave on the slow-wave per period is given by

$$\theta_1 = \beta_o L \qquad (12.11)$$

$\beta_o = \omega/v_o$ is the phase constant of the average beam velocity and L is the period or the pitch. The dc transit time is given by

$$T_o = L/v_o \qquad (12.12)$$

The phase constant of the nth space harmonic is given by

$$\beta_n = \omega/v_o = \beta_o + (2\pi n/L) \qquad (12.13)$$

Here, the axial space-harmonic phase constant is assumed to be synchronized with the beam velocity for interactions between the electron beam and the electric field.

i.e., $\qquad v_{np} = v_o. \qquad (12.14)$

In practice, the dc velocity of the electrons is adjusted to be slightly greater than the axial velocity of the electromagnetic wave for proper energy transfer.

The electrons entering the retarding field are decelerated and those in the accelerating field are accelerated. Hence, they bunch together centered about those electrons that enter the helix during zero electric field. This process is shown in Fig. 12.7. Since the velocity v_o of electrons is slightly greater than the axial wave velocity v_{pn}, more electrons

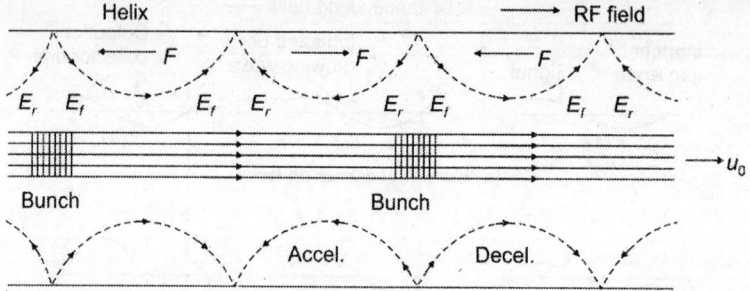

Fig. 12.7: Interaction between electron beam and the electric field

are in the retarding field than in the accelerating field. Hence, large amount of energy is transferred from the beam to the electromagnetic field. Thus, the increased field further amplifies the microwave signal. The bunch continues to become intense and a larger amplification of the signal occurs at the end of the helix.

The magnet produces an axial magnetic field that prevents the spreading of the electron beam as it travels down the tube. An attenuator placed near the center of the helix absorbs all the waves traveling along the helix so that the reflected waves from the mismatched loads cannot reach the input and cause oscillations. The bunched electrons emerging from the attenuator induce a new electric field with the same frequency. In turn, this field induces a new amplified microwave signal on the helix.

12.5.2 Velocity Fluctuations

The motion of electrons in the helix-type traveling-wave tube can be quantitatively analyzed in terms of axial electric field. Assuming the traveling wave is propagating in the z-direction, the z-component of the electric field is given by

$$E_z = E_1 \sin(\omega t - \beta_p z) \qquad (12.15)$$

E_1 is the magnitude of the electric field in the z-direction. Let $t = t_0$, $z = 0$ and the electric field is maximum. The axial phase constant of the microwave is given by

$$\beta_p = \omega / v_p \qquad (12.16)$$

Here, v_p is the axial phase velocity.

The equation of motion of the electron is

$$m \, dv/dt = -eE_1 \sin(\omega t - \beta_p z) \qquad (12.17)$$

v is the velocity of the velocity-modulated electron beam.

Assuming that the velocity of electron is

$$v = v_0 + v_e \cos(\omega_e t + \theta_e) \qquad (12.18)$$

the acceleration is

$$dv/dt = -v_e \omega_e \sin(\omega_e t + \theta_e) \qquad (12.19)$$

Here, v_0 is the dc electron velocity,

v_e is the magnitude of velocity fluctuation in the velocity-modulated electron beam,

ω_e is the angular frequency of velocity fluctuation,

θ_e is the phase angle of the fluctuation.

Substituting the above equation in Eq. (12.17), we obtain

$$mv_e w_e \sin(w_e t + \theta_e) = eE_1 \sin(wt - \beta_p z) \qquad (12.20)$$

For proper interaction and energy transfer between the electrons and the electric field, the velocity of the velocity-modulated electron beam must be approximately equal to the dc electron velocity. Therefore,

$$v \approx v_0 \qquad (12.21)$$

The distance z traveled by the electron at time t is given by

$$z = v_0(t - t_0) \qquad (12.22)$$

Substitution of Eq. (12.22) in Eq. (12.20), we get

$$mv_e \omega_e \sin(\omega_e t + \theta_e) = eE_1 \sin[\omega t - \beta_p v_0(t - t_0)] \qquad (12.23)$$

Comparing both sides of the above equation, we obtain

$$v_e = eE_1/m\omega_e$$

$$\omega_e = \beta_p(v_p - v_o) \text{ since } \omega = \beta_p v_p$$

$$\theta_e = \beta_p v_o t_o \tag{12.24}$$

Thus, the magnitude of the velocity fluctuation v_e of the electron beam is directly proportional to the magnitude of the axial electric field E_1.

12.5.3 Convection Current

With space charge effect, the electron velocity, the charge density, the current density and the axial electric field will perturbate about their average or dc values. These can be expressed mathematically as

$$v = v_o + v_1 e^{j\omega t - \gamma z} \tag{12.25}$$

$$\rho = \rho_o + \rho_1 e^{j\omega t - \gamma z} \tag{12.26}$$

$$J = -J_o + J_1 e^{j\omega t - \gamma z} \tag{12.27}$$

$$E_z = E_1 e^{j\omega t - \gamma z} \tag{12.28}$$

Here, $\gamma = \alpha_e + j\beta_e$ is the propagation constant of the axial waves. The negative sign associated with J_o indicates that J_o is positive in the negative z-direction.

For a weak signal, the electron beam current density is given by

$$J = \rho v = -J_o + J_1 e^{j\omega t - \gamma z} \tag{12.29}$$

$$J_o = -\rho_o v_o \tag{12.30}$$

$$J_1 = \rho_1 v_o + \rho_o v_1 \tag{12.31}$$

$$\rho_1 v_1 \approx 0. \tag{12.32}$$

An axial electric field existing in the slow-wave structure perturbs the electron velocity according to the force equation given by

$$\frac{dv}{dt} = \left(-\frac{e}{m}\right) E_1 e^{j\omega t - \gamma c} = \left(\frac{\partial}{\partial t} + \frac{dz}{dt}\frac{\partial}{\partial z}\right) v$$

$$= (j\omega - \gamma v_o) v_1 e^{j\omega t - \gamma z} \tag{12.33}$$

Here dz/dt is replaced by v_o. Therefore,

$$v_1 = (-e/m)E_1/(j\omega - \gamma v_o) \tag{12.34}$$

The continuity equation is given by

$$\nabla \cdot J + \partial\rho/\partial t = (-\gamma J_1 + j\omega\rho_1) e^{j\omega t - \gamma z}$$

$$= 0 \tag{12.35}$$

Hence,

$$\rho_1 = -j\gamma J_1/\omega \tag{12.36}$$

Substituting Eq. (12.34) and (12.36) in Eq. (12.31), we obtain

$$J_1 = J(\omega/v_o)(e/m) J_o E_1/(j\omega - \gamma v_o)^2 \tag{12.37}$$

Assuming the magnitude of the axial electric field is uniform over the cross-section area of the electron beam, the convection current in the electron beam is given by

$$i = J \frac{\beta_e I_o}{2V_o(j\beta_e - \gamma)^2} E_1 \tag{12.38}$$

$\beta_e = \omega/v_o$ is the phase constant of the velocity-modulated beam and $v_o = \sqrt{2(e/m)V_o}$. The above equation determines the convection current induced by the axial electric field and hence is known as *electronic equation*. If the axial field and all parameters are known, the convection current can be determined from Eq. (12.38).

12.5.4 Axial Electric Field

In the slow-wave structure the convection current in the electron beam induces an electric field. This induced field is in phase with the field already present in the circuit. Because of the increased field, the power increases with the distance. Figure 12.8 shows the relationship between the electron beam and the slow-wave structure.

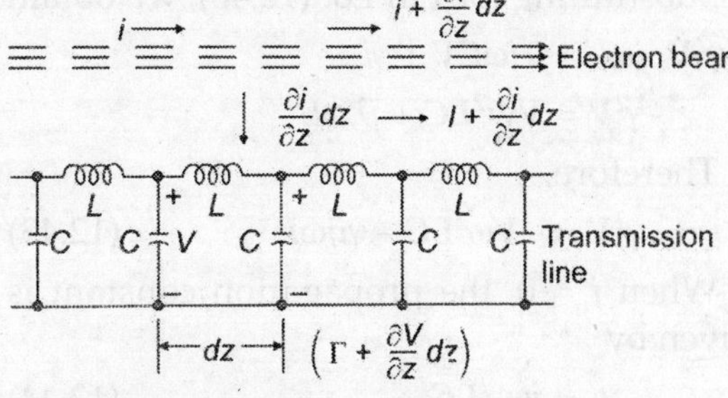

Fig. 12.8: Equivalent circuit of a slow-wave structure and electron beam coupling

The slow-wave helix structure is represented by an equivalent distributed transmission line for simplicity. The transmission line parameters are:

- L is the inductance per unit length
- C is the capacitance per unit length
- I is the alternating current in the transmission line
- V is the alternating voltage in the transmission line
- i is the convection current

The transmission line is coupled to the convection electron-beam current. Hence, a current is induced in the line. The current flowing into a line of length dz is i, and that flowing out of dz is $[i + (\partial i/\partial z)dz]$. Since the net change of current must be zero, the current flowing out of the electron beam into the transmission line must be $(\partial i/\partial z)dz$. Appling transmission line theory and Kirchhoff's current law to the electron beam, it can be shown that

$$\partial I/\partial z = -C\partial V/\partial t - \partial i/\partial z \qquad (12.39)$$

Hence,

$$-\gamma I = -j\omega CV - \gamma i \qquad (12.40)$$

Here, $\partial/\partial z = -\gamma$ and $\partial/\partial t = j\omega$ are substituted. The voltage equation is given by

$$\partial V/\partial z = -L\partial I/\partial t \qquad (12.41)$$

Similarly,

$$-\gamma V = -j\omega LI \qquad (12.42)$$

From Eq. (12.42), we get

$$I = \gamma V/j\omega L$$

Substituting for I in Eq. (12.40), we obtain

$$-\gamma^2 V/j\omega L = -j\omega CV + \gamma i$$

$$-\gamma^2 V = Vw^2 LC + j\lambda\omega L$$

Therefore,

$$\gamma^2 V = -V\omega^2 LC - \gamma ij\omega L \qquad (12.43)$$

When $i = 0$, the propagation constant is given by

$$\gamma_o = j\omega\sqrt{LC} \qquad (12.44)$$

The characteristic impedance of the transmission line is given by

$$Z_o = \sqrt{L/C} \qquad (12.45)$$

With electron beam current is present, the voltage V is given by

$$V = \gamma\gamma_o Z_o i /(\gamma^2 - \gamma_o^2) \qquad (12.46)$$

The axial electric field is given by

$$E_1 = -\gamma^2\gamma_o Z_o i /(\gamma^2 - \gamma_o^2) \qquad (12.47)$$

Equation (12.47) determines how the axial electric field of the slow-wave helix structure is affected by the spatial ac electron beam current and hence is known as *circuit equation*.

12.5.5 Wave Modes of TWT

The simultaneous solution of the electronic and circuit equations for the propagation constants yields the wave modes of a traveling-wave tube. Each solution for the propagation constant is a mode of the traveling wave in the tube. Substituting Eq. (12.38) in Eq. (12.47), we obtain

$$(\gamma^2 - \gamma_o^2)(j\beta_e - \gamma)^2 = -j\gamma^2\gamma_o Z_o\beta_e I_o/2V_o \qquad (12.48)$$

Equation (12.48) is of fourth order in v. Hence, there are four roots and these correspond to four wave modes of traveling wave in the tube. To obtain an approximate solution, we set the dc beam velocity equal to the axial phase velocity. Thus,

$$\gamma_o = j\beta_e \qquad (12.49)$$

Eq. (12.48) becomes

$$(\gamma - j_e^\beta)^3 (\gamma + j\beta_e) = \frac{\gamma^2\beta_e^2 Z_o I_o}{2V_o}$$

$$= 2C^3\gamma^2\beta_e^2 \qquad (12.50)$$

C is the gain parameter of the travelling-wave tube and is given by

$$C = (I_o Z_o/4V_o)^{1/3} \qquad (12.51)$$

From Eq. (12.50), it can be seen that there are *three forward travelling waves* corresponding to $e^{-j\beta_e z}$ and *one backward wave* corresponding to $e^{+j\beta_e z}$. Assume that the propagation constant of the three forward traveling waves is

$$\gamma = j\beta_e - \beta_e C\delta \qquad (12.52)$$

with $C\delta \ll 1$. Substituting Eq. (15.52) in Eq. (12.50), we get

$$(-\beta_e C\delta)^3 (2j\beta_e - \beta_e C\delta)$$

$$= 2C^3 \beta_e^2 [-\beta_e^2 - 2j\beta_e^2 C\delta + (\beta_e C\delta)^2] \tag{12.53}$$

Since $C\delta \ll 1$, the above equation reduces to

$$(-\beta_e C\delta)^3 (2j\beta_e) = 2C^3 \beta_e^2 (-\beta_e^2)$$

$$\delta = (-j)^{1/3} \tag{12.54}$$

The three roots of $(-j)$ are:

For $n = 0$: The first root δ_1 is

$$\delta_1 = e^{-j\pi/6} = \frac{\sqrt{3}}{2} - j\frac{1}{2} \tag{12.55}$$

For $n = 1$: The second root δ_2 is

$$\delta_2 = e^{-j5\pi/6} = -\frac{\sqrt{3}}{2} - j\frac{1}{2} \tag{12.56}$$

For $n = 2$: The third root δ_3 is

$$\delta_3 = e^{-j3\pi/2} = j1 \tag{12.57}$$

The fourth root corresponding to the backward wave is obtained by setting

$$\gamma = -j\beta_e - \beta_e \delta_4 \tag{12.58}$$

Hence, $\delta_4 = -jC^2/4$ \hspace{1em} (12.59)

Therefore, the values of the propagation constants γ are:

$$\gamma_1 = -\beta_e C\sqrt{\frac{3}{2}} + j\beta_e(1 + C/2) \tag{12.60}$$

$$\gamma_2 = -\beta_e C\sqrt{\frac{3}{2}} + j\beta_e\left(1 + \frac{C}{2}\right) \tag{12.61}$$

$$\gamma_3 = j\beta_e(1 - C) \tag{12.62}$$

$$\gamma_4 = -j\beta_e(1 - C^3/4) \tag{12.63}$$

These four propagation constants represent the four different modes of wave propagation in the O-type traveling wave tube. The properties of the wave are:

(i) The wave corresponding to γ_1 is a *forward wave with exponentially increasing amplitude* with distance.

(ii) The wave corresponding to γ_2 is also a *forward wave with exponentially decreasing amplitude* with distance.

(iii) The wave corresponding to γ_3 is also a *forward wave with constant amplitude* with distance.

(iv) The wave corresponding to γ_4 is a *backward wave with constant amplitude* with distance.

Velocity of the growing wave phase is slightly lower than the electron beam velocity. Hence, the energy transferred from the electron beam to the wave of the decaying wave is same as that of the growing wave but the energy flows from the wave to the electron beam. The phase velocity of the constant amplitude is slightly greater than the beam velocity but no energy transfer occurs. The backward wave propagates in the negative z-direction and its phase velocity is slightly greater than the beam velocity. Typical value of the gain parameter $C \approx 0.02$.

12.5.6 Gain Characteristics

For computing gain, let us assume that the slow-wave structure is perfectly matched so that there is no backward wave. The attenuator at the cente of the tube attenuates any reflected wave to a minimum or zero value. Hence, the total circuit voltage is the sum of the three forward voltages corresponding to the forward traveling waves. Thus,

$$V(z) = V_1 e^{-\gamma_1 z} + V_2 e^{-\gamma_2 z} V_3 e^{-\gamma_3 z}$$

$$= \sum_{n=1}^{3} V_n e^{-\gamma_n z} \tag{12.64}$$

From Eq. (12.38), the input current i is given by

$$i(z) = -\sum_{n=1}^{3} \left(\frac{I_o}{2V_o C^2}\right)\left(\frac{V_n}{\delta_n^2}\right) e^{-\gamma_n z} \tag{12.65}$$

The input fluctuating component of the velocity of the total wave is given by

$$v_1(z) = \sum_{n=1}^{3} j\left(\frac{v_o}{2V_o C}\right)\left(\frac{V_n}{\delta_n^2}\right) e^{-\gamma_n z} \tag{12.66}$$

Assume $z = 0$ at the input reference point and the output is at $z = l$. Then, at $z = 0$, the voltage, current and velocity at the input point are given by

$$V(0) = V_1 + V_2 + V_3 \qquad (12.67)$$

$$i(0) = -\left(\frac{I_o}{2V_oC^2}\right)\left(\frac{V_1}{\delta_1^2} + \frac{V_2}{\delta_2^2} + \frac{V_3}{\delta_3^2}\right) \qquad (12.68)$$

$$v_1(0) = -j\left(\frac{v_o}{2V_oC}\right)\left(\frac{V_1}{\delta_1} + \frac{V_2}{\delta_2} + \frac{V_3}{\delta_3}\right) \qquad (12.69)$$

Solving Eqs. (12.67) to (12.69) simultaneously with $v_1 = 0$ and $i = 0$,

$$V_1 = V_2 = V_3 = V(0)/3 \quad (12.70)$$

Substituting the values of δ_1, δ_2 and δ_3 and rearranging, we get

$$V_1\left(\frac{1}{2} + j\frac{\sqrt{3}}{2}\right) + V_2\left(\frac{1}{2} - j\frac{\sqrt{3}}{2}\right) - V_3 = 0$$

Equating the imaginary terms, we have

$$V_1 = V_2$$

The total voltage along the circuit is predominantly due to the growing wave increasing exponentially with distance. When the slow-wave structure length l is sufficiently large, the output voltage is almost equal to the voltage of the growing wave. The output voltage is then given by

$$V(l) = \left[\frac{(V(0)}{3}\right][e^{-\gamma_1 z} + e^{-\gamma_2 z}]$$

$$= \left[\frac{V_1(0)}{3}\right]\exp\left[\left(\sqrt{\frac{3}{2}}\right)\beta_e Cl\right]\exp\left[-j\beta e\left(1 + \frac{C}{2}\right)l\right] \qquad (12.71)$$

$\beta_e l = 2\pi N$ and hence,

$$N = l/\lambda_e \quad \text{and} \quad \beta_e = 2\pi/\lambda_e \qquad (12.72)$$

N is the circuit length in terms of electronic wavelength λ_e.

Then the amplitude of the output voltage is given by

$$V(l) = [V(0)/3] \exp (\sqrt{3}\pi NC) \qquad (12.73)$$

The output power gain in dB is given by

$$A_p = 10 \log |V(l)/V(0)|^2$$

$$= 10\log\left[\frac{1}{3}\cdot\exp(\sqrt{3}\pi NC)\right]^2$$

$$= -10\log 9 + 20\log\left[\exp(\sqrt{3}\pi NC)\right]$$

$$= -9.54 + 47.3\,NC \qquad (12.74)$$

Here N is the circuit length in electronic wave length and is given by $N = l/\lambda_e$ and C is the gain parameter of the circuit and is given by $C = (I_oZ_o/4V_o)^{1/3}$. The power gain is proportional to the circuit length N and gain parameter C. The term (-9.54) dB represents the initial loss at the circuit input due to splitting of signal into three waves of equal magnitude and the growing wave voltage is only one-third of the total input voltage.

Figure 12.9 shows power output and gain characteristics. For low RF inputs, the gain is almost constant. As the RF input increases beyond certain value, the gain decreases. The point at which the RF power output attains a maximum is termed as *saturation point* as shown in Fig. 12.9(a).

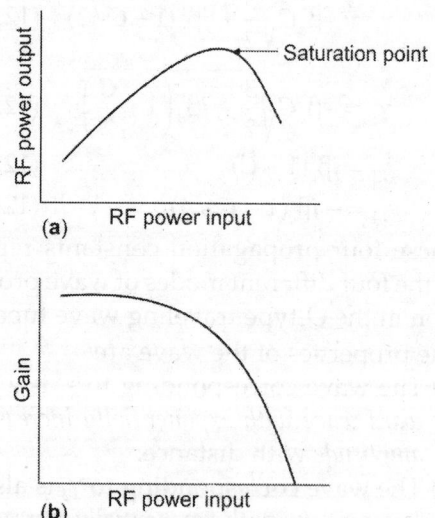

Fig. 12.9: Power output and gain characteristics

The gain of the TWT amplifier varies with frequency because

(i) The velocity of the electric field varies along the axis of the tube.
(ii) The length of the tube in wavelengths varies.
(iii) The strength of the axial electric field is a function of the frequency.
(iv) The terminal impedance of the tube is not perfectly matched at all frequencies.

12.6 SUPPRESSION OF OSCILLATIONS

In order to suppress oscillations from being spontaneously generated in a TWT, it is necessary to prevent internal feedback arising from reflections due to impedance mismatch at the terminals. Thus, the energy reflected at the output terminal will travel back to the input. Upon reflection there, it provides a spurious feedback signal that is further amplified along with the desired signal. It is also necessary to prevent backward-wave oscillations from being generated. This is controlled by introducing an attenuator near the center of the tube as shown in Fig. 12.10. It absorbs any wave propagated along the helix. The attenuator is a conducting coating of Aquadag painted on the glass wall of the tube. The attenuator absorbs the undesired backward or feedback wave.

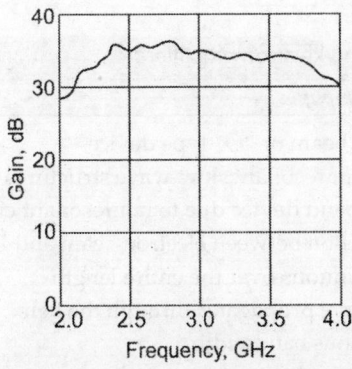

Fig. 12.10: Frequency response of TWT amplifier

12.7 BANDWIDTH

The TWT is inherently a nonresonant device. As a result, it can have enormous bandwidth compared with those obtainable from amplifiers involving resonant circuits. The TWT can have constant amplification within ±3 dB from 2 GHz to 4 GHz as shown in Fig. 12.10.

12.8 DISTORTION

The distortion in the TWT amplifiers is due to

i. harmonic distortion
ii. phase delay distortion.

12.8.1 Harmonic Distortion

This is caused by the nonlinearity of the transfer characteristic of the TWT amplifier. When TWT is operated at or near saturation, intense electron bunching takes place that produces sharp current peaks rich in harmonics. This is known as *harmonic distortion*. The nonlinear characteristic also gives rise to intermodulation distortion.

12.8.2 Phase Delay Distortion

A second form of distortion is due to phase delay between the input and output of a TWT amplifier. When the input is at a fixed level, the time delay between the input and output is negligibly small. At higher input levels, more beam energy is converted into output power. This reduces the average velocity of the beam and hence the delay time is increased. The phase delay is directly proportional to the time delay. Hence, it results in a phase shift at the output relative to the phase shift at the saturation, giving rise to phase delay distortion.

12.9 TYPICAL CHARACTERISTICS

The typical performance characteristics of a TWT amplifier are:

Frequency range: 1 GHz and above
Bandwidth: 0.8 GHz

Efficiency: 20 to 40 %
Power output: Up to 10 KW
Power gain: Up to 60 dB

12.10 APPLICATIONS

The TWT amplifiers are used as
(a) RF amplifiers in microwave broadband receivers.
(b) Repeater amplifiers in wideband communication links.
(c) Low noise front-end amplifiers

12.11 ADVANTAGES

The TWT amplifiers have:
(i) large bandwidth
(ii) very low noise figure

12.12 COMPARISON BETWEEN TWT AND KLYSTRON AMPLIFIERS

The comparison between TWT and klystron amplifiers is given in the Table 12.1

12.13 NUMERICAL EXAMPLES

Example 12.1 A helix TWT operates at 5 GHz with a beam voltage of 9 kV and beam current of 400 mA. If the impedance of helix is 50 ohms and the interaction length is 10 cm, find the power gain in dB.

Solution: Given:

$$V_o = 9 \text{ KV} = 9 \times 10^3 \text{ V}$$
$$I_o = 400 \text{ mA} = 0.4 \text{ A}$$

$$Z_o = 50 \text{ ohms}$$
$$f = 5 \text{ GHz} = 5 \times 10^9 \text{ Hz}$$
$$l = 10 \text{ cm} = 0.1 \text{ m}$$

The electron beam velocity v_o due to V_o is given by

$$v_o = 5.93 \times 10^5 \sqrt{V_o}$$
$$= 5.93 \times 10^5 \sqrt{9 \times 10^3}$$
$$= 56.3 \times 10^6 \text{ m/s}.$$
$$N = l/\lambda_e = l/(v_o/f)$$
$$= 0.1/(56.3 \times 10^6/5 \times 10^9)$$
$$= 8.88$$
$$C = (I_o Z_o/4V_o)^{1/3}$$
$$= (0.4 \times 50/4 \times 9 \times 10^3)^{1/3}$$
$$= 0.082$$
$$\therefore \quad A_p = -9.54 + 47.3 \text{ NC}$$
$$= -9.54 + 47.3 \times 8.88 \times 0.082$$
$$= 24.90 \text{ dB}$$

Example 12.2 A helix TWT operates with a beam current of 250 mA, beam voltage of 4 KV and characteristic impedance of 25 ohms. Compute the length of the helix to give an output power of 40 dB at 10 GHz.

Solution: Given: $I_o = 250 \text{ mA}$, $V_o = 4000 \text{ V}$, $Z_o = 25 \text{ ohms}$, $A_p = 40 \text{ dB}$, $f = 10 \times 10^9$

$$A_p = -9.54 + 47.3 \text{ NC} = 40 \text{ dB}$$
$$47.3 \text{ NC} = 49.54$$
$$NC = 49.54/47.3 = 1.05$$

Table 12.1: Comparison between TWT and klystron amplifiers	
Klystron amplifier	**TWT amplifier**
1. Linear beam or "O" type device	1. Linear beam or "O" type device
2. Uses resonant cavities	2. Uses nonresonant slow-wave structures
3. Narrow band device due to resonant cavities	3. Broadband device due to nonresonant circuits
4. Interaction between electron beam and R.F. field is at cavity gaps only	4. Interaction between electron beam and RF field is continuous over the entire length
5. The wave is not a propagation wave	5. The wave propagates through the helix
6. Moderate bandwidth	6. Enormous bandwidth
7. High-noise figure	7. Low-noise figure

$C = (I_oZ_o/4V_o)^{1/3}$

$= (0.25 \times 25/4 \times 4000)^{1/3}$

$= 0.073$

$N = 1.05/0.073 = 14.38 = l/\lambda_e$

$\lambda_e = v_o/f$

$v_o = 5.93 \times 10^5 \sqrt{V_o}$

$= 5.93 \times 10^5 \sqrt{4 \times 10^3}$

$= 3.75 \times 10^7\,\text{m/s}$

$\lambda_e = v_o/f = 3.75 \times 10^5/10 \times 10^9$

$= 3.75 \times 10^{-3}\,\text{m}$

$l = N\lambda_e = 14.38 \times 3.75 \times 10^{-3}$

$= \textbf{5.39 cm}$

Example 12.3 A TWT operates with $V_o = 4$ kV, $I_o = 4$ mA, $f = 10$ GHz, $Z_o = 25$ ohms $N = 50$. Compute (a) gain parameter C and (b) power gain in dB.

Solution: Given: $V_o = 4$ KV, $I_o = 4$ mA, $f = 10$ GHz, $Z_o = 25$ ohms, $N = 50$

(a) $C = (I_oZ_o/4V_o)^{1/3}$

$= (0.004 \times 25/4 \times 4 \times 10^3)^{1/3}$

$= 0.0184$

(b) $A_p = -9.54 + 47.3\,NC$

$= -9.54 + 47.3 \times 50 \times 0.0184$

$= \textbf{33.98 dB}$

Example 12.4 A TWT amplifier operates with $V_o = 3$ kV, $I_o = 30$ mA, $Z_o = 10$ ohm, $N = 50$, $f = 10$ GHz. Determine (i) gain parameter C, (ii) power gain A_p and all four propagation constants.

Solution: Given: $V_o = 3$ kV, $I_o = 30$ mA, $Z_o = 10$ ohm, $N = 50$, $f = 10$ GHz

(i) The gain parameter is given by

$C = (I_oZ_o/4V_o)^{1/3}$

$= [(30 \times 10^{-3} \times 10)/(4 \times 3 \times 10^3)]^{1/3}$

$= \textbf{2.92} \times \textbf{10}^{-2}$

(ii) The power gain is given by

$A_p = -9.54 + 47.3\,NC$

$= -9.54 + 47.3 \times 50 \times 0.0292$

$= \textbf{59.52 dB}$

(iii) The four propagation constants are

$\beta_e = \dfrac{\omega}{v_o} = \dfrac{2 \times 3.14 \times 10^{10}}{(5.93 \times 10^5 \sqrt{3 \times 10^3})}$

$= 1.93 \times 10^3\,\text{rad}$

$\gamma_1 = -\beta_e C \dfrac{\sqrt{3}}{2} + j\beta_e \left(1 + \dfrac{C}{2}\right)$

$= -1.93 \times 10^3 \times 2.92 \times 10^{-2} \times 0.87 +$ $j1.93 \times 10^3 [1 + (2.92 \times 10^{-2}/2)]$

$= \textbf{-49.03} + \textbf{j1958}$

$\gamma_2 = \beta_e C \dfrac{\sqrt{3}}{2} + j\beta_e \left(1 + \dfrac{C}{2}\right)$

$= \textbf{49.03} + \textbf{j1958}$

$\gamma_3 = j\beta_e(1 - C)$

$= j\,1.93 \times 10^3 [1 - (2.92 \times 10^{-2})]$

$= j\,\textbf{1873.64}$

$\gamma_4 = -j\beta_e(1 - C^3/4)$

$= -j\,1.93 \times 10^3 \times [1 - (2.92 \times 10^{-2})^3/4]$

$= -j\,\textbf{1930}$

KEY POINTS

- The traveling wave tube consists of a long helix slow wave nonresonant microwave guiding structure. It makes use of a distributed interaction between an electron beam and a traveling wave.
- It is used for broadband microwave signal amplification.
- The gain-bandwidth product of a microwave amplifier is limited by the resonant circuit. Hence, the conventional resonators cannot produce large output. Therefore, several nonresonant periodic circuits are used to provide large gain over a wide bandwidth. Such structures are known as slow-wave structures.
- The most commonly used slow-wave structure is a helical coil with concentric conducting cylinder.
- The variation of ω with β for a helical slow-wave structure is known as Brillouin diagram.
- The Floquet's theorem states that "the steady state solutions for the electromagnetic fields of a single propagating mode in a periodic structure have the property that the fields in adjacent cells are related by a complex constant."

- Assuming the magnitude of the axial electric field is uniform over the cross section area of the electron beam, the spatial ac current is given by
  $i = J\beta_e J_o E_1 / [2V_o(j\beta_e - \gamma)^2]$
- There are four wave modes of traveling wave in the tube.
- The output power gain is
  $A_p(dB) = 10 \log |V(l)/V_1(0)|^2 = -9.54 + 47.3NC$
- The principal factors that cause the gain of the TWT to vary with frequency are (i) variation in the velocity of the electric field along the axes of the tube, (ii) variation of length of the tube in wavelengths, (iii) variation in strength of the axial electric field as a function of frequency and (iv) failure to match the terminal impedance of the tube accurately at all frequencies.
- The distortion in the TWT amplifiers is due to (i) harmonic distortion and (ii) phase delay distortion. Harmonic distortion is caused by the nonlinearity of the transfer characteristic of the TWT amplifier. The phase distortion is due to phase delay between the input and output of a TWT amplifier.
- The TWT amplifiers are used as (i) R.F. amplifiers in microwave broadband receivers (ii) repeater amplifiers in wideband communication links and (iii) low noise front-end amplifiers.
- The advantages of TWT amplifiers are its large bandwidth and very low noise figure compared to klystron amplifiers.

FURTHER READING

1. Collins, R.E. (1996) *Foundations of Microwave Engineering*, McGraw Hill, NY.

2. Gandhi, O.P. (1981) *Microwave Engineering and Applications*, Pergamon, NY.

3. Gewartowski, J.W. and Watson, H.A., (1965) *Principles of Electron Tubes*, Van Nostrand, NJ.

4. Liao, S.Y., (1985) *Microwave Solid State Devices*, PH, NJ.

5. Nanavathi, R.P., (1975) *Semiconductor Devices*, Intext Edn., Scranton , PA.

REVIEW QUESTIONS

12.1 What are slow wave structures? Why and where they are used?

12.2 What is a TWT? What are its component parts?

12.3 How are the spurious oscillations suppressed in the TWT amplifier?

12.4 Why is the bandwidth of a TWT amplifier wide?

12.5 Mention the principal factors that affect the gain of a TWT amplifier.

12.6 Write down the expression for power gain of a TWT amplifier.

12.7 Mention the typical characteristics of a TWT amplifier.

12.8 What are the applications of a TWT amplifier?

12.9 Mention the advantages of a TWT amplifier over klystron amplifier.

12.10 Compare klystron and TWT amplifier.

12.11 What is a Brillouin diagram?

12.12 What are the properties of a Brillouin diagram?

12.13 What is a reference electron?

12.14 What is electronic equation?

12.15 What is circuit equation?

12.16 Draw the equivalent circuit of a slow wave structure.

12.17 Mention the transmission line parameters.

12.18 What are wave modes of a TWT?

12.19 What is meant by forward wave and backward wave.

12.20 How are the oscillations in TWT suppressed?

12.21 What are the type of distortions in a TWT amplifier?

12.22 Mention the applications of TWT amplifier.

12.23 Compare TWT and klystron amplifiers.

DESCRIPTIVE QUESTIONS

12.1 Explain, with a neat schematic diagram, the operation of a TWT amplifier.

12.2 Derive the output power and gain equations.

12.3 Show that there are four wave modes and derive the corresponding phase constants.

12.4 (i) Describe the principle of operation of a TWT.

(ii) Explain the need for an attenuator placed midway along the slow-wave structure.

(iii) What is the main advantage of the TWT amplifier compared to klystron amplifier.

12.5 Describe the distortions in a TWT amplifier and their effects on the signal.

12.6 Explain the amplification process and mechanism of energy transfer in TWT amplifier.

12.7 Derive the expression for the convection current in the electron beam of a TWT amplifier.

12.8 Derive the expression for the axial electric field in a TWT amplifier.

12.9 Describe the wave modes of TWT amplifier.

12.10 Derive the expression for the output power and gain of a TWT amplifier.

12.11 (i) Mention the factors that cause the gain of the TWT to vary with the frequency.

(ii) Explain how the unwanted oscillations are suppressed in a TWT amplifier.

12.12 Describe the structure of an O-type TWT and its characteristics. Explain its working.

PRACTICE PROBLEMS

12.1 A helix TWT operates at 4 GHz with beam voltage of 10KV and beam current of 500 mA. If the impedance of helix is 25 ohms and the interaction length is 20 cm, find the power gain in dB.

[**Ans:** 15.3 dB]

12.2 A helix TWT operates with a beam current of 300 mA, beam voltage of 5KV and characteristic impedance of 20 ohms. Compute the length of the helix to give an output power of 50 dB at 10 GHz.

[**Ans:** 12.9 cm]

12.3 A TWT amplifier operates with $V_o = 3$ kV, $I_o = 3$ mA, $f = 10$ GHz, $Z_o = 25\ \Omega$ and $N = 50$. Find A_p.

[**Ans.** $C = 0.042$, $A_p = 89.73$ dB]

12.4 A TWT amplifier operates with $V_o = 2$ kV, $I_o = 4$ mA, $f = 8$ GHz, $Z_o = 20\ \Omega$ and $N = 50$. Calculate gain parameter C and power gain in dB.

[**Ans.** $C = 0.022$, $A_p = 42.49$ dB]

12.5 A TWT amplifier operates with $V_o = 2.5$ kV, $I_o = 50$ mA, $f = 8$ GHz, $Z_o = 6.75\ \Omega$ and $N = 45$. Determine the gain parameter C and power gain dB.

[**Ans.** $C = 0.069$, $A_p = 137.33$ dB]

REFERENCE

1. Bethe HA (1942). *Theory of the Boundary Layer of Crystal Rectifiers*, MIT Rep., pp 43–52.

2. Das A and Das SK (2004). *Microwave Engineering*, TMH, New Delhi.

3. Davis WA (1984). *Microwave Semiconductor Circuit Design*, Van Nostrand, NY,

4. Johnson JB et al. (1965). *A Silicon Diode Microwave Oscillator*, Bell Sys. Tech. J., vol. 44, pp 369–372.

5. Mead CA (1966). *Schottky Barrier Gate Field Effect Transistor*, Proc. IEEE ED-2, pp 307–308.

6. Navon DH (1986). *Semiconductor Micro-devices and Materials*, HRW, NY.

7. Pozar DM (1990). *Microwave Engineering*, Addison-Wesley, Mass.

8. Pulfrey DL and Tarr NG (1989). *Introduction to Microelectronic Devices*, PH. N.J.

9. Reich HJ et al. (1953). *Microwave Theory and Techniques*, Van Nostrand, N.J.

10. Roy SK and Mitra M (2003). *Microwave Semiconductor Devices*, PHI, New Delhi.

11. Saad T and Hansen RC (1971). *Microwave Engineer's Handbook*, vol. I, Artech., Mass.

12. Sze SM (1985). *Semiconductor Devices: Physics and Technology*, John Wiley, NY.

13. Sze SM (Ed.) (1983). *VLSI Technology*, John Wiley, NY

14. Terman FE (1955). *Electronic and Radio Engineering*, McGraw-Hill, Intl.

15. IEEE Trans Electron Devices (1980 Feb.). Special Issue on Microwave Solid State Devices, ED-27, No.2.

16. IEEE Trans. Electron Devices, (1980 June) Special Issue on Microwave Solid State Devices, ED-27, No.6.

17. IEEE Trans. Electron Devices, (1981 Feb.) Special Issue on Microwave Solid State Devices, ED-28, No.2.

18. IEEE Trans. Electron Devices, (1981 Aug.) Special Issue on Microwave Solid State Devices, ED-28, No.8.

19. Kennedy G and Davis B (1999). *Electronic Communication Systems*, TMH, New Delhi.

Magnetron Oscillator

Objectives

- Classify the magnetron tubes.
- Know the structure of magnetron tube.
- Understand the principle of operation.
- Study the Hull cut-off voltage.
- Explain the mode separation method.
- Determine the power output and efficiency.
- Know the applications of magnetron oscillator.

13.1 INTRODUCTION

The microwave tubes are broadly classified as

   (i) *Linear-beam* or *O*-type tubes

  (ii) *Cross-field* or *M-type* tubes.

In linear-beam tubes, the dc magnetic and dc electric fields are in parallel. The dc magnetic field is used to focus the beam. In cross-field tubes, the fields are mutually perpendicular to each other. The dc magnetic field plays a direct role in the RF interaction process.

Cross-field tubes are so called because the dc magnetic and dc electric fields are mutually perpendicular to each other. In a cross-field tube, the electric field accelerates the electrons emitted from the cathode and the electrons gain velocity. The dc magnetic field that is perpendicular to the electric field bends the path of electrons so that they take curved paths. If an RF field is applied to the anode circuit, electrons entering the circuit during the retarding filed are decelerated and they transfer some of their energy to the RF field. Hence, their velocity is decreased. Because of cross-field interactions, only those electrons that have transferred sufficient energy to the RF field travel all the way to the anode. This phenomenon makes the cross-field devices relatively efficient. Electrons that enter the circuit during the accelerating filed are accelerated as they receive energy from the RF field and are returned back to the cathode. The bombardment of the cathode by the returning electrons produces heat in the cathode and the operational efficiency is decreased.

In this chapter, we shall discuss the constructional features, operating principles and application of cylindrical, coaxial and voltage-tunable magnetrons.

13.2 TYPES OF CROSS-FIELD TUBES

The common types of microwave tubes are:

1. *Cylindrical magnetron*: This is the most commonly used magnetron.
2. *Coaxial magnetron*: The coaxial magnetron is that in which a stabilizing cavity is integrated with the magnetron geometry.
3. *Voltage-tunable magnetron*: The cathode-anode cylindrical geometry of the voltage-tunable magnetron is same as the conventional magnetron but its anode can easily be tuned by varying the anode voltage.
4. *Inverted magnetron*: This magnetron has the inverted geometry of the conventional magnetron. Its cathode is placed on the outside surrounding the anode and microwave circuit.
5. *Forward-wave cross-field amplifier*: This is an *M*-type forward-wave amplifier.
6. *Amplitron*: This is an *M*-type backward-wave cross-field amplifier. It is a broadband, high power, high gain and high efficiency microwave tube. It is used in airborne radar systems and space-borne communication systems.
7. *Carcinotron*: This is a *M*-type backward-wave cross-field oscillator. In this magnetron, the conventional cylindrical cathode of the magnetron is replaced by an injection type cathode.

13.3 MAGNETRON OSCILLATORS

The magnetron oscillator was the first microwave device that was capable of generating large powers (up to 40 kW) at microwave frequency. Rapid development of this device took place during World War II because of urgent need for high power microwave generators for microwave radar transmitters.

All magnetrons consist of some form of anode and cathode. They are operated in a mutually perpendicular dc magnetic field and the dc electric filed in the anode-cathode space. The electrons emitted from the cathode are influenced by the cross-field to move in curved paths. If the dc magnetic field is strong enough, the electrons will be turned back towards the cathode. Hence, the anode current is cut off and the oscillations cease.

13.4 CYLINDRICAL MAGNETRON OSCILLATORS

Figure 13.1 shows the essential elements of a typical cylindrical magnetron oscillator. It consists of a cylindrical cathode surrounded by an anode structure. The anode structure has cavities opening into cathode-anode space or an interaction space through slots. Output power is obtained by means of a coupling loop. The external magnetic field with flux lines parallel to the axis of the cathode is usually provided by permanent magnets. The dc magnetic field and the dc

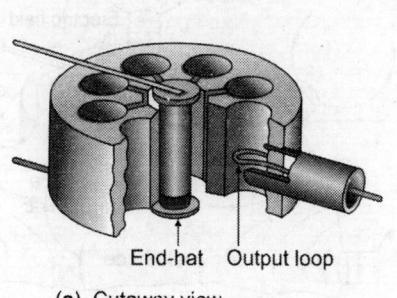

(a) Cutaway view

End-hat   Output loop

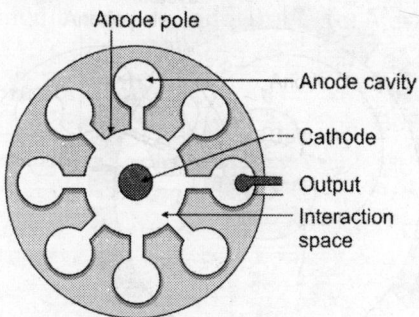

Anode pole

Anode cavity

Cathode

Output

Interaction space

(b) Cross-section perpendicular to axis of cathode

Fig. 13.1: Cylindrical magnetron oscillator

electric field are mutually perpendicular to each other.

13.4.1 Mechanism of Operation

To understand the mechanism of operation of a magnetron oscillator, one has to examine the behaviour of the electrons emitted from the cathode under radial electric and axial magnetic fields.

An electron emitted from the cathode is accelerated by the radial electric field due to the anode voltage. In the absence of magnetic field, the electron would traverse directly towards the anode along the path *a* as shown in Fig. 13.2. If the axial magnetic field is present, it exerts a force on it. If the magnetic field is weak, the electrons take the path *b* as shown in Fig. 13.2. If the intensity of the magnetic field is sufficiently increased, the electrons are turned back to cathode before reaching the anode as illustrated by paths *c* and *d*. The magnetic field that just turns the electrons back to the cathode before reaching the anode is known as *Hull cut-off field*. When the magnetic field exceeds the cut-off value, then in the absence of oscillations, all the emitted electrons are returned to the cathode and the anode current is zero. Hence, there is no oscillation.

Let us assume that oscillations exist in the resonant cavities. Then, when the magnetic field exceeds the cut-off value, an interaction takes place between the electrons and the electric field. This, under favourable conditions, causes the oscillations to receive energy from the electrons in the interaction space. Consider oscillations corresponding to π-mode where the phase difference between adjacent anode poles is π radians. They produce RF fringing fields extending into the interaction space as shown in Fig. 13.3. In the absence of RF field, electrons *a* and *b* would traverse paths shown by dotted lines. However, the presence of RF filed associated with the oscillations act on the electrons and modify their orbits. Thus, the electron *a* is so situated with respect to these fields that its tangential velocity is opposed by the field. This electron is slowed down by the oscillations, delivers energy to the oscillations and its velocity is decreased. Moreover, since the electron *a* has lost velocity, the deflecting force exerted on it by the axial magnetic field is reduced. As a result, this electron moves towards the anode as shown by the solid path, instead of being turned back to the cathode. If the relationship between the dc anode voltage and the magnetic field is such that the tangential velocity of the electrons makes the time required by electron *a* to travel from position 1 to 2 in Fig. 13.3 is approximately a half cycle of the RF oscillations, then, when electron *a* reaches point 2 in Fig. 13.3, the electric field

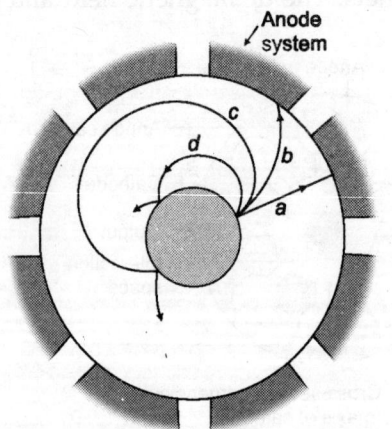

Fig. 13.2: Electron trajectory in a magnetron

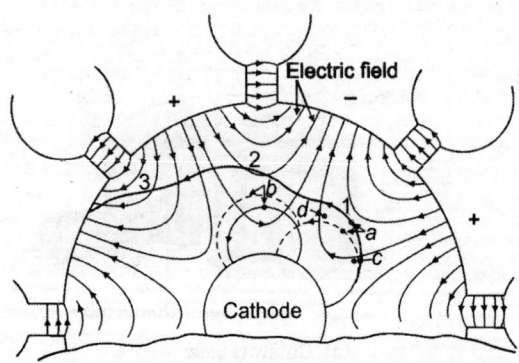

Fig. 13.3: Trajectory of electrons in a magnetron under oscillating conditions

would have reversed. Hence the electron *a* is further slowed down and drifts towards the anodes. Having delivered to the oscillations a large part of the energy represented as kinetic energy due to cathode-anode potential, the working electron *a* is ultimately collected by the anode.

On the other hand, consider the electron *b* shown in Fig. 13.3. It is emitted under circumstances such that the RF field accelerates it. This electron gains velocity and is therefore reflected more sharply by the axial magnetic field. As a result, this electron follows the solid path *b*. It is turned backward and returns to the cathode more quickly. This electron is harmful because it abstracts energy from the oscillations and causes "*back heating*" of the cathode. Thus, about 5 percent of the anode power is used in back heating the cathode.

13.4.2 Phase Focusing

The focusing mechanism in the magnetron tends to keep the working electrons such as *a* in step with the fields in the interaction space so that the working electrons deliver maximum possible energy to the oscillation. For example, consider electron *c* in Fig. 13.3. It delivers some energy to the oscillations since it was emitted a little too late to be in the correct position to make maximum contribution. This electron is acted upon by the radial and the tangential components of the field. The direction of the radial field is such that it aids the anode voltage. This increases the velocity of electron *c* and therefore assists it in catching up with electron *a* that is in the optimum position. Similarly, the electron *d* that is advanced beyond the optimum position encounters a radial field that opposes the anode voltage acting on it. This causes the electron *d* to slow down in its motion and thereby fall back towards optimum position. This focusing action is equivalent to velocity modulation that causes electrons such as *c* and *d* to form

a bunch centered about electron *a*. The end result of these actions is to cause the orbit of electrons to be confined to *spokes*, one spoke for each two anodes as shown in Fig. 13.4. In the case of π-mode, these spokes rotate at an angular velocity that corresponds to two poles per cycle. A certain fraction of the electrons emitted from the cathode travel out through the spokes and continuously deliver energy to the oscillations until these electrons reach the anode and disappear. Electrons emitted in the portions of the cathode between spokes are however returned to the cathode very quickly. These are harmful electrons and absorb some energy from the oscillations. It is small compared with the energy delivered by the electrons in the spokes. Thus, the oscillations receive a substantial net energy from the electrons.

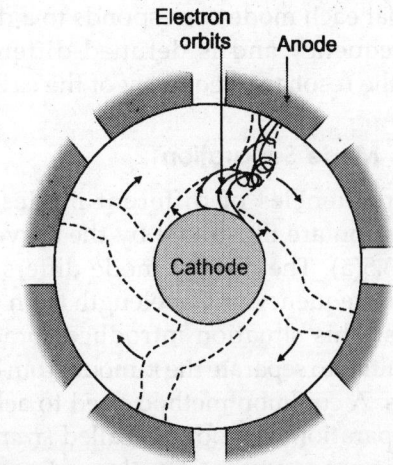

Fig.13.4: Confinement of electron orbits into spokes

13.4.3 Modes

The anode cavities, together with the spaces at the top and the bottom of the anode block, form the resonant system of the magnetron oscillator. The resonant system possesses a series of the resonant frequencies or *modes*. The number of modes is equal to the number of cavities because the resonant system may be regarded as consisting of a number of individual resonators, one for each cavity, that are all coupled together. When two resonant circuits are coupled together it produces two resonant frequencies or modes. Similarly, when *n* resonant cavities are coupled together, they produce *n* resonant frequencies or modes.

The magnetron is normally operated in π-mode in which the phase difference between the adjacent anode poles is π-radians. Other modes have some other value of phase difference between adjacent poles. The total phase shift around the periphery of the interaction space must always be some integer multiple of 2π. For π-mode, the total phase difference is ± 8π radians for the eight cavity magnetron. For other modes, it may be ± 6π, ± 4π and ± 2π radians that correspond to progressive phase difference of ± 135°, ± 90° and ± 45° respectively. The phase differences arise from the fact that each mode corresponds to a different frequency and is detuned differently from the resonant frequency of the cavities.

13.4.4 Mode Separation

The frequencies of different modes in a magnetron are illustrated by the curve *a* in Fig. 13.5(a). The desired mode differs very little in frequency or wavelength from other modes. This situation introduces practical difficulties to separate the π-mode from other modes. A common method used to achieve the separation of modes is called *strapping*. Two rings are arranged in the end space as shown in Fig. 13.5(b). One ring is connected to even numbered anode poles and the other to odd numbered anode poles. In π-mode, all parts of each ring are at the same potential, but the two rings are of opposite potential as indicated by '+' and '–'signs. They form a capacitance between the rings and add capacitive loading to the resonator cavities, thereby lowering the frequency of the π-mode. For other modes, there exists a phase difference between the successive poles connected to a given ring. This causes current

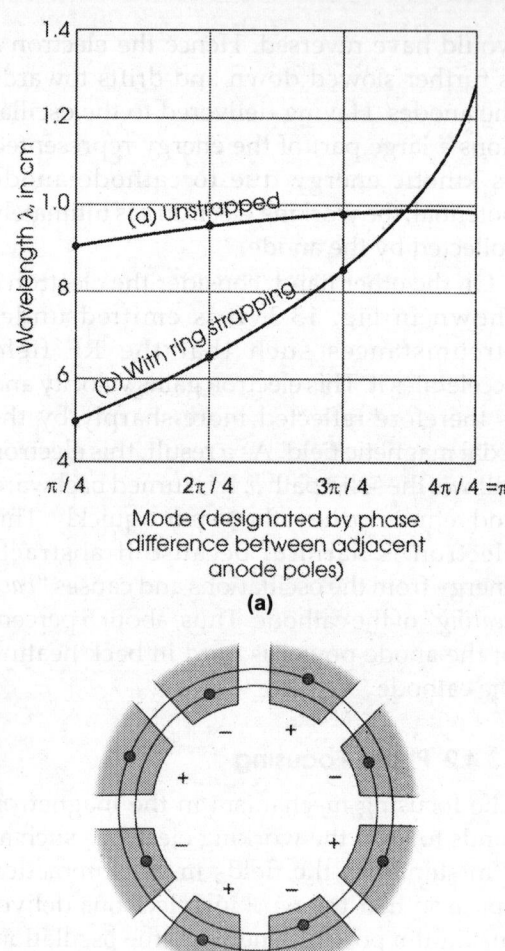

(a)

(b)

Fig. 13.5: (a) Mode separation obtained experimentally (b) Mode separation by ring strapping

to flow along the rings or straps. Since the rings have inductive reactance, this places inductive shunts in parallel with the equivalent resonant circuit of the cavity, thus raising the frequency for these modes. Thus, the π-mode is separated from other modes as shown by curve *b* in Fig. 13.5(a).

13.4.5 Resonant Frequency Variation or Tuning

The resonant frequency of the magnetron can be varied by employing a "C" ring as shown in Fig. 13.6. This adds capacitance between the straps of a ring-strapped magnetron. This

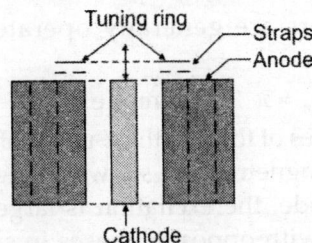

Fig. 13.6: C-ring tuning of a magnetron

lowers the resonant frequency of the π-mode by an amount depending on the position of the "C" ring. Another method is to closely couple a tunable high-Q resonant cavity to one of the anode cavities.

13.4.6 Equation of Electron Motion

The equation of motion of electrons in a cylindrical magnetron is given by

$$\frac{d^2r}{dr^2} - r\left(\frac{d\varphi}{dt}\right)^2 = \left(\frac{e}{m}\right)E_r - \left(\frac{e}{m}\right)rB_z\left(\frac{d\varphi}{dt}\right) \quad (13.1)$$

$$\left(\frac{1}{r}\right)\frac{\left(\frac{r^2 d\varphi}{dt}\right)}{d/dt} = \left(\frac{e}{m}\right)B_z\left(\frac{dr}{dt}\right) \quad (13.2)$$

(e/m) is the charge-to-mass ratio of the electron and is equal to 1.76×10^{11} C/kg.

The magnetic flux density B_z is assumed to be in the positive z-direction. Rearranging Eq. (13.2), we obtain

$$\frac{\left(\frac{r^2 d\varphi}{dt}\right)}{d/dt} = \left(\frac{e}{m}\right)rB_z\left(\frac{dr}{dt}\right) = \frac{1}{2}\omega_c\left[\frac{d(r)^2}{dt}\right]$$

$$(13.3)$$

Here, $\omega_c = (e/m)B_z$ is the *cyclotron angular frequency*. Integrating Eq. (13.3), we get

$$r^2 d\varphi/dt = \frac{1}{2}\omega_c r^2 + \text{constant} \quad (13.4)$$

At $r = a$, where a is the radius of the cylindrical cathode, $d\varphi/dt = 0$. Hence, the constant of integration is $(-\frac{1}{2}\omega_c a^2)$. Therefore the angular velocity is given by

$$d\varphi/dt = \frac{1}{2}\omega_c(1 - a^2/r^2) \quad (13.5)$$

As the magnetic field has no effect on the electrons, the kinetic energy of the electrons is given by

$$\frac{1}{2}m\mathcal{V}^2 = eV \quad (13.6)$$

$\mathcal{V}$ is the tangential electron velocity. The electron velocity has r-components $\mathcal{V}_r$, and φ-component $\mathcal{V}_\phi$ such that

$$V^2 = (2e/m)V$$
$$= \mathcal{V}_r^2 + \mathcal{V}_\phi^2 = (dr/dt)^2 + (r\,d\varphi/dt)^2$$
$$(13.7)$$

At $r = b$, where b is the radius from the center of the cathode to the edge of the anode, when the electrons just graze the anode, $V = V_0$ and $dr/dt = 0$. Hence, Eq. (13.5) becomes

$$d\varphi/dt = \frac{1}{2}\omega_c(1 - a^2/b^2) \quad (13.8)$$

From Eq. (13.7), we get

$$b^2(d\varphi/dt)^2 = (2e/m)V_0 \quad (13.9)$$

Substituting Eq. (13.8) in Eq. (13.9), we obtain

$$b^2[\frac{1}{2}\omega_c(1 - a^2/b^2)]^2 = (2e/m)V_0 \quad (13.10)$$

Thus the electron acquires a tangential and a radial velocity. Whether the electron will just graze the anode and return to the cathode depends on the relative amplitudes of V_0 and B_0.

13.4.7 Hull Cut-off Magnetic Field and Voltage

For a given anode voltage V_0, if the magnetic field is increased, we reach a critical magnetic field B_c at which all electrons return to the cathode and no electron will reach the anode. This critical axial magnetic field B_c is obtained from Eq. (13.10).

$$b[\frac{1}{2}\omega_c(1 - a^2/b^2)] = (2e\,V_0/m)^{1/2}$$

Substituting $\omega_c = (e/m)B_c$, we get

$$b[\frac{1}{2}(e/m)B_c(1 - a^2/b^2)] = (2e\,V_0/m)^{1/2}$$

$$\therefore \quad B_c = (8V_0 m/e)^{1/2}/[b(1 - a^2/b^2)] \quad (13.11)$$

Here a is the radius of the cathode and b is the radius of the cylindrical anode. The equation is known as *Hull cut-off magnetic equation* and B_c is known as *Hull cut-off magnetic flux density.* Hence, the dc axial magnetic field B_o *should be always less than or equal to* B_c for proper operation of the magnetron oscillator.

Similarly, for a given axial magnetic field B_o, there is a critical anode voltage V_{oc} at which all electrons are returned to the cathode and no electron reaches the anode. The critical anode voltage V_{oc} is obtained from Eq. (13.10). Substituting $V_o = V_{oc}$, Eq. (13.10) becomes

$$b^2[\tfrac{1}{2}(e/m)B_o(1 - a^2/b^2)]^2 = 2V_{oc}e/m$$

$$\therefore \quad V_{oc} = (e/8m)(B_o b)^2 [1 - a^2/b^2]^2 \quad (13.12)$$

The above equation is known as *Hull cut-off voltage equation.* Therefore V_o *should always be greater than or equal to* V_{oc} *for normal operation.*

13.4.8 Cyclotron Frequency

Since the dc magnetic field is perpendicular to the dc electric field, the electrons travel in a cycloidal path. Hence, the outward centrifugal force is equal to the pulling force. Therefore

$$m\mathcal{V}^2/R = e\mathcal{V}B \quad (13.13)$$

where R is the radius of the cycloid path and $\mathcal{V}$ is the tangential electron velocity.

The cyclotron angular frequency of the circular motion of the electron is given by

$$\omega_c = \mathcal{V}/R = (e/m)B \quad (13.14)$$

The period of one complete revolution is given by

$$T = 2\pi/\omega_c = 2\pi m/(eB) \quad (13.15)$$

Since the slow-wave structure is a reentrant type, *oscillations exist only if the total phase shift around the structure is an integral multiple of 2π radians.* Assuming that there are N reentrant cavities in the anode structure, the phase shift ϕ_n between two adjacent cavities is given by

$$\phi_n = 2\pi n/N \quad [n = 0, \pm 1, \pm 2, ...] \quad (13.16)$$

Oscillations are produced when the anode dc voltage is adjusted so that the average rotational velocity of the electrons corresponds to the phase velocity of the field in the slow-wave structure. Since, magnetron

oscillators are generally operated in the π-mode,

$$\phi_n = \pi \quad \text{for } \pi\text{-mode} \quad (13.17)$$

The lines of force in the π-mode of an eight-cavity magnetron are shown in Fig. 13.7. In the π-mode, the excitation is largely in the cavities with opposite phases in successive cavities. The successive rise and fall of adjacent anode cavity fields may be considered as a traveling wave along the surface of the slow-wave structure so that the energy is transferred from the moving electrons to the traveling field. When they pass through each anode cavity, a retarding field decelerates the electrons.

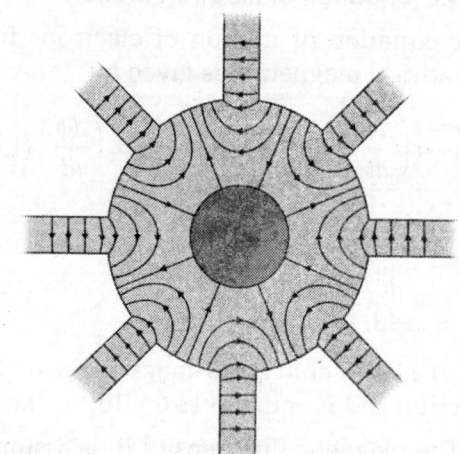

Fig. 13.7: Lines of force in π-mode of eight-cavity magnetron

Let L be the mean separation between cavities. Then the phase constant β_o of the fundamental-mode field is given by

$$\beta_o = 2\pi n/(NL) \quad (13.18)$$

The angular velocity of the fundamental mode of the traveling field around the structure is given by

$$d\phi/dt = \omega_c/\beta_o \quad (13.19)$$

The interaction between the electrons and the field occurs when the cyclotron frequency is equal to the angular frequency of the field and the energy is transferred. Thus,

$$\omega_c = \beta_o \, d\phi/dt \quad (13.20)$$

13.4.9 Equivalent Circuit

The equivalent circuit of one resonator cavity of the magnetron oscillator is shown in Fig.13.8. The circuit parameters are:

Y_e is the electronic admittance of the electron beam,

V is the RF voltage across the vane tips,

C is the capacitance at the vane tips,

L is the inductance of the resonator,

G_r is the conductance of the resonator, and

G_l is the load conductance per resonator

Each resonator is a separate resonant circuit as shown in Fig. 13.8.

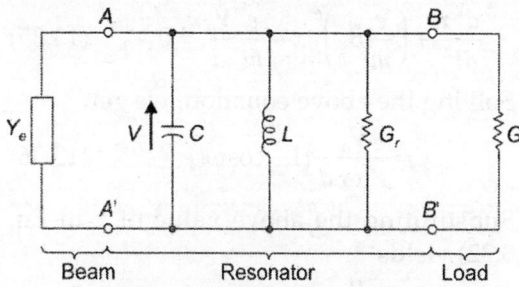

Fig. 13.8: Equivalent circuit

The unloaded quality factor is given by

$$Q_o = \omega_o C / G_r \qquad (13.21)$$

Here ω_o is the angular resonant frequency. The external quality factor of the load circuit is given by

$$Q_{ex} = \omega_o C / G_l \qquad (13.22)$$

The loaded quality factor of the resonant circuit is given by

$$Q_l = Q_o + Q_{lx} = \omega_o C / (G_l + G_r) \quad (13.23)$$

13.4.10 Power Output

The electrons moving towards the anode transfer energy to the resonant cavity. Thus the RF power generated is given by

$$P_{gen} = V_o I_o - P_{lost} \qquad (13.24)$$

$$= V_o I_o - I_o \left(\frac{m}{2e}\right)\left(\frac{\omega_o^2}{\beta^2}\right) + \frac{E_{max}^2}{B_z^2} \qquad (13.25)$$

$$= \tfrac{1}{2} N |V|^2 \omega_o C / Q_l \qquad (13.26)$$

Here,

N = the total number of resonators,

V = the RF voltage across the resonator gap,

$E_{max} = M_1 |V| / L$ is the maximum electric field,

$M_1 = \sin(\beta_n \delta / 2)/(\beta_n \delta / 2) = 1$ for small δ, is the gap factor for π-mode operation,

β = the phase constant,

B_z = the magnetic flux density, and

L = the center-to-center spacing of the vane tips.

Substituting $|V| = E_{max} L / M_1$ in Eq. (13.26) and rearranging, we get

$$P_{gen} = (NL^2 \omega_o C / 2M_1^2 Q_l)\, E_{max}^2 \quad (13.27)$$

Here power generated is simplified to Eq. (13.27).

13.4.11 Efficiency

The electronic efficiency of the magnetron oscillator is defined as the ratio of the output power to the input dc power. Thus

$$\eta_e = P_{gen}/V_o I_o = (V_o I_o - P_{lost})/V_o I_o$$

$$= \frac{1 - \left(\dfrac{m\omega_0^2}{2eV_o\beta^2}\right)}{1 + \left(\dfrac{I_o m M_1^2 Q_l}{B_z e N L^2 \omega_o C}\right)} \qquad (13.28)$$

13.4.12 Typical Characteristics

The typical performance characteristics of a magnetron oscillator are:

Frequency range : 500 MHz to 70 GHz
Power output : 800 kW
(average)
Power output (peak) : 40 MW at 10 GHz
Efficiency : 40 % to 70 %

13.4.13 Applications

The magnetron oscillator is used in
(a) Radar transmitters
(b) Microwave ovens
(c) Industrial heating.

13.5 LINEAR MAGNETRON

Figure 13.9 shows the schematic diagram of a linear magnetron. In this, the electric field

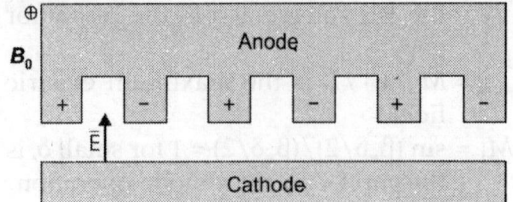

Fig. 13.9: Schematic diagram of a linear magnetron

E_x is in the positive x-direction. The magnetic flux density B_z in the positive z-direction. The differential equations of motion of electrons in the crossed-electric and magnetic fields are

$$\frac{d^2x}{dt^2} = -\frac{e}{m}\left(E_x + B_z\frac{dy}{dt}\right) \quad (13.29)$$

$$\frac{d^2y}{dt^2} = \frac{e}{m}B_z\frac{dx}{dt} \quad (13.30)$$

$$\frac{d^2z}{dt^2} = 0 \quad (13.31)$$

Here, $e/m = 1.759 \times 10^{11}$ C/kg is the charge to mass ratio of an electron, B_z is the magnetic flux density in the positive z-direction and E_x is the electric field in the positive x-direction.

The presence of space charge causes the field to be nonlinear function of the distance x. The complete solution of Eqs (13.29) to (13.31) is very difficult. However, Eq. (13.30) can be integrated directly. Assuming that the electrons are emitted from the cathode surface with zero initial velocity, origin of electrons is the cathode surface and that the Eq. (13.30) becomes

$$\frac{dy}{dt} = \frac{e}{m}B_z x \quad (13.32)$$

Equation (13.32) indicates that, regardless of space charges, the electron velocity parallel to the cathode surface is proportional to the distance x of the electron from the cathode and the magnetic flux density B_z. The distance x depends on B_z and the variation of the potential V with x. This, in turn, depends on the space charge distribution, anode potential and electrode spacing.

Assuming that the space charge is negligible, that the cathode potential is zero and

the anode potential is V_o, the differential electric field becomes

$$\frac{dV}{dx} = \frac{V_o}{d} \quad (13.33)$$

where V_o is the anode potential and d is the distance between cathode and anode in meters.

Substituting Eq. (13.33) into Eq. (13.29), we get

$$\frac{d^2x}{dt^2} = \frac{e}{m}\left(\frac{V_o}{d} - B_z\frac{dy}{dt}\right) \quad (13.34)$$

Combining Eq. (13.32) and Eq. (13.34), we obtain

$$\frac{d^2x}{dt^2} + \left(\frac{e}{m}B_z\right)^2 x - \frac{e}{m}\frac{V_o}{d} = 0 \quad (13.35)$$

Solving the above equation, we get

$$x = \frac{V_o}{B_z\omega_c d}[1 - \cos\omega t] \quad (13.36)$$

Substituting the above value of x in Eq. (13.32) yields

$$y = \frac{V_o}{B_z\omega_c d}[\omega_c t - \sin\omega t] \quad (13.37)$$

$$z = 0 \quad (13.38)$$

where $\omega_c = \frac{e}{m}B_z$ is the cyclotron angular frequency, $f_c = 2.8 \times 10^{11}$ is the cyclotron frequency in Hz.

13.5.1 Cut-off Condition

Equation (13.36) to (13.38) are the equations of a cycloid, generated by a point on a circle of radius $(V_o/B_z\omega_c d)$ rolling on the plane of the cathode with angular frequency ω_c. The maximum distance d_{max} the electrons move in a direction normal to the cathode is

$$d_{max} = \frac{2V_o}{[B_z^2(e/m)d]} \quad (13.39)$$

when $d_{max} = d$, the electrons grace the anode surface and the anode current is cut-off. Then, the cut-off condition is

$$d_{max} = \frac{2V_o}{[B_z^2(e/m)d]} = d \quad (13.40)$$

Let us define a factor K. K is given by

$$K = \frac{d^2 B_z^2}{V_0} = \frac{2}{(e/m)} = 1.14 \times 10^{11} \quad (13.41)$$

When $K < 1.14 \times 10^{11}$, electrons strike the anode and the anode current flows. When $K > 1.14 \times 10^{-11}$, the electrons return to the cathode and no anode current flows. The electron path in a linear magnetron is shown in Fig. 13.10.

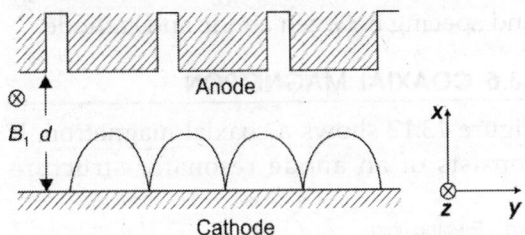

Fig. 13.10: Electron path in a linear magnetron

13.5.2 Hull Cut-off Voltage

From Eq. (13.40), the Hull cut-off voltage V_{oc} for a linear magnetron is

$$V_{oc} = \frac{1}{2} \frac{e}{m} B_0^2 d^2 \quad (13.42)$$

where $B_0 = B_z$ is the magnetic flux density in the positive z-direction. Thus, if $V_0 < V_{oc}$ for a given B_0, the electrons will not reach the anode and no anode current flows.

13.5.3 Hull Cut-Off Magnetic Flux Density

The Hull cut-off magnetic flux density for a linear magnetron is given by

$$B_{oc} = \frac{1}{d} \sqrt{\frac{2V_0}{(e/m)}} \quad (13.43)$$

Thus, if $B_0 > B_{oc}$ for a given V_y, the electrons will not reach the anode.

13.5.4 Hartree Anode Voltage

Figure 13.11 shows the linear model of a magnetron. The electron beam lies within a region extending a distance h from the cathode. h is known as hub thickness. The spacing between the anode and cathode is d.

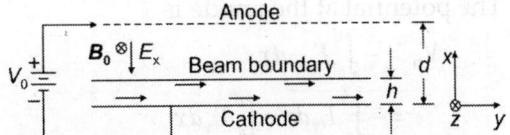

Fig. 13.11: Linear model of a magnetron

Assume the electron motion in the positive y-direction with a velocity of V is given by

$$V_y = -\frac{E_x}{B_0} = \frac{1}{B_0} \frac{dV}{dx} \quad (13.44)$$

where $B_0 = B_z$ is the magnetic flux density in the positive z-direction and V is the potential.

From the principle of energy conversion, we have

kinetic energy = potential energy

$$\frac{1}{2} m V_y^2 = eV \quad (13.45)$$

Substituting for V_y from Eq. (13.44) into Eq. (13.45), we get

$$\left(\frac{dV}{dx}\right)^2 = 2\left(\frac{e}{m}\right) V B_0^2 \quad (13.46)$$

$$\frac{dV}{dx} = \sqrt{2\frac{e}{m} V} \, B_0$$

$$dx = \frac{1}{\sqrt{2\frac{e}{m}} B_0} \cdot V^{-1/2} dV$$

Integrating, we get

$$x = \frac{1}{\sqrt{2\frac{e}{m}} B_0} \cdot 2V^{1/2}$$

or $\quad V^{1/2} = \frac{x}{2} \sqrt{2\frac{e}{m}} \cdot B_0$

$$\therefore \quad V = \frac{x^2}{4} \cdot 2 \frac{e}{m} B_0^2 = x^2 \frac{e}{2m} B_0^2 \quad (13.47)$$

where the constant of integration is zero $V = 0$ at $x = 0$.

The potential at the hub surface is given by

$$V(h) = \frac{e}{2m} B_0^2 h^2 \quad (13.48)$$

The electric field at the hub surface is given by

$$E_x = -\frac{dV}{dx} = -\frac{e}{m} B_0^2 h \quad (13.49)$$

The potential at the anode is

$$V_0 = -\int_o^d E_x \cdot dx$$

$$= -\int_o^h E_x dx - \int_h^d E_x dx$$

$$\lambda = \frac{e}{2m} B_0^2 h^2 + \frac{e}{m} B_0^2 h (d-h)$$

$$= \frac{e}{m} B_0^2 h \left[\frac{h}{2} + (d-h) \right]$$

$$= \frac{e}{m} B_0^2 h \left(d - \frac{h}{2} \right) \qquad (13.50)$$

The electron velocity at the hub surface is

$$\mathcal{V}_y(h) = \frac{1}{B_o} \frac{dV}{dx} = \frac{e}{m} B_o h \qquad (13.51)$$

To obtain synchronism, the phase velocity (ω/β) of the slow-wave structure must be equal to the electron velocity. Thus

$$\frac{\omega}{\beta} = \frac{e}{m} B_o h \qquad (13.52)$$

For the π-mode of operation, the anode potential is finally given by

$$V_{oh} = \frac{\omega B_o d}{\beta} - \frac{m}{2e} \frac{\omega^2}{\beta^2} \qquad (13.53)$$

This voltage is known as *Hartree anode voltage*. It is a function of magnetic flux density and spacing between anode and cathode.

13.6 COAXIAL MAGNETRON

Figure 13.12 shows a coaxial magnetron. It consists of an anode resonator structure

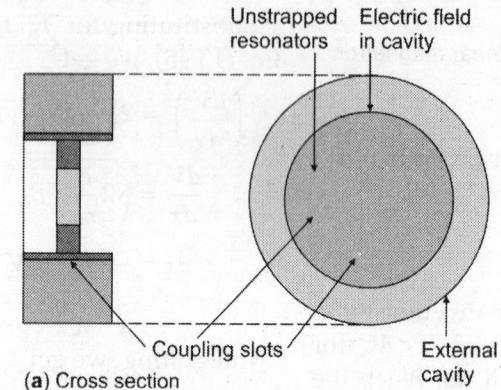

(a) Cross section

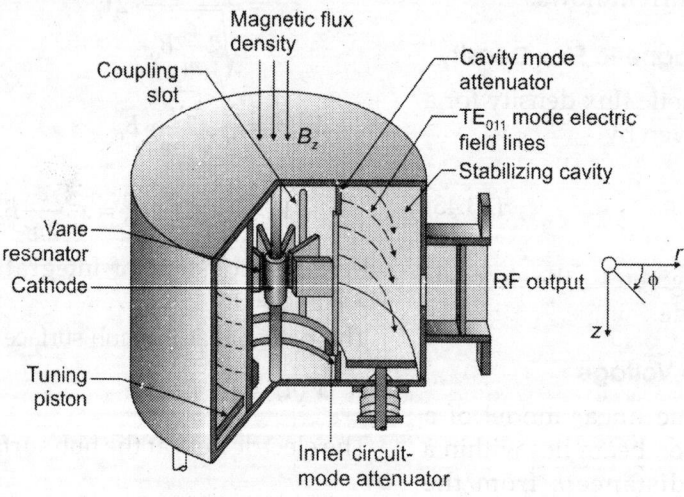

(b) Cut away view

Fig. 13.12: Coaxial magnetron

surrounded by an inner-single high-Q cavity operating in TE_{011} mode. These are slots in the back walls of alternate cavities of the anode resonator structure. These tightly couples the electric fields in the resonators to the surrounding cavity. In the π-mode operation, the electric field in every other cavity is in phase. Hence, they couple the electric field in the same direction into the surrounding cavity. Thus, the surrounding coaxial cavity stabilizes the desired π-mode operation.

In the desired TE_{011} mode, the electric fields follow a circular path within the cavity and become zero at the walls of the cavity. Current flow in the TE_{011} mode is in the walls of the cavity in circular paths about the axis of the tube. The unwanted modes are attenuated by the attenuator within the inner slotted cylinder near the ends of the coupling slots. The tuning mechanism is simple and reliable. Since the straps are not required, the anode resonator for the coaxial magnetron can be larger and less complex than strapped magnetrons. Thus, cathode loading is lower and voltage gradients are reduced.

13.6.1 Typical Characteristics

The coaxial magnetron is a typical X-band magnetron. Its minimum peak power is 400 kW at a frequency range from 8.9 GHz to 9.6 GHz. The nominal anode voltage is 32 kV and the duty cycle is 0.0013.

13.7 VOLTAGE-TUNABLE MAGNETRON

Figure 13.13 shows a voltage-tunable magnetron. It is a broadband oscillator. Its frequency can be changed by varying the voltage applied between the anode and the sole. The electron beam is emitted from a short cylindrical cathode situated at one end of the device. Electrons are formed into a hallow beam by the electric and magnetic forces near the cathode and are accelerated outward from the cathode. Then, the electron beam is injected into the region between the sole and anode and it rotates about the sole at a rate controlled by the axial magnetic field and the applied dc voltage between the anode and the sole. The voltage-tunable magnetron uses a low-Q resonator. Its

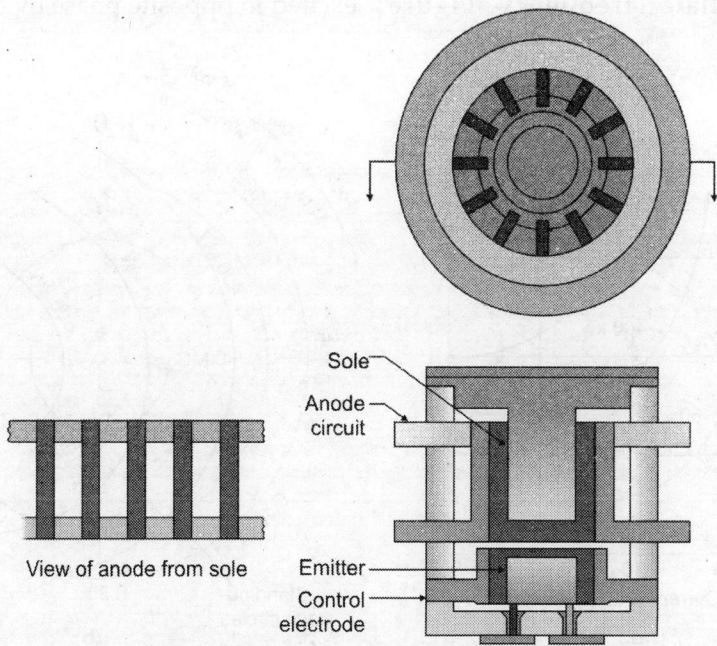

Sole
Anode circuit
View of anode from sole
Emitter
Control electrode

Fig. 13.13: Voltage-tunable magnetron

bandwidth is about 50% at low-power levels. In the π-mode operation, the bunching process of the hollow beam occurs in the resonator. The rotational velocity of the electron beam determines the frequency of oscillation. Thus, frequency of oscillation is controlled by varying the applied dc voltage between the anode and the sole. The power output can be adjusted to some extent by the use of the control electrode in the electron gun. At high power levels and high frequencies, the bandwidth is limited whereas at low power and low frequencies, the bandwidth may approach 70%.

13.8 RIEKE DIAGRAM

The performance of a magnetron is relatively sensitive to the strength of the dc magnetic field, dc anode voltage and the load impedance. Variation in any of these quantities will affect the output power, the efficiency and the frequency to a marked extent. The frequency of the magnetron oscillator is varied by changing the anode voltage. This alters the orbital velocity of the electrons and hence the oscillator frequency. Figure

13.14(a) shows the *performance chart*. This presents the magnetron performance for a given load impedance. The magnetron performance as a function of anode voltage and magnetic field strength is given by *Rieke diagram* shown in Fig. 13.14(b). The Rieke diagram is similar to a Smith chart on which the standing-wave circles and radial lines are drawn with the curvilinear impedance or admittance coordinates omitted. It can be seen that the frequency of the magnetron is quite sensitive to changes in load impedance. The variation in oscillator frequency due to variation in load impedance is called *frequency pulling* and the variation in oscillator frequency due to variation in anode voltage for a given load impedance and magnetic filed is known as *frequency pushing*.

13.9 AMPLITRON (BWCFA)

The amplitron is a backward-wave cross-field amplifier (BWCFA). Figure 13.15 shows the schematic diagram of an amplitron. The anode cavity and pins form the resonator circuits. A cavity and a pair of pins are excited in opposite phase by the input strap

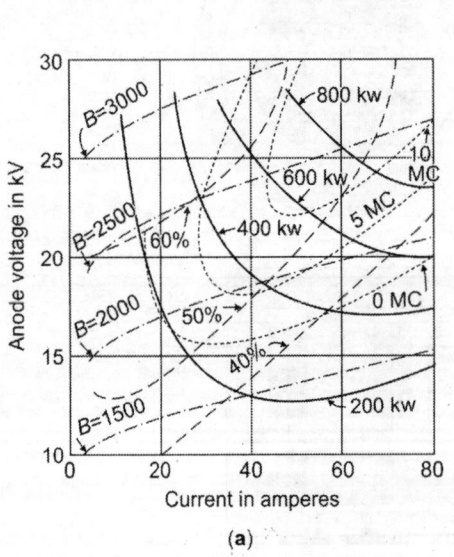

(a)

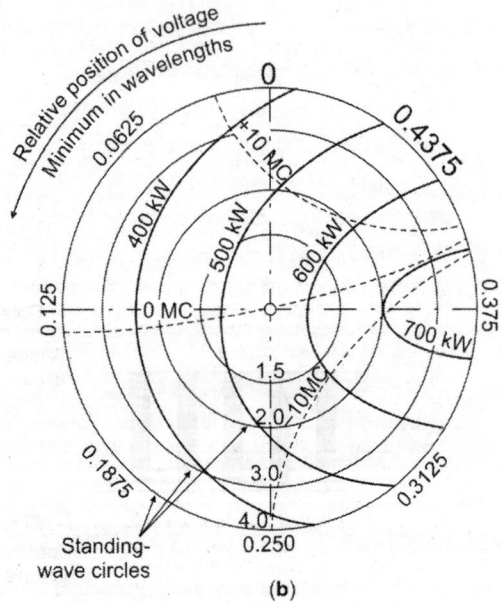

(b)

Fig. 13.14: Magnetron oscillator (a) Performance chart (b) Rieke diagram

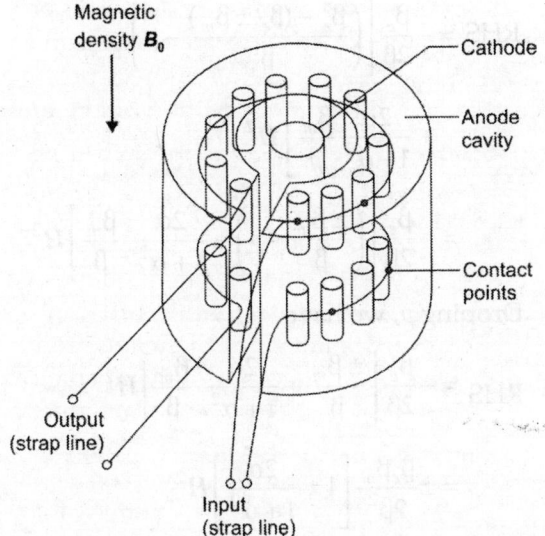

Magnetic
density B_0

Cathode

Anode
cavity

Contact
points

Output
(strap line)

Input
(strap line)

Fig. 13.15: Schematic diagram of amplitron

line. The electron beam and the EM waves interact in the resonator circuits.

The basic secular equation including the effect of space-charge is

$$(\gamma^2 - \gamma_o^2)(j\beta_e - \gamma)[(jp_e - \gamma)^2 + \beta_m^2]$$

$$= -j\beta_e\gamma_o\gamma^2\left[(j\beta_e - \gamma) + j\frac{2\alpha}{1+\alpha^2}B_m\right]H_z^2$$

(13.54)

Here, γ_o is the circuit propagation constant,

γ is the harmonic wave propagation constant,

$\beta_e (= \omega/\mathcal{V}_o)$ is the electron-beam phase constant,

$\mathcal{V}_o[\sqrt{2e/m})V_o]$ is the dc electron-beam velocity,

$\beta_m [(\omega_c/\gamma_o) = (e/\mathcal{V}_o^2 m)B_o]$ is the cyclotron angular frequency,

β_o is the cross-magnetic flux density

$H^2 = 2(1 + \alpha^2)\phi^2 C^3$,

$C [= (I_oZ_o/4V_o)^{1/3}]$ is the gain parameter,

$\phi [=A \exp(-j\gamma y) + B \exp(j\gamma y)]$ is the wave equation, and

$$\alpha = \left[\frac{A\exp(-j\gamma y) - B\exp(j\gamma y)}{\phi} = j\frac{1}{\gamma\phi}\frac{d\phi}{dt}\right]$$

a factor.

In general, γ has five solutions from Eq. (13.54). Let

$$\gamma_o = j\beta \tag{13.55}$$

$$\gamma = j\beta(1 + p) = \gamma_o(1 + p) \tag{13.56}$$

where $p \ll 1$.

Substitution of Eqs (13.55) and (13.56) in Eq. (13.54), each term yields

$$(\gamma^2 - \gamma_o^2) = \gamma_o^2(1+p)^2 - \gamma_o^2$$

$$= \gamma_o^2(1 + 2p + p^2) - \gamma_o^2$$

$$= 2p\gamma_o^2 + p^2\gamma_o^2$$

$$\simeq 2p\gamma_o^2 = -2p\beta^2 \text{ since } p \ll 1$$

$$(j\beta_e - \gamma) = [j\beta_e - j\beta(1+p) = j\beta_e - j\beta - jp\beta$$

$$= j\beta\left[\frac{\beta_e}{\beta} - 1 - p\right] = j\beta \cdot x$$

where $x = \left[\frac{\beta_e}{\beta} - 1 - p\right]$

$$(j\beta_e - \gamma)^2 + \beta_m^2 = -\beta^2 x^2 + \beta_m^2$$

$$= -\beta^2\left[x^2 - \left(\frac{\beta_m}{\beta}\right)^2\right]$$

$$= -\beta^2(x^2 - a^2)$$

where $a = \beta_m/\beta$

$$-j\beta_e\gamma_o\gamma^2 = -j\beta_e j\beta[j\beta(1+p)]^2$$

$$= \beta_e\beta[-\beta^2(1 + 2p + p^2)]$$

$$= -\beta^3\beta_e \text{ since } p \ll 1$$

$$\therefore \quad \text{LHS} = \text{RHS}$$

$$(-2p\beta^2)(j\beta x) \cdot -\beta^2(x^2 - a^2)]$$

$$= -\beta^3\beta_e \cdot \left[cj\beta x + j\frac{2\alpha}{1+\alpha^2}\beta_m\right]H^2$$

$$j2p\beta^5(x)(x^2 - a^2)$$

$$= \left[-\beta^3\beta_e \, j\beta\left(x + \frac{2\alpha}{1+\alpha^2}\frac{\beta_m}{\beta}\right)\right]H^2$$

$$px(x^2 - a^2)$$

$$= -\frac{\beta_e}{2\beta}\left[x + \frac{2\alpha}{1+\alpha^2}\frac{\beta_m}{\beta}\right]H^2 \quad (13.57)$$

The right hand side of Eq. (13.57) is small. Hence, either one of the two terms in the LHS is also to be small. The first factor $x = \left(\frac{\beta_e}{\beta} - 1 - p\right)$ is small if $\beta_e \simeq \beta$. Then p is given by

$$-p^2 = -\frac{1}{2}\left[-p + \frac{2\alpha}{1+\alpha^2}\frac{\beta_m}{\beta}\right]H^2$$

$$= -\frac{\alpha}{1+\alpha^2}\frac{\beta_m}{\beta}H^2 \text{ since } p \ll 1$$

$$p = \pm\left(\frac{\alpha}{1+\alpha^2}\right)^{1/2}\left(\frac{\beta}{\beta_m}\right)^{1/2}H \quad (13.58)$$

The second factor is small if $\beta_e \pm \beta_m = \beta$

$$-\left(\frac{\beta_m}{\beta}\right)^2\left(\frac{\beta_e}{\beta} - 1 - p\right)^2$$

$$= \frac{\beta_e}{2\beta}\left[\left(\frac{\beta_e}{\beta} - 1 - p\right) + \frac{2\alpha\beta_m}{(1+\alpha^2)\beta}\right]H^2$$

$$\text{LHS} = \left[\frac{\beta_e - (\beta_e \pm \beta_m)}{\beta} - p\right]^2 - \left(\frac{\beta_m}{\beta}\right)^2$$

$$= \left(\frac{\pm\beta_m}{\beta} - p\right)^2 - \left(\frac{\beta_m}{\beta}\right)^2$$

$$= \left(\frac{\beta_m}{\beta}\right)^2 \pm \frac{2\beta_m}{\beta}p + p^2 - \left(\frac{\beta_m}{\beta}\right)^2$$

$$= \pm 2\frac{\beta_m}{\beta}p + p^2$$

$$\simeq p^2 \text{ (droping } p\text{)}$$

$$\text{RHS} = -\frac{\beta_e}{2\beta}\left(\left(\frac{\beta_e - (\beta_e \pm \beta_m)}{\beta} - p\right)\right.$$

$$\left. + \frac{2\alpha}{1+\alpha^2}\frac{\beta_m}{p}\right]H^2$$

$$= -\frac{\beta_e}{2\beta}\left[\left(\frac{\pm\beta_m}{\beta} - p\right) + \frac{2\alpha}{1+\alpha^2}\cdot\frac{\beta_m}{\beta}\right]H^2$$

Droping p, we have

$$\text{RHS} = -\frac{\beta_e}{2\beta}\left[\frac{\pm\beta_m}{\beta} + \frac{2\alpha}{1+\alpha^2}\cdot\frac{\beta_m}{\beta}\right]H^2$$

$$= \pm\frac{\beta_e\beta_m}{2\beta^2}\left[1 \pm \frac{2\alpha}{1+\alpha^2}\right]H^2$$

$$= \left[\frac{(1\pm\alpha)^2}{1+\alpha^2}\right]$$

$$\therefore \quad p^2 = \pm\frac{1}{4}\left[\frac{(1\pm\alpha)^2}{1+\alpha^2}\right]$$

$$\left(\text{since } \beta_e\beta_m = \frac{\beta^2}{2}\right)$$

In the above equation, p is imaginary when $\beta_e + \beta_m = \beta$ and α is less than unity. Therefore,

$$p = \pm\frac{1}{2}\frac{1-\alpha}{(1+\alpha)^{1/2}}H$$

13.9.1 Typical Characteristics

The characteristics of the highly successful QK434 amplitron are

Anode voltage	: up to 25 kV
Anode current	: 4 A
Gain	: 16 dB
Power output	: upto 3 MW
Frequency	: 8 GHZ
Efficiency	: 60% to 76%
Bandwidth	: 50 MHz

The characteristics of two-stage super power amplitron are

Anode voltage	: up to 25 kV
Anode current	: up to 5A
Gain	: 9 dB

Power output	: up to 425 kW
Frequency	: 8 GHz
Efficiency	: 76%
Bandwidth	: 150 MHz

13.9.2 Applications

The amplitron is commonly used in
  (i) Air surveillance radar
  (ii) Military pulsed radar
  (iii) High data rate transmitters

13.10 CARCINOTRON (BWCFO)

The carcinotron is a backward-wave cross-field oscillator (BWCFO). The BWCFO of M-carcinotron has two following configurations:

  (i) Linear M-carcinotron
  (ii) Circular M-carcinotron

13.9.1 Linear M-Carcinotron

The M-carcinotron oscillator is an M-type backward-wave oscillator. The interaction between the slow-wave structure and the electrons takes place in a space of crossed field (Fig. 13.16).

The slow-wave structure is in parallel with the sole electrode. An electric field is maintained between the negative sole electrode and the grounded slow-wave structure. A dc magnetic field is directed into the page. The magnetic field bents the electrons emitted from the cathode by 90°. The electrons interact with a backward space harmonic of

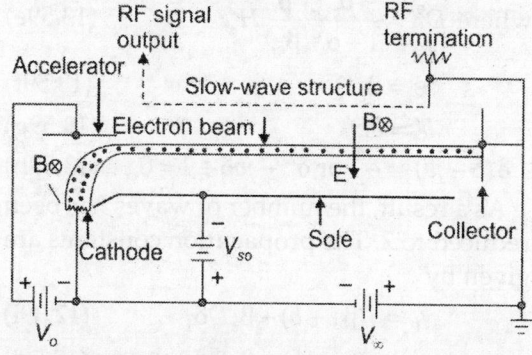

Fig. 13.16: Linear model of M-carcinotron oscillator

the circuit. The energy in the circuit flows opposite to the direction of the electron motion. The slow-wave structure is terminated at the oscillator end. The RF output signal is obtained at the electron gun end.

Figure 13.17 shows the perturbed electrons moving in synchronism with the wave in a linear M-carcinotron. Electrons at A near the beginning of the circuit are moving towards the circuit whereas electrons at B are moving towards the sole. Further down the circuit, electrons at C are closer to the circuit. The electrons at D are closer to the sole. Electrons at C have departed from the unperturbed path a greater distance than the electrons at D. Thus, the electrons have lost a net amount of potential energy. This energy has been transferred to the RF field. The electrons closer to the circuit are in stronger RF fields and hence the displacement is greater. Electrons at G have moved far from the unperturbed position so that some of them are intercepted on the circuit. The length from A to G is a half cycle of the electron motion.

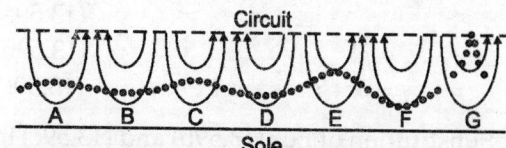

Fig. 13.17: Beam electrons movement in a linear M-carcinotron

13.9.2 Circular M-Carcinotron

Figure 13.18 shows the general construction of the M-carcinotron in the circular reentrant form. The sole and the slow-wave structure are circular and nearly reentrant to conserve the magnet weight. The sole has the appearance of the cathode in a magnetron.

In the circular configuration, the delay line is terminated at the collector end by spraying attenuator material on the surface of the conductors. The output RF signal is taken from the gun end of the delay line. The delay

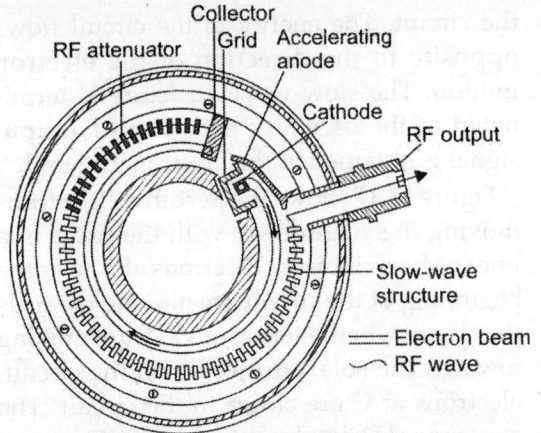

Fig. 13.18: Circular M-carcinotron

line is an inter-digital line. In this case, the electron drift velocity has to be in synchronism with a backward-space harmonic.

In the circuit equation, the only modification is a change of sign. This change is incorporated in Eq. (13.54). Thus

$$(\gamma^2 - \gamma_o^2)(j\beta_e - \gamma)[(j\beta_e - \gamma)^2 + \beta_m^2$$

$$= j\beta_e\gamma_o\gamma^2\left[(j\beta_2 - \lambda) + j\frac{2\alpha}{1+\alpha^2}\beta_m\right]^2 \tag{13.59a}$$

$$\gamma_o = j\beta \tag{13.59b}$$

$$\gamma = jk + \varepsilon \quad \varepsilon \ll 1 \tag{13.59c}$$

Substitution of Eqs (13.59b) and (13.59c) in Eq. (13.59a), each term yields

$$(\gamma^2 - \gamma_o^2) = (jk + \varepsilon)^2 + \beta^2$$

$$= (-k^2 + 2jk\varepsilon + \varepsilon^2) + \beta^2$$

$$= \beta^2 - k^2 + 2jk\varepsilon \quad \text{since } \varepsilon \ll 1$$

$$(j\beta_e - \gamma) = (j\beta_e - jk - \varepsilon) = j(\beta_e - k) - \varepsilon$$

$$(j\beta_e - \gamma)^2 + \beta_m^2 = (j\beta_e - jk - \varepsilon^2 + \beta_m^2$$

$$= [\beta_m^2 - (\beta_e - k)^2 - j2(\beta_e - k)$$

$$= 2j\varepsilon(k - \beta_e) +$$

$$2\beta_e k - \beta_o^2 + \beta_m^2 + k^2$$

$$\text{since } \varepsilon \ll 1$$

$$j\beta_e\gamma_o\gamma^2 = j\beta_e(j\beta)(jk+\varepsilon)^2$$

$$= -\beta\beta_e(-k^2 + 2jk\varepsilon + \varepsilon^2)$$

$$= -\beta\beta_e(k^2 + 2jk\varepsilon) = \beta$$

$$\left((j\beta_e - \gamma) + j\frac{2\alpha}{1+\alpha^2}\beta_m\right)H^2$$

$$= \left[(j\beta_e - jk - \varepsilon) + j\frac{2\alpha}{1+\alpha^2}\beta_m\right]H^2$$

LHS = RHS

$$(\beta^2 - k^2 + 2jk\varepsilon)[j(\beta_e - k) - \varepsilon][-2j\varepsilon(\beta_e - k) - (\beta_e - k)^2 + \beta_m^2$$

$$= \beta\beta_e(k^2 - 2jk\varepsilon)\left[j(\beta_e - k) - \varepsilon + j\frac{2\alpha}{1+\alpha^2}\beta_m\right]H^2$$

$$= j\beta\beta_e k^2\left(\beta_e - k + \frac{2\alpha}{1+\alpha^2}\beta_m\right)H^2 \tag{13.59d}$$

To obtain a solution of Eq. (13.59d), let $\beta = \beta_e$ and $\beta_e - k = \beta_e b'$, where b' is a small so that b'^2 and $b'\varepsilon$ can be neglected. This yields

$$2jk\varepsilon(j\beta_e b' - \varepsilon)\beta_m^2$$

$$= j\beta\beta_e k^2\frac{2\alpha}{1+\alpha^2}\frac{1}{\beta_m}H_2$$

after dropping negligible terms.

$$2\varepsilon(j\beta_e b' - \varepsilon)$$

$$= \left(\beta\beta_e k\frac{2\alpha}{1+\alpha^2}\frac{1}{\beta_m}\right)H^2$$

$$= \beta_e k\frac{2\alpha}{1+\alpha^2}\frac{\beta}{\beta_m}H^2$$

$$= 2\beta_e k D^2$$

where $D^2 = \dfrac{\alpha}{1+\alpha^2}\dfrac{\beta}{\beta_m}H^2 \tag{13.59e}$

$$\varepsilon = \beta_e D\delta \tag{13.59f}$$

$$b' = bD \tag{13.59g}$$

$$\delta(\delta - jb) = -1 \text{ or } \delta^2 - jb\delta + 1 = 0 \tag{13.59h}$$

As a result, the number of waves has been reduced to 2. The propagation constants are given by

$$\gamma_1 = j(\beta_o + b) + \beta_e D\delta_1 \tag{12.39i}$$

$$\gamma_2 = j(\beta_e + b) + \beta_e D\delta_2 \tag{13.59j}$$

where the δ's are given by

$$\delta_1 = j\frac{b - \sqrt{b^2 + 4}}{2} \qquad (13.59k)$$

$$\delta_2 = j\frac{b + \sqrt{b^2 + 4}}{2} \qquad (13.59l)$$

To obtain the amplification of the growing waves, the input and output reference points are set at $y = 0$ and $y = l$ respectively. At $y = 0$, the voltage at the input point is

$$V_1(o) + V_2(o) = V(o) \qquad (13.59m)$$

$$\frac{V_1(o)}{\delta_1} + \frac{V_2(o)}{\delta_2} = 0 \qquad (13.59n)$$

The simultaneous solutions of the above two equations yields

$$V_1(o) = \frac{V(o)}{1 - \frac{\delta_2}{\delta_1}} = \frac{\delta_1 V(o)}{\delta_1 - \delta_2} \qquad (13.59o)$$

$$V_2(o) = \frac{-V(o)}{1 - \frac{\delta_1}{\delta_2}} = -\frac{\delta_2 V(o)}{\delta_2 - \delta_1} \qquad (13.59p)$$

The voltage at the output point $y = l$ is given by

$$V(o) = V_1(o)\exp(-\gamma_1 l) + V_2(o)\exp(-\gamma_2 l) \qquad (13.59q)$$

$$= V(o)\frac{\delta_1 \exp(-\gamma_1 l) - \delta_2 \exp(-\gamma_2 l)}{\delta_1 - \delta_2}$$

$$= \frac{V(o)}{A_G/(\delta_1 - \delta_2)}$$

The voltage gain A_G is given by

$$A_G = \frac{1}{\delta_1 \exp(-\gamma_1 l) - \delta_2 \exp(-\gamma_2 l)} \qquad (13.59r)$$

The condition to be satisfied for the oscillations to take place is

$$A_G = \infty$$

or $\quad \delta_1 \exp(-\gamma_1 l) = \delta_2 \exp(-\gamma_2 l) \qquad (13.59s)$

$$\therefore \qquad \delta_1/\delta_2 = \exp(\gamma_1 - \gamma_2)\, l \qquad (13.59t)$$

From Eqs (13.59k) and (13.59l), we have

$$\delta_1/\delta_2 = \frac{b - \sqrt{b^2 + 4}}{b + \sqrt{b^2 + 4}} \qquad (13.59u)$$

and $\delta_2 - \delta_1 = j\sqrt{b^2 + 4} \qquad (13.59v)$

$$\therefore \quad \delta_1/\delta_2 = \exp{-(j\beta_e Dl\sqrt{b^2 + 4})} \quad (13.59w)$$

Equations (13.59t) and (13.59v) will be simultaneously satisfied only if $b = 0$ and $d_1 = -d_2$. This yields

$$2\beta_e Dl = (2n + 1)\pi \qquad (13.59x)$$

where n is any integer number. Substituting $\beta_e l = 2\pi N$, the oscillation condition becomes

$$DN = \frac{2n + 1}{4} \qquad (13.59y)$$

13.11 NUMERICAL EXAMPLES

Example 13.1 A cylindrical magnetron is operated with $V_o = 20$ kV, $I_o = 20$ mA, $B_o = 0.34$ Wb/m², radius of cylindrical cathode 5 cm and radius of cylindrical anode 10 cm. Calculate (a) cyclotron angular frequency, (b) cut-off voltage and (c) cut-off flux density.

Solution: Given: $V_o = 20$ kV, $I_o = 20$ mA, $B_o = 0.34$ Wb/m², $a = 5$ cm, $b = 10$ cm

(a) Cyclotron angular frequency

$$\omega = eB_o/m = 1.759 \times 10^{11} \times 0.34$$
$$= \mathbf{59.81 \times 10^9}\ \mathbf{rad.}$$

(b) Cut-off voltage

$$V_c = \left(\frac{eB_0^2 b^2}{8m}\right)\left[1 - \left(\frac{a}{b}\right)^2\right]^2$$

$$= \left(\frac{1.759 \times 10^{11} \times 0.34^2 \times 10^{-4}}{8}\right)\left[1 - \left(\frac{5}{10}\right)^2\right]^2$$

$$= \mathbf{142.87\ kV}$$

(c) Cut-off magnetic field density B_{oc} is given by

$$B_{oc} = (8V_o m/e)^{1/2}/[b(1 - a^2/b^2)]$$

$$= \frac{\left(\dfrac{8 \times 20 \times 10^3}{1.759 \times 10^{11}}\right)^{1/2}}{[0.1(1 - 0.25)]} = \mathbf{12.72\ mWb/m^2}$$

Example 13.2 A cylindrical magnetron is operated at 5 GHz with $a = 3$ cm, $b = 5$ cm, $N = 16$, $V_0 = 30$ kV and $B_0 = 0.05$ tesla. Compute (a) Hull cut-off voltage, and (b) cut-off magnetic field.

Solution: Given: $f = 5 \times 10^9$, $a = 3$ cm, $b = 5$ cm, $N = 16$, $V_0 = 30000$ V, $B_0 = 0.05$ T

(a) Cut-off voltage V_c **is given by**

$$V_c = \left(\frac{eB_0^2 b^2}{8m}\right)\left[1 - \left(\frac{a}{b}\right)^2\right]^2$$

$$= \frac{1.759 \times 10^{11} \times 0.05^2 \times 25 \times 10^{-4}}{8}\left[1 - \frac{9}{25}\right]^2$$

$$= \mathbf{56.3 \ kV}$$

(b) Cut-off magnetic field density B_{oc} is given by

$$B_{oc} = (8V_0 m/e)^{1/2}/[b(1 - a^2/b^2)]$$

$$= \frac{\left(\dfrac{8 \times 30000}{1.759 \times 10^{11}}\right)^{1/2}}{\left[0.05\left(1 - \dfrac{9}{25}\right)\right]}$$

$$= \mathbf{57.04 \ mWb/m^2}$$

Example 13.3 An X-band pulsed cylindrical magnetron has $V_0 = 30$ kV, $I_0 = 80$ mA, $B_0 = 0.01$ Wb/m², $a = 3$ cm, $b = 5$ cm. Compute (a) the cyclotron angular frequency, (b) cut-off voltage and (c) cut-off magnetic flux density.

Solution: Given: $V_0 = 30000$, $I_0 = 0.08$, $B_0 = 0.01$, $a = 3$ cm, $b = 5$ cm

(a) Cyclotron angular frequency

$$\omega_c = (e/m)B_0$$
$$= 1.759 \times 10^{11} \times 0.01$$
$$= \mathbf{1.759 \times 10^9 \ rad}$$

(b) Cut-off voltage

$$V_c = \left(\frac{eB_0^2 b^2}{8m}\right)\left[1 - \left(\frac{a}{b}\right)^2\right]^2$$

$$= \frac{1.759 \times 10^{11} \times 0.01^2 \times 25 \times 10^{-4}}{8}\left[1 - \frac{9}{25}\right]^2$$

$$= \mathbf{2.25 \ kV}$$

(c) Cut-off magnetic field density B_{oc} is given by

$$B_{oc} = (8V_0 m/e)^{1/2}/[b(1 - a^2/b^2)]$$

$$= \frac{\left(\dfrac{8 \times 30000}{1.759 \times 10^{11}}\right)^{1/2}}{\left[0.05\left(\dfrac{1 - 9}{25}\right)\right]} = \mathbf{18.04 \ mWb/m^2}$$

Example 13.4 A cylindrical magnetron is operated at 3 GHz with $V_0 = 3.2$ kV, $a = 0.6$ m, $b = 0.8$ m, $N = 16$ and $B_0 = 0.06$ T. Calculate the average drift velocity in the cathode-anode region.

Solution: Given: $f = 3 \times 10^9$, $V_0 = 3.2$ kV, $a = 0.6$ m, $b = 0.8$ m, $N = 16$, $B_0 = 0.06$ T.

Average drift velocity

$$v_\varphi = E_r/B_z = [V_0/(b - a)]/B_0$$
$$= (3200/0.2)/0.06 = \mathbf{2.67 \times 10^5 \ m/s}$$

Example 13.5 A pulsed cylindrical magnetron has $V_0 = 30$ kV and $I_0 = 30$ A, $B_0 = 0.336$ Wb/m², $a = 5$ cm and $b = 10$ cm. Determine (a) the cyclotron angular frequency, (b) the cut-off voltage and (c) the cut-off magnetic flux density for a fixed V_0.

Solution: Given: $V_0 = 30000$, $I_0 = 30$ A, $B_0 = 0.336$ Wb/m², $a = 5$ cm, $b = 10$ cm

(a) Cyclotron angular frequency

$$\omega_c = (e/m)B_0 = 1.759 \times 10^{11} \times 0.336$$
$$= \mathbf{5.91 \times 10^{10} \ rad}$$

The cut-off voltage is

$$V_c = \left(\frac{eB_0^2 b^2}{8m}\right)\left[1 - \left(\frac{a}{b}\right)^2\right]^2$$

$$= \frac{1.759 \times 10^{11} \times 0.036^2 \times 100 \times 10^{-4}}{8}\left[1 - \frac{25}{100}\right]^2$$

$$= \mathbf{2.25 \ kV}$$

(c) Cut-off magnetic field density B_{oc} is given by

$$B_{oc} = (8V_0 m/e)^{1/2}/[b(1 - a^2/b^2)]$$

$$= \frac{\left(\dfrac{8 \times 30000}{1.759 \times 10^{11}}\right)^{1/2}}{\left[10 \times 10^{-2}\left(\dfrac{1 - 25}{100}\right)\right]} = \mathbf{15.57 \ mWb/m^2}$$

Example 13.6: A linear magnetron has $V_0 = 10$ kV, $I_0 = 1$A, $B_0 = 0.01$ Wb/m² and $d = 5$ cm. Determine (i) Hull cut-off voltage for a fixed B_0 and (ii) Hull cut-off magnetic flux density for a fixed value of V_0.

Solution: Given $V_0 = 10 \times 10^3$ V, $I_0 = 1$ A, $B_0 = 0.01$ Wb/m², $d = 5$ cm

(i) Hull cut-off voltage is

$$V_{oc} = \frac{1}{2}\frac{e}{m}B_0^2 d^2$$
$$= \frac{1}{2} \times 1.759 \times 10^{11} \times (0.01)^2 \times (5 \times 10^{-2})^2$$
$$= 22 \text{ kV}$$

(ii) Hull cut-off magnetic flux density is

$$B_{oc} = \frac{1}{d}\sqrt{\frac{2V_o}{e/m}}$$
$$= \frac{1}{5 \times 10^{-2}}\sqrt{\frac{2 \times 10 \times 10^3}{1.759 \times 10^{11}}}$$
$$= 6.74 \text{ mWb/m}^2$$

Example 13.7: A circular carcinotron operates at $V_0 = 20$ kV, $I_0 = 3.5$ A, $B_0 = 0.3$ Wb/m², $f = 4$ GHz, $Z_0 = 50$ ohms, $D = 0.8$ and $b = 0.5$. Calculate (i) the dc electron velocity, (ii) the electron beam phase constant, (iii) the delta differentials, (iv) the propagation constants and (v) the oscillation condition.

Solution: Given $V_0 = 20 \times 10^3$ V, $I_0 = 3.5$A, $B_0 = 0.3$ Wb/m², $f = 4 \times 10^9$ Hz, $Z_0 = 50$ ohms, $D = 0.8$, $b = 0.5$.

(i) The dc electron velocity is
$$\mathcal{V} = 5.93 \times 10^5 (20 \times 10^3)^{1/2}$$
$$= 0.8386 \times 10^6 \text{ m/s}$$

(ii) The electron beam phase constant is
$$\beta_e = \omega/\mathcal{V}_o$$
$$= \frac{2\pi \times 4 \times 10^9}{0.8386 \times 10^6} = 300 \text{ rad/m}$$

(iii) The delta differentials are
$$\delta_1 = j\frac{0.5 - \sqrt{(0.5)^2 + 4}}{2} = -j0.78$$
$$\delta_2 = j\frac{0.5 + \sqrt{(0.5)^2 + 4}}{2} = -j1.78$$

(iv) The propagation constants are
$$\gamma_1 = j(\beta_e + b) + \beta_e D\delta_1$$
$$= j(300 + 0.5) + 300 \times 0.8 \times (-j0.78)$$
$$= j113.3$$
$$\gamma_2 = j(\beta_e + b) + \beta_e D\delta_2$$
$$= j(300 + 0.5) + 300 \times 0.8 \times j1.28$$
$$= j607.7$$

(v) The oscillations occur at
$$DN = \frac{2n + 1}{4} = 1.25 \text{ for } n = 1$$
$$\therefore \quad N = \frac{1.25}{D} = \frac{1.25}{0.8} = 1.5625$$
$$l = \frac{2\pi N}{\beta_e} = \frac{2 \times 3.14 \times 1.5625}{300}$$
$$= 3.27 \text{ cm}$$

KEY POINTS

- The microwave tubes are broadly classified as: (i) linear-beam or O-type tubes and (ii) cross-field or M-type tubes.
- In linear-beam tubes, the dc magnetic and dc electric fields are in parallel, and the dc magnetic field is used to focus the beam.
- In cross-field tubes, the dc magnetic and dc electric fields are perpendicular to each other, and the dc magnetic field plays a direct role in the RF interaction process.
- Cross-field tubes are so called because the dc magnetic and dc electric fields are perpendicular to each other.
- The common types of microwave tubes are: (i) Cylindrical magnetron, (ii) Coaxial magnetron, (iii) Voltage-tunable magnetron, (iv) Inverted magnetron, (v) Forward-wave cross-field amplifier, (vi) Backward-wave cross-field oscillator.
- All magnetrons consist of some form of anode and cathode operated in a dc magnetic field that is normal to the electric filed between the anode and cathode.
- There is also a focusing mechanism that tends to keep the working electrons in step with the fields in the interaction space in such a way that the working electrons deliver maximum possible energy to the oscillation.
- The magnetron is normally operated in π-mode in which the phase difference between the adjacent anode poles is π-radians.

- A "C" ring is used to vary the resonant frequency of the magnetron.
- This focusing action is equivalent to velocity modulation that causes electrons to form a bunch centered about the reference electron. The end result of various actions that take place is to cause the orbit of electrons to be confined to spokes, one for each two anodes.
- The variation in oscillator frequency due to variation in anode voltage is known as frequency pushing and the variation in oscillator frequency due to variation in load impedance is called frequency pulling.
- For a given anode voltage V_0, there exists a critical magnetic field B_c at which all electrons return to the cathode and no electron will reach the anode. This critical axial magnetic field B_c is known as Hull's cut-off magnetic flux density.
- Similarly, for a given axial magnetic field B_0, there is a critical anode voltage V_{oc} at which all electrons are returned to the cathode and no electron reaches the anode. The critical anode voltage V_{oc} is known as Hull's cut-off voltage.
- The oscillations for π-mode start at a critical beam voltage and this voltage is known as *Hartree voltage*.
- Since the dc magnetic field is perpendicular to the dc electric field, the electrons travel in a cycloidal path with outward centrifugal force equal to the pulling force. The frequency of the circular motion of the electron is known as cyclotron angular frequency.
- A coaxial magnetron consists of an anode resonator structure surrounded by an inner-single high-Q cavity resonator operating in TE_{011} mode.
- A voltage-tunable magnetron is a broadband oscillator and its frequency can be changed by varying the voltage applied between the anode and the sole.

FURTHER READING

1. Atwater HA (1962). *Introduction to Microwave Theory*, McGraw Hill, NY.
2. Collins RE (1996). *Foundations of Microwave Engineering*, McGraw Hill, NY.
3. Gandhi OP (1981). *Microwave Engineering and Applications*, Pergamon, NY.
4. Gilmour AS Jr (1986). *Microwave Tubes*, Artech., Massachussetts.
5. Howes MJ and Morgan DV (1976). *Microwave Devices*, John Wiley, NY.

REVIEW QUESTIONS

13.1 What are the two types of microwave tubes?

13.2 Mention the various types of cross field tubes.

13.3 What is Amplitron?

13.4 What is Carcinotron?

13.5 Mention the essential parts of a magnetron.

13.6 What is Hull cut-off field?

13.7 What are modes? How is the π-mode separated from other modes in a magnetron oscillator?

13.8 What is strapping? Explain.

13.9 How can the frequency of a magnetron oscillator be varied?

13.10 What is meant by frequency pulling and pushing?

13.11 Define Hull cut-off voltage.

13.12 Write down the expression for Hull cut-off magnetic field and the anode voltage.

13.13 Draw the equivalent circuit of one resonant cavity of a magnetron oscillator.

13.14 Write down the expression for power output of a magnetron oscillator.

13.15 Define the efficiency of a magnetron oscillator.

13.16 Mention the typical characteristics of a magnetron oscillator.

13.17 Give the applications of a magnetron oscillator.

13.18 What is cyclotron frequency?

13.19 What is a coaxial magnetron?

13.20 What is a tunable magnetron?

13.21 What is Rieke diagram?

13.22 Write down the Hull cut-off voltage of a linear magnetron.

13.23 Write down the Hull cut-off magnetic flux density of a linear magnetron.

13.24 Give an expression for Hartree anode voltage.

13.25 What is an amplitron?

13.26 What is the power output of the amplitron?

13.27 What is BW amplitrons?

13.28 What is the efficiency of amplitron.

13.29 What is the power output of the two stage amplitron?

13.30 What is BW of the two stage amplitrons?

13.31 What is the efficiency of of the two stage amplitron.

13.32 Mention applications of amplitron.

13.33 What is a carcinotron?

13.34 Mention the two configurations of carcinotron.

DESCRIPTIVE QUESTIONS

13.1 Describe the construction and working of a magnetron.

13.2 Derive Hull cut-off magnetic field and voltage equations of a magnetron oscillator.

13.3 Explain the process of generation of microwaves by a cavity magnetron operated on π-mode. Explain briefly its applications.

13.4 Describe the π-mode of oscillation in a magnetron.

13.5 With necessary theory, explain the mechanism of oscillations in a multi-cavity magnetron.

13.6 Discuss the various modes of oscillations and their separation by means of straps in magnetron oscillators. Obtain an expression for the efficiency of this oscillator. How would you represent its operating characteristics graphically?

13.7 Describe the construction and working of a magnetron oscillator. Show that in a magnetron oscillator, the angular velocity of electrons is related with the frequency of oscillation by the relation $\omega_o = 2\pi f/(m + nN)$.

13.8 Describe the construction and working of a coaxial magnetron.

13.9 Describe the construction and working of a voltage tunable magnetron.

13.10 Explain the Rieke diagram?

13.11 Derive the Hull cut-off field in a magnetron.

PRACTICE PROBLEMS

13.1 An X-band pulsed cylindrical magnetron has $V_o = 30$ KV, $I_o = 80$ mA, $B_o = 0.01$ Wb/m^2, $a = 4$ cm, $b = 8$ cm. Compute (a) the cyclotron angular frequency, (b) cut-off voltage and (c) cut-off magnetic flux density.
[**Ans:** (a) 1.759×10^9, (b) 7.92 kV, (c) 19.46 mWb/m^2]

13.2 A cylindrical magnetron is operated at 3 GHz with $V_o = 1.6$ KV, $a = 0.6$ m, $b = 0.8$ m, $N = 16$ and $B_o = 0.06$ T. Calculate the average drift velocity in the cathode-anode region.
[**Ans:** 1.33×10^5 m/s]

13.3 A pulsed cylindrical magnetron has $V_o = 26$kV and $I_o = 27$ A, $B_o = 0.336$ Wb/m^2, $a = 5$ cm and $b = 10$ cm. Determine (a) the cyclotron angular frequency, (b) the cut-off voltage and (c) the cut-off magnetic flux density for a fixed V_o.
(**Ans:** 5.91×10^{10} rad, 139.5 kV, 14.495 mWb/m^2)

13.4 A pulsed cylindricl magnetron has $V_o = 25$ kV, $I_o = 25$A, $B_o = 0.34$ Wb/m^2, radius of cathode cylinder = 5 cm, radius of anode cylinder = 10 cm. Determine (i) the angular frequency, (ii) cut-off voltage and (iii) the cut-off magnetic flux density.
(**Ans:** 5.981×10^{10} rad, 142.97 kV, 14.22 mWb/m^2)

13.5 A pulse conventional magnetron has $V_o = 5.5$ kV, $I_o = 4.5$A, $f = 9$ GHz, $G_r = 2 \times 10^{-4}$ mho, $G_e = 2.5 \times 10^{-5}$ mho, $C = 2.5$ pF, $DC = 0.002$ and $P_{loss} = 18.5$ kW. Find (i) angular resonant frequency, (ii) unloaded quality factor, (iii) loaded quality factor, (iv) external quality factor, (v) circuit efficiency and (vi) electronic efficiency.
(**Ans:** 5.655×10^{10} rad, 707, 628, 5655, 11.11%, 25.25%)

13.6 A linear magnetron has $V_o = 15$ kV, $I_o = 1.2$A, $f = 8$ GHz, $B_o = 0.015$ Wb/m^2, $h = 2.77$ cm and $d = 5$ cm. Calculate (i) electron velocity at the hub surface, (ii) phase velocity for synchronism and (iii) Hartree anode voltage.
(**Ans:** 0.73×10^3 m/s, 0.73×10^8 m/s, $V_{oc} = 39.60$ kV.

REFERENCE

1. Gentile C (1987). *Microwave Amplifiers and Oscillators*, McGraw Hill, NY.

2. Ghose RN (1963). *Microwave Circuit Theory and Analysis*, McGraw Hill, NY.

3. Terman FE (1955). *Electronic and Radio Engineering*, McGraw Hill, Intl.

4. Collins GB (1948). *Microwave Magnetrons*, McGraw Hill, NY.

5. Hamilton DR et al (1948). *Klystron and Microwave Triodes*, McGraw Hill, NY.

6. Harvey AF (1963). Microwave Engineering, Acad. Press, NY.

7. Gewartowski JW and Watson HA (1965). Principle of Microwave Engineering, IEEE Proc. Vol.61, No.3, Mar. (1973) Special Issue on High Power Microwave Tubes.

Microwave Crystal, Schottky and PIN Diodes

Objectives

- Classify microwave diodes.
- Know the constructional details.
- Understand the operating principle.
- Learn their applications.

14.1 INTRODUCTION

For proper operation, microwave tubes require high anode voltage, high magnetic fields and special type of electron guns. These requirements tend to increase the weight and cost of the devices. Recent advances in semiconductor technology had made it possible to design solid-state generators at microwave frequencies using semiconductor devices. These devices generally require low voltages for operation. They do not require an electron gun or focusing system. Hence, solid state devices are small in size, light in weight, highly reliable and compact. For space applications, they are well suited. They are easily incorporated into microwave integrated circuits. Silicon and gallium arsenide (GaAs) are the primarily used semiconductors. The most commonly used semiconductor devices are microwave diodes and transistors. They are efficient, highly reliable and develop continuous and pulsed power required at microwave frequencies.

In this chapter, we shall discuss the construction, operation and applications of crystal, Schottky and PIN diodes.

14.2 CLASSIFICATION OF MICROWAVE DIODES

Microwave diodes are classified according to their applications as

(a) Crystal and Schottky diodes for *mixing and detection.*
(b) PIN diodes for *modulation, switching, phase shifting, limiting and attenuation.*
(c) Varactor diodes for *frequency multiplication, parametric amplification and tuning.*
(d) Tunnel and Gunn diodes for *oscillations.*
(e) Read diodes for *amplification and oscillations.*

14.3 CRYSTAL DIODE

A typical silicon crystal diode is shown in Fig. 14.1(a). It consists of a pointed tungsten wire made in the form of a spring and a silicon wafer doped suitably with impurities. The tungsten spring presses against the surface of the doped silicon wafer. Rectification occurs at the contact point. The *V-I* characteristic of the crystal diode is shown in Fig. 14.1(c).

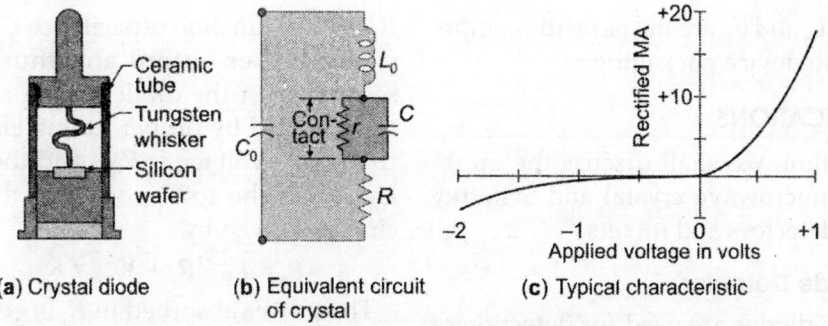

(a) Crystal diode   (b) Equivalent circuit   (c) Typical characteristic
of crystal

Fig. 14.1: Crystal diode (a) Structure (b) Equivalent circuit (c) *V-I* characteristic

14.3.1 Principle of Operation

The equivalent circuit of a crystal diode is shown in Fig. 14.1(b). It is used for analysis and design. In this circuit, R is the *spreading resistance*. It represents the resistance that the body of the crystal offers to the current flowing away from the region of the point contact. The non-linear resistance r gives rise to rectification. This resistance r is *small* when the diode is conducting and *large* in the reverse direction. Capacitance C represents the barrier layer capacitance. The inductance L_o of the tungsten wire and the capacitance C_o of the crystal holder can be used as a part of the resonant system associated with crystal diode. Thus, their only effect is to modify slightly the conditions for resonance. In contrast, r, R and C are related to the rectifying action. Hence affect the ability of the crystal mixer to operate satisfactorily at microwave frequencies. Typical values of R and C of a crystal mixer operating at a wavelength of 10 cm are 30 ohms and 0.3 pF respectively.

14.4 SCHOTTKY DIODE

Figure 14.2(a) shows the construction details of a Schottky diode. It is a metal-semiconductor barrier diode. It is constructed on a thin n^+ type silicon substrate by growing epitaxially on an n-type active layer of about 2 micron thickness. Over the active layer, a thin SiO_2 layer is grown thermally. By depositing metals such as *gold, silver* or

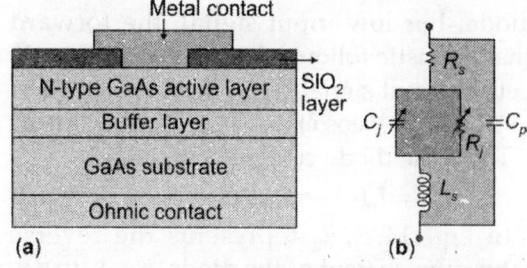

Fig. 14.2: Schottky diode (a) Structure (b) Equivalent circuit

platinum over SiO_2, a metal-semiconductor junction is formed.

14.4.1 Principle of operation

In the Schottky diode, the majority carriers are *electrons*. When the diode is *unbiased*, electrons on the n-side have lower energy levels than the electrons in the metal. Hence they cannot surmount the junction barrier and cross over to the metal. Therefore, the diode is also known as *Schottky barrier diode*. When the diode is *forward-biased*, electrons from highly doped n-semiconductor material are injected into the metal. When it is *reverse-biased*, the barrier height becomes too high for the electrons to cross and no conduction takes place.

For purpose of analysis and design, the equivalent circuit of Schottky diode is represented as shown in Fig. 14.2(b). In this circuit, R_s represents losses in ohmic contacts, substrate and undepleted epitaxial layer. C_j is the voltage dependent junction capacitance and R_j is the current dependent junction resistance. L_s and C_p are the parasitic components due to device packaging.

14.5 APPLICATIONS

In this section, we shall discuss the applications of microwave crystal and Schottky diodes as detectors and mixers.

14.5.1 Diode Detector

Microwave diodes are used for detection of microwave signals. Fig. 14.3 shows the forward *V–I* characteristic of a microwave diode. For low input signal, the forward characteristic follows the *square law*: $I \propto V^2$. Let the input signal be

$$v = V \cos \omega t \qquad (14.1)$$

Then, the diode current is given by

$$i = I_0(e^{aV} - 1) \qquad (14.2)$$

In Eq. (14.2), I_o represents the reverse saturation current of the diode, $a = 1/(\eta V_T)$, η is a constant and equals to 1.1 for Schottky diodes and 1.4 for crystal diodes.

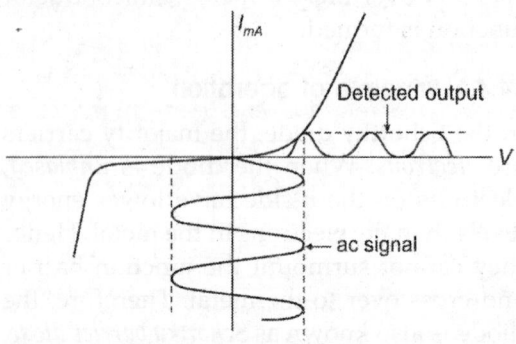

Fig. 14.3: Diode detector

V_T is the equivalent thermal voltage and equal to 26 mV at room temperature. The Fourier series expansion of Eq. (14.2) gives

$$i = I_0[aV \cos \omega t + (a^2V^2/4)(1 + \cos 2 \omega t)] \qquad (14.3)$$

It has a dc diode current I_{dc} given by

$$I_{dc} = I_0 a^2 V^2/4 \qquad (14.4)$$

It is proportional to the square of the amplitude of the signal voltage. Hence, known as *square-law* detector. The detector circuit filters out the ac components. The series resistance

R_s and the junction capacitance C_j reduce the signal power output and thus, limit the sensitivity of the diode detector. L_s and C_p are matched by proper tuning circuit. If the rms signal voltage is V_{rms} and the current is I_{rms}, then the total power in the detector circuit is given by

$$P_t = I_{rms}{}^2 R_s + V_{rms}^2 / R_j \qquad (14.5)$$

The power absorbed in R_j is given by

$$P_a = V_{rms}^2 / R_j \qquad (14.6)$$

The power loss is defined as the ratio of the power absorbed to the total power. Thus,

Power loss

$$= P_a/ P_t$$
$$= \frac{(V_{rms}^2 / R_j)}{(I_{rms}^2 R_s + V_{rms}^2 / R_j)}$$
$$= 1/[1 + (I_{rms}/V_{rms})^2 R_s R_j]$$
$$= 1/[1 + |Y_j|^2 R_s R_j]$$
$$= 1/[1 + \omega^2 C_j^2 R_s R_j] \qquad (14.7)$$

since $Y_j = \omega C_j$.

The microwave detector diodes are sensitive and operate without any external dc bias. The diodes are usually mounted in a wave guide or a coaxial cable which has the matching elements so that the VSWR < 1.3. The microwave power is absorbed without appreciable reflection. An RF bypass capacitor is included in the output circuit so that the microwave signal is not coupled to the measuring instruments such as VSWR meter. The detector circuit is matched using short-circuit stub.

14.5.2 Harmonic Mixer

Figure 14.4 shows the schematic circuit of a harmonic generator. Crystal diodes such as 1N21B or 1N23B mounted in a waveguide or coaxial cable are employed. In order to compromise between low conversion loss and minimum noise, a standard signal level of 1 V is used. The RF choke provides the dc return path. The RF bypass capacitor prevents RF signal leakage to the IF circuit. The

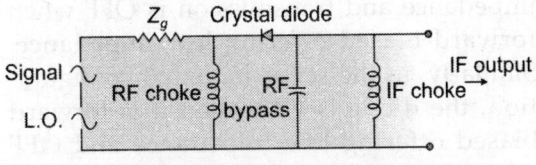

Fig. 14.4: Harmonic mixer

IF choke provides the dc return-path for IF circuit. The local oscillator voltage $V_p \cos \omega_p t$ generates current in the diode. This current is rich in harmonics. An incoming RF signal beats with these frequencies and produces difference frequencies $n\omega_p \pm \omega_s$. The IF amplifier can be tuned to the required harmonic difference frequencies. Thus, the harmonic frequencies can be used with low frequency local oscillator to generate IF.

For optimum performance, there should be reasonably good impedance matching between the crystal unit, microwave signal source and load impedance Z_{if} at IF. The input and output impedances depend on the amplitude of the local oscillator signal. Hence, the signal amplitude of the local oscillator should be properly adjusted.

The efficiency of conversion is the ratio of RF input power to IF output power at the difference frequency and it is known as *conversion loss* and is given by

Conversion loss (dB)

$$L_c = 10 \log (\text{IF output power}/ \text{RF input power}) \quad (14.8)$$

The IF output power is the IF power delivered to the load whose impedance is the *conjugate of Z_{if}* of the mixer. Typical conversion loss ranges from 4.5 dB to 7.5 dB for fundamental frequency. It is higher for higher harmonic mixing.

The output noise of diode mixers affects the operation of the receiver. This is measured in terms of output noise ratio N_r given by

$$N_r = \frac{\text{IF output noise}}{\text{Thermal or Johnson's noise power}}$$

$$= N_0/kTB_{if} \quad (14.9)$$

The corresponding noise temperature T_n is given by

$$T_n = N_r T = N_0/kB_{if} \quad (14.10)$$

14.6 PIN DIODE

Figure 14.5 shows a PIN diode. It consists of a heavily doped p-region and a heavily doped n-region separated by an un-doped intrinsic region i. The thickness of i-region is usually in the range of 10–200 µm. The intrinsic layer has a resistivity of 1000 ohm-cm. In actual practice, the i-region is either a high resistivity p-layer, known as π-type or a high resistivity n-layer, known as v-type. The resistance of the intrinsic layer is very high in the reverse bias and decreases in the forward bias.

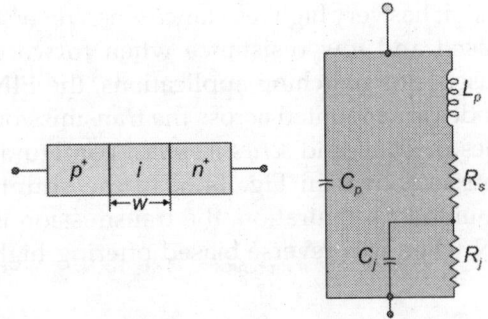

Fig. 14.5: PIN diode (a) Structure (b) Equivalent circuit

14.6.1 Equivalent Circuit

The equivalent circuit of a PIN diode is shown in Fig. 14.5(b). R_j is the variable junction resistance. C_j is the constant junction capacitance and is equal to 0.2 pF at frequencies higher than 1 GHz. R_s is the bulk and contact resistance of the p^+ and n^+ layers and is equal to 1 ohm. L_p and C_p are the package inductance and capacitance respectively.

The admittance of the PIN diode is given by

$$Y = [1/(R_s + j\omega L_s + 1/j\omega C_j)] + j\omega C_p$$

Neglecting L_s, the admittance is given by

$$Y = [1/(R_s + 1/j\omega C_j)] + j\omega C_p$$
$$= [j\omega C_j/(1 + j\omega C_j R_s)] + j\omega C_p$$

$$= \frac{j\omega C_j(1 - j\omega C_j R_s)}{1 + (\omega C_j R_s)^2} + j\omega C_s$$

Assuming $(j\omega C_j R_s)^2 \ll 1$, the admittance reduces to

$$Y = j\omega C_j(1 - j\omega C_j R_s) + j\omega C_p$$
$$= \omega^2 C_j^2 R_s + j\omega(C_j + C_p)$$
$$= G_r + jB_r$$

where $G_r = \omega^2 C_j^2 R_s$ and $B_r = \omega(C_j + C_p)$

14.7 PIN DIODE APPLICATIONS

In this section, we shall study the various applications of PIN diodes.

14.7.1 Single Pole Single Throw (SPST) Switch

PIN diode is used as a microwave switch since it has very high resistance when reverse biased and low resistance when forward biased. For switching applications, the PIN diodes are mounted across the transmission lines in *shunt* and *series mounted* configuration as shown in Fig. 14.6. In the shunt-mounted configuration, the transmission is ON when it is reverse biased offering high impedance and transmission is OFF when forward biased offering low impedance. Similarly, in the series-mounted configuration, the diode is ON when it is forward biased offering low impedance and OFF when reverse biased offering high impedance.

14.7.2 Single Pole Double Throw (SPDT) Switch

Figure 14.7 shows a SPDT switch configuration using two PIN diodes. The distance between the location of the diodes and the junction point J are quarter-wave length each at the center frequency. When the diode A is forward biased and the diode B is reverse biased, port 2 is shorted and port 3 is open-circuited. Hence, transmission takes place from port 1 to port 3. Similarly, if the diode A is reverse biased and the diode B is forward biased, transmission takes place from port 1 to port 2. The short-circuited branch with the forward biased diode appears as a quarter-wave stub. Because of this feature, the switch characteristics vary with frequency even when the diodes are ideal.

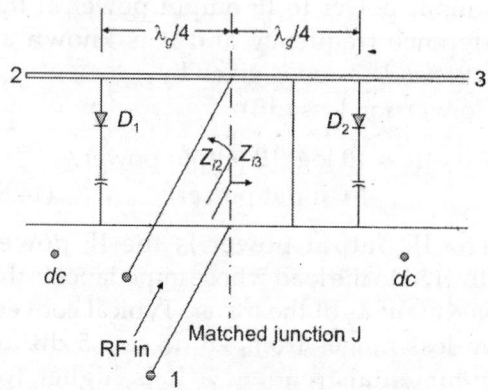

Fig. 14.7: PIN diode as SPDT switch

14.7.3 Digital Phase Shifter

Several basic designs are used to construct a digital or electronically controlled phase shifter. In all these designs, PIN diodes are used to switch the circuit elements in and out of the transmission path. Each switching

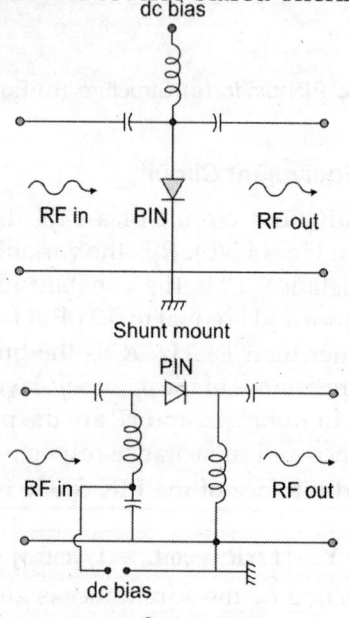

Fig. 14.6: PIN diode as SPST switch

operation adds or subtracts a finite phase shift such as $\pm11.25°$, $\pm22.5°$, $\pm45°$, $\pm90°$ etc.

The simplest digital phase shifter is shown in Fig. 14.8. It consists of PIN diode switches to switch one of the two alternate transmission line lengths into the transmission path of the signal. The bias current is supplied by connections at the midpoint of a half wave open-circuited stub as shown in Fig 14.8. The first quarter-wave section is a low impedance stub. It transforms the open circuit impedance to a low impedance or a short circuit at the point where the bias line is connected. The second quarterwave section uses a high impedance line. It transforms the low impedance of the mid point into high impedance that produces negligible loading on the main transmission line. The dc return for the bias current is obtained by connecting the input and output lines to the ground plane through a short circuited high impedance quarterwave line sections as shown in Fig. 14.8.

Let the lengths of the two transmission lines be l_1 and l_2. Then when line 2 is switched in to replace line 1, the incremental phase change is $\Delta\varphi = \beta\,(l_2 - l_1)$ where β is the phase constant. At a specified frequency, this type of phase shifter produces incremental changes in phase that is proportional to the difference in length of the two transmission paths. By cascaded transmission paths, a full range of $0°$ to $180°$ phase shift can be obtained.

14.7.4 PIN Diode Attenuator

PIN diodes are also used in electronically controlled attenuator. An important characteristic of a variable attenuator is that its input impedance Z_{in} should remain constant so that the attenuator stays matched over its operating range. One way of realizing this is shown in Fig. 14.9. It consists of three PIN diodes for R_1, R_3 and R_1 respectively. The impedance ZA to the right of AA' is given by

$$Z_A = R_3 + (R_1 Z_0 / R_1 + Z_0) \quad (14.11)$$

For the input impedance matching, $Z_{in}(= R_1 \| Z_A)$ must be equal to Z_0. Hence

$$1/Z_0 = (1/R_1) + (1/Z_A) \quad (14.12)$$

We have $E_1 = I_1 Z_A$ and $E_2 = I_1 R_1 Z_0/(R_1 + Z_0)$. Therefore the attenuation ratio $k = E_1/E_2$ is

$$k = E_1/E_2 = Z_A/[(R_1 Z_0/\ (R_1+Z_0)] \quad (14.13)$$

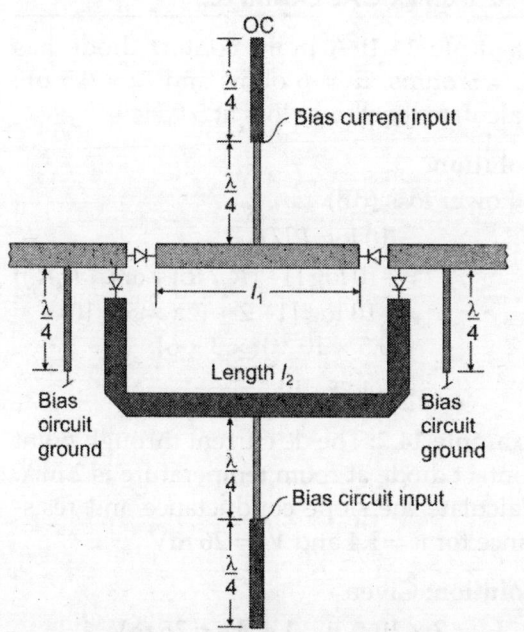

Fig. 14.8: Digital phase shifter

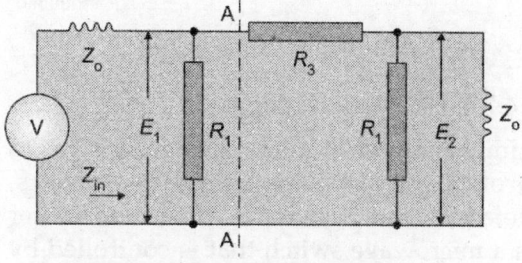

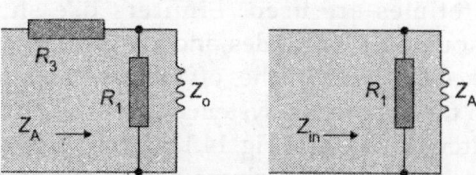

Fig. 14.9: PIN diode attenuator

Substituting for Z_A from Eq. (14.12), we get

$$k = E_1/E_2 = (R_1 + Z_0)/(R_1 - Z_0) \quad (14.14)$$

From Eq. (14.14), we can express R_1 as

$$R_1 = Z_0(k+1)/(k-1) \quad (14.15)$$

From Eq. (14.11),

$$R_3 = Z_0(k^2 - 1)/2k \quad (14.16)$$

Equations (14.15) and (14.16) give the variation of PI-arm resistance or PIN diode resistances relative to input–output ratio k.

14.7.5 PIN Diode Modulator

PIN diode modulators are 3 port devices. One port is for the modulating signal and the other two ports are RF ports. The unmodulated RF input is connected to one of the two ports and the modulated output is obtained at the other port. When a PIN modulator is connected as shown in Fig. 14.10 along a transmission line, sine wave, square wave and pulse modulations can be obtained by varying currents through the PIN diodes suitably.

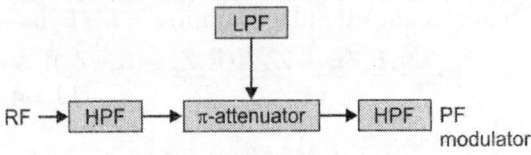

Fig. 14.10: PIN modulator

14.7.6 PIN Diode Limiters

Limiters are used in microwave systems to protect the sensitive amplifiers, mixers, detectors, samplers etc. A PIN diode limiter is a microwave switch that is controlled by self-bias. PIN diodes with very short carrier lifetimes are used. Limiters use shunt mounted PIN diodes and the presence of excess power switches off the power applied to the microwave systems. A typical limiter circuit is shown in Fig. 14.11. Two PIN diodes are connected in shunt across the transmission line. The diodes are placed

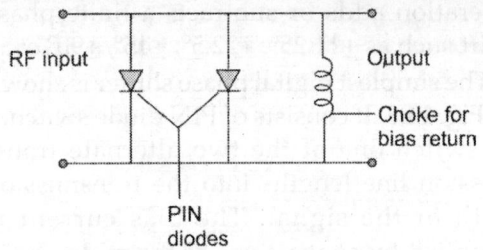

Fig. 14.11: PIN limiter

$\lambda/4$ apart so that the reflections are cancelled and low VSWR is obtained.

The limiting characteristic curve is shown in Fig. 14.11. At the limiting point, the threshold voltage across the diode is equal to the built-in junction voltage V_j. At high voltage levels, the voltage across the diode exceeds V_j and the diode resistance becomes very low. Thus, the circuit acts as a closed switch and the incident power is reflected back. The input-output characteristic of a practical limiter deviates from the ideal characteristic because the transition from high reverse to low forward resistance is not abrupt.

14.8 NUMERICAL EXAMPLES

Example 14.1: A point contact diode has $R_j = 3$ ohms, $R_s = 6$ ohms and $C_j = 0.5$ pF. Calculate the power loss at 5 GHz.

Solution:

Power loss (dB)

$$= 10 \log P_a/P_t$$
$$= -10 \log [1 + (R_s/R_j) + \omega^2 C_j^2 R_s R_j)]$$
$$= -10 \log [1 + 2 + (2\pi \times 5 \times 10^9 \times 0.5 \times 10^{-12})^2 \times 3 \times 6]$$
$$= \mathbf{-4.78 \ dB}$$

Example 14.2: The dc current through point contact diode at room temperature is 2 mA. Calculate the slope conductance and resistance for $n = 1.4$ and $V_T = 26$ mV.

Solution: Given

$$I_{dc} = 2 \times 10^{-3}, n = 1.4, V_T = 26 \text{ mV}$$
$$I = I_0(e^{aV} - 1)$$

$G_{ac} = dI/dV = I_o e^{aV}/a$

$a = 1/nV_T = 1/(1.4 \times 26 \times 10^{-3}) = 27.5$

$G_{ac} = dI/dV = I_o e^{aV}/a = (I_{dc} + I_o)/a$

$\approx I_{dc}/a = 2 \times 10^{-3}/2.75$ since $I_o << I_{dc}$

$= 727.3$ µmhos.

$R_{ac} = 1/G_{ac} = \textbf{1.375}$ k ohms.

Example 14.3 A sinusoidal microwave signal with peak voltage of 100 mV is applied to a microwave diode having $I_o = 1$µA, $n = 1.4$ and $V_T = 26$ mV. Compute I_{dc}.

Solution: Given $I_o = 1$µA, $V = 100$ mV, $n = 1.4$ and $V_T = 26$ mV

$I_{dc} = I_o a^2 V^2/4$

$a = 1/nV_T = 1/(1.4 \times 26 \times 10^{-3})$

$= 27.5$

$I_{dc} = 10^{-6} \times 27.5^2 \times (0.1/\sqrt{2})^2/4$

$= \textbf{0.945 µA}$

Example 14.4 A point contact diode detector has $I_o = 1$ µA, $n = 1.4$ and $V_T = 26$ mV. Find the detector current when the signal amplitude is 0.5 V at room temperature.

Solution: Given: $I_o = 1$ µA, $V = 500$ mV, $n = 1.4$ and $V_T = 26$ mV.

$I = I_o (e^{aV} - 1)$

$a = 1/nV_T = 1/(1.4 \times 26 \times 10^{-3})$

$= 27.5$

$aV = 27.5 \times 0.5 = 13.75$

$I = I_o (e^{aV} - 1) = 10^{-6} \times (e^{13.75} - 1)$

$= \textbf{0.94 A}$

Example 14.5: A shunt mounted PIN diode in a **TEM** transmission with $Z_o = 50$ ohms can be represented by $Z = 0.2 - j1990$. Compute the insertion loss and isolation at 2 GHz

Solution: Given: $Z_o = 50$ ohms, $Z = 0.2 - j1990$

$Z_f = R_j = 0.2$ ohm for forward bias,

$Z_r = 1/\omega C_j = 1990$ ohms for forward bias.

Insertion loss for forward bias

$= 20 \log (1/|T|^2)$

Transmission coefficient $T = 1 + \Gamma$

Reflection coefficient

$\Gamma = (Z_L - Z_o)/(Z_L + Z_o)$

Effective load

$Z_L = Z_f Z_o/(Z_f + Z_o)$

$= (0.2 \times 50)/(0.2 + 50)$

$= 0.1992$ ohm for forward bias

$\Gamma = (Z_L - Z_o)/(Z_L + Z_o)$

$= (0.1992 - 50)/(0.1992 + 50)$

$= -0.992$

Transmission coefficient

$T = 1 + \Gamma = (1 - 0.992)$

$= 0.008$

Insertion loss for forward bias

$= 10 \log (1/|T|^2)$

$= 10 \log [1/(0.008)^2]$

$= \textbf{41.94 dB}$

Isolation for reverse bias

$= 20 \log [(1 + (Z_o/Z_r)]$

$= 20 \log [1+(50/1990)]$

$= \textbf{0.216 dB}$

KEY POINTS

- The most commonly used semiconductor devices at microwave frequencies are microwave diodes and transistors. They are efficient, highly reliable and develop continuous and pulsed power required at microwave frequencies.
- These devices are small in size, light in weight, highly reliable and compact. For space applications, they are well suited. They are easily incorporated into microwave integrated circuits.
- Microwave diodes are classified as (i) crystal and Schottky diodes for mixing and detection, (ii) PIN diodes for modulation, switching, phase shifting, limiting and attenuation, (iii) varactor diodes for frequency multiplication, parametric amplification and tuning, (iv) Tunnel and Gunn diodes for oscillation, (v) Read diodes for amplification and oscillations.
- A typical silicon crystal diode consists of a pointed tungsten wire made in the form of a spring and a silicon wafer doped suitably with impurities.

- The applications of microwave crystal and Schottky diodes are as microwave detectors and mixers.
- A PIN diode consists of a heavily doped *p*-region and a heavily doped *n*-region separated by an undoped intrinsic region *i*.
- The application of PIN diodes are (i) SPST Switch (ii) SPDT Switch, (iii) digital phase shifter, (iv) attenuator,(v) limiter and (vi) modulator.

FURTHER READING

1. Collins RE (1996). *Foundations of Microwave Engineering*, McGraw Hill. NY.
2. Gandhi OP (1981). *Microwave Engineering and Applications*, Pergamon, NY.
3. Gewartowski JW and Watson HA (1965). *Principles of Electron Tubes*, Van Nostrand, NJ.
4. Liao SY (1985). *Microwave Solid State Devices*, PH. NJ.
5. Nanavathi RP (1975). *Semiconductor Devices*, Intext Edn., Scranton , PA.

REVIEW QUESTIONS

14.1 What are the limitations of microwave tubes?

14.2 Mention the advantages of microwave solid-state devices.

14.3 Mention the various classifications of microwave diodes.

14.3 Draw the equivalent circuit of a crystal diode

14.4 Draw the equivalent circuit of the Schottky diode.

14.5 Give the applications of microwave diodes.

14.6 Describe a square-law detector.

14.7 What is a harmonic mixer?

14.8 Define conversion loss of a harmonic mixer.

14.9 What is a PIN diode?

14.10 Draw the equivalent circuit of a PIN diode.

14.11 Give two applications of PIN diode.

14.12 Draw shunt and series mounted PIN diode configurations.

DESCRIPTIVE QUESTIONS

14.1 With neat sketch, explain the construction and working of a microwave crystal diode.

14.2 Explain in detail two applications of crystal diodes.

14.3 Describe a square-law detector. What is a harmonic mixer? Explain.

14.4 With neat sketch, explain the construction and working of a Schottky diode.

14.5 With neat sketch, explain the construction and working of a microwave crystal diode.

14.6 Explain PIN diode SPST and SPDT switches.

14.7 Explain PIN diode phase shifter.

14.8 Explain the PIN attenuator.

14.9 Explain PIN diode limiter.

14.10 Explain PIN diode modulator.

PRACTICE PROBLEMS

14.1 A point contact diode has $R_j = 2$ ohms, $R_s = 5$ ohms and $C_j = 0.5$ pF. Calculate the power loss at 5 GHz.
[**Ans:** −5.4 dB]

14.2 The dc current through point contact diode at room temperature is 1.5 mA. Calculate the slope conductance and resistance for $n = 1.4$ and $V_T = 26$ mV.
[**Ans:** 54.5 μmhos, 18.3 K ohms]

14.3 A sinusoidal microwave signal with peak voltage of 50 mV is applied to a microwave diode having $I_o = 1$ μA, $n = 1.4$ and $V_T = 26$ mV. Compute I_{dc}.
[**Ans:** 0.236 μA]

14.4 A point contact diode detector has $I_o = 1$ μA, $n = 1.4$ and $V_T = 26$ mV. Find the detector current when the signal amplitude is 0.1 V at room temperature.
[**Ans:** 14.64 μA]

14.5 A shunt mounted PIN diode in a **TEM** transmission with $Z_o = 50$ ohms can be represented by $Z = R_j + jX_c$. Compute the insertion loss and isolation at 2 GHz. Assume $R_j = 0.1$ ohm and $C_j = 0.02$ pF.
[**Ans:** 47.96 dB, 0.108 dB]

14.6 For a PIN diode, $C_c = 0.32$ pF, $C_j = 0.15$ pF and $R_s = 0.25$ ohm. Neglecting the series inductance, calculate the admittance of the diode at 3 GHz.
[**Ans:** 2 + j8860 μmhos]

REFERENCE

1. Bethe HA (1942). *Theory of the Boundary Layer of Crystal Rectifiers*, MIT Rep., p 43–52.
2. Das A and Das SK (2004). *Microwave Engineering*, TMH, New Delhi.

3. Davis WA (1984). *Microwave Semiconductor Circuit Design*, Van Nostrand, NY.

4. Johnson JB et al (1965). A silicon diode microwave oscillator, Bell Sys. Tech. J., Vol.44, p369–372.

5. Mead CA (1966). Schottky Barrier Gate Field Effect Transistor, Proc. IEEE ED-2, p 307–308.

6. Navon DH (1986). *Semiconductor Micro-devices and Materials*, HRW, NY.

7. Pozar DM (1990). *Microwave Engineering*, Addison-Wesley, Massachuttes.

8. Roy SK and Mitra M (2003). *Microwave Semiconductor Devices*, PHI, New Delhi.

9. Seeger JA (1988). *Microwave Theory Components and Devices*, PH, NJ.

10. Sze SM (1985). *Semiconductor Devices: Physics and Technology*, John Wiley, NY.

11. Terman FE (1955). *Electronic and Radio Engineering*, McGraw-Hill, Intl.

12. Kennedy G and Davis B (1999). *Electronic Communication Systems*, TMH, New Delhi.

Transferred Electron (Gunn) Devices

Objectives

- Understand the bulk negative resistance property.
- Know the Gunn effect and Gunn diode.
- Discuss the RWH theory and its application.
- Explain the principle of operation of Gunn diode.
- Learn the methods of microwave generation and amplification.

15.1 INTRODUCTION

The common characteristic of all the active two terminal solid-state microwave devices is their negative resistance. The real part of the impedance is negative over a range of frequencies. The current through a positive resistance and the voltage across it are in phase. The voltage drop across a positive resistance is positive and a power of I^2R is dissipated in the form of heat in the resistance. However, the current through a negative resistance and the voltage across it are out of phase by 180°. The voltage drop across a negative resistance is negative, and the power is $(-I^2R)$ Thus, the negative resistance generates a power of I^2R. In other words, *positive resistances absorb power* and hence, they are passive devices, whereas *negative resistances generate power* and hence, they are active devices.

Transferred electron devices are commonly used microwave diodes that exhibit negative resistance property. They are:

(i) Bulk devices with no junctions or gates

(ii) Fabricated from compound semiconductors such as *gallium arsenide* (GaAs), *indium phosphide* (InP) or *cadmium telluride* (CdTe). They operate with "hot" carriers whose energy is very much greater than the thermal energy. The continuous, average and peak power of these devices at higher microwave frequencies are very high.

15.2 BULK NEGATIVE RESISTANCE

Gunn diode is a transferred electron device. This device was studied by the scientist J.B. Gunn in 1963 and is named after him. He observed a periodic fluctuation of current passing through the *n*-type GaAs specimen when the applied voltage exceeded a certain critical value. In 1965, B.C. DeLoach, R.C. Johnson and B.G. Cohen discovered the impact ionization avalanche transit-time (IMPATT) mechanism in silicon. This employs the avalanching and transit-time properties of the diode to generate microwave frequencies. In later years, the limited space-charge accumulation (LSA) diode and the Indium Phosphide (InP) diode and Cadmium Telluride (CdTe) were successfully developed. They are bulk devices. The microwave amplifications and oscillations are derived from the bulk negative resistance property of uniform semiconductors rather than from junction negative resistance property between two different semiconductors as in the tunnel diode.

15.2.1 Background Material

Schokley, one of the inventors of the transistor, suggested in 1954 that two-terminal semiconductor negative resistance devices have advantages at high frequencies over the transistors. In 1961, Ridley and Watkins described a method of obtaining negative differential mobility in semiconductors. The principle is to heat carriers in a light-mass, high-mobility sub-band, with electric field so that they can transfer to a heavy-mass, low-mobility, higher-energy sub-band when they have high enough temperature. Ridley and Watkins also said that Ge-Si alloys and some III-V compounds have suitable sub-band structures in the conduction bands. In 1962, Hilsum had taken a further step in the theory of achieving negative differential mobility in bulk semiconductors by transferring electrons from high-mobility energy bands to low-mobility energy bands. He calculated carefully the transferred electron effect in several III-V compounds. He was the first to use the terms *transferred electron amplifiers* (**TEAs**) and *transferred electron oscillators* (**TEOs**). He accurately predicted that a **TEA** bar of semi-insulation GaAs would be operated at 373° K at an electric field of 3200 V/cm. His attempts to verify the theory experimentally could not succeed because the GaAs diode available at that time was not having sufficient high quality.

15.3 GUNN EFFECT AND GaAs DIODE

In 1963, J.B. Gunn, while studying the noise properties of semiconductors, discovered the so-called Gunn effect from thin disks on *n*-type GaAs and *n*-type InP specimens. In the same year, Ridley, Watkins and Hilsum predicted that the field domain is continually moving down through the crystal, disappearing at the anode and then reappearing at a favoured nucleation center, and staring the whole cycle once again. Finally, Kroemer stated that (i) the origin of the negative differential mobility is Ridley-Watkins-Hilsum's mechanism of electron transfer into the satellite valleys that occur in the conduction bands of both *n*-type GaAs and *n*-type InP and (ii) the properties of the Gunn effect are the current oscillations caused by the periodic nucleation and disappearance of traveling space-charge instability domain. Thus, the correlation between the theory of transferred electron devices and experimental discoveries was established.

Gunn diode is a transferred electron device. Figure 15.1 shows the schematic diagram of a uniform *n*-type GaAs Gunn diode with ohmic contacts at the end surfaces. This *n*-type GaAs bulk diode was studied extensively by the scientist J.B. Gunn in 1963 and is named in his honour. His observations were presented in his first research paper on this device as

"Above some critical voltage, corresponding to an electric field of 2000-4000 V/cm, the current in every specimen became a fluctuating function of time. In the GaAs specimens, this fluctuation took the form of

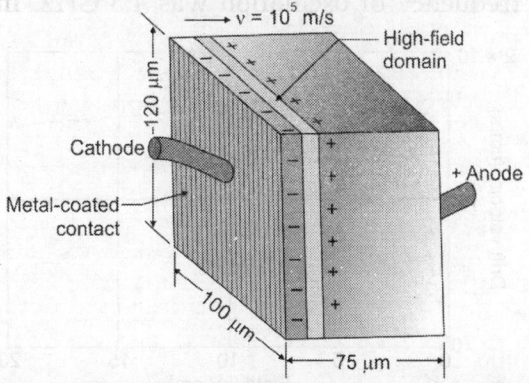

Fig. 15.1: Schematic diagram for *n*-type GaAs diode

a periodic oscillation superimposed upon the pulse current. The frequency of oscillation was determined mainly by the specimen, and not by the external circuit. The period of oscillation was usually inversely proportional to the specimen length and closely equal to the transit time of electrons between the electrodes, calculated from their estimated velocity of slightly over 10^7 cm/s.... The peak pulse microwave power delivered by the GaAs specimen to a matched load was measured. Value as high as 0.5 Q at 1 Gc/s, and 0.15 W at 3 Gc/s, were found, corresponding to 1–2% of the pulse input power."

The observation of periodic fluctuation of current passing through a uniform *n*-type GaAs specimen when the applied voltage exceeded a certain critical or threshold value is known as *Gunn effect*.

During the study, it was observed that the carrier drift velocity is linearly increased from zero to a maximum when the electric field is varied from zero to a *threshold* value. When the electric field is increased beyond the threshold value of 3000 V/cm for the *n*-type GaAs, the drift velocity is decreased and the diode exhibits *negative resistance*. Figure 15.2 shows this variation. The fluctuations in current are shown in Fig. 15.3. The current waveform is generated on the application of a voltage pulse of 16 V amplitude with duration of 10 ns to a specimen of *n*-type GaAs 2.5×10^{-3} cm in length. The frequency of oscillation was 4.5 GHz. In

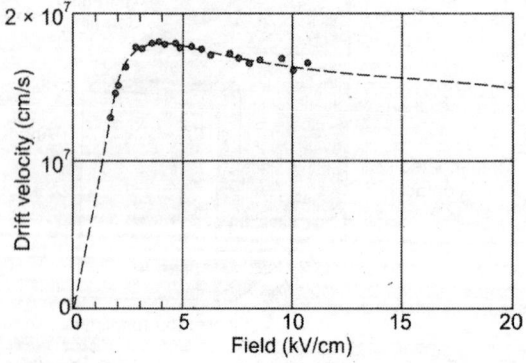

Fig. 15.2: Drift velocity versus electric field

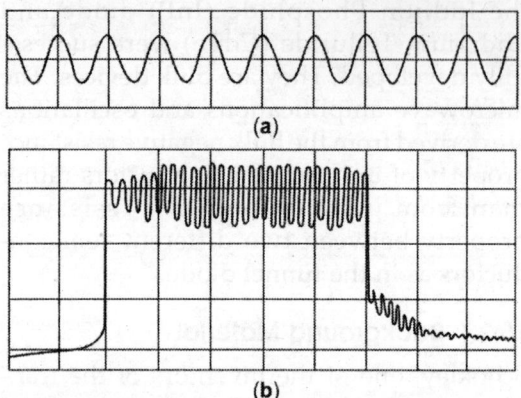

Fig. 15.3: (a) Expanded view (b) Current waveform of *n*-type GaAs

Fig 15.3(a), the x-axis is 2 ns/cm and the y-axis is 0.23 A/cm. Figure 15.3(b) is the expanded view of Fig. 15.3(a). It is observed that the period of these oscillations are equal to the transit time of the electrons through the specimen, calculated from the threshold current. It is also observed that the threshold electric field E_{th} varied with the length and type of material. Gunn developed an elaborate capacitive probe for plotting the electric field distribution within the *n*-type GaAs of length $L = 210$ μm and a cross-sectional area of 3.5×10^{-3} cm^2 with a low field resistance of 16 ohms. Current instabilities occurred at specimen voltages above 59 V, which implies that the threshold electric field is

$$E_{th} = V/L \qquad (15.1)$$
$$= 59/(210 \times 10^{-6} \times 10^2) = 2810 \text{ V/cm}$$

15.4 RIDLEY-WATKINS-HILSUM (RWH) THEORY

In 1964, Kroemer suggested the Gunn's observations were in complete agreement with Ridley-Watkins-Hilsum theory.

15.4.1 Differential Negative Resistance

The fundamental concept of RWH theory is based on the fact that the differential negative resistance is developed in a bulk solid-state III-V compound when either a voltage (or electric field) or current is applied to its terminals of the sample. The negative resistance devices have two modes:

(i) Voltage-controlled mode
(ii) Current-controlled mode

as shown in Fig. 15.4(a) and (b) respectively.

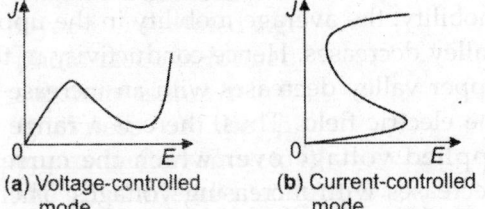

(a) Voltage-controlled mode   **(b)** Current-controlled mode

Fig. 15.4: Negative resistance device (a) Voltage-controlled (b) Current-controlled

In the voltage-controlled mode, the current density is *multi-valued* whereas in the current-controlled mode, the voltage is *multi-valued*. The major effect of this is to render the sample electrically unstable. As a result of this, the initially homogeneous sample becomes electrically heterogeneous in an attempt to reach stability. In the voltage-controlled mode, high field domains are formed, separating two low-field regions. The interfaces that separate the two domains lie along equipotentials. Thus, they are in planes normal to the current direction as shown in Fig. 15.5(a). In the current-controlled mode, splitting the sample results in high-current filaments running along the field direction as shown in Fig. 15.5(b).

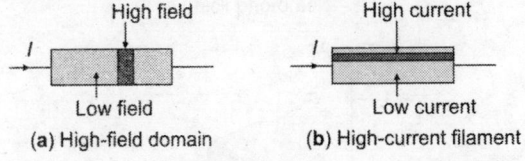

(a) High-field domain   **(b)** High-current filament

Fig. 15.5: (a) High-field domains (b) High current filaments

The negative resistance of the sample at a particular region can be expressed mathematically as

$$\text{negative resistance} = dV/dI$$
$$= dE/dJ \qquad (15.2)$$

If an electric field E_0 (or a voltage V_0) is applied to the sample, the current density J_0 is produced. As the applied electric field (or a voltage) is decreased to E_1 (or V_1), the current density is increased to J_1. When the applied electric field (or voltage) is increased to E_2 (or V_2), the current density is decreased to J_2. This results in a negative resistance. This is shown in Fig. 15.6(a). Similarly, for current-controlled mode, the negative resistance profile is shown in Fig. 15.6(b).

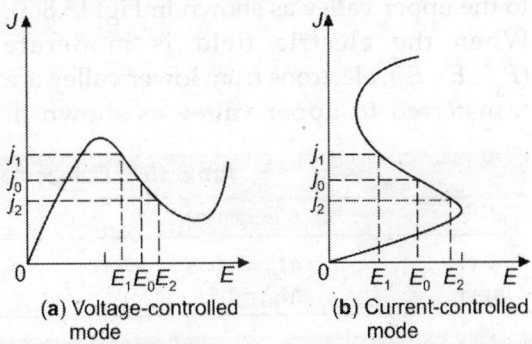

(a) Voltage-controlled mode   **(b)** Current-controlled mode

Fig. 15.6: Negative resistance profile (a) Voltage controlled mode (b) Current-controlled mode

15.4.2 Two-Valley Model Theory

The *n*-type GaAs has two closely spaced energy valleys in the conduction band. The high-mobility lower valley is separated by an energy gap of 0.36 eV from the low-mobility upper valley as shown in Fig. 15.7.

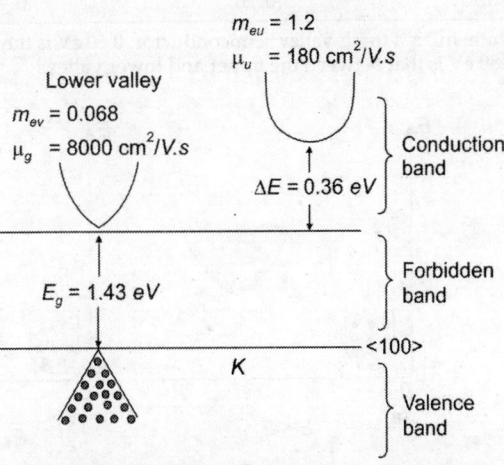

Fig. 15.7: Two-valley model for *n*-type GaAs

The data for the two valleys in the *n*-type GaAs is given in Table 15.1 and the data for the two valley semiconductors is given in Table 15.2. Electron densities in the lower and upper valleys remain the same under equilibrium conditions. When a dc voltage is applied across the device, an electric field is established. If the electric field is lower than the electric field of the lower valley $(E < E_g)$, most of the electrons remain in the lower valley and no electron is transferred to the upper valley as shown in Fig. 15.8(a). When the electric field is moderate $(E_g < E < E_u)$, electrons from lower valley are transferred to upper valley as shown in Fig. 15.8(b). At higher electric fields $(E > E_u)$, all the electrons are transferred to the upper valley as shown in Fig. 15.8(c). In the upper valley, the effective electron mass is larger and hence the electron mobility is lower than what it is in the lower valley. Since the conductivity is directly proportional to the mobility, the average mobility in the upper valley decreases. Hence conductivity in the upper valley decreases with an increase in the electric field. Thus, there is a range of applied voltage over which the current decreases with increasing voltages. Therefore, the device displays a negative resistance characteristic. This is known as *transferred*

Table 15.1: Data for two valleys in *n*-type GaAs

Valley	Effective mass M_e	Mobility μ	Separation
Lower	$M_{el} = 0.068$	$\mu_l = 8000 \text{ cm}^2/\text{V·s}$	$\Delta E = 0.36 \text{ eV}$
Upper	$M_{eu} = 1.2$	$\mu_u = 180 \text{ cm}^2/\text{V·s}$	$\Delta E = 0.36 \text{ eV}$

Table 15.2: Data for two-valley semiconductors

Semi-conductor	Gap energy (at 300 K) E_g	Separation energy between two valleys ΔE (eV)	Threshold field E_{th} (kV/cm)	Peak velocity v_p (10^7 cm/s)
Ge	0.80	0.18	2.3	1.4
GaAs	1.43	0.36	3.2	2.2
InP	1.33	0.60	10.5	2.5
		0.80		
CdTe	1.44	0.51	13.0	1.5
InAs	0.33	1.28	1.60	3.6
InSb	0.16	0.41	0.60	5.0

Note: InP is a three-valley semiconductor. 0.60 eV is the separation energy between the middle and the lower valleys. 0.80 eV is that between the upper and lower valleys

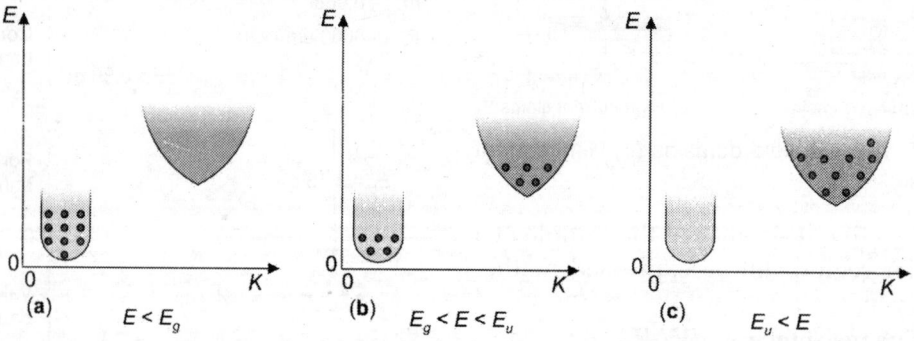

(a) $E < E_g$ **(b)** $E_g < E < E_u$ **(c)** $E_u < E$

Fig.15.8: Transfer of electron densities in the valleys

electron effect. The devices using this property are known as *transferred effect devices.*

Let the electron densities in the lower and upper valleys be n_l and n_u. Then, the conductivity of n-type GaAs is given by

$$\sigma = e(\mu_l n_l + \mu_u n_u) \quad (15.3)$$

where

e is the electron charge,

μ is the electron mobility,

When the applied electric field is sufficiently high enough, the electrons are accelerated and their effective temperature rises above the lattice temperature. Moreover, the lattice temperature also increases. Thus, electron density n and electron mobility μ are functions of the electric field. Differentiating Eq. (15.3) with respect to the electric field E, we obtain

$$d\sigma/dE = e(\mu_l\, dn_l/dE + \mu_u\, dn_u/dE) +$$
$$e(n_l\, d\mu_l/dE + n_u\, d\mu_u/dE) \quad (15.4)$$

The total electron density is $n = n_l + n_u$. Since the total electron density n is constant,

$$dn/dE = d\,(n_l + n_u)/dE = 0 \quad (15.5)$$
$$\therefore\ dn_l/dE = -dn_u/dE \quad (15.6)$$

Let us assume that μ_l and μ_u are proportional to E^p where p is a constant. Then,

$$d\mu/dE \propto dE^p/\,dE = pE^{p-1}$$
$$= pE^p/E \propto p\mu E = \mu p/E \quad (15.7)$$

since $\mu \propto E^p$.

Substituting Eq. (15.5) to (15.7) in Eq. (15.4), we get

$$d\sigma/dE = e(\mu_l - \mu_u)\, dn_l/dE + e(n_l\mu_l + n_u\mu_u)p/E \quad (15.8)$$

The current density J is given by

$$J = \sigma E \quad (15.9)$$

Differentiating Eq. (15.9) with respect to E, we obtain

$$dJ/dE = \sigma + (d\sigma/dE)E \quad (15.10)$$

Equation (15.10) can be written as

$$(1/\sigma)\, dJ/dE = 1 + (d\sigma/dE)/(\sigma/E) \quad (15.11)$$

For the resistance to be negative, the current density J must decrease with increasing electric field E or dJ/dE must be negative. This will be the case if the right-hand term in Eq. (15.11) is negative. Therefore the condition for negative resistance is

$$(dJ/dE)/(\sigma/E) < -1 \quad (15.12)$$

Substituting Eqs (15.6) and (15.8) in Eq. (15.12), we get

$$\frac{e(\mu_l - \mu_u)\dfrac{dn_l}{dE} + e(n_l\mu_l + n_u\mu_u)\dfrac{p}{E}}{e(n_l\mu_l + n_u\mu_u)/E} > 1$$

or

$$\left[\frac{(\mu_l - \mu_u)}{(\mu_l + \mu_u f)}\left(-\frac{E}{n_l}\right)\left(\frac{dn_l}{dE}\right) - p \right] > 1 \quad (15.13)$$

where $f = n_u/n_l$.

The exponent p is a function of the scattering mechanism and it should be negative. Impurity scattering is quite undesirable because, when it is dominant, its mobility increases and the exponent is positive. When lattice scattering is dominant, p is negative and depends on the lattice and carrier temperature. In order to satisfy the inequality, the first term in Eq. (15.13) must be positive. Thus, $\mu_l > \mu_u$. Initially, electrons must be in low-mass valley and then transferred to high-mass valley when they are heated by the electric field. The maximum value of the first term in Eq. (15.13) must be unity, i.e., $\mu_l \gg \mu_u$. The term dn_l/dE is negative as n_l is decreasing. This quantity represents the rate of carrier density with electric field at which electrons transfer to the upper valley. This rate depends on differences between electron densities, electron temperature and gap energies in the two valleys.

Based on the RWH theory, the band structure of a semiconductor must satisfy the following three criteria in order to exhibit negative resistance:

(i) The separation energy ΔE between the bottoms of the lower and the upper valleys must be several times larger than the thermal energy (0.026 eV) at room temperature. That is $\Delta E \gg kT$ or $\Delta E \gg 0.026$ eV.

(ii) The separation energy between valleys must be smaller than the gap energy between the conduction and valence bonds. That is $\Delta E < E_g$. Otherwise, the semiconductor will break down and become highly conductive before the electrons are transferred to the upper valley because hole-electron pairs are created.

(iii) Electrons in the lower valley must have high mobility, small effective mass and low density of state, whereas those in the upper valley must have low mobility, large effective mass and high density of state. That is the electron velocities must be larger in the lower valleys compared to those in the upper valleys.

Selenium and germanium do not satisfy all the above criteria. Some compound semiconductors such as gallium arsenide (GaAs), indium phosphide (InP) and cadmium telluride (CdTe) do satisfy these criteria and hence extensively used. Fig. 15.9 shows the negative resistance characteristic of a two-valley semiconductor.

The magnitude of the current density in a semiconductor is given by

$$J = qnv \tag{15.14}$$

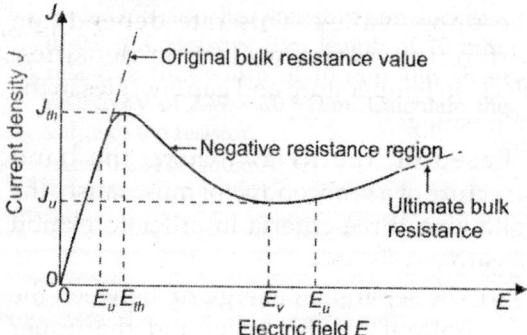

Fig. 15.9: Current density–electric field characteristic

where q is the charge of electron

n is the electron density

v is the average electron velocity.

Differentiating the above equation with respect to the electric field E, we obtain

$$dJ/dE = qn \, dv/dE \tag{15.15}$$

The condition for negative differentiial conductance is

$$dv/dE = \mu_n < 0 \tag{15.16}$$

where μ_n is the negative mobility. Fig. 15.10 shows this negative mobility.

15.4.3 High-Field Domain

We explained in the last section how differential resistance can occur when an electric field of a certain range is applied to a multivalley n-type GaAs. In this section, we describe how a decrease in drift velocity with increasing electric field forms a high-field domain for microwave generation and amplification.

In the n-type GaAs diode, the majority carriers are electrons. When a low voltage is applied to the GaAs diode, the electric field and current density are uniform throughout the diode. At low voltages, the GaAs diode behaves like a resistor since the drift velocity of the electrons is proportional to the electric field. This is shown in Fig. 15.2. The conduction current density in the diode is given by

$$J = \sigma E_x = (\sigma V/L) \, U_x = \rho v_x U_x \tag{15.17}$$

where

J is the conduction current density

σ is the conductivity

E_x is the electric field in the x-direction

V is the applied voltage

L is the length of the diode

U_x is the unit vector in the x-direction

ρ is the charge density

v_x is drift velocity

The current is due to the free electrons drifting through a fixed positive charge. The positive charge is due to donor atoms and is

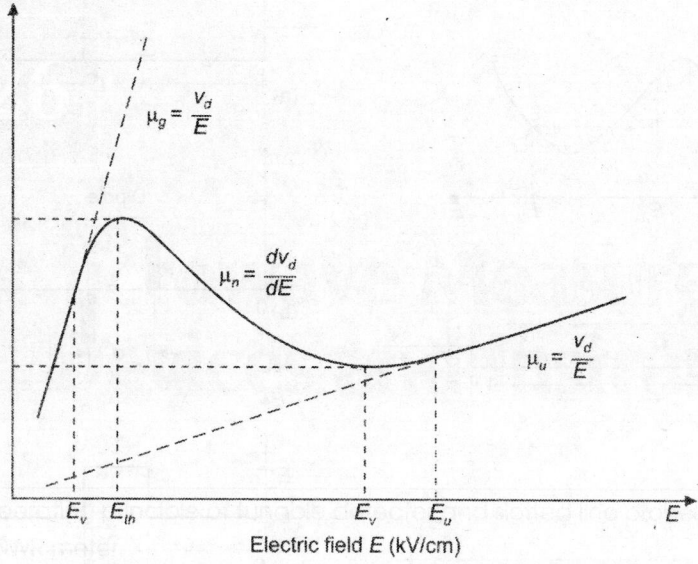

Fig. 15.10: Variation of electron drift velocity with electric field

sometimes reduced by acceptor atoms. As long as fixed charge is positive, the semi-conductor is *n*-type as the principal carriers are electrons. The difference between the densities of donors and acceptors is termed *doping*. When the space charge is zero, the carrier density is equal to the doping.

When the applied voltage is above the threshold value, a *high-field domain* is formed near the cathode. This reduces the electric field in the rest of the diode and causes the current to drop to about two-thirds of its maximum value. This occurs because the applied voltage is given by

$$V = -\int_0^L E_x dx \qquad (15.18)$$

For a constant voltage *V*, an increase in the electric field within the specimen is accompanied by a decrease in the electric field in the rest of the diode. Then, the high-field domain drifts with carrier stream across the electrodes and disappears at the anode. When the electric field increases the electron drift velocity decreases and the GaAs exhibits negative resistance.

15.4.3.1 Gunn Diode Characteristics

The typical *V-I* characteristic of a Gunn diode is shown in Fig. 15.11(a). Let us assume that at point *A* on the *J-E* plot in Fig. 15.11(b) there exists an excess or accumulation of negative charge caused by a random noise fluctuation or by a permanent non-uniform doping in the *n*-type GaAs diode. The excess charge creates an electric field as shown in Fig. 15.11(d). The electric field to the left of *A* is lower than that to the right. If the GaAs diode is biased at point E_A on the *J-E* plot, this implies that the carriers or the current flowing into *A* are greater than those flowing out of *A*, thereby increasing the excess negative charge at *A*. Moreover, when the electric field to the left of *A* lower than it was earlier, the field to the right is then greater than the original one. This results in an even greater space charge accumulation. This process continues until the low and high fields reach values outside the differential negative resistance region and settle at points 1 and 2 as shown in Fig. 15.11(a) where the current in the two field regions are same as explained in the previous section. As a result of this, a traveling space charge accumulation

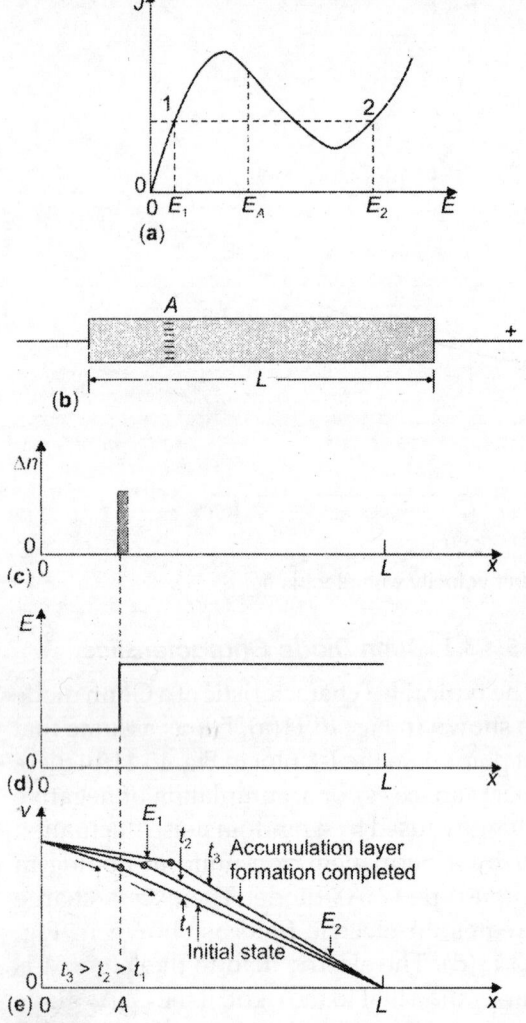

Fig. 15.11: Formation of electron accumulation layer in GaAs

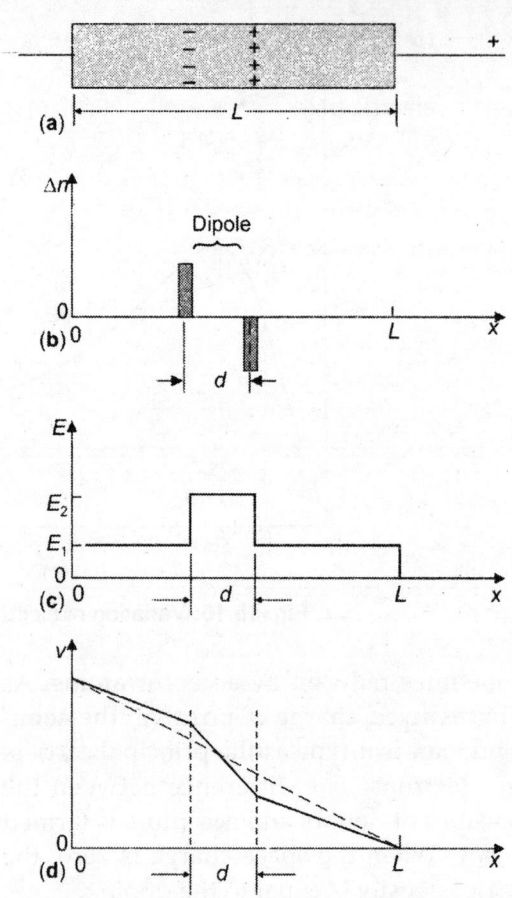

Fig. 15.12: Formation of electron dipole layer in GaAs

is formed. It is assumed that the number of electrons inside the diode is large enough to allow the necessary amount of space charge to be built during the transit time of the space charge layer.

When positive and negative charges are separated by a small distance, a *dipole domain* is formed as shown in Fig. 15.12. The electric field inside the dipole domain would be greater than the fields on the other side of the dipole. This is shown in Fig. 15.12(c). Because of the differential negative resistance, the current in the low-field side would

be greater than that in the high-field side. The two field values tend towards equilibrium conditions outside the differential negative resistance region, where the low and high field currents are equal. When the dipole field reaches a stable condition, it moves through the specimen of GaAs towards the anode. When the high-field domain disappears at the anode, a new dipole is formed at the cathode and the process is repeated.

15.4.3.2 Properties of High Field Domain

The general properties of the high-field domain are:

(i) A domain will be formed whenever the electric field in a region of the sample increases above the threshold electric field and will drift with the carrier stream through the device. When the electric field increases, the electron drift velocity decreases and the GaAs diode exhibits negative resistance.

(ii) When the applied voltage to a device containing a domain is increased, the size of the domain increases and it absorbs more voltage than was added and the current decreases.

(iii) A domain disappears only on reaching the anode. It may disappear before reaching the anode if the voltage is dropped appreciably below the threshold value.

(iv) A slight decrease in the applied voltage below the threshold value prevents the formation of a new domain.

(v) As the domain passes through the regions of different doping and cross-sectional area, it may modulate the current through the device or disappear.

(vi) The length of a domain is inversely proportional to the doping. Hence, devices with the same doping-length product will behave similarly in terms of frequency-length product, voltage / length and efficiency.

(vii) As a domain passes a point in the device, the voltage changes suddenly. Hence, it can be detected with a capacitive probe. The presence of domain anywhere in a device can be detected by a decreased current or by a change in differential impedance.

Properties (iii) and (vi) are valid only when the length of the domain is much longer than the thermal diffusion length for carriers. For GaAs, it is about 1 μm for a doping of $10^{16}/cm^3$ and about 10 μm for a doping of $10^{14}/cm^3$.

15.5 EQUIVALENT CIRCUIT

The equivalent circuit of a Gunn diode is shown in Fig. 15.13. In this circuit, C_j is the

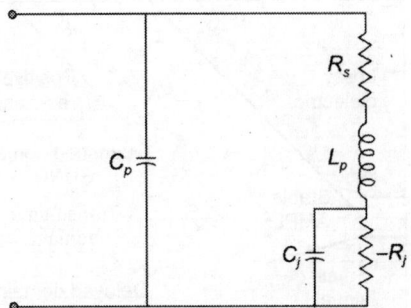

Fig. 15.13: Equivalent circuit of a GaAs diode

junction capacitance of the diode. The negative resistance R_j is the total resistance of the lead, ohmic contacts and the bulk resistance of the Gunn diode. L_p and C_p are the package inductance and capacitance respectively. The range of negative resistance is from −5 ohms to −20 ohms.

15.6 MODES OF OPERATION

After the discovery of the Gunn effect, various modes of operation have been developed depending on the material parameters and operating conditions. The formation of a strong space-charge instability depends on the conditions that (i) enough space charge is available in the diode, (ii) the specimen is long enough so that the necessary amount of space charge can be built up within the transit time of the electrons. This requirement sets up a criterion for the various modes of operation of bulk negative differential resistance devices. The four modes of operation of uniformly doped bulk diodes with low-resistance contacts are:

(i) Gunn oscillator mode or transit time mode

(ii) Stable amplification mode

(iii) LSA oscillation mode

(iv) Bias-circuit oscillation mode

These modes are shown in Fig. 15.14.

15.6.1 Criterion for Classifying Modes of Operation

The Gunn-effect diodes are basically made from an n-'ype GaAs. The concentration of

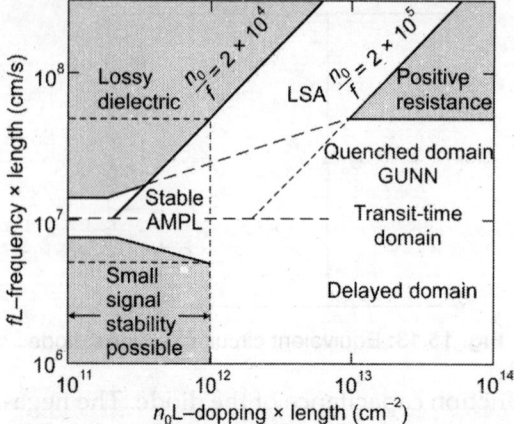

Fig. 15.14: Modes of operation for Gunn diodes

free electrons in *n*-type GaAs ranges from 10^{14} to $10^{17}/\text{cm}^3$ at the room temperature. Its typical dimensions are 150×150 μm in cross-section and 30 μm long. The time rate of growth of the space-charge layers during the early stages of space-charge accumulation is given by

$$Q(x, t) = Q(x - vt, 0) \exp (t/\tau_d) \quad \text{(i)}$$

where $\tau_d = \varepsilon/\sigma = \varepsilon/[en_0|\mu_n|]$ is the magnitude of the negative dielectric relaxation time, ε is the semiconductor dielectric permittivity, n_0 is the doping concentration, μ_n is the negative mobility, *e* is the electronic charge and σ is the conductivity.

If Eq. (i) is valid throughout the entire transit time of the space-charge layer, the maximum growth factor is given by

$$\text{Max. growth factor} = \frac{Q(L, L/v)}{Q(0, 0)}$$

$$= \exp\left(\frac{L}{v\tau_d}\right)$$

$$= \exp\left(\frac{Ln_0e|\mu_n|}{\varepsilon v}\right) \quad \text{(ii)}$$

It is assumed that the layer starts at the cathode at $t = 0$, and $x(0)$, and arrives at the anode at $t = L/v$ and $x = L$. For a large space-charge growth, the growth factor must be larger than unity. Therefore

$$n_0L > \varepsilon v/(e|\mu_n|) \quad \text{(iii)}$$

This is the criterion for the classification of the modes of operation of the Gunn-effect diodes. For an *n*-type GaAs, the value of $\varepsilon v/(e|\mu_n|)$ is about $10^{12}/\text{cm}^2$ where $|\mu_n|$ is assumed to be 150 cm²/Vs.

15.6.2 Gunn Oscillation or Transit Time (TT) Mode

When the applied voltage across the Gunn diode exceeds the threshold value E_m, a region of electron concentration and depletion, known as a *dipole domain*, is formed near the cathode. Since the applied voltage is constant, the electric field across the domain is greater than the average field. Across the rest of the diode, the electric field remains below the threshold level. This prevents the formation of further domains. The current in the presence of the domain also decreases. The dipole domain sweeps across the device. When it arrives at the anode, the device is in a high-mobility state and a new dipole domain is formed at the cathode and moves towards the anode. This mechanism is self-repeating and the period of oscillation is equal to transit time. This mode of operation has a low efficiency for microwave generation.

This mode is defined in the region where the frequency-length product is about 10^7 cm/s and the doping-length product is greater than $10^{12}/\text{cm}^2$. The device in this region is unstable because of the cyclic formation of either the accumulation layer or the high-field domain. In a relatively low impedance circuit, the device operates in the high-field domain mode. The oscillation frequency is near the intrinsic frequency. When the device is operated in a relatively high-Q cavity and coupled properly to the load, the domain is *quenched* or *delayed* (or both) before nucleating. The oscillation frequency is almost entirely determined by the resonant frequency of the cavity and is several times the intrinsic frequency.

The various modes of operation of Gunn diodes can be classified based on the time in which various operations occur. These times are defined as τ_t, domain transit time; τ_d, the dielectric relaxation time at low field; τ_g, the domain growth time and τ_0, the natural period of oscillation of a high-Q external electric circuit.

15.6.3 Stable Amplification Mode

This mode is defined in the region where the frequency-length product is about 10^7 cm/s and the doping-length product n_0L is between 10^{11} and 10^{12}/cm². When the $n_0L < 10^{12}$/cm², the derive exhibits amplification at the transit-time frequency rather than spontaneous oscillation. This occurs because the negative conductance is utilized without domain formations. There are too few carriers for domain formation within the transit time. Hence, amplification of signals near the transit-time frequency can be accomplished.

15.6.4 Limited Space-charge Accumulation (LSA) Mode

In the LSA mode, the Gunn diode is incorporated as a part of a resonant circuit as shown in Fig. 15.15(a). The resonant circuit is tuned to a frequency several times greater than that of *TT* mode. As a result, dipole domains do not have sufficient time to form and the device operates as a negative resistance device. The dc voltage is adjusted to a value greater than the threshold voltage and nearly at the midpoint of the negative resistance region. The RF oscillation voltage will build up to a peak-to-peak value approximately equal to the voltage increment over which the device resistance is negative as shown in Fig. 15.15(b). The resonator load represented by R_L is adjusted to a value about 20% greater than the maximum negative resistance of the device to ensure that the oscillations start and attain a stable steady state. The amplitude of the oscillations builds up until the average negative resistance of the Gunn diode becomes equal to the resonator resistance R_L and then becomes steady. This mode is defined in the region where the frequency-length product is about 10^7 cm/s and the ratio of doping/frequency is between 2×10^4 and 2×10^5.

15.6.5 Bias-circuit Oscillation Mode

This mode occurs only when there is either Gunn or LSA oscillation. It is usually at the region where the frequency-length product is too small. When a bulk diode is biased to threshold, the Gunn oscillation begins and the average current drops suddenly. This drop in current at the threshold leads to oscillations in the bias circuit that are typically 1 kHz to 100 MHz.

15.7 LSA DIODES

LSA stands for *limited space-charge accumulation* mode of the Gunn diode. If the product

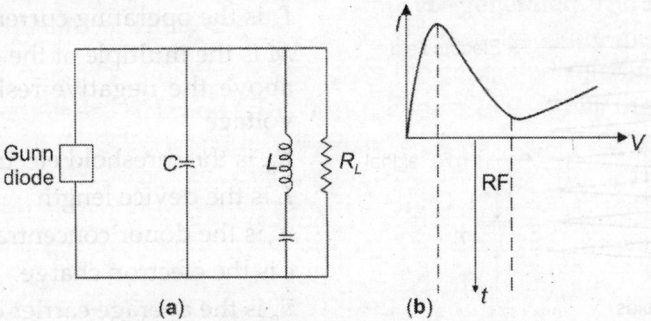

Fig. 15.15: Gunn diode in LSA mode

of doping and length n_oL is greater than $10^{12}/cm^2$ and the ratio of doping/frequency is between 2×10^4 and 2×10^5, the high-field domains and the space charge layers do not have sufficient time to build up. In order to dissipate the space charge, the magnitude of the RF voltage must be large enough to drive the diode below threshold during each cycle but also small enough, when the RF voltage is above threshold during the portion of each cycle, in order to prevent the domain formation and space-charge accumulation. The primary accumulation layer forms near the cathode. The rest of the sample remains fairly homogeneous. Thus, *with limited space-charge formation*, the remainder of the specimen appears as a series negative resistance that increases the frequency of oscillation in the resonant circuit.

In the LSA mode, the diode is placed in a resonator tuned to an oscillation frequency of f_o given by

$$f_o = 1/\tau_o \qquad (15.19)$$

The device is biased to several times the threshold value as shown in Fig. 15.16.

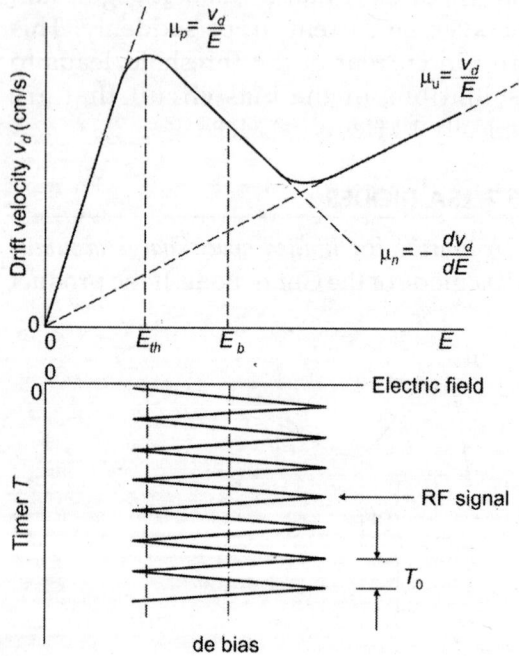

Fig. 15.16: LSA mode operation of a Gunn diode

As the RF voltage swings beyond the threshold value, the space charge starts building up at the cathode. The oscillation period τ_o of the RF signal is less than the domain-growth time constant τ_g. Hence the total voltage swings below the threshold before the domain can form. Moreover, τ_o is much larger than the dielectric relaxation time τ_d. Hence, the accumulated charge is drained in a very small fraction of the RF cycle. Therefore, the device for the most of the RF cycle is in the negative resistance region, and the space charge is not allowed to build up. The frequency of oscillation in the LSA mode is independent of the transit time of the carriers. It is solely determined by the external circuit. The output power in the LSA mode is greater than that in other modes.

15.7.1 Limitations of LSA Mode

The limitations of LSA mode are:
  (i) It is very sensitive to load conditions, temperatures and doping fluctuations
  (ii) The RF field must allow the field to build up quickly in order to prevent domain formation

15.7.2 Output Power of LSA Oscillator

The power output of an LSA oscillator is given by

$$P = \eta V_o I_o = \eta (ME_{th}L)(n_o e v_o A) \qquad (15.20)$$

where
  η is the dc-to-RF conversion efficiency
  V_o is the operating voltage
  I_o is the operating current
  M is the multiple of the operating voltage above the negative-resistance threshold voltage
  E_{th} is the threshold electric field
  L is the device length
  n_o is the donor concentration
  e is the electron charge
  v_o is the average carrier drift velocity
  A is the device area

For an LSA oscillator, n_0 is mainly determined by the desired operating frequency f_0 so that, for a properly designed circuit, peak power output is directly proportional to the volume (LA) of the active layer. Active volume cannot be increased indefinitely because of practical considerations. The power capabilities of LSA oscillators vary from 6 kW of pulse power at 1.75 GHz to 400 W of pulse power at 51 GHz.

15.8 InP DIODES

Basically both the GaAs diode and InP diode operate the same way in a circuit with dc voltages applied to the electrodes. The two-valley model theory is the basis for explaining the electrical behaviour of GaAs Gunn diode. However, the InP and alloys of indium gallium antimonide work as three-level devices. Figure 15.17 shows the three-valley model of InP. It is seen that InP has an upper valley energy level and a lower-valley energy level similar to n-type GaAs and also has a third middle-valley energy level.

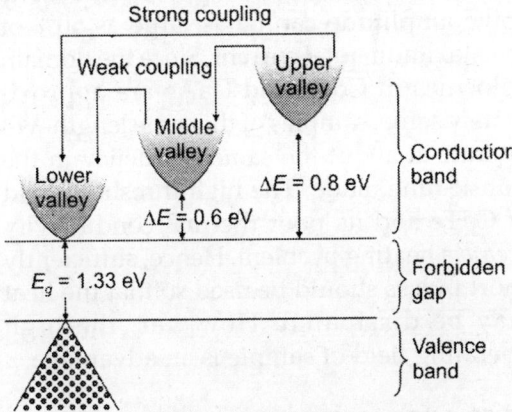

Fig.15.17: Three-valley model of InP diode

In GaAs, the electron transfer process from the lower valley to the upper valley is comparatively slow. At a particular voltage above the threshold, current flow consists of a larger contribution of electrons from the lower valley. Because of this larger contribution, relatively low peak-to-valley current ratio results. This is shown in Fig. 15.18.

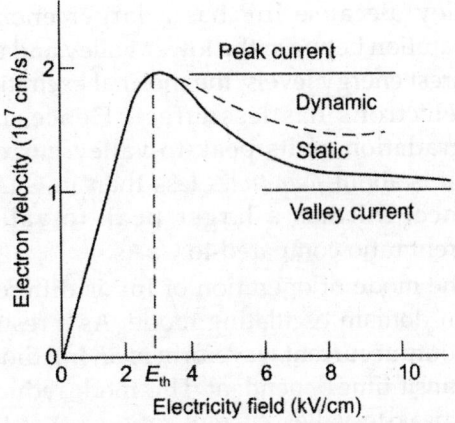

Fig. 15.18: Peak-to-valley current for n-type GaAs

Figure 15.19 shows the peak-to-valley current ratio of the InP diode. It has a larger peak-to-valley current ratio because an electron transfer occurs rapidly as the field increases. This is because the coupling between the lower and upper valley in InP is weaker than in GaAs. The middle-valley energy level provides the additional energy loss mechanism required to avoid breakdown caused by the high energies acquired by lower-valley electrons from the weak coupling. From Fig. 15.17, it can be seen that the lower valley is weakly coupled to the middle valley but strongly coupled to the upper valley to prevent breakdown, this ensures that under normal operating conditions, electrons concentrate in the middle

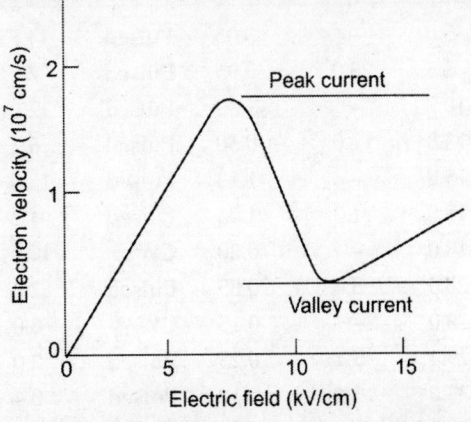

Fig. 15.19: Peak-to-valley current for n-type InP

valley. Because InP has a larger energy separation between the lower valley and the nearest energy levels, the thermal excitation of electrons has less effect. Hence, the degradation of its peak-to-valley current ratio is about *four times* less than in GaAs. Hence, InP has a larger peak-to-valley current ratio compared to GaAs.

The mode of operation of InP is different from domain oscillating mode. As a result, the output current waveform of an InP diode is transit-time dependent. This mode reduces the peak-to-valley current ratio so that the efficiency is reduced. Because of this, it is operated in a mode where charge domains are not formed. The three-valley model of InP inhibits the formation of domains because the stronger coupling increases the electron diffusion coefficient. Experimentally it was found that the epitaxial InP oscillators operate through a transit-time phenomenon and do not oscillate in a bulk mode of the LSA type. By adjusting the cavity size, the InP oscillator can be tuned over a large frequency range, bounded only by the thickness. Table 15.3 summarizes the highest power and efficiencies for InP diodes.

Table 15.3: Performance characteristics of InP diode

Fre-quency GHz	Thick-ness μm	Power W	Operation	Effi-ciency %
5.5	–	3.05	Pulsed	14.7
8.5	28.0	0.95	Pulsed	7.0
10.75	–	1.33	Pulsed	12.0
13.8	11.0	0.50	Pulsed	6.3
15.0	–	1.13	Pulsed	15.0
18.0	11.0	1.05	Pulsed	4.2
18.0	–	0.20	CW	10.2
25.0	5.4	0.65	Pulsed	2.6
26.0	–	0.15	CW	6.0
29.4	5.4	0.23	Pulsed	2.0
33.0	5.4	0.10	Pulsed	0.4
37.0	–	0.01	CW	1.0

15.9 CdTe DIODES

In 1963, Gunn observed the Gunn effect. Since then, the same effect has been observed in *n*-type InP, *n*-type CdTe, alloys of *n*-GaAs and *n*-GaP and in InAs. In *n*-type cadmium telluride, the Gunn effect was observed in samples of 250 to 300 μm long with carrier concentration of $5 \times 10^{14}/cm^3$ and a room temperature mobility of 1000 cm²/Vs. Extensive studies of Gunn effect on CdTe over a wide range of sample doping levels and lengths have confirmed that the Gunn effect occurs in CdTe in the same manner as in GaAs. From the two-valley model theory of CdTe, the <000> minimum is the lowest in energy. The effective mass $m_e = 0.11m$ (electron mass) and the intrinsic mobility $\mu \approx 1100$ cm²/V·s. The <111> minima are the next lowest energy, being 0.51 eV higher than <000> minimum. A major difference between CdTe and GaAs is a higher threshold field of about 13 kV/cm for CdTe compared to 3 kV/cm for GaAs. The ratio of peak-to-valley current is higher in CdTe. The spike amplitude can be as large as 50% of the maximum total current. Since the domain velocities in CdTe and GaAs are approximately same, samples of the same length will operate at about the same frequency in the transit-time mode. The high threshold field of CdTe and its poor thermal conductivity create a heating problem. Hence, sufficiently short pulses should be used so that the heat may be dissipated. However, the high operating field of sample is an advantage.

15.10 MICROWAVE GENERATION AND AMPLIFICATION

If the applied electric field is less than the threshold, the Gunn diode sample is stable. However, if the electric field is greater than the threshold value, the sample is unstable and divides up into two domains of different conductivity and different electric field but of the same drift velocity. Figure 15.20 shows the stable and unstable regions of a Gunn

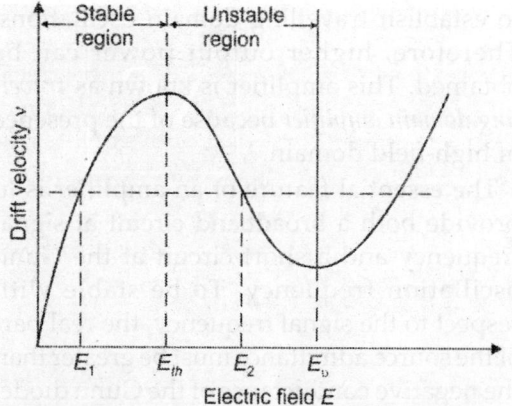

Fig. 15.20: Stable and unstable regions of a Gunn diode

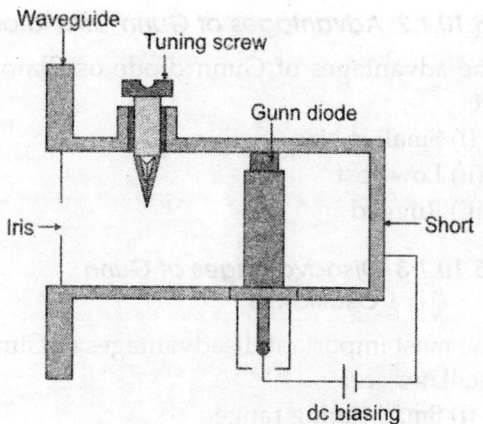

Fig.15.21: Gunn diode oscillator

diode. Initially when the accumulation layer is formed near the cathode, the electric field to the left of the layer decreases and that to its right increases. This process continues as the layer travels from the cathode towards the anode. After the anode collects the layer, the electric field in the whole sample is higher than the threshold. A new dipole field is formed again near the cathode and the process is repeated.

15.10.1 Microwave Generation— Gunn Diode Oscillator

Gunn diode oscillator circuits consist of (i) a resonant cavity, (ii) an input-coupling arrangement, (iii) a diode bias circuit and (iv) an output-coupling arrangement. The most widely used Gunn diode oscillator circuit is the postcoupled rectangular waveguide cavity. The waveguide cavity is terminated with an adjustable short at one end and by an iris at the other end as shown in Fig. 15.21. The diode is mounted at the center perpendicular to the broad wall where the electric field component is the maximum under the dominant TE_{10} mode. The intrinsic frequency f_o of the oscillations depends on the electron drift velocity v_d and the effective length L. Thus,

$$f_o = v_d/L \qquad (15.21)$$

$v_d = 10^7$ cm/sec for GaAs. The cavity is normally tuned to f_o by adjusting the position of the short. A tuning screw is provided perpendicularly at the center of the broad wall for fine frequency tuning. The total resistive loading R_L from the cavity and external load should be around 20% higher than the Gunn diode resistance $-R_j$ such that the net resistance $-R_L R_j/(R_L - R_j)$ is negative. The cavity transforms the high impedance of the output waveguide to the required value for the Gunn diode. The Gunn diode is placed on a metal post. The top of the post is insulated from the waveguide to provide RF bypass capacitance and the dc bias voltage is applied to the post. The degree of output coupling is adjusted by selecting proper dimensions of the iris. The output power of a Gunn oscillator is limited by the heat dissipation from the small chip. It delivers 10 W at 30 to 40 GHz and a pulsed power of 100 to 200 W.

15.10.1.1 Typical Characteristics

The characteristics of the Gunn diode oscillators are:
   (i) Frequency of operation: 20 to 100 GHz
  (ii) Efficiency (Pulse): 29%
                        (CW): 5.2%
 (iii) Continuous power: 10 W at 20–40 GHz
 (iv) Pulsed power: 100 W to 200 W

15.10.1.2 Advantages of Gunn Oscillators

The advantages of Gunn diode oscillators are:

(i) Small in size

(ii) Low cost

(iii) Rugged

15.10.1.3 Disadvantages of Gunn Oscillators

The most important disadvantages of Gunn oscillator are:

(i) Small tuning range

(ii) High noise

(iii) Low efficiency at $f_0 > 10$ GHz

(iv) Large dependence of frequency on temperature

15.10.1.4 Applications

The Gunn diode oscillators are used in

(i) Radar transmitters

(ii) Low and medium power oscillators

(iii) Parametric amplifiers as pump source

(iv) Broadband linear amplifiers

15.10.2 Microwave Amplification

When an RF signal is applied to a Gunn oscillator, amplification occurs provided that the signal frequency is low enough to allow the space charge in the domain to readjust itself. There is a critical value of fL above which the device will not amplify. Below this frequency limit, the sample has an impedance with negative real part and is utilized for amplification. If $n_oL < 10^{12}/cm^2$, domain formation is inhibited. The device exhibits a non-uniform field distribution that is stable with respect to time and space. Such a diode can amplify signals in the vicinity of transit-time frequency and its harmonics without any oscillation. However, the power output of a stable amplifier is quite low.

The Gunn diode must oscillate at the transit-time frequency while it is amplifying the signal at some other frequency. The value of n_oL must be greater than $10^{12}/cm^2$ in order to establish travelling domain oscillations. Therefore, higher output power can be obtained. This amplifier is known as *travelling domain amplifier* because of the presence of high-field domain.

The essential feature of an amplifier is to provide both a broadband circuit at signal frequency and a short circuit at the Gunn oscillation frequency. To be stable with respect to the signal frequency, the real part of the source admittance must be greater than the negative conductance of the Gunn diode. Figure 15.22 shows the simplest circuit satisfying this condition. The gain between 5.5 GHz and 6.5 GHz is about 3 dB.

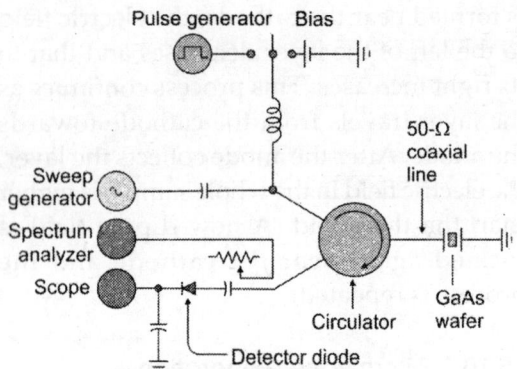

Fig. 15.22: Gunn diode amplifier circuit

15.10.2.1 Typical Characteristics of Gunn Diode Amplifier

The typical characteristics of a Gunn diode amplifier are:

(i) It can be used in conjunction with circulator-coupled networks

(ii) The gain-bandwidth product is greater than 10 dB from 4 to 16 GHz.

(iii) Linear gains of 6 to 12 dB per stage is achievable.

Table 15.4 lists the performance of several amplifiers.

15.11 NUMERICAL EXAMPLES

Example 15.1: The drift velocity of electrons in a Gunn diode is 3×10^7 cm/sec. The length

Table 15.4: CW Gunn diode amplifier performance in different frequency of band

Frequency band	3 dB band width GHz	Small signal gain dB	Power gain dB	Efficiency %
C	4.5–8.0	8	3.0	3.0
X	7.5–10.75	12	1.65	2.3
	8.0–12.0	6	1.8	2.5
Ku	12.0–16.0	6	1.5	2.5
	13.0–15.0	8	0.36	2.0

of the active region is 12×10^{-4} cm. Calculate the natural frequency of the diode and the critical voltage. Assume a critical electric field of 3.2 kV/cm.

Solution: Given: $v_d = 3 \times 10^7$, $L = 12 \times 10^{-4}$

(a) The natural frequency f_0 of the diode is given by
$$f_0 = v_d/L = 3 \times 10^7/12 \times 10^{-4}$$
$$= 25 \text{ GHz}$$

(b) The critical voltage V_c is given by
$$V_c = L \times \text{critical electric field}$$
$$= 12 \times 10^{-4} \times 3.2 \times 10^3$$
$$= 3.84 \text{ V}.$$

Example 15.2: A Gunn diode has $L = 0.5$ mm and $v_d = 10^7$ m/s. The critical electric field is 3.2 kV/cm. Calculate the natural frequency of the diode and the critical voltage.

Solution: Given: $v_d = 10^7$, $L = 5 \times 10^{-4}$, $E_c = 3.2 \times 10^3$ V/cm

(a) The natural frequency f_0 of the diode is given by
$$f_0 = v_d/L = 10^7/5 \times 10^{-4}$$
$$= 20 \text{ GHz}$$
The critical voltage V_c is given by
$$V_c = L \times \text{critical electric field}$$
$$= 5 \times 10^{-4} \times (3.2 \times 10^3)$$
$$= 1.6 \text{ V}$$

Example 15.3: A Gunn diode in transit time mode operates at 10 GHz. The drift velocity is 10^7 cm/s. Calculate the length of the device.

Solution: Given: $f = 10^{10}$, $v_d = 10^7$ cm/s
$$L = v_d/f = 10^7/10^{10} = 10^{-3} \text{ cm}$$
$$= 0.01 \text{ mm}$$

Example 15.4: A Gunn diode oscillator operates at 10 GHz with $v_d = 10^7$ cm/s. Find the length of the active region and the required dc voltage for oscillations for a critical electric field of 3.2 kV/cm.

Solution: Given: $f = 10^{10}$, $v_d = 10^7$ cm/s, $E_c = 3.2$ kV/cm.

(a) $L = v_d/f = 10^7/10^{10} = 10^{-3}$ cm
$$= 0.01 \text{ mm}$$

(b) $V_c = L \times E_c = 10^{-3} \times (3.2 \times 10^3)$
$$= 3.2 \text{ V}$$

Example 15.5: A Gunn diode operating at 10 GHz, generates 100 mW RF output with 3% efficiency. Assume $E_c = 3.2$ kV/cm and $v_d = 10^5$ m/s. Find L, V_c, V_{bias}, P_{dc}, power dissipated as heat and I_{bias}.

Solution: Given: $f = 10$ GHz, $v_d = 10^5$ m/s, $E_{th} = 3.2$ kV/cm, $P_{rf} = 100$ mW, $\eta = 0.03$

(a) $L = v_d/f = 10^5/10 \times 10^9$
$$= 10^{-5} \text{ m} = 10^{-3} \text{ cm} = 0.01 \text{ mm}$$

(b) $V_c = E_c L = 3200 \times 10^{-3} = 3.2$ V

(c) $V_{bias} \approx 3 V_c = 9.6$ V

(d) $P_{dc} = P_{rf}/\eta = 100 \times 10^{-3}/0.03 = 3.3$ W

(e) $I_{bias} = P_{dc}/V_{bias} = 3.3/9.6 = 0.344$ A

(f) $P_d = P_{dc} - P_{rf} = 3.3 - 0.1 = 3.2$ W

Example 15.6: An *n*-type GaAs diode has $\mu_l = 8000 \times 10^{-4}$, $\mu_u = 180 \times 10^{-4}$, $n_l = 10^{16}/\text{cm}^3$, $n_u = 10^{14}/\text{cm}^3$ and $T = 300$ °K. Find the conductivity of the diode.

Solution: Given: $\mu_l = 8000 \times 10^{-4}$, $\mu_u = 180 \times 10^{-4}$, $n_l = 10^{16}/\text{cm}^3$, $n_u = 10^{14}/\text{cm}^3$ and $T = 300$ K.

The conductivity
$$\sigma = e(\mu_l n_l + \mu_u n_u)$$
$$= 1.6 \times 10^{-19} \times (8000 \times 10^{-4} \times 10^{16} + 180 \times 10^{-4} \times 10^{14})$$
$$= 1.6 \times 10^{-19} \times 8000 \times 10^{-4} \times 10^{16},$$
since $n_l \gg \mu_u n_u$
$$= 1.28 \text{ m mhos}$$

Example 15.7: An LSA oscillator has the conversion efficiency $\eta = 0.06$, multiplication factor $M = 3.5$, threshold field $E_{th} = 320$ kV/m, device length $L = 10$ μm, donor concentration $n_o = 10^{21}$ m^3, average carrier velocity $v_o = 1.5 \times 10^5$ m/s and area $A = 3 \times 10^{-8}$m^2. Find the output power.

Solution: Given: $\eta = 0.06$, $M = 3.5$, $E_{th} = 320$ kV/m, $L = 10$ μm, $n_o = 10^{21}$ m^3, $v_o = 1.5 \times 10^5$ m/s, area $A = 3 \times 10^{-8}$m^2.

The output power is given by

$P = \eta(ME_{th}L)(n_o ev_o A)$

$= 0.06 \times (3.5 \times 320 \times 10^3 \times 10 \times 10^{-6}) \times$

$\quad (10^{21} \times 1.6 \times 10^{-19} \times 1.5 \times 10^5 \times 3 \times 10^{-8})$

$= 0.06 \times (11.2) \times (7.2 \times 10^{-1})$

$= \mathbf{484\ mW}$

KEY POINTS

- The common characteristic of all the active two terminal solid-state microwave devices is their negative resistance.
- Transferred electron devices that exhibit negative resistance property are: (i) bulk devices with no junctions or gates; (ii) fabricated from compound semiconductors such as Gallium Arsenide (GaAs), Indium Phosphide (InP) or Cadmium Telluride (CdTe).
- Gunn effect is the periodic fluctuation of current passing through a uniform n-type GaAs specimen when the applied voltage is exceeded a certain critical or threshold value.
- The fundamental concept of RWH theory is that the differential negative resistance is developed in a bulk solid-state III-V compound when either a voltage (or electric field) or current is applied to the terminals of the sample.
- Based on the RWH theory, the band structure must satisfy the following three criteria in order to exhibit negative resistance:
  (i) The separation energy between the bottoms of the lower and the upper valleys must be several times larger than the thermal energy (0.026 eV) at room temperature. That is $\Delta E \gg kT$ or $\Delta E \gg 0.026$ eV.
  (ii) The separation energy between valleys must be smaller than the gap energy between the conduction and valence bonds. That is $\Delta E < E_g$.
  (iii) Electrons in the lower valley must have high mobility, small effective mass and low density of state whereas those in the upper valley must have low mobility, large effective mass and high density of state.
- The four modes of operation of uniformly doped bulk diodes with low-resistance contacts are: (i) Gunn oscillator mode or transit time mode, (ii) Stable amplification mode, (iii) Limited Space-charge Accumulation mode and (iv) Bias-circuit oscillation mode.
- The limitations of LSA mode are: (i) It is very sensitive to load conditions, temperature and doping fluctuations and (ii) The RF field must allow the field to build up quickly in order to prevent domain formation
- The typical characteristics of the Gunn diode oscillators are: (i) Frequency of operation is 20 to 100 GHz, (ii) Efficiency (Pulse) is 29% and for CW is 5.2%, (iii) Continuous power is 10 W at 20 to 40 GHz and (iv)Pulsed power is 100 W to 200 W.
- The advantages of Gunn diode oscillators are: (i) Small in size, (ii) Low cost and (iii) Rugged.
- The disadvantages of Gunn diode oscillators are: (i) Small tuning range, (ii) High noise, (iii) Low efficiency above 10 GHz and (iv) Large dependance of operating frequency on temperature.
- The Gunn diode oscillators are used in (i) Radar transmitters, (ii) Low and medium power oscillators, (iii) Parametric amplifiers as pump source and (iv) Broad-band linear amplifiers.

FURTHER READING

1. Liao SY (1990). *Semiconductor Electron Devices*, PH, NJ.
2. Collins RE (1996). *Foundations of Microwave Engineering*, McGraw Hill, NY.
3. Eastman LF (1973). *Gallium Arsenide Microwave Bulk and Transit Time Devices*, Artech, Mass.
4. Hilsun C (1962). Transferred Electron Amplifiers and Oscillators, Proc. IEEE, vol. 50, pp 185–189.
5. Navon DH (1986). *Semiconductor Microdevices and Materials*, HRW, NY.
6. Soohoo RF (1971). *Microwave Electronics*, Addison-Wesley, Mass.
7. Streetman BG (2000). *Solid State Electronic Devices*, PH, NJ.
8. Sze SM (1985). *Semiconductor Devices: Physics and Technology*, John Wiley, NY.

REVIEW QUESTIONS

15.1 What is the common characteristic of all active solid-state devices for use as microwave generators?

15.2 What is the difference between a positive resistor and a negative resistor?

15.3 Define Gunn effect.

15.4 State the RWH theory.

15.5 Mention the two modes of negative resistance devices.

15.6 What is two-valley model theory?

15.7 Why Si and Ge are not used as negative resistance devices?

15.8 What is high field domain? When is it formed?

15.9 State two properties of high-field domain.

15.10 What are the four modes of Gunn diode?

15.11 Draw the equivalent circuit of a Gunn diode.

15.12 Draw the V-I characteristic of a Gunn diode.

15.13 Give the performance characteristics of a Gunn diode.

15.14 What are the advantages of a Gunn diode?

15.15 What are the disadvantages of a Gunn diode?

15.16 Give the applications of a Gunn diode.

15.17 What is an LSA diode?

15.18 What are the limitations of LSA diode?

15.19 What is a three-valley model theory?

15.20 What is the difference between InP and GaAs diode?

15.21 Mention two advantages of Gunn diode amplifier.

DESCRIPTIVE QUESTIONS

15.1 What is Gunn effect? Describe construction and operation of a Gunn diode

15.2 Explain the RWH theory.

15.3 Explain the two-valley model theory.

15.4 What are the properties of high-field domain?

15.5 Explain the four modes of operation of Gunn diodes.

15.6 Explain the operation of LSA diode.

15.7 Explain the three-valley model theory.

15.8 Draw the circuit of a Gunn diode oscillator and explain its operation.

15.9 Draw the circuit of a Gunn diode amplifier and explain its operation.

PRACTICE PROBLEMS

15.1 The drift velocity of electrons in a Gunn diode is 2×10^7 cm/sec. The length of the active region is 10×10^{-4} cm. Calculate the natural frequency of the diode and the critical voltage. $E_c = 9.2/2$ kV.
[**Ans:** 20 GHz, 3.2 V]

15.2 A Gunn diode has $l = 1$ mm and $v_d = 10^7$ m/s. The critical electric field is 3 kV/cm. Calculate the natural frequency of the diode and the critical voltage.
[**Ans:** 10 GHz, 3 V]

15.3 A Gunn diode in transit time mode operates at 12 GHz. The drift velocity is 10^5 m/s. Calculate (a) the length of the device. (b) Can the device work at 10 and 14 GHz? (c) Which is the mode of operation in each case?
[**Ans:**(a) 8.33 m, (b) (i) Delayed mode, (ii) Quenched mode]

15.4 A Gunn diode oscillator operates at 8 GHz with $V_d = 10^7$ m/s. Find the length of the active region and the required dc voltage for oscillations for a critical electric field is 3 kV/cm.
[**Ans:** 1.25 mm, 3.75 V]

15.5 A Gunn diode operating at 5 GHz generates 200 mW RF output with 3% efficiency. Assume $E_{th} = 3$ kV/cm and $v_d = 10^7$ cm/sec. Find L, V_{th}, V_{bias}, P_{dc}, power dissipated as heat and I_{bias}.
[Ans: $L = \mathbf{0.02}$ **mm**, $V_{th} = \mathbf{6}$ **V**, $V_{bias} = \mathbf{18}$ **V**, $P_{dc} = \mathbf{6.7}$ **W**, $I_{bias} = \mathbf{0.372}$ **A**, $P_d = \mathbf{6.5}$ **W**]

15.6 An LSA oscillator has the conversion efficiency $\eta = 0.06$, multiplication factor $M = 3.5$, threshold field $E_{th} = 320$ kV/m, device length $L = 12$ μm, donor concentration $n_o = 10^{21}$ m^3, average carrier velocity $v_o = 1.5 \times 10^5$ m/s and area $A = 3 \times 10^{-8}$ m^2. Find the output power (**Ans:** 581 mW)

15.7 For a transit-time domain mode, the domain velocity is equal to the carrier drift velocity and is about 10^7 cm/sec. Calculate the drift length of the diode at a frequency of 8 GHz. (**Ans:** 1.25 mm)

REFERENCE

1. Berenz JJ et al (1978). Ion implanted *p-n* junction indium phosphide IMPATT, *Electron. Lett.*, vol. 34, p 683–684.

2. Das A and Das SK (2004). *Microwave Engineering*, TMH, New Delhi.

3. Esaki L (1958). New phenomenon in narrow Ge *p-n* junction, *Phys. Rev.*, Vol. 109, p 603.

4. Gunn JB (1963). Microwave Oscillations of Current in III–IV Semiconductors, Solid State Comm., Vol.1, p 88–91.

5. IEEE Proc. Vol.70, No.1, Jan., 1962. Special Issue on Very Fast Solid State Technology.

6. IEEE Trans. Electron Devices, (1980 Feb.) Special Issue on Microwave Solid State Devices, ED-27, No. 2.

7. IEEE Trans. Electron Devices, (1980 Jun.) Special Issue on Microwave Solid State Devices, ED-27, No. 6.

8. IEEE Trans. Electron Devices, (1981 Feb.) Special Issue on Microwave Solid State Devices, ED-28, No. 2.

9. IEEE Trans. Electron Devices, (1981 Aug.) Special Issue on Microwave Solid State Devices, ED-28, No.8.

10. De Loach, B.C. Jr., (1967) Recent advances in solid state microwave generators, *Advances in Microwaves*, Vol. 2, Academic Press, NY.

11. Milnes, A.G., (1980) *Semiconductor Devices and Integrated Electronics*, Van Nostrand, NY.

12. Kroemer, H., (1959) The Physical Principles of Amplifier, Proc. IRE, Vol.47, p 397–406, Mar.

13. Gunn, J.B., (1966) Effect of domain and circuit properties on oscillations in GaAs, *IBMJ, Res. Dev.*, p 310–320.

14. Copland, J.A., (Jan.,1967) Continuous wave operation of LSA oscillator diodes – 44-88 GHz, *Bell Sys. Tech. J.*, Vol. 46, p 284–287.

15. Wilson, W.E., (1971 Aug.) Pulsed LSA and TRAPATT sources for microwave systems, *Microwave J.*, Vol. 46, p 87–90.

Avalanche Transit Time Devices

Objectives

- Classify the ATTDs.
- Explain the principle of operation of ATTDs.
- Understand their applications.
- Compare their characteristics.

16.1 INTRODUCTION

Ever since the development of modern semi-conductor device theory, scientists were carrying out research works to develop a two-terminal negative resistance device. The first such practical device realized was the tunnel diode. Its operation depends on the properties of a forward-biased *p-n* junction in which both *p* and *n* regions are heavily doped. The other two devices are the transferred electron devices and the ava-lanche transit-time devices. In the previous chapter, we have studied in detail the transferred electron devices. In this chapter, we shall discuss the avalanche transit-time devices.

16.2 AVALANCHE TRANSIT TIME DEVICES (ATTD)

The avalanche transit time devices are *pn* junction diodes with heavily doped *p* and *n* regions operated under the reverse bias condition. Its operation depends on the effect of breakdown across the reverse biased

junction to produce a supply of electrons and holes.

The transferred electron device or Gunn oscillator operates by the application of a dc voltage to a bulk semiconductor specimen. There is no *p-n* junction in this device. Its frequency is a function of the load and of natural frequency of the circuit.

The avalanche diode oscillator uses a carrier impact ionization and drift in the high-field region of a semiconductor junction to produce negative resistance. This device was first proposed in 1958 by Read in a theoretical paper in which he analyzed the negative resistance proper-ties of an idealized n^+-p-i-p^+ diode. Two distinct modes of avalanche oscillator are the *impact ionization avalanche transit-time* (IMPATT) mode and the other *trapped plasma avalanche triggered transit* (TRAPATT) mode. In the IMPATT mode, the typical dc-to-RF conversion efficiency with silicon diodes is 5% to 10% and frequency of operation is as high as 100 GHz. In the TRAPATT mode, the typical dc-to-RF conversion efficiency is 20% to 75% and the frequency of operation is up to 10 GHz.

Another type of active microwave device is the *barrier injected transit-time* (BARITT) diode. It has long drift regions similar to those of IMPATT diodes. The carriers traversing the drift region of BARITT diodes are generated by minority carrier injection from forward-biased junctions.

16.2.1 Types of ATTDs

The four types of ATTDs are:
  (i) Read diode
 (ii) Impact avalanche transit time (IMPATT) devices
(iii) Trapped plasma avalanche triggered transit time (TRAPTT) devices
(iv) Barrier injection transit time (BARITTT) devices

16.3 READ DIODE

Read diode is the first avalanche diode theoretically proposed by Read in 1958. However, the experimental diode was developed in 1965. A study of this diode will be of much help in understanding the basic operating principle of the IMPATT diode. Fig. 16.1 shows the structure, field distribution and doping profile of a Read diode.

16.3.1 Physical Description

The Read diode is an n^+-p-i-n^+ structure. The *plus* sign indicates very high doping and i or v refers to intrinsic material. This device consists of essentially two regions. One is the thin p region at which avalanche multiplication occurs. Hence, this region is known as *avalanche region* or *high-domain region*. The other region is the i or v region through which the generated holes must drift while moving to the p^+ contact. This region is known as *drift region* or *intrinsic region*. The space between the n^+-p junction and the i-p^+ junction is known as *the space charge region*. The Read diode can also be a p^+-n-i-p^+ structure.

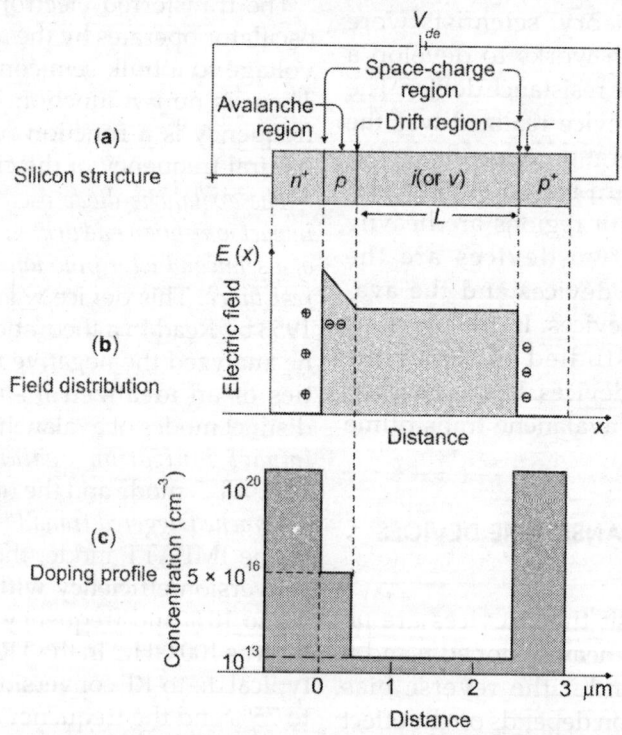

Fig. 16.1: Read diode structure, field distribution and doping profile

The Read diode oscillator consists of an n^+-p-i-n^+ diode reverse-biased and mounted in a microwave cavity. The impedance of the diode is mainly capacitive and that of the cavity is inductive. They are matched together to form a resonant circuit. The device produces a negative resistance that delivers power from the dc bias voltage to the oscillation.

16.3.2 Avalanche Multiplication

When the reverse-biased voltage is much above the breakdown or punch-through voltage, the space charge region extends from the n^+-p region through the p and i regions to the i-p^+ junction. Fig. 16.1(b) shows the fixed charges in the various regions. A positive charge gives a rising field in moving from left to right. The maximum field that occurs at the n^+-p junction is about several hundred kilovolts per centimeter. Carriers or holes moving in the high field near the n^+-p junction acquire enough energy to knock the valence electrons to the conduction band and produces electron-hole pairs. The rate of electron-hole pair production is known as *avalanche multiplication*. It is sensitive non-linear function of the electric field. By proper doping, the electric field can be given a sufficiently sharp peak so that the avalanche multiplication is confined to a very narrow region at the n^+-p junction. The electrons move into the n^+ region and the holes drift through the space charge region to the p^+ region with a constant velocity v_d of about 10^7 cm/s for silicon. The electric field throughout the space charge region is about 5 kV/cm.

The transit time of a hole across the drift i-region of length L is given by

$$\tau = L/v_d \tag{16.1}$$

The avalanche multiplication factor is given by

$$M = 1/[1 - (V/V_b)^n] \tag{16.2}$$

where

V is the applied voltage

V_b is the avalanche breakdown voltage

n is a numerical factor that depends on the doping of p^+-n or n^+-p junction and ranges from 3 to 6 for silicon.

The avalanche breakdown voltage for a silicon p^+-n junction is given by

$$|V_b| = (\rho_n \mu_n \varepsilon_s |E_{b\max}^2|/2) \tag{16.3}$$

where

ρ_n is the resistivity

μ_n is the electron mobility

ε_s is the semiconductor permittivity

$E_{b\max}^2$ is the maximum breakdown electric field

Fig. 16.2 shows the avalanche breakdown voltage for several semiconductors as a function of impurity at a p^+-n junction.

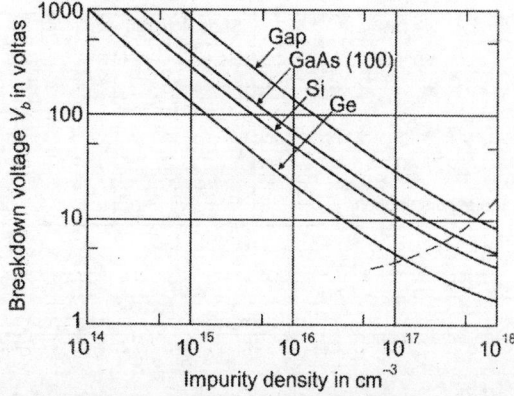

Fig. 16.2: Breakdown voltage versus doping

16.3.3 Carrier Current and External Current

Figure 16.3 shows the structure, field distribution and currents in a Read diode The Read diode is mounted in a microwave resonant circuit. At a given frequency, an ac voltage is maintained in the circuit. The total field across the diode is the sum of the ac and dc fields. If the total field is above the breakdown voltage, it causes breakdown at the p^+-n junction during the positive half cycle of the ac voltage. The carrier or hole current $I_0(t)$ is generated at the n^+-p junction by avalanche multiplication and it grows exponentially with time while the field continues to be above the critical value. During the negative half cycle, the field is below the breakdown voltage and the carrier current $I_0(t)$ decays exponentially to a small steady-state value. The carrier current $I_0(t)$ is the current at the junction only and is in the form of a pulse of very short duration as shown in Fig. 16.3(d). Hence, the carrier current $I_0(t)$ reaches the maximum value in the middle of the ac voltage cycle or 90° later than the voltage. The generated holes, under the influence of the electric field, are injected into the space-charge region towards the negative terminal. As the injected holes traverse the drift space, they induce a current $I_e(t)$ in the external circuit as shown in Fig. 16.3(d).

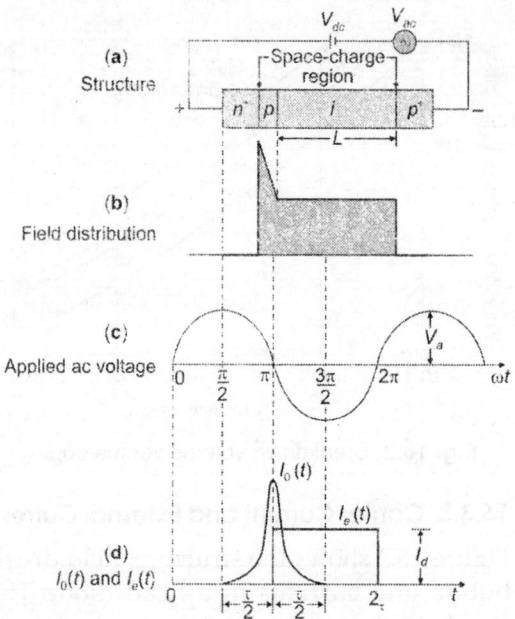

Fig. 16.3: Structure, field distribution and currents in Read diode

When the holes generated at n^+-p junction drifts through the space-charge region, they reduce the field in accordance with the Poisson's equation

$$dE/dx = -\rho/\varepsilon_r \qquad (16.4)$$

where ρ is the volume charge density and ε_r is the semiconductor permittivity. The drift velocity of the holes in the space-charge region is constant. Hence, the induced current $I_e(t)$ in the external circuit is equal to

$$I_e(t) = Q/\tau = v_d Q/L \qquad (16.5)$$

where

Q is the total charge of the moving holes
v_d is the hole drift velocity
L is the length of the drift i region.

The induced current $I_e(t)$ in the external circuit is equal to the average current in the space-charge region. When the pulse of hole current $I_0(t)$ is suddenly generated at the n^+-p junction, a constant current $I_e(t)$ starts flowing in the external circuit. It continues to flow during the time τ in which the holes are moving across the space-charge region. Because of moving holes, on the average, the external current $I_e(t)$ is delayed by $\tau/2$ or 90° relative to the pulsed carrier current $I_0(t)$ generated at the n^+-p junction. The carrier current is delayed by a quarter of a cycle or 90° relative to ac voltage, the external current $I_e(t)$ is then delayed 180° relative to the voltage as shown in Fig. 16.3(d). Hence, the resonator cavity should be tuned to give a resonant frequency of $2\pi f = \pi/\tau$. The frequency is given by

$$f = 1/2\tau = v_d/2L \qquad (16.6)$$

Thus, the external current $I_e(t)$ and the applied ac voltage are out of phase by 180°. Therefore, negative conductance occurs. Hence, the Read diode can be used for microwave oscillation and amplification. Assuming $v_d = 10^7$ cm/s for silicon, the optimum frequency for a Read diode with an i-region of length 2.5 μm is 20 GHz.

16.3.4 Output Power and Quality Factor

The external current $I_e(t)$ is negligible during the positive half cycle of the ac voltage and constant during the negative half cycle. Hence, it is almost a *square wave*. The direct current I_d supplied by the dc bias voltage is the average external or conductive current. Therefore, the amplitude of variations in $I_e(t)$ is approximately equal to I_d. If V_a is the amplitude of the ac voltage, the ac power delivered is given by

$$P = 0.707 V_a I_d \quad \text{W/unit area} \quad (16.7a)$$

The quality factor Q of a circuit is defined as

$$Q = \omega \frac{\text{Maximum stored energy}}{\text{Average dissipated power}} \quad (16.7b)$$

Since the Read diode supplies ac energy, it has a negative Q in contrast to the positive Q of the cavity circuit. As the amplitude of the ac voltage increases, the stored or oscillation energy increases faster than the energy delivered per cycle. This is the condition to be satisfied for stable operation of the Read diode.

16.4 IMPATT DIODES

IMPATT is the acronym for **IMP**act **A**valanche **T**ransit **T**ime. The IMPATT diodes exhibit a differential negative resistance by two different effects:

(i) The impact ionization avalanche effect. This causes the carrier current $I_0(t)$ and the ac voltage to be out of phase by 90°.

(ii) The transit-time effect. This further delays the external current $I_e(t)$ by 90° relative to ac voltage.

The IMPATT diodes are used for a wide range of frequency spectrum. Therefore, they have emerged as very powerful solid-state sources of microwaves, millimeter waves and sub-millimeter waves. The frequency ranges from 6 GHz to 450 GHz. The CW power output of an IMPATT diode is quite high. It can supply 12 W at 6 GHz, 1 W at 94 GHz and 2.2 mW at 412 GHz. The wide frequency range and high power output make the IMPATT diode a highly suitable device for present day communication needs.

IMPATT diodes may be n^+pip^+, p^+pnn^+, p^+nn^+ abrupt junction or p^+ip^+ structure. They are shown in Fig. 16.4 along with the doping profiles. These diodes may be fabricated

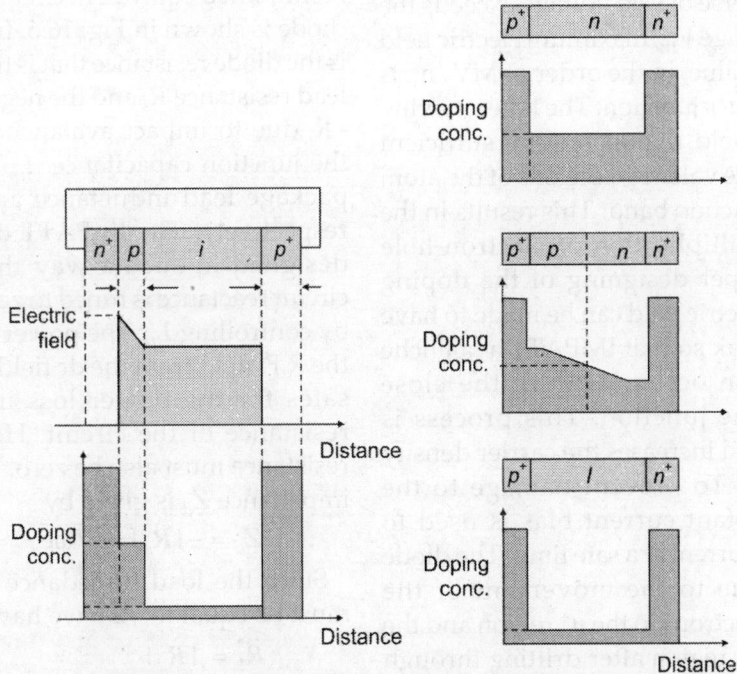

Fig. 16.4: IMPATT diode types and doping profile

from Ge, Si, GaAs or InP. However, GaAs provides highest efficiency, highest operating frequency and least noise figure. But the manufacturing process is more difficult and expansive than Si.

Figure 16.5 shows the typical constructional details of an p^+nn^+ IMPATT diode. It consists of a heavily doped p^+ region, a normally doped n region and heavily doped n^+ region. A metallized cathode and plated heat sink as anode are also provided.

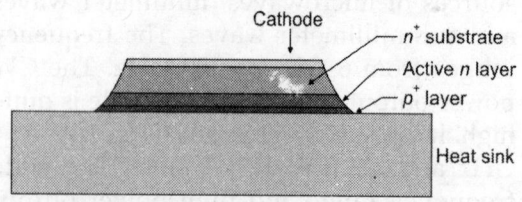

Fig. 16.5: Constructional details of an p^+nn^+ IMPATT diode

16.4.1 Mechanism of Operation

Figure 16.3 shows the electric field distribution, MW voltage and the external carrier flow when the n^+pip^+ diode is reverse biased. When the reverse biased voltage exceeds the threshold voltage V_{th}, maximum electric field of very high value, in the order of MV/m, is formed at the n^+p junction. The holes moving in this high field region acquire sufficient energy to excite valence electrons of the atom into the conduction band. This results in the avalanche multiplication of electron-hole pairs. By proper designing of the doping profile, the electric field can be made to have very sharp peak so that IMPATT avalanche multiplication occurs only in the close vicinity of the junction. This process is cumulative and increases the carrier density very rapidly. To prevent damage to the diode, a constant current bias is used to maintain the current at a safe limit. The diode current is due to the movement of the conduction electrons to the n^+ region and the holes to the p^+ region after drifting through the intrinsic space region.

The drift time τ is given by

$$\tau = L/v_d \qquad (16.8)$$

Here v_d is the drift velocity of the holes that is approximately equal to 10^5 m/sec. and L is the length of the drift region. If L is equal to 2 µm, then $\tau = 20$ ps. Thus, in the IMPATT diode negative resistance arises from two types of delays that cause the current to lag behind the applied voltage. The two types of delays are:

(i) Avalanche delay caused by finite build-up time of Avalanche current.

(ii) Transit time delay due to the finite time taken by the carriers to cross the drift region.

When these two delays add up to 180°, the diode electronic resistance becomes negative corresponding to that frequency.

IMPATT diodes are mounted in coaxial lines, wave-guides or micro-strip lines to form MW circuits for oscillation and amplification.

16.4.2 Equivalent Circuit

A simplified equivalent circuit of an IMPATT diode is shown in Fig. 16.6. In the circuit, R_d is the diode resistance that is the sum of series lead resistance R_s and the negative resistance $-R_j$ due to impact avalanche process. C_j is the junction capacitance. L_p and C_p are the package lead inductance and capacitance respectively. The IMPATT diode mount is designed in such a way that the overall circuit reactance is tuned to zero at resonance by controlling L_p. The power is extracted by the R.F. field from the dc field. This compensates for the power loss in the positive resistance of the circuit. Hence, the total resistance must also be zero. The diode chip impedance Z_d is given by

$$Z_d = -|R_d| - j/\omega C_j \qquad (16.9)$$

Since the load impedance $Z_L = R_L + jX_L$ must be equal to $-Z_d$, we have

$$R_L = |R_d| \qquad (16.10)$$

$$X_L = 1/\omega C_j \qquad (1611)$$

R_d varies with both signal current and bias voltage. Therefore, for a given load and bias voltage, stable oscillations are obtained when $|R_d| = R_L$. The corresponding peak R.F. current determines the load power. Since R_d is low (about 10 ohms), for the oscillations to be sustained, multi-section quarter-wave transformers are used for impedance matching between the diode circuit and the load as shown in Fig. 16.6.

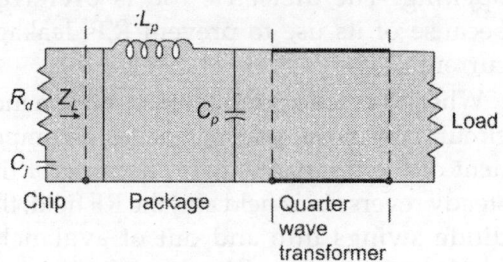

Fig. 16.6: Equivalent circuit

16.4.3 Power Output and Efficiency

Semiconductor materials and the attainable impedance levels in microwave circuitry limit the maximum output power of a single diode at a given frequency. For a uniform avalanche, the maximum voltage that can be applied across the diode is given by

$$V_m = E_m L \qquad (16.12)$$

where L is the depletion length and E_m is the maximum electric field. The breakdown voltage limits the maximum applied voltage. Moreover, the avalanche breakdown process also limits the maximum current that can be carried by the diode, because the current in the space-charge region causes an increase in the electric field. The maximum current is given by

$$I_m = J_m A = \sigma E_m A = \varepsilon_t E_m A/\tau$$
$$= v_d \varepsilon_s E_m A/L \qquad (16.13)$$

Hence, the upper limit of the power is given by

$$P_m = I_m V_m = E_m^2 \varepsilon_s v_d A \qquad (16.14)$$

The capacitance across the space charge region is given by

$$C = \varepsilon_s A/L \qquad (16.15)$$

Substituting $\varepsilon_s A = CL$ from Eq. (16.15) in Eq. (16.14) we get

$$P_m = E_m^2 v_d\, CL$$

Multiplying and dividing by v_d and substituting $L/v_d = \tau$, we get

$$P_m = E_m^2 v_d^2 \frac{CL}{v_d} = E_m^2 v_d^2 C\tau$$

Multiplying numerator and denominator by $(2\pi f)^2$ and substituting $2\pi f\tau = 1$, we obtain

$$P_m = E_m^2 v_d^2 (2\pi f)^2\, \tau \frac{C}{(2\pi f)^2}$$

$$= E_m^2 v_d^2 \frac{(2\pi fC)}{(2\pi f)^2}$$

$$= \frac{E_m^2 v_d^2}{(2\pi f)^2 X_c} \quad \text{since } 2\pi fC = \frac{1}{X_c} \quad (16.16)$$

Thus, the maximum power that can be given to mobile carriers decreases as $1/f^2$. This limitation is dominant for silicon at frequencies as high as 100 GHz.

The efficiency of the IMPATT diode is given by

$$\eta = P_{ac}/P_{dc} = V_a I_a/V_d I_d \qquad (16.17)$$

For an ideal IMPATT diode, $V_a/V_d = 0.5$ and $I_a/I_d \approx 2/\pi$. Hence, $\eta = 1/\pi = 0.318$.

The efficiency is more than 30%. In practice, the η is usually less than 30% because of (i) space charge effect, (ii) the reverse saturation current effect, (iii) high-frequency skin effect and (iv) the ionization-saturation effect.

16.4.4 IMPATT Power Amplifier

The IMPATT diode is used as a power amplifier by incorporating a circulator in the basic oscillator circuit arrangement as shown in Fig. 16.7, and making $R_L > |R_d|$. One port of the circulator is terminated with the

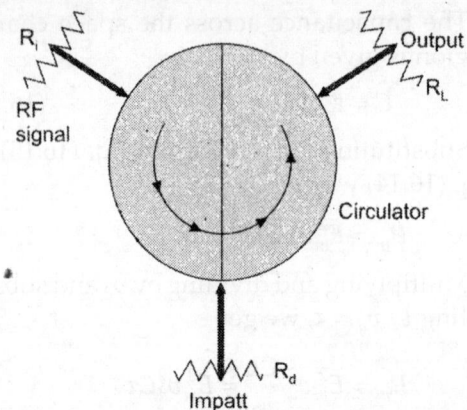

Fig. 16.7: IMPATT diode amplifier

negative resistance and the other port is connected to the load. The input RF power is fed through the third port. Because of the negative resistance, the voltage reflection coefficient at the port is greater than unity. Thus, the average power P_{av} from the source circulates to the negative resistance port and the reflected power is greater than the incident power. The reflected power is delivered to the load. The power gain G_p is given by

$$G_p = |\Gamma|^2 P_{av}/P_{av} = |\Gamma|^2 > 1$$

$$= \left[\frac{-R_d - R_L}{-R_d + R_L}\right]^2 \quad (16.18)$$

If the diode resistance $R_d = -2$ ohms and $R_L = 3$ ohms, then $G_p = |-5/1|^2 = 25$.

16.4.5 IMPATT Diode Oscillator

Figure 16.8 shows a coaxial cavity oscillator and a waveguide cavity oscillator. The frequency of the coaxial cavity oscillator is adjusted by inserting a tuning screw through the sidewall. The loading is adjusted by rotating the coupling loop of the load. The frequency of the wave-guide cavity oscillator is adjusted by inserting a dielectric or metallic rod and the loading is adjusted by window opening. The dielectric rod is preferred because of its use to prevent R.F. leakage current.

When the diode is mounted in a resonance circuit, any noise voltage excites a component of the resonant circuit. Because of the steady reverse bias field and the RF field, the diode swings into and out of avalanche condition. Since the drift time of the hole is very short, carriers drift to the end before the RF voltage swings the diode out of the avalanche condition. The RF field therefore absorbs energy from the carriers or, in effect, from the dc bias. Thus, the RF voltage builds up in the IMPATT diode oscillator.

Due to the RF field, the hole current increases exponentially to a maximum value and then decays exponentially to zero. The oscillator is so designed that the hole current lags behind the RF voltage by 90°. During the hole drifting process, a constant electron current is induced into the external circuit

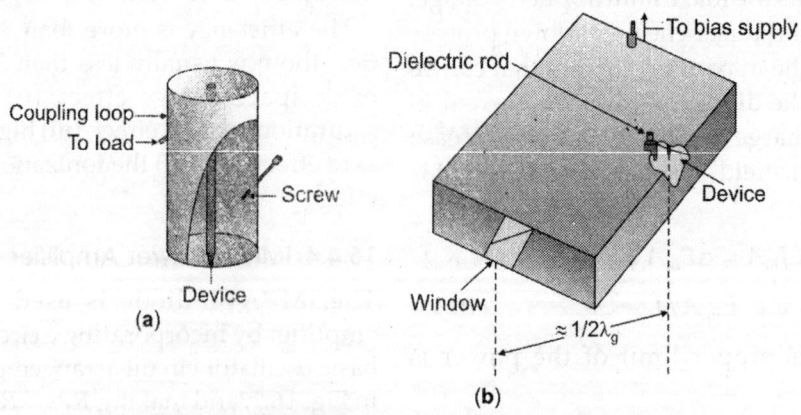

Fig. 16.8: (a) Coaxial cavity (b) Waveguide cavity oscillator

that is equal to the average current in the space-charge region. Thus, the dc power is obtained from the reverse bias. This electron current starts flowing when the hole current reaches its peak. It continues to flow for a half-cycle corresponding to the negative swing of the RF voltage. Thus, 180° phase shift between the external current and the RF voltage provides the negative resistance for sustained oscillations. The maximum value of the negative resistance occurs at a drift transit angle of $\theta_d = \omega\tau = \pi$. Hence, the oscillation frequency is given by

$$\omega\tau = \omega L / v_d = \pi \qquad (16.19a)$$
$$\therefore \quad f = \pi v_d / 2\pi L = v_d / 2L \qquad (16.19b)$$

16.4.6 Typical Characteristics

The typical characteristics of IMPATT diode oscillators are
  (i) Frequency of operation: 6 GHz to 450 GHz
  (ii) Efficiency: Less than 30% for continuous power 60% for pulsed power
  (iii) Continuous power: 1 W
  (iv) Pulsed power: 400 W

Advantages

The advantages of IMPATT diodes are that they are:
  (i) Reliable
  (ii) Compact
  (iii) Inexpensive
  (iv) Moderately efficient.

Disadvantages

The disadvantages of IMPATT diode oscillators are
  (i) Low efficiency (30 %)
  (ii) High noise (30dB)

16.4.7 Applications

The IMPATT diodes are used in
  (i) MW generators
  (ii) Modulated output oscillators
  (iii) MW receivers as local oscillators
  (iv) Parametric amplifiers as pump source
  (v) Negative resistance amplifiers.
  (vi) Radars for civilian purposes.
  (vii) Missiles for defense systems.

16.5 TRAPATT DIODES

TRAPATT is the acronym for **TRA**pped **P**lasma **A**valanche **T**riggered **T**ransit. It is capable of producing *very high MW power in pulsed operation*. The TRAPATT diodes are fabricated from Silicon. They have p^+nn^+ or n^+pp^+ configuration. Figure 16.9 shows the p^+nn^+ configuration. The PN junction is reverse biased beyond the avalanche breakdown region so that the current density is higher. The depletion region width varies from 2.5 µm to 12.5 µm. The p^+ region is kept as thin as possible at 2.5 µm to 7.5 µm. The diameter of these diodes ranges from 50 µm for continuous wave operation to 750 µm at lower frequencies for high peak power. The TRAPATT diode is mounted inside a coaxial cavity resonator at the position where the RF voltage is the maximum.

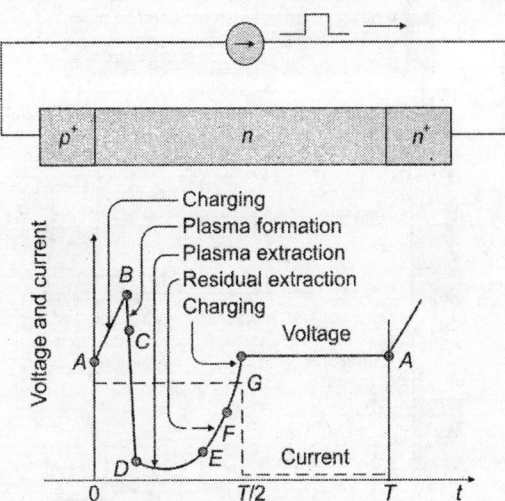

Fig. 16.9: p^+nn^+ configuration of TRAPATT diode

16.5.1 Principle of Operation

Approximate analysis of TRAPATT diodes have shown that a high-field avalanche zone propagates through the diode. It fills the depletion layer with dense plasma of electrons and holes. These get trapped in the low-field region behind the zone. Fig. 16.10 shows a typical waveform of TRAPATT mode of avalanche p^+nn^+ diode that operates with a square wave current excitation. At point A, the electric field is uniform throughout the diode. Its magnitude is large but less than the avalanche breakdown value. The current density is given by

$$J = \varepsilon_s dE/dt \tag{16.20}$$

where ε_s is the dielectric permittivity of the semiconductor diode. The diode current is turned on at the instant of time at A. The only charge carriers that are present are those caused by thermal generation. Hence, the diode charges initially like a linear capacitor. This drives the magnitude of the electric field above the breakdown voltage to point B. With sufficient number of carriers generated, the current exceeds the external current. The

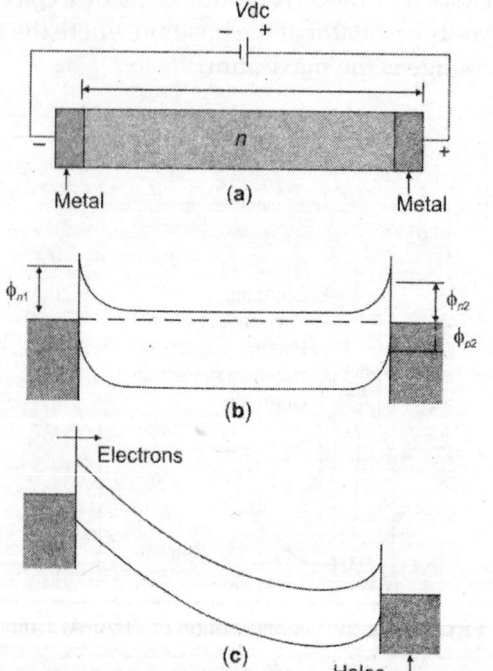

(a)

(b)

(c)

Fig. 16.10: BARITT diode (a) *M-n-M* diode, (b) Energy band diagram in thermal equilibrium, (c) Energy band under bias condition

electric field is depressed throughout the depletion region causing the voltage to decrease from B to C. During this period, the electric field is sufficiently large for avalanche to continue, and a dense-plasma of electrons and holes is created. Some of the electrons and holes drift out of the ends of the depletion layer and the electric field is further depressed and traps the remaining plasma decreasing the voltage to D. Because the total plasma charge is large compared to charge per unit time in the external current, a long time is required to remove the plasma. At E, the plasma is removed. But a residual charge of electrons remains in one end of the depletion layer and a residual charge of holes at the other end. As the residual charge is removed, the voltage increases to F. At F, all charges that are generated internally have been removed. This charge must be greater than or equal to that supplied by the external current. Otherwise, the voltage will exceed that at point A. The diode charges as a capacitor and the voltage increases to G. At G, the diode drive-current falls to zero for half a period and the voltage remains constant at V_A until the current comes on. Then, the cycle is repeated.

The electric field can be expressed as

$$E(x,t) = E_m - (qN_A/\varepsilon_s)x + Jt/\varepsilon_s \tag{16.21}$$

where N_A is the doping concentration of the *n*-region and *x* is the distance. Thus, the value of *t* at which the electric field reaches E_m at a given distance *x* into the depletion region is obtained by setting $E(x,t) = E_m$. It is given by

$$t = (qN_A/J)x \tag{16.22}$$

Differentiating the above equation with respect to time, we get

$$v_z = dx/dt = J/qN_A \tag{16.23}$$

where v_z is the velocity in the avalanche zone. Thus, the avalanche zone quickly sweeps across most of the diode and leaves the diode filled with highly conducting plasma of electrons and holes. This space charge depresses the voltage to low values. Because the drift velocity depends on the electric field, electrons and holes drift at velocities determined by the low-field mobilities. The total transit time is the sum of the delay time in releasing the trapped plasma and the drift time. The total transit time is longer due to low voltage and, hence, the operating frequency of TRAPATT diodes is limited to 10 GHz. Since the current pulse is associated with low voltage, the power loss is low and hence, the efficiency is high.

16.5.2 Power Output and Efficiency

The TRAPATT diode is mounted inside a coaxial cavity resonator at the position where the RF voltage is the maximum. The main function of this circuit is to match the diode effective negative resistance to the load at the output frequency to ensure TRAPATT operation and to deliver power to the load. Five diodes in series can deliver 1.2 kW of pulse power at 1.1 GHz. The highest efficiency is 75% at 0.6 GHz.

16.5.3 Typical Characteristics

The typical characteristics of a TRAPATT diode are:
  (i) Frequency of operation: Up to 10 GHz
  (ii) Efficiency: 15% to 75%
  (iii) Continuous power: Up to 3 W
  (iv) Pulsed power: 1.2 kW
  (v) Noise figure: >30 dB

16.5.4 Disadvantages

The major disadvantages of TRAPATT diodes are
  (i) High noise Figure (> 30 dB)
  (ii) Strong harmonics because of short duration current pulse.

16.5.5 Applications

The TRAPATT diodes are used in
  (i) Low power radars
  (ii) Radar local oscillators
  (iii) MW beam landing systems
  (iv) Radio altimeters
  (v) Phased antenna arrays

16.6 BARITT DIODES

BARITT is an acronym for **BAR**rier **I**njection **T**ransit **T**ime. BARITT diodes are formed with forward biased PN junction. They have p^+np^+, *pnip*, *pn-metal* and *metal-n-metal* (*m-n-m*) configurations. They have long drift regions as in IMPATT diodes. Minority carriers or holes are injected in the drift region by forward biased P-N junction. The transit time through the drift region provides the required phase shift between the current and voltage in order to obtain the negative resistance. The BARITT diode is usually mounted in a resonator.

16.6.1 Principle of Operation

Figure 16.10(a) shows a schematic diagram of *metal-n-metal* BARITT diode and Fig. 16.10(b) shows the energy band diagram at thermal equilibrium. φ_{n1} and φ_{n2} are the barrier heights for the metal-semiconductor contacts respectively and are equal to 0.85 eV for PtSi-Si-PtSi structure. The hole-barrier height φ_{p2} for a forward biased contact is 0.15 eV. Fig. 16.10(c) shows the energy band diagram with external voltage applied.

The mechanisms responsible for microwave oscillations are:
  (i) The rapid increase of the carrier injection process that is caused by the decreasing potential barrier of a forward biased metal-semiconductor contact.
  (ii) An apparent $3\pi/2$ transit angle of the injected carrier traversing semiconductor depletion region.

When the applied voltage is above 30 V, the depletion layer of the reverse-biased contact reaches through the entire device thickness and the terminal current rapidly increases due to thermionic hole-injection into the semiconductor. The critical voltage is given by

$$V_c = qNL^2/2\varepsilon_s \qquad (16.24)$$

where

N is the doping concentration

L is the thickness of the semiconductor

e_s is the dielectric permittivity of the semi-conductor.

Typical device parameters are: $L = 10 \ \mu m$, $N = 4 \times 10^{14} \ cm^3$, $\varphi_{n1} = \varphi_{n2} = 0.85 \ eV$ and area $= 5 \times 10^{-4} \ cm^2$.

The frequency is given by

$$f = (3/4)\tau = 3v_d/4L$$

Here, τ is the drift time, v_d is the drift velocity and L is the drift length.

16.6.2 Typical Characteristics

The typical characteristics of the BARITT diodes are:

(i) Frequency of operation: 4 GHz to 8 GHz

(ii) Efficiency: 2%

(iii) Continuous power: Up to 50 mW at 4.9 GHz

(iv) Noise figure: <15 dB

16.7 COMPARISON BETWEEN TED AND ATTD

Table 16.1 shows a comparison of the performance characteristics of TEDs and ATTDs.

Table 16.1: Comparison of TEDs and ATTDs

Characte-ristic	Gunn diode	IMPATT diode	TRAPATT diode	BARITT diode
Frequency	1–100 GHz	6–100 GHz	1–10 GHz	4–8 GHz
Bandwidth	2% of f_c	10% of f_c	–	Narrow
CW power	10 W	1 W	3 W	50 mW
Pulsed power	200 W	400 W	100 W	1 W
Efficiency	2%	3%	15–75%	2%
Noise figure	–	30 dB	<30 dB	<15 dB

(f_c is the center frequency)

16.8 NUMERICAL EXAMPLES

Example 16.1: An IMPATT diode amplifier has $R_d = -1$ ohms and $R_L = 5$ ohms. Calculate the power gain.

Solution: Given: $R_d = -1 \ \Omega$, $R_L = 5 \ \Omega$

Power gain $= | (-R_d - R_L)/(-R_d + R_L)]^2$

$= [(-1 - 5)/(-1 + 5)]^2$

$= 2.25$

Example 16.2: An IMPATT diode amplifier has $v_d = 2 \times 10^7 cm/sec$, drift length of 8 μm, maximum operating voltage $V_{dc \ max} = 150$ V, maximum operating current $I_{dc \ max} = 250$ mA, breakdown voltage is 100 V and $\eta = 20\%$. Calculate (a) the maximum continuous output power and (b) the resonant frequency.

Solution: Given $v_d = 2 \times 10^7$ cm, $L = 8 \times 10^{-4}$ cm, $V_{dc \ max} = 150$ V, $I_{dc \ max} = 250 \times 10^{-3}$ A, $V_b = 100$ V, $\eta = 20\%$.

(a) $\eta = P_o/P_{dc}$

$\therefore \quad P_o = \eta P_{dc}$

$= (20/100) \times 150 \times 250 \times 10^{-3}$

$= 7.5$ W

(b) $f_r = v_d/2L$

$= 2 \times 10^7/(2 \times 8 \times 10^{-9})$

$= 12.5$ GHz

Example 16.3: An IMPATT diode with normal frequency of 10 GHz has $C_j = 0.4$ pF, $L_p = 0.4$ nH and $C_p = 0.2$ pF. The breakdown bias is 75 V for the bias current of 75 mA and current is 0.60 A for $R_d = -2$ ohms. Determine (a) the resonant frequency of the oscillation and (b) the efficiency.

Solution: Given: $f = 10$ GHz; $C_j = 0.4$ pF, $L_p = 0.4$ nH and $C_p = 0.2$ pF, $V_b = 75$ V, $I_f = 75 \times 10^{-3}$, $I_B = 0.60$ A, $R_d = -2 \ \Omega$.

(a) The resonant frequency: For sustained oscillations,

$$R_L = |Z_d| = 2 \text{ ohms.}$$

The effective load impedance

$$Z_L = j\omega L_p + [R_L/(1 + j\omega C_p R_L)]$$

$$= j\omega L_p + \left[R_L / \sqrt{1 + (\omega C_p R_L)^2} \right]$$

At $f = 10$ GHz:

$\omega L_p = 2 \times 3.14 \times 10 \times 10^9 \times 0.4 \times 10^{-9}$

$= 25.12$ ohm

$\omega C_p R_L = 2 \times 3.14 \times 10 \times 10^9 \times 0.2 \times 10^{-12} \times 2$

$= 0.0251$ ohm

$\varphi = \tan^{-1} \omega C_p R_L$

$= 1.43°$

Since $\omega C_p R_L \ll 1$,

$Z = R_L + j\omega L_p$

Hence,

$f_r = 1/[2\pi\sqrt{L_p C_j}]$

$= \dfrac{1}{2 \times 3.14 \times \sqrt{0.4 \times 10^{-9} \times 0.4 \times 10^{-12}}}$

$= \textbf{12.59 GHz}$

(b) Resonant efficiency

$\eta = P_L/P_{dc}$

$=$ output power/input power

$P_L = I_{rf}^2 R_L/2 = 0.6^2 \times 2/2 = 0.36$

$P_{dc} =$ Breakdown voltage $\times$

dc bias current

$= 75 \times 75 \times 10^{-3} = 5.63$ W

$\eta = P_L/P_{dc} = (0.36/5.63) \times 100$

$= \textbf{6.39\%}$

Example 16.4: An IMPATT diode has a pulsed operating voltage of 120 V and pulsed operating current of 0.8 A. The efficiency of operation is 15%. Find (a) the output power and (b) the duty cycle, if the pulsed width is 0.01 ns and the frequency is 10 GHz.

Solution: Given: $V = 120$ V, $I = 0.8$ A, $\eta = 15\%, f = 10$ GHz

(a) The efficiency is given by

$\eta = P_o/P_i$

$P_o = \eta P_i$

$= 0.15 \times 120 \times 0.8$

$= \textbf{14.4 W}$

(b) Duty cycle $=$ Pulse duration/pulse repetition time

$= \tau/T = \tau f$

$= 0.01 \times 10^{-9} \times 10 \times 10^9$

$= \textbf{10\%}$

Example 16.5: The equivalent circuit parameters of an IMPATT diode oscillator are: $R_j = -2$ ohms, $C_j = 0.5$ pF at a breakdown voltage of 60 V with $L_p = 0.55$ nH and

$C_p = 0.3$ pF. The oscillator operates into a resistive load of 2 ohms connected across C_p under a bias current of 60 mA. Calculate (a) the resonant frequency, (b) the average power output, (c) the average power input and (d) the conversion efficiency for a peak R.F. current of 0.4 A.

Solution: Given: $R_d = -2$, $C_j = 0.5$ pF, $V_b = 60$ V, $I_{bias} = 60$ mA, $L_p = 0.55$ nH and $C_p = 0.3$ pF,

$I_{RF} = \left(\dfrac{0.4}{\sqrt{2}}\right)$ A.

(a) The resonant frequency is given by

$f_o = \dfrac{1}{(2\pi\sqrt{L_p C_j})}$

$= \dfrac{1}{(6.28 \times \sqrt{0.55 \times 10^{-9} \times 0.5 \times 10^{-12}})}$

$= \textbf{9.6 GHz}$

(b) The output power is given by

$P_o = I_{RF}^2 R_L / 2$

$= 0.4^2 \times 2/2$

$= \textbf{0.16 W}$

(c) The input power is given by

$P_i = P_{dc} = V_b \times I_{bias}$

$= 60 \times 60 \times 10^{-3}$

$= \textbf{3.6 W}$

(d) Efficiency is given by

$\eta = P_o/P_i$

$= 0.16/3.6$

$= \textbf{4.4\%}$

Example 16.6: An IMPATT diode amplifier has an $R_d = -2$ ohms. It is operated into a load of 4 ohms. What is the power gain in dB at resonant frequency?

Solution: Given: $R_d = -2$ and $R_L = 4$.

The power gain is given by

$A_p = [\,|\,(-R_d - R_L)/(-R_d + R_L)\,|\,]^2$

$= |\,(-2 - 4)/(-2 + 4)\,|^2$

$= 9$

The power gain in dB is given by

$P_{dB} = 10 \log A_p$

$= \textbf{9.54 dB}$

Example 16.7: A TRAPATT diode has $N_A = 2 \times 10^{14}/\text{cm}^3$ and $J = 20\text{kA}/\text{cm}^2$. Find the avalanche-zone velocity.

Solution: Given: $N_A = 2 \times 10^{14} /\text{cm}^3$,

$J = 20 \text{ kA }/\text{cm}^2.$

The avalanche-zone velocity v_z is given by

$$v_z = J/qN_A$$
$$= 20 \times 10^3/(1.6 \times 10^{-19} \times 2 \times 10^{15})$$
$$= \textbf{6.25} \times \textbf{10}^7 \textbf{ cm/s}$$

Example 16.8 The drift velocity of a BARITT diode is 10^5 m/s and width is 7 μm. Find frequency of oscillation.

Solution: Given: $v_d = 10^5$m/s, $L = 7$ μm.

$$f = 3v_d/4L$$
$$= 3 \times 10^5/4 \times 7 \times 10^{-6}$$
$$= \textbf{10.71 GHz}$$

Example 16.9 A BARITT diode has $\varepsilon_r = 11.8$, $N = 3 \times 10^{21}$ and $L = 6$ μm. Find (a) the breakdown voltage and (b) the breakdown electric field.

Solution: Given: $\varepsilon_r = 11.8$, $N = 3 \times 10^{21}$, $L = 6$ μm

(a) The breakdown voltage is

$$V_{bd} = qNL^2/\varepsilon_r$$

$$= 1.6 \times 10^{-19} \times 3 \times 10^{21} \times \frac{(6 \times 10^{-6})^2}{8.854 \times 10^{-12} \times 11.8}$$

$$= \textbf{165.68 V}$$

(b) The breakdown electric field is

$$E_{bd} = V_{bd}/L = 165.68/(6 \times 10^{-6})$$
$$= \textbf{2.76} \times \textbf{10}^7 \textbf{ V/cm}$$

KEY POINTS

- Two-terminal negative resistance devices are the tunnel diode, the transferred electron devices and the avalanche transit-time devices.
- Two distinct modes of avalanche oscillator are the impact ionization avalanche transit-time (IMPATT) mode and the other trapped plasma avalanche triggered transit (TRAPATT) mode.
- The Read diode is an n^+-p-i-n^+ structure. The plus sign indicates very high doping and i or v refers to intrinsic material.

- IMPATT is the acronym for IMPact Avalanche Transit Time. The IMPATT diodes exhibit a differential negative resistance by two effects: (i) The impact ionization avalanche effect. This causes the carrier current $I_o(t)$ and the ac voltage to be out of phase by 90°.(ii) The transit-time effect. This further delays the external current $I_e(t)$ by 90° relative to ac voltage.
- The oscillation frequency of IMPATT oscillator is given by $f = \pi v_d /2\pi L = v_d /2L$.
- The efficiency of the IMPATT diode is given by $\eta = V_a I_a / V_d I_d$.
- The advantages of IMPATT diodes are that they are (i) reliable, (ii) compact, (iii) inexpensive and (iv) moderately efficient.
- The disadvantages of IMPATT diode oscillators are (i) Low efficiency (30%) and (ii) High noise (30dB).
- The IMPATT diodes are used in (i) MW generators, (ii) Modulated output oscillators, (iii) MW receivers as local oscillators, (iv) Parametric amplifiers as pump source, (v) Negative resistance amplifiers (vi) Radars for civilian purposes and (vii) Missiles for defense systems.
- TRAPATT is the acronym for TRApped Plasma Avalanche Triggered Transit. It is capable of producing very high MW power in pulsed operation. The TRAPATT diodes are fabricated from Silicon. They have p^+nn^+ or n^+pp^+ configuration.
- The major disadvantages of TRAPATT diodes are (i) High noise Figure (> 30 dB) and (ii) Strong harmonics because of short duration current pulse.
- The TRAPATT diodes are used in (i) Low power radars, (ii)Radar local oscillators, (iii) MW beam landing systems, (iv) Radio altimeters and (v) Phased antenna arrays
- BARITT is an acronym for BARrier Injection Transit Time. BARITT diodes are formed with forward biased p-n junction. They have p^+np^+, $pnip$, pn-metal and metal-n-metal (m-n-m) configurations. They have long drift regions as in IMPATT diodes.
- The mechanisms responsible for microwave oscillations are (i) The rapid increase of the carrier injection process caused by the decreasing potential barrier of a forward biased metal-semiconductor contact and (ii) An apparent $3\pi/2$ transit angle of the injected carrier that traverses the semiconductor depletion region.
- The frequency is given by $f = 3/4\tau = 3v_d/4L$.

FURTHER READING

1. Collins RE (1996). Foundations of Microwave Engineering, McGraw Hill, NY.
2. Das A and Das SK (2004). Microwave Engineering, TMH, New Delhi.
3. Gibbons G (1973). Avalanche Diode Microwave Oscillators, Clarendon Press, Oxford.
4. Liao SY (1990). Semiconductor Electron Devices, PH. NJ.
5. Sze SM (1985). Semiconductor Devices: Physics and Technology, John Wiley, N.Y.

REVIEW QUESTIONS

16.1 What is an ATTD?

16.2 Mention three types of ATTDs.

16.3 What is an IMPATT diode?

16.4 Mention the delays in IMPATT diode that give rise to negative resistance.

16.5 Draw the equivalent circuit of an IMPATT diode.

16.6 Give the applications of an IMPATT diode.

16.7 Give the performance characteristics of an IMPATT diode.

16.8 Mention the advantages and limitations of IMPATT diode.

16.9 What is a TRAPATT diode?

16.10 How is plasma formed in a TRAPATT diode?

16.11 Give the performance characteristics of a TRAPATT diode.

16.12 Give the applications of TRAPATT diodes.

16.13 Mention the disadvantages or limitations of TRAPATT diodes.

16.14 What is a BARITT diode?

16.15 Give the performance characteristics of BARITT diode.

16.16 What are the necessary conditions for an IMPATT diode to produce oscillations?

16.17 Compare Gunn diode with IMPATT diode.

16.18 Compare BARITT diode with IMPATT diode.

16.19 Expand the terms IMPATT, TRAPATT and BARITT.

DESCRIPTIVE QUESTIONS

16.1 Describe the constructional details and operation of an IMPATT diode.

16.2 With a neat circuit, explain the operation of IMPATT diode amplifier

16.3 With a neat circuit, explain the operation of IMPATT diode oscillator.

16.4 Describe the constructional details and operation of a TRAPATT diode.

16.5 Describe a Read diode and Avalanche multiplication.

16.6 Explain the structure, field distribution and currents in a Read diode.

16.7 Describe the constructional details and operation of a BARITT diode.

16.8 With a neat circuit, explain the operation of BARITT diode oscillator.

16.9 Compare the TEDs with ATTDs.

PRACTICE PROBLEMS

16.1 An IMPATT diode amplifier has $V_d = 2 \times 10^7$ cm/sec, drift length of 6 mm, maximum operating voltage $V_{dc\,max} = 100$ V, maximum operating current $I_{dc\,max} = 200$ mA, breakdown voltage is 90 V and $\eta = 15\%$. Calculate (a) the maximum continuous output power and (b) the resonant frequency.
[**Ans:** 3 W, 16.67 GHz]

16.2 An IMPATT diode with normal frequency of 10 GHz has $C_j = 0.5$ pF, $L_p = 0.5$ nH and $C_p = 0.3$ pF. The breakdown bias is 80 V and the bias current is 0.065 A for $R_d = -2$ ohms. Determine (a) the resonant frequency of the oscillation and (b) the efficiency is $I_{rf} = 0.6$ A peak.
[**Ans:** 13 GHz, 6.9%]

16.3 The equivalent circuit parameters of an IMPATT diode oscillator are: $R_j = -2$ ohms, $C_j = 0.5$ pF at a breakdown voltage of 80 V with $L_p = 0.55$ nH and $C_p = 0.3$ pF. The oscillator operates into a resistive load of 2 ohms connected across C_p under a bias current of 80 mA. Calculate (a) the resonant frequency, (b) the average power output, (c) the average power input and (d) the conversion efficiency for a peak RF current of 0.6 A.
[**Ans:** (a) 9.6 GHz, (b) 0.36 W, (c) 6.4 W, (d) 5.6%]

16.4 An IMPATT diode amplifier has an $R_d = -3$ ohms. It is operated into a load of 5 ohms. What is the power gain in dB at resonant frequency?
[**Ans:** 12.04 dB]

16.5 An IMPATT diode has $v_d = 10^5$ m/s and $L = 5$ μm. Calculate the oscillation frequency.
[**Ans:** 10 GHz]

16.6 An IMPATT diode has $v_d = 1.5 \times 10^5$ m/s, $L = 8$ μm, $I_{max} = 180$ mA, $V_{max} = 90$ V and

$\eta = 10\%$. Calculate (i) the maximum CW output power and (ii) the frequency.

[**Ans:** 1.62 W, 9.375 GHz]

16.7 An IMPATT diode has a pulsed operating voltage of 150 V and pulsed operating current of 0.5 A. The efficiency of operation is 10%. Find (a) the output power and (b) the frequency, if the pulsed width is 0.02 ns and the duty cycle is 10%.

[**Ans:** (a) 7.5 W, (b) 5 GHz]

16.8 The drift velocity of a BARITT diode is 10^5 m/s and width is 5 μm. Find frequency of oscillation.

[**Ans:** 15 GHz]

16.9 A BARITT diode has $e_r = 11.8$, $N = 2.8 \times 10^{21}$ and $L = 6$ μm. Find (a) the breakdown voltage and (b) the breakdown electric field.

(**Ans:** 154.63 V, 2.58×10^5 V/cm)

REFERENCE

1. Ahmed, S. and Freyer, J., (1977) High power Pt Schottky BARITT diode, *Electron. Lett.*, Vol. 12, p 238–239.

2. Berenz, J.J. *et al*, (1978) Ion implanted p-n junction indium phosphide IMPATT, *Electron. Lett.*, Vol. 34, p 683–684.

3. Chang, K. *et al*, (1981) GaAs read type IMPATT diode for 130 GHz CW operation, *Electron. Lett.*, Vol. 17, pp 471–472.

4. Chlorofeine, A.S. *et al*, (1969) A theory for high-efficiency mode of oscillation in avalanche diodes, *RCA Rev.*, Vol. 3, pp 397–421.

5. Fong, T.T. and H.J. Kumo, (1979) Millimeter Wave IMPATT Sources, IEEE MTT-27.

6. Iglesius, D.E. *et al*, (1975) 10 W and 12 W GaAs IMPATTs, *IEEE Trans.* ED-22, p 200.

7. Ishibashi,T. et al (1977) Liquid Nitrogen Cooled Sub-millimeter Wave Silicon IMPATT Diodes, Electron. Lett., vol.13, p 299-3000.

8. Konyan, O.E. *et al*, (1976) Microwave BARITT diode, *Solid State Electron*. Vol. 19, p 795.

9. Midford, T.K. and Bernick, R.L., (1979) Milli-meter Wave IMPATT Diodes and Oscillators, IEEE Trans. MTT-27.

10. Sze, S.M.(Ed.)., (1983) *VLSI Technology*, John Wiley, NY.

11. Kennedy, G and Davis, B., (1999.) *Electronic Communication Systems*, TMH, New Delhi.

12. Prager, H.S. *et al*, (1967) High Power High Efficiency Silicon Avalanche Diodes at Ultra high Frequencies, Proc. IEEE, Vol. 55, p 586–587.

13. Read, W.T., (1958) A proposed high-frequency negative resistance diode, *Bell Sys.Tech. J.*, Vol. 37, p 407–446.

14. De Loach, BC Jr. and Scharfetter, D.L., (1970) Device Physics of TRAPATT Oscillators, IEEE Trans. Electron Devices, ED –17, p 9-21, Jan.

15. Haddaad, G.I. et al. (1973) Avalanche Transit Time Devices, Artec h.,Mass.

16. Haddaad, G.I., *et al.*, (1970) Basic Principles and Properties of Avalanche Transit Time Devices, IEEE Trans. MTT –18, No. 11, p 752-772, Nov.

17. Milnes, A.G. (1980) *Semiconductor Devices and Integrated Electronics*, Van Nostrand, NY

18. Wilson, W.E., (1971 Aug.) Pulsed LSA and TRAPATT Sources for Microwave systems, *Microwave J.*, vol.46, p 87-90.

Tunnel Diodes

- Understand the operation of tunnel diode.
- Study the characteristics and applications.
- Compare tunnel diode with *pn* junction diode.

17.1 INTRODUCTION

In a conventional *p-n* junction diode, the doping is in the order of 1 part in 10^8. It creates a depletion layer of 5 micron width around the junction. This depletion layer forms the potential barrier at the junction. This prevents the flow of carriers across the junction. If the concentration of impurity atoms is greatly increased, the device characteristics are completely changed. In 1958, Esaki discovered this phenomenon. Hence, it is also known as *Esaki diode*.

17.2 TUNNEL DIODE

A tunnel diode is a *p-n* junction diode with both *p* and *n* sides being heavily doped with impurities of the order of $10^{19}/cm^3$. Compared to conventional *pn* junction diodes, the doping in tunnel diode is many times that of conventional junction diodes. Because of heavy doping, the depletion layer is extremely thin, of the order of 0.01 µm. Due to the extremely thin depletion layer, the *electrons tunnel* through the potential barrier

at a relatively low voltage less than 0.05 V. Hence, it is known as *tunnel diode*.

Tunnel diodes are fabricated from Ge, GaAs and GaSb. Figure 17.1 shows the *V-I* characteristic of a Ge and GaAs tunnel diode. The tunnel diode has a negative resistance characteristic over a part of its V-I characteristic. The negative resistance is due to the electrons tunneling across the extremely thin barrier layer of the diode. Tunnel diodes are also known as *Esaki diodes* in honour of its inventor.

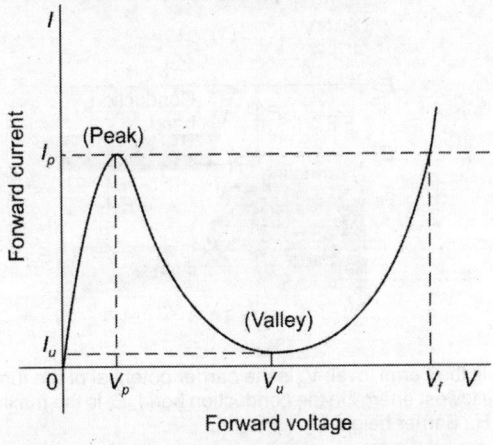

Fig. 17.1: *V-I* characteristics of tunnel diode

17.2.1 Principle of Operation

Figure 17.2(a) shows the upper energy levels of conduction electrons in the *n*-region and the upper energy levels of holes in the *p*-region under *zero bias* condition. Both are at the same Fermi level. Hence, there is no charge flow in either direction and the current is zero as shown in Fig. 17.2(a). When the tunnel diode is forward biased with a voltage that is greater than zero but less than the peak value V_p, the potential barrier is decreased by the magnitude of the applied forward bias. The resulting energy diagram is as shown in part (1) of Fig. 17.2(b). Thus a difference in Fermi-level on both sides is created. Therefore, the electrons tunnel through the barrier from *n*-region to *p*-region. A forward tunneling current flows from the *p*-region to the *n*-region. As the forward bias voltage is increased to the peak value V_p, all conduction band electrons in the *n*-region cross over to the valence band in the *p*-region. This is because the two regions are exactly aligned. Hence, maximum or

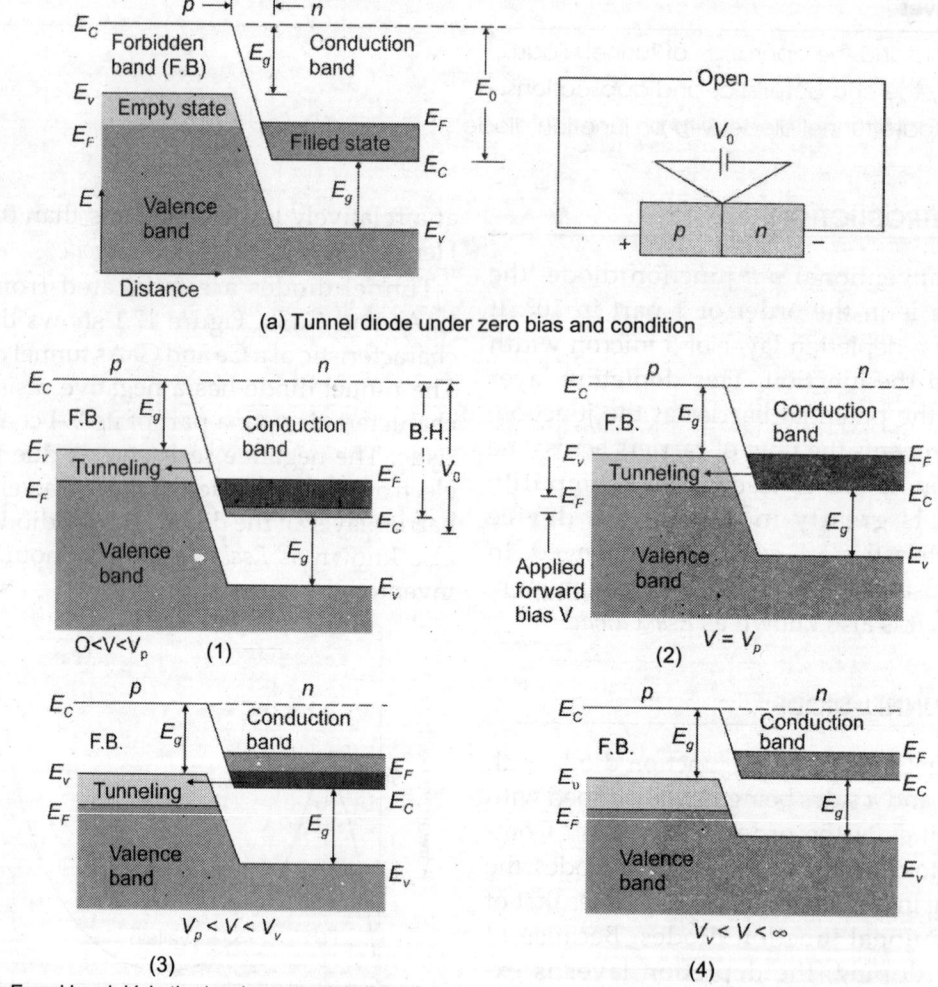

(a) Tunnel diode under zero bias and condition

$O<V<V_p$ (1)

$V=V_p$ (2)

$V_p<V<V_v$ (3)

$V_v<V<\infty$ (4)

E_f is the Fermi level; V_o is the barrier potential of the function; E_g is the energy required to break a covalent bond; E_c is the lowest energy in the conduction bond; E_v is the maximum energy in the valence band; V is the applied forward bias; B.H.: Barrier height

Fig. 17.2: Tunnel diode energy levels

peak current I_p flows in the circuit. The energy band diagram under this condition is shown in part (2) of Fig. 17.2(b). When the forward bias voltage is further increased, current decreases because, the two bands gradually get out of alignment. This is shown in part (3) of Fig. 17.2(b). The current reaches a minimum value I_v, known as *valley current*, when the two bands are totally out of alignment. This is shown in part (4) of Fig. 17.2(b). The forward voltage at the valley point is known as *valley voltage* V_v. As the forward voltage is increased beyond V_v, the current again increases as in the case of conventional *p-n* diode.

17.2.2 Equivalent Circuit

Figure 17.3 shows the equivalent circuit of a tunnel diode. The capacitance C_j is the junction diffusion capacitance. It is in the range of 1 to 10 pF. R_j is the negative resistance of the tunnel diode. It is in the range of −20 to −100 ohms. L_s is the lead inductance and is in the range of 0.1 to 4 nH. R_s is the resistance due to leads, ohmic contacts and the bulk resistance. These limit the upper frequency of operation and switching speed.

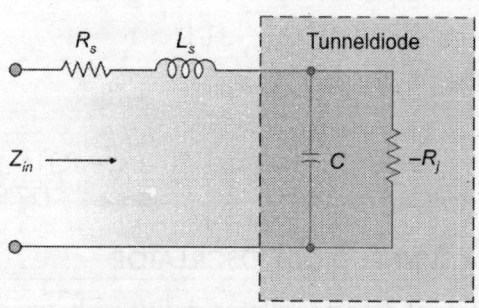

Fig. 17.3: Equivalent circuit

The input impedance Z_{in} of the tunnel diode is given by

$$Z_{in} = R_s + j\omega L_s + \left[\frac{R_j(j/\omega C_j)}{(-R_j - j/\omega C_j)}\right]$$

$$= R_s - \frac{R_j}{1+(\omega C_j R_j)^2}$$

$$+ j\left(\omega L_s - \frac{\omega C_j R_j^2}{1+(\omega C_j R_j)^2}\right) \quad (17.1)$$

Two important frequencies can be obtained from Eq. (17.1). They are resistive cut-off frequency and self-resonance frequency. For resistive cut-off frequency, the real part of Z_{in} is zero. Thus,

$$Re\{Z_{in}\} = 0 \quad (17.2)$$

Hence, the resistive cut-off frequency f_r is given by

$$f_r = \left[\frac{1}{(2\pi C_j R_j)}\right]\sqrt{\left(\frac{R_j}{R_s}\right)-1} \quad (17.3)$$

For self-resonance frequency, the imaginary part of Z_{in} is zero. Thus,

$$\pm Im\{Z_{in}\} = 0 \quad (17.4)$$

The self-resonance frequency f_o is given by

$$f_o = \left[\frac{1}{(2\pi C_j R_j)}\right]\sqrt{\frac{R_j^2 C_j}{L_s}-1} \quad (17.5)$$

17.2.3 Parallel Load

The tunnel diode amplifier can be connected either in parallel or in series with a resistive load. The equivalent circuit of tunnel diode amplifier with parallel load is shown in Fig. 17.4(a).

The output power in the load resistance R_l is given by two parts:

(i) the power $P_{in} (= V^2/AR_j)$ generated by the low input voltage V through the tunnel diode amplifier with gain A and

(ii) the power $P_n (= V^2/R_j)$ generated by the negative resistance R_j. Thus, $P_o = V^2/R_j = P_{in} + P_n = V^2/AR_l + V^2/R_j$. Hence, $1/R_l = 1/AR_l + 1/R_j$. Therefore the **gain** of the tunnel diode amplifier is given by

$$A = R_j/(R_j - R_l) \quad (17.6)$$

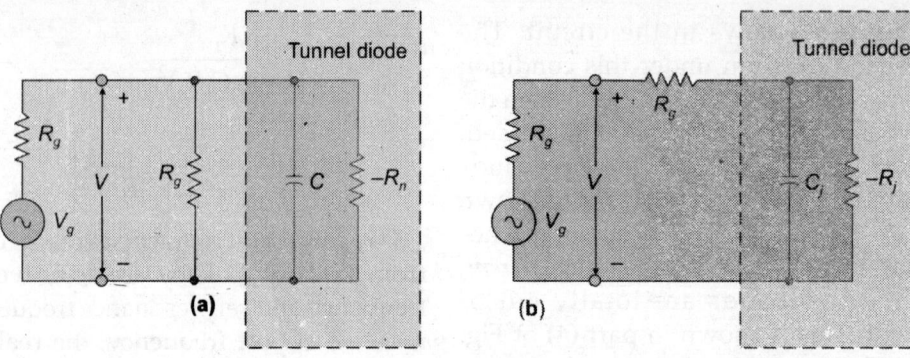

Fig. 17.4: Equivalent circuit with (a) Parallel load (b) Series load

17.2.4 Series Load

The equivalent circuit of tunnel diode amplifier with series load is shown in Fig. 17.4(b). The output power in the series load resistance R_l is given by two parts:

(i) the power $P_{in}\,(= I^2 R_l/A)$ generated by the low input through the tunnel diode amplifier with gain A

(ii) the power $P_n\,(= I^2/R_j)$ generated by the negative resistance R_n. Thus, $P_o = I^2 R_l = P_{in} + P_n = I^2 R_l/A + I^2 R_j$. Hence, $R_l = R_l/A + 1/R_j$. Therefore the gain of the tunnel diode amplifier is given by

$$A = R_j/(R_l - R_j) \qquad (17.7)$$

17.3 TUNNEL DIODE AMPLIFIER

Figure 17.5 shows a tunnel diode connected to a circulator. This arrangement acts as a negative resistance tunnel diode amplifier. The circulator is a 3-port junction. The power flows from port 1 to port 2 to port 3 in the direction indicated in the figure. If the circulator is loss-less and has a positive characteristic impedance $Z_o = R_o$, then the reflection coefficient is given by

$$\Gamma = [(Z_{in}/Z_o) - 1]/[(Z_{in}/Z_o) + 1]$$
$$= (Z_{in} - Z_o)/(Z_{in} + Z_o)$$
$$= (-R_j - R_o)/(-R_j + R_o) \qquad (17.8)$$

By setting $R_j = R_o$, the gain becomes *infinity*. Usually, R_o must be greater than R_j so that the gain is *finite and stable*.

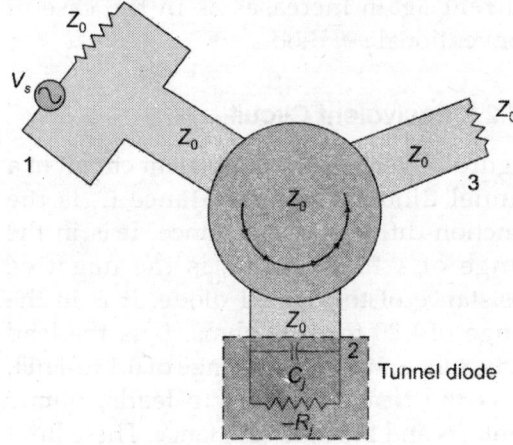

Fig. 17.5: Tunnel diode amplifier

The output load power P_L is given by

$$P_L = |\Gamma|^2 P_{in}, \quad |\Gamma|^2 > 1$$

The power gain A_p is

$$A_p = P_L/P_{in}$$
$$= |\Gamma|^2 = |(R_o + R_j)/(R_o - R_j)|^2 \qquad (17.9)$$

17.4 TUNNEL DIODE OSCILLATOR

A tunnel diode oscillator circuit is shown in Fig. 17.6. It consists of a voltage divider bias circuit R_1-R_2, a tank circuit L-C coupled to the diode by means of capacitive divider network C_1-C_2. The tunnel diode is so biased that it operates in the negative resistance region. The operating point is fixed at the midpoint of the negative resistance region.

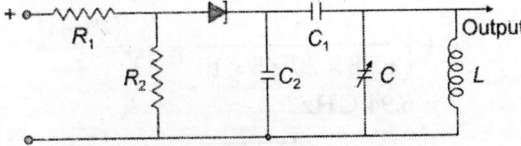

Fig. 17.6: Tunnel diode oscillator

When the dc power is switched on, a surge current generates oscillations in the resonant tank circuit. As the voltage V_T across the tunnel diode increases beyond V_p, tunnel diode is driven into the negative resistance region and its negative resistance starts increasing. Hence V_T increases further until it is equal to V_v, the valley voltage. Any further increase in V_T drives the tunnel diode into the positive resistance region and the current increases. This increase in current increases the voltage drop across R_1 and hence V_T decreases. This pulls back the tunnel diode in the negative resistance region. The decrease in V_T increases the circuit current till V_T equals V_p. This describes one cycle of operation. Thus, the circuit will continue to oscillate back and forth through the negative resistance region between V_p and V_v in the V-I characteristic curve.

Advantages

The advantages of tunnel diodes are:

(i) It requires low dc power

(ii) It has a broad bandwidth

(iii) It has low noise figure (<5 dB at 10 GHz)

(iv) It operates up to 100 GHz

(v) It is immune to nuclear radiation

(vi) It is immune to solar radiation

(vii) It is suitable for space communication applications.

Disadvantages

The major disadvantages of tunnel diodes are:

(i) Its operating voltage is very low (1 V dc or less)

(ii) There is no isolation between input and output circuits

17.5 COMPARISON BETWEEN TUNNEL DIODE AND PN JUNCTION DIODE

The difference between tunnel diode and the conventional PN junction diode are given in Table 17.1.

Table 17.1: Comparison between tunnel diode and *pn* junction diode

Tunnel diode	*PN Junction diode*
1. *p*- and *n*-sides are heavily doped	1. Doping is normal on both sides
2. Tunneling current is due to majority carriers (electrons) from *n*-to *p*-side	2. Diode current is due to minority carriers (holes) from *p*- to *n*- side
3. Majority carrier current responds rapidly to voltage changes	3. Majority carrier current responds slowly to voltage changes
4. It is used as switches at MW frequencies	4. It is used as switches at low frequencies
5. At low reverse bias, large current flows because of considerable overlap between the conduction and valence bands	5. At low reverse bias, the current I_o is extremely small up to considerable reverse bias; then abruptly increases to a very high value at the breakdown voltage
6. It is used as a frequency converter	6. It is used as rectifiers
7. It has a negative resistance region	7. It has no negative resistance region
8. Used as a negative resistance amplifier	8. It is used as detectors and mixers
9. It is a low noise device	9. It is a moderate noise device
10. Preferred semiconductors for tunnel diodes are Ge and GaAs	10. Preferred semiconductors for junction diodes are Ge and Si

17.6 APPLICATIONS

The tunnel diodes are used as
   (i) MW oscillators.
   (ii) MW amplifiers.
   (iii) Ultra high-speed switches.
   (iv) Relaxation oscillators.
   (v) Logic memory devices.

17.7 NUMERICAL EXAMPLES

Example 17.1 A tunnel diode has $R_j =$ 50 ohms, $R_s =$ 10 ohms, $C_j =$ 0.6 pF and $L_s =$ 1 nH. Compute (a) the resistive cut-off frequency and (b) self-resonant frequency.

Solution: Given: $R_j =$ 50 ohms, $R_s =$ 10 ohms, $C_j =$ 0.6 pF and $L_s =$ 1 nH

(a) $f_r = (1/2\pi R_j C_j) [(R_j/R_s) - 1]^{1/2}$

$= (6.28 \times 50 \times 0.6 \times 10^{-12})^{-1} \times$
$[(50/10) - 1]^{1/2}$

$= \mathbf{10.62\ GHz}$

(b) $f_o = \dfrac{1}{2 \times 3.14 \times 50 \times 0.6 \times 10^{-12}}$

$\sqrt{\dfrac{50 \times 50 \times 0.6 \times 10^{-12}}{1 \times 10^{-9}} - 1}$

$= \dfrac{10^{12}}{188.4} \sqrt{1500 \times 10^{-3}} = \dfrac{10^{12}}{188.4} \sqrt{\dfrac{15}{10}}$

$= \dfrac{10^{12}}{188.4} \times \dfrac{3.8730}{3.1623}$

$= \mathbf{6.5\ GHz.}$

Example 17.2 A tunnel diode has a negative resistance of 20 ohms, series resistance of 1 ohm, junction capacitance of 5 pF and series inductance of 1 μH. Compute (a) the resistive cut-off and (b) resonance frequencies.

Solution: Given: $R_j =$ 20, $R_s =$ 1, $C_j =$ 5 pF and $L_s =$ 1 μH

The resistive cut-off frequency

$$f_r = \left[\dfrac{1}{2\pi R_j C_j}\right] \sqrt{\dfrac{(R_j - R_s)}{R_s}}$$

$= \left(\dfrac{1}{6.28 \times 20 \times 5 \times 10^{-12}}\right) \sqrt{\dfrac{(20 - 1)}{1}}$

$= \mathbf{6.94\ GHz}$

$$f_o = \dfrac{1}{2\pi R_j C_j} \sqrt{\dfrac{R_j^2 C_j}{L_s} - 1}$$

$= \dfrac{1}{2 \times 3.14 \times 20 \times 5 \times 10^{-12}}$

$\sqrt{\dfrac{20 \times 20 \times 5 \times 10^{-9}}{1 \times 10^{-6}} - 1}$

$= \dfrac{10^{12}}{628} \sqrt{2000 \times 10^{-3} - 1}$

$= 1.59 \times 10^9 \sqrt{2 - 1}$

$= \mathbf{1.59\ GHz}$

Example 17.3 A tunnel diode amplifier has a negative resistance of 20 ohms. A load of 24 ohms is connected (i) in parallel and (ii) in series. Find the gains.

Solution: Given: $R_j =$ 20 Ω, $R_l =$ 24 Ω. The gain with parallel load is

$A = R_j/(R_j - R_c)$

$= 20/(20 - 24) = -5$

The gain with series load is

$A = R_l/(R_l - R_j)$

$= 24/(24 - 20) = \mathbf{6}$

Example 17.4 A tunnel diode has a negative resistance of 26 ohms, series resistance of 1 ohm, series inductance of 1 nH and a resistive cut-off frequency of 8 GHz. Find (i) the junction capacitance and (ii) the self-resonance frequency.

Solution: Given: $R_j =$ 26, $R_s =$ 1, $L_s =$ 1 nH and $f_r =$ 8 GHz.

The resistive cut-off frequency

$$f_r = \left(\dfrac{1}{2\pi R_j C_j}\right) \sqrt{\dfrac{(R_j - R_s)}{R_s}} = 8 \times 10^9$$

The junction capacitance

$$C_j = \frac{1}{2\pi f_r R_j}\left[\frac{(R_j - R_s)}{R_s}\right]^{1/2}$$

$$= \left(\frac{1}{6.28 \times 26 \times 8 \times 10^9}\right)\sqrt{\frac{(26-1)}{1}}$$

$$= 3.83 \text{ pF}$$

$$f_o = \frac{1}{2\pi R_j C_j}\sqrt{\frac{R_j^2 C_j}{L_s} - 1}$$

$$= \frac{1}{6.28 \times 26 \times 3.83 \times 10^{-12}} \times$$

$$\sqrt{\frac{26 \times 26 \times 3.83 \times 10^{-12}}{1 \times 10^{-9}} - 1}$$

$$= 1.599 \times 10^9 \sqrt{2.589 - 1}$$

$$= 1.599 \times 10^9 \times 1.261$$

$$= 2.02 \text{ GHz}$$

KEY POINTS

- A tunnel diode is a PN junction diode with both p and n sides being heavily doped with impurities of the order of $10^{19}/\text{cm}^3$. Because of heavy doping, the depletion layer is extremely thin, of the order of 0.01 μm. Due to the extremely thin depletion layer, the electrons tunnel through the potential barrier at relatively low voltage less than 0.05 V. Hence, it is known as tunnel diode.

- Tunnel diodes or Esaki diodes are fabricated from Ge, GaAs and GaSb.

- The tunnel diode has a negative resistance characteristic over a part of its V-I characteristic due to the electrons tunneling across the extremely thin barrier layer of the diode.

- The advantages of tunnel diodes are: (i)It requires low D.C. power, (ii) It has a broad bandwidth, (iii) It has low noise figure (< 5 dB at 10 GHz), (iv) It operates up to 100 GHz, (v) It is immune to nuclear radiation, (vi) It is immune to solar radiation, and (vii) It is suitable for space communication applications.

- The major disadvantages of tunnel diodes are: (i) Its operating voltage is very low (1 V dc or less) and (ii) There is no isolation between input and output circuits

- The tunnel diodes are used as (i) MW oscillators. (ii) MW amplifiers, (iii) Ultra high-speed switches, (iv) Relaxation oscillators and (v) Logic memory devices.

FURTHER READING

1. Esaki, L., (1958) New phenomenon in narrow **Ge p-n junction,** *Phys. Rev.*, Vol.109, p 603.
2. Tunnel Diode Manual, GEC, (1961) Semiconductor Products Department, N.Y.
3. Tunnel Diode Manual, TD-30, RCA, (1963) Semiconductor Materials Division, N.J.

REVIEW QUESTIONS

17.1 What is a tunnel diode?

17.2 Draw the V-I characteristic of a tunnel diode.

17.3 Draw the equivalent circuit of a tunnel diode.

17.4 Give the applications of tunnel diodes.

17.5 Mention the advantages of tunnel diodes.

17.6 Mention the limitations of tunnel diodes.

DESCRIPTIVE QUESTIONS

17.1 Explain the construction and operation of a tunnel diode oscillator.

17.2 Explain with a neat circuit the operation of a tunnel diode amplifier.

17.3 Draw the *V-I* characteristic and the equivalent circuit of a tunnel diode and explain.

17.4 Mention the applications, advantages and limitations of tunnel diodes.

17.5 Compare tunnel diode with the conventional PN junction diode.

17.6 Derive down the expression for resistance cutoff frequency.

17.7 Derive down the expression for self-resonance frequency.

17.8 Derive down the expression for the gain of a tunnel diode amplifier.

17.9 Derive down the expression for the gain of a tunnel diode amplifier with series load.

17.10 Draw the equivalent circuit of a tunnel diode and explain.

17.11 Draw the equivalent circuit of a tunnel diode amplifier with parallel load.

17.12 Draw the equivlent circuit of a tunnel diode amplifier with series load.

PRACTICE PROBLEMS

17.1 A tunnel diode has $R_j = 60$ ohms, $R_s = 9$ ohms, $C_j = 0.6$ pF and $L_s = 1$ nH. Compute (a) the resistive cut-off frequency and (b) self-resonant frequency.

[**Ans:** (a) 25.08 GHz, (b) 20.1 GHz]

17.2 A tunnel diode has a negative resistance of 26 ohms, series resistance of 1 ohm, junction capacitance of 5 pF and series inductance of 1 mH. Compute (a) the resistive and (b) reactive cut-off frequencies.

[**Ans:** (a) 6.12 GHz, (b) 2.0 GHz)]

17.3 A tunnel diode amplifier has a negative resistance of 26 ohms. A load of 24 ohms is connected (i) in parallel and (ii) in series. Find the gains.

[**Ans:** (i) 13, (ii) 12]

17.4 A tunnel diode has a negative resistance of 18 ohms, series resistance of 2 ohm, series inductance of 1 nH and a resistive cut-off frequency of 8 GHz. Find (i) the junction capacitance and (ii) the resonance frequency.

[**Ans:** (i) 3.13 pF, (ii) 0.138 GHz]

REFERENCE

1. Watson A (Ed.), (1969). *Microwave Semiconductor Devices and Their Applications*, McGraw Hill, NY.

2. Bahl IJ and Bhatia P (1988), *Microwave Solid State Circuit Design*, John Wiley, NY.

3. Chang KKN (1964). *Parametric and Tunnel Diodes*, PH, NJ.

4. Collins RE (1996). *Foundations of Microwave Engineering*, McGraw Hill, NY.

5. De Loach BC Jr (1967). *Recent Advances in Solid State Microwave Generators, Advances in Microwaves*, vol.2, Academic Press, NY.

Varactor Diode

* Know the principle of operation of varactor diode.
* Derive the equivalent circuit.
* Understand the operation of varactor diode frequency multiplier and tuner.
* Explain the applications of varactor diode.

18.1 INTRODUCTION

Another important device for microwave applications is the varactor diode. It is a *p-n* junction diode operated with reverse bias. In this chapter, we describe the structure of a varactor diode and its operating principle. Its application as frequency multiplier and tuner are also discussed.

18.2 PRINCIPLE OF OPERATION

The term varactor means a *variable reactor*. The varactor diode is *p-n* junction diode operated with reverse bias voltage. The junction or *transition capacitance* C_j is dependent on the reverse bias voltage and hence, its reactance is variable. It is therefore known as *varicap*, *voltacap* or *voltage variable capacitor* (VVC) diode. Basically, it is just a reverse biased junction diode. When a *p*-n junction is formed, initially the carriers diffuse across the junction and a *depletion* region is formed as shown in Fig. 18.1(a). The electric field set up by the exposed donor and accepter centers establishes an equilibrium condition that limits the diffusion of carriers.

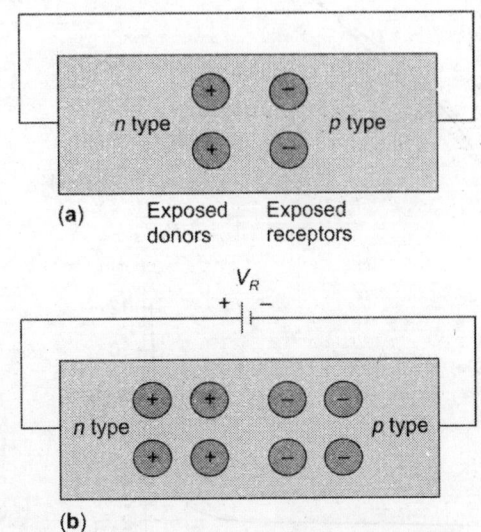

(a)

(b)

Fig 18.1: Diode depletion region (a) zero bias (b) reverse bias

When the *p-n* diode is short-circuited, no external current flows because the contact potential between the external *p* and *n* contacts exactly balances the internal potential. When it is reverse biased as in Fig. 18.1(b), the depletion region is increased and hence the exposed charge is also increased. This is similar to the action of a capacitor with positive side of the battery connected to the positively charged side of the depletion region. The charge increases as the reverse bias V_R is increased. On the negative side, an equal and opposite charge is maintained. Figure 18.2(a) shows how the charge and voltage are related in an ordinary or linear capacitor. In a linear capacitor, the capacitor charge is proportional to the voltage, the constant of proportionality being the capacitance C. Thus,

$$Q = CV \qquad (18.1)$$

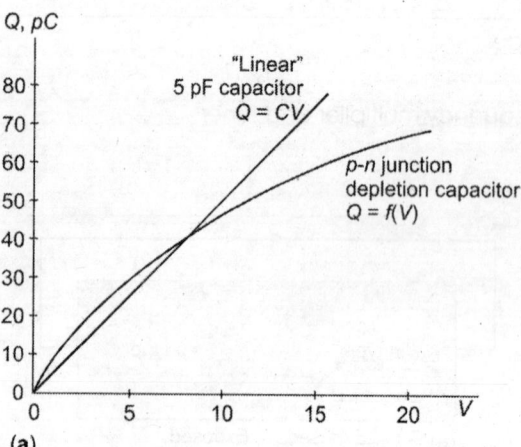

(a)

of a *p-n* junction diode is also shown on the same graph. Here, the charge is the change relative to equilibrium condition, i.e., the charge is zero when the applied voltage is zero.

The junction capacitance is given by the slope of the Q–V curve but varies from point to point along the curve. Hence, the junction capacitance is given by

$$C_j = dQ/dV \qquad (18.2)$$

The theoretical equation for junction or transition capacitance C_j is given by

$$C_j = C_o[1 + (V_R/V_B)]^{-n} \qquad (18.3)$$

Here C_o is the junction capacitance for zero bias, V_R is the reverse bias voltage below breakdown voltage and V_B is the barrier potential. The constant $n = 0.5$ for *abrupt p-n junction* and $1/3$ for *linearly graded junction*. As the magnitude of the reverse bias is increased, the depletion-layer width w increases. Hence, the junction capacitance decreases, as it is inversely proportional to the width of the depletion layer. Thus,

$$C_j \propto 1/w \qquad (18.4)$$

Figure 18.2(b) shows the variation of capacitance with bias voltage.

18.3 STRUCTURE AND EQUIVALENT CIRCUIT

The typical structure of a varactor diode along with its equivalent circuit is shown in Fig. 18.3. In this circuit, R_j is the reverse biased junction resistance, C_j is the junction capacitance. R_s is the diode bulk resistance. L_s is the series inductance of the leads. Since R_j is very large and L_s is negligible, the

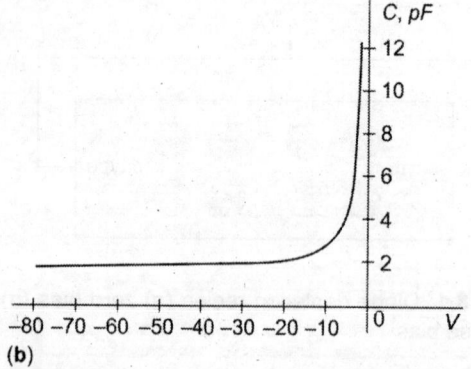

(b)

Fig. 18.2: (a) Charge-voltage relationship for linear capacitor and *p-n* junction diode (b) Capacitance voltage relationship

The capacitance is given by the slope of the Q–V line. For the example shown, the capacitance is 5 pF. The charge-voltage graph

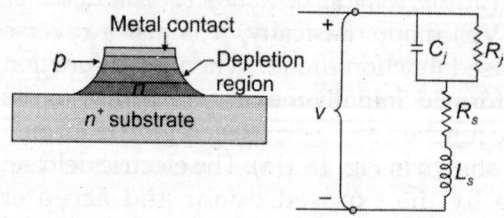

Fig. 18.3: Structure of a varactor diode and equivalent circuit

simplified model is a series combination of R_s and C_j. The varactor diode has a wide capacitance variation.

At a given reverse bias, the cut-off frequency of operation f_c is given by

$$f_c = 1/2\pi R_s C_j \qquad (18.5)$$

Due to skin effect, R_s increases with frequency. Hence, the varactor diode is normally used at frequencies below $0.2f_c$. Varactor diodes, fabricated with GaAs, have high operating frequency up to 90 GHz.

18.4 VARACTOR DIODE FREQUENCY MULTIPLIER

Figure 18.4 shows the variation of capacitance of a varactor diode with ac pump voltage. When an ac pumping voltage $v = V_p \sin w_p t$ is applied to a reverse biased varactor diode, the junction capacitance C_j varies according to Eq. (18.6).

$$C_j(t) = C_o[1 + (V_R + V_P \sin \omega_p t)/V_B]^{-n} \qquad (18.6)$$

Expanding Eq. (18.6) in harmonic series, we get

$$C_j(t) = C_o - C_1 \sin \omega_p t + C_2 \sin 2\omega_p t - C_3 \sin 3\omega_p I + ... \qquad (18.7)$$

The varactor diode current due to the varying $C_j(t)$ can be expressed as

$$i(t) = I_1 \cos \omega_p I + I_2 \cos 2\omega_p t + I_3 \cos 3\omega_p t + ... \qquad (18.8)$$

Equation (18.8) shows that the varactor diode can be used as a frequency multiplier or harmonic generator.

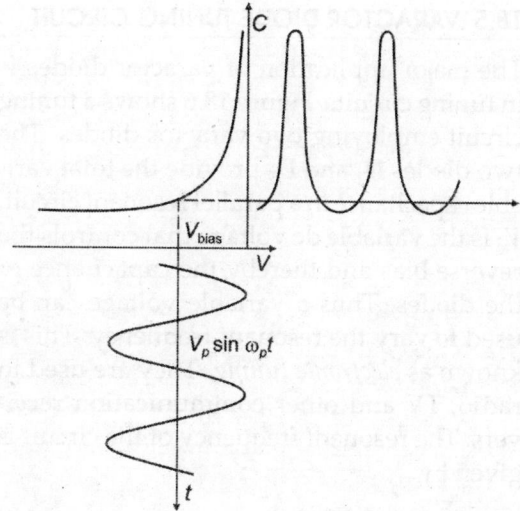

Fig. 18.4: Capacitance variation with ac pump voltage

Figure 18.5 shows that the input signal at frequency f is fed from a stable crystal oscillator to the reverse biased varactor diode represented by R_s and C_j in series through a buffer amplifier. The input resonant circuit 1 prevents unwanted frequencies reaching the varactor diode and isolates the input circuit from the varactor diode circuit. The output resonant circuit 3 is tuned to the third harmonic to produce an output at the triple frequency $3f$. The intermediate resonant circuit 2, called the *idler*, eliminates the heterodyning between the input and output frequencies. Since the harmonic current is capacitive, power loss is negligible. Hence, varactor diode multiplier operates at high efficiency without excessive noise generated.

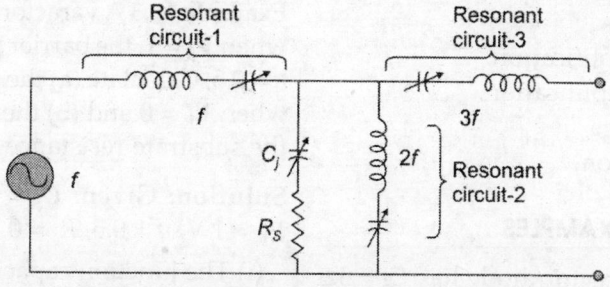

Fig. 18.5: Varactor diode frequency tripler

18.5 VARACTOR DIODE TUNING CIRCUIT

The major application of varactor diodes is in tuning circuits. Figure 18.6 shows a tuning circuit employing two varactor diodes. The two diodes D_1 and D_2 provide the total variable capacitance in a parallel resonant circuit. V_c is the variable dc voltage that controls the reverse bias and thereby the capacitance of the diodes. Thus a variable voltage can be used to vary the resonant frequency. This is known as *electronic tuning*. They are used in radio, TV and other communication receivers. The resonant frequency of the circuit is given by

$$f_0 = 1/(2\pi LC) \qquad (18.9)$$

Here L is the inductance of the tank circuit and C is the net capacitance equal to $C_1 C_2/(C_1 + C_2)$. C_1 and C_2 are the maximum and the minimum capacitance of the varactor diode.

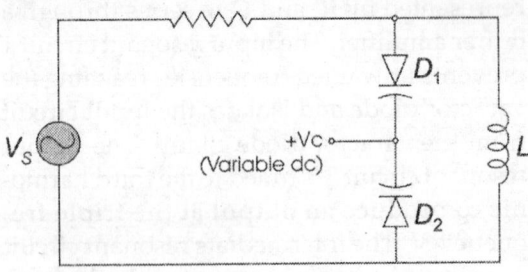

Fig. 18.6: Varactor diode tuning circuit

18.6 APPLICATIONS

The varactor diodes are used for the following purposes:

   (i) Harmonic generation.
   (ii) Tuning circuits.
   (iii) Low noise amplification.
   (iv) Parametric amplification.
   (v) Active filtering.
   (vi) F.M. modulation.

18.7 NUMERICAL EXAMPLES

Example 18.1 A varactor diode has $C_j = 0.5$ pF when $V_R = 0$, the barrier potential is 1.1 V and $n = 0.3$, Calculate (a) the junction capacitance and (b) the cut-off frequency for a reverse voltage of 1 V, if the substrate resistance is 0.7 ohm.

Solution: Given: $C_j = 0.5$ pF, $n = 0.3$, $V_R = 1$V, $V_B = 1.1$ V, $R_s = 0.7\Omega$

   (i) The junction capacitance is given by
$$C_j = C_0[1 + (V_R/V_B)]^{-n}$$
$$= 0.5 [1 + (1/1.1)]^{-0.3}$$
$$= 0.5 \times 0.842$$
$$= \mathbf{0.421 \ pF}$$

   (ii) The cut-off frequency is given by
$$f_c = 1/2\pi R_s C_j$$
$$= 1/(6.28 \times 0.7 \times 0.421 \times 10^{-12})$$
$$= \mathbf{540.3 \ GHz}$$

Example 18.2 A varactor diode has $C_j = 0.5$ pF when $V_R = 0$, the barrier potential is 1.1 V and $n = 0.5$, Calculate (a) the junction capacitance and (b) the cut-off frequency for a reverse voltage of 1 V, if the substrate resistance is 0.7 ohm.

Solution: Given: $C_j = 0.5$ pF, $n = 0.5$, $V_R = 1$ V, $V_B = 1.1$ V, $R_s = 0.7$ W

   (i) The junction capacitance is given by
$$C_j = C_0[1 + (V_R/V_B)]^{-n}$$
$$= 0.5 [1 + (1/1.1)]^{-0.5}$$
$$= 0.5 \times 0.724$$
$$= \mathbf{0.362 \ pF}$$

   (ii) The cut-off frequency is given by
$$f_c = 1/2\pi R_s C_j$$
$$= 1/(6.28 \times 0.7 \times 0.362 \times 10^{-12})$$
$$= \mathbf{628.4 \ GHz}$$

Example 18.3 A varactor diode has $C_j = 0.5$ pF when $V_R = 1$, the barrier potential is 1.1 V and $n = 0.5$, Calculate (a) the junction capacitance when $V_R = 0$ and (b) the cut-off frequency, if the substrate resistance is 0.7 ohm.

Solution: Given: $C_j = 0.5$ pF, $V_B = 1.1$ V, $V_R = 1$ V, $n = 0.5$, $R_s = 0.7$

   (i) The junction capacitance is given by
$$C_j = C_0[1 + (V_R/V_B)]^{-n}$$

$$C_o = C_j [1 + (V_R/V_B)]^n$$
$$= 0.5 [1 + (1/1.1)]^{0.5}$$
$$= 0.5 \times 1.382$$
$$= \mathbf{0.691 \ pF}$$

(ii) The cut-off frequency is given by

$$f_c = 1/2\pi R_s C_j$$
$$= 1/(6.28 \times 0.7 \times 0.691 \times 10^{-12})$$
$$= \mathbf{329.2 \ GHz}$$

Example 18.4: A varactor diode has $C_j = 0.5$ pF when $V_R = 0.8$ V, the barrier potential is 1.1 V and $n = 0.3$, Calculate (a) the junction capacitance when $V_R = 0$ and (b) the cut-off frequency, if the substrate resistance is 0.7 ohm.

Solution: Given: $C_j = 0.5$ pF, $V_R = 0.8$, $V_B = 1.1$, $n = 0.3$, $R_s = 0.7 \ \Omega$.

(i) The junction capacitance is given by

$$C_j = C_o[1 + (V_R/V_B)]^{-n}$$
$$C_o = C_j [1 + (V_R/V_B)]^n$$
$$= 0.5 [1 + (0.8/1.1)]^{0.3}$$
$$= 0.5 \times 1.178$$
$$= \mathbf{0.589 \ pF}$$

(ii) The cut-off frequency is given by

$$f_c = 1/2\pi R_s C_j$$
$$= 1/(6.28 \times 0.7 \times 0.589 \times 10^{-12})$$
$$= \mathbf{386.2 \ GHz}$$

KEY POINTS

• The term varactor means a variable reactor. The varactor diode is a *p-n* junction diode operated with reverse bias voltage. The junction or transition capacitance C_j is dependent on the reverse bias voltage and hence, its reactance is variable. It is therefore known as varicap, voltacap or voltage variable capacitor (VVC) diode.

• The theoretical equation for junction or transition capacitance C_j is given by $C_j = C_o[1 + (V_R/V_B)]^{-n}$. The constant $n = 0.5$ for abrupt *p-n* junction and 1/3 for linearly graded junction.

• At a given reverse bias, the cut-off frequency of operation f_c is given by $f_c = 1/2\pi R_s C_j$.

• The varactor diodes are used for (i) Harmonic generation, (ii) Tuning circuits, (iii) Low noise amplification, (iv) Parametric amplification, (v) Active filtering and (vi) FM modulation.

FURTHER READING

1. Johnson JB et al (1965). A Silicon Diode Microwave Oscillator, Bell Sys. Tech. J., vol.44, pp 369–372.
2. Liao SY (1985). Microwave Solid State Devices, PH, NJ.
3. Read WT (1958). A Proposed High-frequency Negative Resistance Diode, Bell Sys.Tech. J., vol.37, pp 407–446.
4. Reinfield P and Rafuse P (1962). Varactor Applications, MIT, Mass.

REVIEW QUESTIONS

13.1 What is a varactor diode?

13.2 Draw the equivalent circuit of a varactor diode.

13.3 Mention the applications of a varactor diode.

13.4 Draw Q vs V curve of a varactor diode.

13.5 Draw C vs V curve of a varactor diode.

13.6 Give the relationship between C_j and C_o.

13.7 Give expression for the cutoff frequency of operation of a varactor diode.

13.8 Give the expression for the resonant frequency of the varactor diode tuning circuit and explain.

DESCRIPTIVE QUESTIONS

18.1 Explain the operation of a varactor diode and its equivalent circuit.

18.2 Explain the variation of junction capacitance with pump voltage.

18.3 Explain, with a circuit, the operation of a varactor diode frequency multiplier.

18.4 Explain, with a circuit, the operation of a varactor diode tuning circuit.

PRACTICE PROBLEMS

18.1 A varactor diode has $C_j = 0.5$ pF when $V_R = 0$, the barrier potential is 1.1 V and $n = 0.3$, Calculate (a) the junction capacitance and (b) the cut-off frequency for a reverse voltage of 0.8 V, if the substrate resistance is 0.7 ohm. (**Ans:** 0.425 pF, 535 GHz)

18.2 A varactor diode has $C_j = 0.5$ pF when $V_R = 0$, the barrier potential is 1.1 V and $n = 0.5$, Calculate (a) the junction capacitance and (b) the cut-off frequency for a reverse voltage of 0.8 V, if the substrate resistance is 0.7 ohm. (**Ans:** 0.380 pF, 598.6 GHz)

18.3 A varactor diode has $C_j = 0.5$ pF when $V_R = 0.8$, the barrier potential is 1.1 V and $n = 0.5$, Calculate (a) the junction capacitance when $V_R = 0$ and (b) the cut-off frequency, if the substrate resistance is 0.7 ohm.

(**Ans:** 0.657 pF, 346.2 GHz)

18.4 A varactor diode has $C_j = 0.5$ pF when $V_R = 1$ V, the barrier potential is 1.1 V and $n = 0.3$, Calculate (a) the junction capacitance when $V_R = 0$ and (b) the cut-off frequency, if the substrate resistance is 0.7 ohm.

(**Ans:** 0.607 pF, 374.8 GHz)

18.5 The capacitance of a varactor diode is varied from 5 pF to 50 pF. Determine the range of tuning if $L = 10$ mH.

(**Ans:** 10.06 kHz to 31.85 kHz)

REFERENCE

1. Roy SK and Mitra M (2003). *Microwave Semiconductor Devices*, PHI, New Delhi.

2. Sims GD and Stephen IM (1963). *Microwave Tubes and Semiconductor Devices*, Inter-Science Publication, NY.

3. Streetman BG (2000). *Solid State Electronic Devices*, PH, NJ.

4. Sze SM (1985). *Semiconductor Devices: Physics and Technology*, John Wiley, NY.

5. Watson A (Ed.) (1969). *Microwave Semiconductor Devices and Their Applications*, McGraw Hill, NY.

6. Gentile C (1987). *Microwave Amplifiers and Oscillators*, McGraw Hill, NY.

7. De Loach BC Jr (1967). *Recent Advances in Solid State Microwave Generators, Advances in Microwaves*, Vol. 2, Academic Press, NY.

8. Hess K (1988). *Advanced Theory of Semiconductor Devices*, PH, NJ.

9. IEEE Trans. Electron Devices, (1980). Special Issue on Microwave Solid State Devices, ED-27, No. 2.

10. IEEE Trans. Electron Devices (1980). Special Issue on Microwave Solid State Devices, ED-27, No. 6.

11. IEEE Trans. Electron Devices, (1981). Special Issue on Microwave Solid State Devices, ED-28, No. 2.

12. IEEE Trans. Electron Devices (1981). Special Issue on Microwave Solid State Devices, ED-28, No. 8.

Parametric Amplifiers

- Know the principle of operation of parametric amplifier.
- Derive the Manley-Rowe power equation.
- Classify the parametric amplifiers.
- Explain the applications of parametric amplifier.

19.1 INTRODUCTION

In this chapter, we shall first discuss the operating principle of a parametric amplifier and derive the Manley-Rowe power relation. Then, we shall describe the various types of parametric amplifiers such as up-converter, down-converter, negative resistance amplifier and degenerative amplifier and finally their merits and limitations.

19.2 PRINCIPLE OF PARAMETRIC AMPLIFIER

A parametric amplifier utilizes the variation of a device-parameter for its operation, such as capacitance of a varactor diode. Hence it is known as *parametric amplifier*. The capacitance of a varactor diode is varied by a suitable R.F. signal, called *pump signal*. If a pump signal at a frequency f_p and a small input signal at frequency f_s are applied together to a varactor diode, the input signal is amplified due to the time varying capacitance of the varactor diode. The power required for amplification is provided by the pump signal. The output power is either at

the input signal frequency f_s or at the sum and difference frequency $f_i = f_p \pm f_s$. The frequency f_i is known as the *idler frequency*. Thus, in a parametric amplifier three frequencies are present. They are:

(i) The signal frequency f_s
(ii) The pump frequency f_p
(iii) The idler frequency f_i.

19.3 MANLEY-ROWE POWER RELATIONS

A set of general energy relations regarding power flowing into and out of an ideal nonlinear reactance were derived by Manley-Rowe. These energy relations are used in predicting the power gain in parametric amplifiers. Figure 19.1 shows the equivalent circuit for deriving Manley-Rowe power relations. An input signal at a frequency f_s and a pump signal at a frequency f_p along with associated series resistances R and band-pass filters are applied to a nonlinear capacitor $C(t)$. The filter resonance circuits are designed to reject power at all frequencies other than the respective signal frequencies. Because of two applied frequencies f_s and f_p,

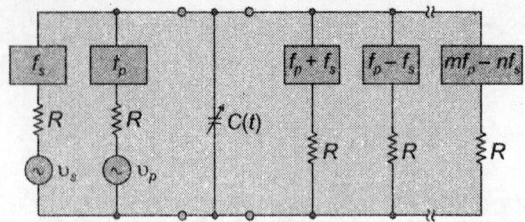

Fig. 19.1: Equivalent circuit for Manley-Rowe power relation

an infinite number of resonant frequencies of $mf_p \pm nf_s$ are generated, where m and n are any *integer* from zero to infinity.

Assumptions: The assumptions in deriving the Manley-Rowe power relations are:

(i) The resonating circuits are ideal.

(ii) The power loss by the nonlinear susceptances is negligible.

This implies that, due to nonlinear interaction, the power entering the nonlinear capacitance at the pump frequency f_p is equal to the power leaving the capacitance at the other frequencies.

The power relations between the input power at the frequencies f_s and f_p, and the output power at other frequencies $mf_p \pm nf_s$ have been established by Manley–Rowe.

The total voltage across the nonlinear capacitor $C(t)$ can be expressed as

$$v = v_p + v_s$$

$$= (\tfrac{1}{2}V_p)(e^{j\omega_p t} + e^{-j\omega_p t}) + (\tfrac{1}{2}V_s)(e^{j\omega_s t} + e^{-j\omega_s t}) \tag{19.1}$$

The general expression for the charge Q on the capacitor is given by

$$Q = \sum_{m=-\infty}^{\infty} \sum_{n=-\infty}^{\infty} Q_{mn}\, e^{j(m\omega_p t \pm n\omega_s t)} \tag{19.2}$$

The total voltage v can be expressed as a function of Q. A Taylor series expansion of $v(Q)$ shows that

$$v = \sum_{m=-\infty}^{\infty} \sum_{n=-\infty}^{\infty} V_{mn}\, e^{j(m\omega_p t \pm n\omega_s t)} \tag{19.3}$$

The current i flowing through $C(t)$ is given by

$$i = dQ/dt$$

$$= \sum_{m=-\infty}^{\infty} \sum_{n=-\infty}^{\infty} j(m\omega_p t \pm n\omega_s t)\, Q_{mn}\, e^{j(m\omega_p t \pm n\omega_s t)}$$

$$= \sum_{m=-\infty}^{\infty} \sum_{n=-\infty}^{\infty} I_{mn}\, e^{j(m\omega_p t \pm n\omega_s t)} \tag{19.4}$$

where $I_{mn} = j(m\omega_p t \pm n\omega_s t))Q_{mn}$. The capacitance $C(t)$ is assumed to be a pure reactance. Hence, the average power at the frequencies $mf_p \pm nf_s$ is given by

$$P_{mn} = (V_{mn}I_{mn}^* + V_{mn}^* I_{mn}) \tag{19.5}$$

then the conservation of power is given by

$$\sum_{m=-\infty}^{\infty} \sum_{n=-\infty}^{\infty} P_{mn} = 0 \tag{19.6}$$

Multiplication and division of the above equation by $(mw_p + nw_s)$ and rearranging the result into parts yield

$$\sum_{m=-\infty}^{\infty} \sum_{n=-\infty}^{\infty} \frac{mP_{mn}}{(m\omega_p + n\omega_s)} + \frac{nP_{mn}}{(mn_p + n\omega_s)} = 0 \tag{19.7}$$

For any choice of frequencies f_p and f_s, the external resonating circuit can be adjusted such that the currents keep all the voltage amplitudes V_{mn} constant. Hence, the frequencies f_p and f_s can be arbitrarily adjusted so that

$$\sum_{m=-\infty}^{\infty} \sum_{n=-\infty}^{\infty} \frac{mP_{mn}}{(m\omega_p + n\omega_s)} = 0 \tag{19.8}$$

and

$$\sum_{m=-\infty}^{\infty} \sum_{n=-\infty}^{\infty} \frac{nP_{mn}}{(m\omega_p + n\omega_s)} = 0 \tag{19.9}$$

Eq. (19.8) can be expressed as

$$\sum_{m=-\infty}^{\infty} \sum_{n=-\infty}^{\infty} \frac{mP_{mn}}{(m\omega_p + n\omega_s)} - \frac{nP_{mn}}{(m\omega_p + n\omega_s)} = 0 \tag{19.10}$$

or

$$\sum_{m=-\infty}^{\infty} \sum_{n=-\infty}^{\infty} \frac{-mP_{mn}}{-(m\omega_p + n\omega_s)} = 0 \tag{19.11}$$

Hence,

$$\sum_{m=-\infty}^{\infty} \sum_{n=-\infty}^{\infty} \frac{-mP_{mn}}{-(m\omega_p + n\omega_s)} = 0 \tag{19.12}$$

Similarly,

$$\sum_{m=-\infty}^{\infty} \sum_{n=-\infty}^{\infty} \frac{-nP_{mn}}{-(m\omega_p + n\omega_s)} = 0 \tag{19.13}$$

Here ω_p and ω_s are replaced by f_p and f_s respectively.

Equations (19.12) and (19.13) are known as *Manley–Rowe* power relations. The term P_{mn} is the real power flowing into or leaving from the nonlinear capacitor at a frequency of $mf_p + nf_s$. It is assumed that the power flowing into $C(t)$ or the power coming from the two voltage generators is positive, whereas the power leaving from $C(t)$ or the power flowing into the load resistance is negative.

19.4 POWER OUTPUT

Let us consider the case where power output flow is at a frequency $(f_p + f_s)$. All other harmonics are open-circuited. Then, the currents at the f_p, f_s and $f_p + f_s$ frequencies are the only ones existing. Under these conditions, m and n vary from -1 to $+1$. Hence, Eq. (19.12) and (19.13) reduce to

$$P_{10}/f_p + P_{11}/(f_p + f_s) = 0 \qquad (19.14)$$

$$P_{01}/f_s + P_{11}/(f_p + f_s) = 0 \qquad (19.15)$$

P_{10} and P_{01} are the power supplied by the two voltage sources at frequencies f_p and f_s respectively and are positive. The power P_{11} flowing from the reactance into the resistive load at the frequency $(f_p + f_s)$ is negative.

19.5 POWER GAIN

The power gain of a parametric amplifier is defined as the ratio of the power delivered by the capacitor at a frequency $(f_p + f_s)$ to the power absorbed by the capacitor at the frequency f_s. Thus,

$$\text{Power gain} = P_{11}/P_{01}$$
$$= (f_p + f_s)/f_s = f_0/f_s \qquad (19.16)$$

Here $(f_p + f_s) = f_0$ and $f_0 > f_p > f_s$. Thus, the maximum gain is the ratio of the output frequency to the input frequency. The output frequency f_0 is the sum of the pump and signal frequencies. Such a parametric ampli-

fier is known as *up-converter* or *sum frequency amplifier*.

If the signal frequency is the sum of the pump and the output frequencies, then the output power must move out from the signal generator circuits. This implies that the power gain in this case is

$$\text{Power gain} = P_{01}/P_{11} = f_s/(f_p + f_s) \qquad (19.17)$$

Here $f_s = (f_p + f_0)$. The gain is actually a *loss*. Such a parametric amplifier is known as *down-converter*.

If the signal frequency is f_s, the pump frequency is f_p and the output frequency $f_0 = (f_p - f_s)$, the power P_{11} supplied at the frequency f_p is positive. Both P_{01} and P_{10} are negative. This implies that the capacitor delivers power to the signal generator at the frequency f_s instead of absorbing the power. Hence the power gain may become infinite. This is an unstable condition and the circuit may oscillate both at f_s and f_0. Such a parametric amplifier is known as *negative resistance amplifier*.

19.6 PARAMETRIC AMPLIFIERS

In a super-heterodyne radio receiver, the R.F. incoming signal is mixed with a local oscillator signal in a mixer circuit to generate the sum and difference frequencies. In a parametric amplifier, a pumping generator, such as a reflex klystron, replaces the local oscillator, and the nonlinear capacitor, such as a varactor diode, replaces the mixer circuit, This is shown in Fig. 19.2. The signal frequency f_s and the pump frequency f_p are mixed in the nonlinear capacitor $C(t)$. A voltage at the fundamental frequencies f_s and f_p and the sum and difference frequencies $(mf_p \pm nf_s)$ appears across $C(t)$. If a load resistance is connected across the idler circuit, an output voltage is generated across the load at f_0. The output circuit that does not require external excitation is known as *idler circuit*. The output or idler frequency f_0

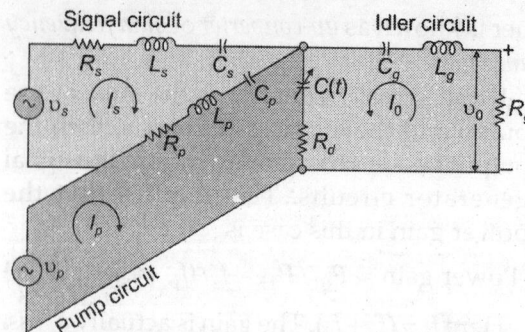

Fig. 19.2: Parametric amplifier

is expressed as the sum and difference frequencies of f_s and f_p. Thus,

$$f_o = (mf_p \pm nf_s) \qquad (19.18)$$

Here m and n are positive integers from zero to infinity. If $f_o > f_s$, then the parametric amplifier is known as *up-converter* and if $f_o < f_s$, then the parametric amplifier is known as *down-converter*.

19.7 UP-CONVERTER

The important properties of an up-converter are:

(i) The output frequency f_o is the sum of the signal frequency f_s and the pump frequency f_p. Thus $f_o = f_s + f_p$.

(ii) There is no power flow at frequencies other than, f_s, f_p and f_o.

19.7.1 Power Gain

The maximum power gain A_p of an up-converter is given by

$$A_p = \left(\frac{f_o}{f_s}\right)\left[\frac{x}{(1 + \sqrt{1+x})^2}\right] \qquad (19.19)$$

where

$f_o = (f_p + f_s)$

$x = (f_s / f_o)(\gamma Q)^2$

$Q = 1/(2\pi f_s C R_d)$

R_d = the series resistance of the p-n junction diode

γQ = the figure of merit of the nonlinear capacitor.

The quantity $x/(1 + \sqrt{1+x})^2$ is the *gain degradation factor*. As R_d approaches zero, γQ tends to infinity and the gain degradation factor becomes equal to unity. As a result of this, the power gain of the up-converter for a loss-less diode is equal to f_o/f_s as predicted by Manley-Rowe power relations. In a typical microwave diode, $\gamma Q = 10$. If $f_o/f_s = 15$, the power gain A_p is 7.3 dB.

19.7.2 Noise Figure

The parametric amplifiers have low noise figure because a pure reactance does not generate *thermal* or *Johnson* noise. The noise figure F of an up-converter is given by

$$F = 1 + (2T_d/T_o)[1/(\gamma Q) + 1/(\gamma Q)^2] \qquad (19.20)$$

where

T_d is the diode temperature in degrees Kelvin,

T_o is the ambient temperature, 300 K

γQ is the figure of merit of the nonlinear capacitor.

In a typical microwave diode, $\gamma Q = 10$. If $f_o/f_s = 10$ and $T_d = 300°K$, then $F = 0.86$ dB.

19.7.3 Bandwidth

The bandwidth of the up-converter is related to γ and the ratio f_o/f_s. Thus, the bandwidth B of the up-converter is given by

$$B = 2\gamma\sqrt{\frac{f_o}{f_s}} \qquad (19.21)$$

If $\gamma = 0.2$ and $f_o/f_s = 10$, then the bandwidth $B = 1.265$.

19.8 DOWN-CONVERTER

If the operation of a parametric amplifier as down-converter is required, then $f_s = (f_p + f_o)$. This means that the input power must be fed into the idler circuit and the output power must move out from the signal circuit. The down-converter gain is actually a loss and is given by

$$\text{Power loss} = \left(\frac{f_s}{f_o}\right)\left[\frac{x}{(1 + \sqrt{1+x})^2}\right] \qquad (19.22)$$

19.9 NEGATIVE RESISTANCE PARAMETRIC AMPLIFIER

Figure 19.3 shows the equivalent circuit of a negative resistance parametric amplifier. The varactor diode, represented by the series continuation of C_j and R_s, provides the necessary negative resistance at the signal frequency for amplification of the signal. If significant power flows only at the signal frequency f_s, the pump frequency f_p and the idler frequency $f_i = (f_p - f_s)$, a regenerative condition with a possibility of oscillations at both f_s and f_i will occur. When the diode is operated below the threshold of oscillation, the parametric amplifier behaves as a *bilateral negative resistance parametric amplifier*. The external tuned circuit and band-pass filters shown in Fig. 19.3 allow currents at frequencies f_s, f_p and f_i. The output is obtained across the load resistance R_L in the idler circuit. Since the fundamental frequencies only are passed, we have

$$C_j(t) = C_0 - C_1 \sin \omega_p t \qquad (19.23)$$

$$i_s = I_s \sin \omega_s t \qquad (19.24)$$

$$i_i = I_i \sin \omega_i t \qquad (19.25)$$

The diode current i is given by

$$i = i_s + i_i + i_p \qquad (19.26)$$

Since i_p involves only the pump frequency, its contribution towards signal current is negligibly small. Hence,

$$i = i_s + i_i = I_s \sin \omega_s t + I_i \sin \omega_i t \quad (19.27)$$

The signal voltage V_d across the diode is given by

$$V_d = \left(\frac{I}{C_j}\right) \int i\, dt \qquad (19.28)$$

$$\int i\, dt = -\left[\left(\frac{I_s}{\omega_s}\right)\cos\omega_s t + \left(\frac{I_i}{\omega_i}\right)\cos\omega_i t\right] \quad (19.29)$$

Substituting for C_j and $\int i\, dt$ in Eq. (19.28), we get

$$V_d = -\left(\frac{1}{C_0}\right)\left[\frac{\left(\frac{I_s}{\omega_s}\right)\cos\omega_s t + \left(\frac{I_i}{\omega_i}\right)\cos\omega_i t}{\left[1 - \left(\frac{C_1}{C_0}\right)\sin\omega_p t\right]}\right]$$

Since C_1/C_0 is comparatively smaller than 1, $(1/C_0)$ $[1 - (C_1/C_0)\sin\omega_p t]$ is replaced by $(1/C_0)$ $[1 + (C_1/C_0)\sin w_p t]$. Thus,

$$V_d = -\left[\left(\frac{I_s}{\omega_s}\right)\cos\omega_s t + \left(\frac{I_i}{\omega_i}\right)\cos\omega_i t\right]$$

$$\left\{\frac{1}{C_0}\left[1 + \left(\frac{C_1}{C_0}\right)\sin\omega_p t\right]\right\} \quad (19.30)$$

The voltage term contains f_s, f_p, f_o, $f_p \pm f_s$ and $f_p \pm f_o$ frequencies. The product terms result in signal voltage components at frequencies $f_p \pm f_s$ and $f_p \pm f_o$. Because of the resonant circuits, only $f_p - f_o = f_s$ contributes to the signal voltage across the diode. Hence, the signal frequency voltage is given by

$$V_{ds} = -\left(\frac{1}{C_0}\right)\left[\left(\frac{I_s}{\omega_s}\right)\cos\omega_s + \left(\frac{C_1}{C_0}\right)\left(\frac{\frac{1}{2}I_i}{\omega_i}\right)\sin\omega_s t\right] \quad (19.30a)$$

The factor ½ appears in the second term of the above equation since $(\sin\omega_p t \cdot \cos\omega_p t) = \frac{1}{2}[\sin(\omega_p + \omega_o)t + \sin\omega_s t]$. Since $|V_s| < |V_p|$, the signal voltage V_{ds} across the diode is mostly due to the second term only. Thus,

$$V_{ds} = -\left(\frac{1}{C_0^2}\right)\left[\left(\frac{\frac{1}{2}C_1 I_i}{\omega_i}\right)\sin\omega_s t\right]$$

$$= -\left(\frac{1}{C_0^2}\right)\left[\left(\frac{C_1}{2\omega_i}\right)\left(\frac{I_i}{I_s}\right)I_s \sin\omega_s t\right]$$

$$= -K I_s \sin\omega_s t \qquad (19.31)$$

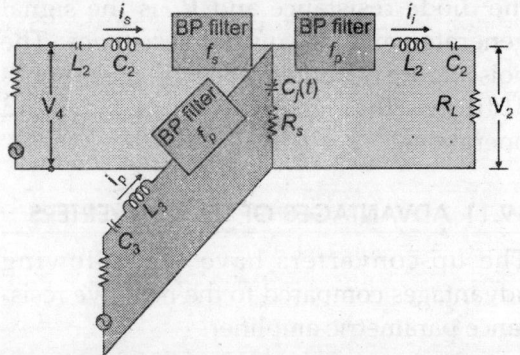

Fig. 19.3: Equivalent circuit of negative resistance parametric amplifier

where $K = \left(\dfrac{1}{C_0^2}\right)\left(\dfrac{C_1}{2\omega_i}\right)\left(\dfrac{I_i}{I_s}\right)$

Thus, the voltage V_{ds} is out of phase with the signal current giving rise to the negative resistance. The negative resistance R_n of the varactor diode at f_s is given by

$$R_n = (C_1 I_i)/(2C_0\omega_i I_s) \qquad (19.32a)$$

The total input resistance R_{in} of the input loop is

$$R_{in} = R_s + R_n \qquad (19.32b)$$

19.9.1 Power Gain

The output power is taken across the resistance R_i at f_0. The power gain A_p is given by

$$A_p = (4f_i/f_s)\,(R_g R_i/R_{Ts}R_{Ti})\,[a/(1-a)^2] \qquad (19.33)$$

where

R_g is the output resistance of the signal generator,

R_i is the output resistance in the idler circuit,

R_{Ts} is the total series resistance at f_s,

R_{Ti} is the total series resistance at f_i

a is R/R_{Ts}

R is $\gamma^2/(\omega_s\omega_i C^2 R_{Ti})$

19.9.2 Noise Figure

The optimum noise figure of a negative resistance parametric amplifier is given by

$$F = 1 + 2\,(T_d/T_o)\,[(1/\gamma Q) + 1/(\gamma Q)^2] \quad (19.34)$$

Here γQ is the figure of merit of the capacitor, T_o is the ambient temperature, $300°K$ and T_d is the diode junction tempe-rature in $°K$. In a typical microwave diode, $\gamma Q = 10$. If $f_0/f_s = 10$ and $T_d = 300°K$, then $F = 0.90$ dB.

19.9.3 Bandwidth

The maximum bandwidth of a negative resistance parametric amplifier is given by

$$B = \left(\dfrac{\gamma}{2}\right)\sqrt{\dfrac{f_i}{f_s G}} \qquad (19.35)$$

G is the gain of the amplifier. If $G = 20$ dB, $f_0/f_s = 4$ and $\gamma = 0.3$, the bandwidth for a single-tuned circuit is 0.03.

19.10 DEGENERATE PARAMETRIC AMPLIFIER

The degenerate parametric amplifier or oscillator is defined as a negative resistance parametric amplifier with $f_s = f_i$. Since the idler frequency $f_i = f_p - f_s$, the signal frequency $f_s = f_p/2$.

19.10.1 Power Gain and Bandwidth

The power gain and bandwidth characteristics of degenerate parametric amplifiers are exactly same as those of the up-converter. With $f_s = f_i$ and $f_p = 2f_s$, the power transferred from f_p to f_s is equal to the power transferred from f_p to f_i. At high gain, the total power at f_s is almost equal to the total power at f_i. Hence, the total power in the pass-band will have 3 dB more gain.

19.10.2 Noise Figure

The noise figure F of a single-sideband and double-sideband of the degenerate parametric amplifier is given by

$$F_{ssb} = 2 + (2T_{id}R_d/T_o R_g) \qquad (19.36)$$
$$F_{dsb} = 1 + (T_{id}R_d/T_o R_g)$$
$$= F_{ssb}/2 \qquad (19.37)$$

Here, T_d is the diode temperature in K, T_o is the ambient temperature, 300 K, R_d is the diode resistance and R_g is the signal generator external output resistance. The noise figure of double-sideband operation is 3 dB less than that for single-sideband operation.

19.11 ADVANTAGES OF UP-CONVERTERS

The up-converters have the following advantages compared to the negative resistance parametric amplifier.

(i) The input impedance is positive.

(ii) It is absolutely stable.

(iii) Power gain is independent of source impedance.

(iv) No circulator is required for proper operation.

(v) It has a larger bandwidth.

19.12 ADVANTAGES AND LIMITATIONS OF PARAMETRIC AMPLIFIERS

The parametric amplifiers have the following advantages:

(i) Noise figure is low (< 2 dB).

(ii) It has wide range of operating frequency (40 to 200 GHz).

The limitations are:

(i) The gain is limited to 20 to 80 dB.

(ii) The bandwidth is narrow.

19.13 APPLICATIONS

The applications of the parametric amplifiers are:

(i) As front-end highly sensitive, low noise MW amplifiers in MW receivers.

(ii) As MW amplifiers in radar systems.

19.14 NUMERICAL EXAMPLES

Example 19.1 In an up-converter parametric amplifier, the figure of merit of the diode nonlinear capacitor is 10 and the ratio of the output frequency to the signal frequency is also 10. The diode temperature is 300°K. Determine (a) Power gain, (b) noise figure and (c) bandwidth for $\gamma = 0.2$. Assume the room temperature to be 27°C.

Solution: Given: $(f_o/f_s) = 10$, $T_d = 300°K$, $\gamma = 0.2$, $T_o = 300°K$, $\gamma Q = 10$.

(a) Power gain

$$= \left(\frac{f_o}{f_s}\right)\left[\frac{x}{(1+\sqrt{1+x})^2}\right]$$

$$x = \left(\frac{f_s}{f_o}\right)(\gamma Q)^2 = \left(\frac{1}{10}\right)10^2 = 10$$

∴ Power gain

$$= \left(\frac{f_o}{f_s}\right)\left[\frac{x}{(1+\sqrt{1+x})^2}\right]$$

$$= \left(\frac{10 \times 10}{(1+\sqrt{1+10})^2}\right) = 5.37$$

Power gain in dB

$$= 10 \log 5.37 = 7.3 \text{ dB}$$

(b) Noise figure

$$F = 1 + [2(T_d/T_o)][1/(\gamma Q) + 1/(\gamma Q)^2]$$
$$= 1 + [(2 \times 300)/(300)][1/10 + 1/100]$$
$$= 1.22 = 0.86 \text{ dB}$$

(c) Bandwidth

$$B = 2\gamma\sqrt{\left(\frac{f_o}{f_s}\right)} = 2 \times 0.2 \times \sqrt{10} = 1.265$$

Example 19.2 An up-converter parametric amplifier has a ratio of the output frequency to the signal frequency of 25, figure of merit γQ of 10 and factor of merit figure γ of 0.4. The diode temperature is 300°K. Find (a) the power gain in dB, (b) the noise figure in dB and (c) the bandwidth. Assume the room temperature to be 27°C.

Solution: Given: $f_o/f_s = 25$, $\gamma Q = 10$, $\gamma = 0.4$, $T_d = 300°K$, $T_o = 300°K$

(a) Power gain

$$= (f_o/f_s)[x/(1+\sqrt{1+x})^2]$$

$$x = (f_s/f_o)(\gamma Q)^2 = (1/25)10^2 = 4$$

Power gain

$$= (f_o/f_s)[x/(1+\sqrt{1+x})^2]$$

$$= 25 \times 4/[(1+\sqrt{1+4})^2] = 9.55$$

Power gain in dB

$$= 10 \log 9.55 = 9.8 \text{ dB}$$

(b) Noise figure

$$F = 1 + [2(T_d/T_o)][1/(\gamma Q) + 1/(\gamma Q)^2]$$
$$= 1 + [(2 \times 300)/(300)][1/10 + 1/100]$$
$$= 1.22$$
$$= 10 \log 1.22 = 0.864 \text{ dB}$$

(c) Bandwidth

$$B = 2\gamma \sqrt{\left(\frac{f_0}{f_s}\right)} = 2 \times 0.4 \times \sqrt{25} = 4$$

Example 19.3 An up-converter parametric amplifier has a ratio of the output frequency to the signal frequency of 8, figure of merit γQ of 8 and factor of merit figure $\gamma = 0.2$. The diode temperature is 300°K. Find (a) the power gain in dB, (b) the noise figure in dB and (c) the bandwidth. Assume the room temperature to be 27°C.

Solution: Given: $f_0/f_s = 8$, $\gamma Q = 8$, $\gamma = 0.2$, $T_d = 300°K$, $T_0 = 300°K$

(a) Power gain

$$= (f_0/f_s)[x/(1+\sqrt{1+x})^2]$$

$$x = (f_s/f_0)(\gamma Q)^2 = (1/8)\, 8^2 = 8$$

Power gain

$$= (f_0/f_s)[x/(1+\sqrt{1+x})^2]$$

$$= 8 \times 8/[(1+\sqrt{1+8})^2] = 4$$

Power gain in dB

$$= 10 \log 4 = \textbf{6.02 dB}$$

(b) Noise figure

$$F = 1 + [2(T_d/T_o)]\,[1/(\gamma Q) + 1/(\gamma Q)^2]$$

$$= 1 + [(2 \times 300)/(300)]\,[1/8 + 1/64]$$

$$= 1.28$$

$$= 10 \log 1.28 = \textbf{1.072 dB}$$

(c) Bandwidth

$$B = 2\gamma \sqrt{\left(\frac{f_0}{f_s}\right)} = 2 \times 0.2 \times \sqrt{8}$$

$$= 1.13$$

Example 19.4 A negative resistance parametric amplifier has $f_s = 2\,\text{GHz}$, $f_p = 12\ \text{GHz}$, $f_i = 10\ \text{GHz}$, $R_g = 1\ \text{k}\Omega$, $R_i = 1\ \text{k}\Omega$, $R_{Ts} = 1\ \text{k}\Omega$, $R_{Ti} = 1\ \text{k}\Omega$, $\gamma = 0.35$, $\gamma Q = 10$ and $C = 0.01\ \text{pF}$. The diode temperature is 300°K. Find (a) the power gain in dB, (b) the noise figure in dB and (c) the bandwidth. Assume the room temperature to be 27°C.

Solution: Given: $f_s = 2\ \text{GHz}$, $f_p = 12\ \text{GHz}$, $f_i = 10\ \text{GHz}$, $R_g = 1\ \text{k}\Omega$, $R_i = 1\ \text{k}\Omega$, $R_{Ts} = 1\ \text{k}\Omega$, $R_{Ti} = 1\ \text{k}\Omega$, $\gamma Q = 10$, $\gamma = 0.35$, $T_d = 300°K$, $T_o = 300°K$, $C = 0.01\ \text{pF}$.

(a) Power gain

$$G = (4f_i/f_s)\,(R_g R_i/R_{Ts} R_{Ti})\,[a/(1-a)^2]$$

$$a = R/R_{Ts}$$

$$R = \gamma^2/\omega_s \omega_i\, C^2\, R_{Ti})$$

$$= 0.35^2/[6.28 \times 2 \times 10^9 \times 6.28 \times$$

$$10 \times 10^9 \times (0.01 \times 10^{-12})^2 \times 1 \times 10^3)$$

$$= 1.553\ \text{k}\Omega$$

$$a = R/R_{Ts} = 1.553/1 = 1.553$$

$$G = (4f_i/f_s) - (R_g R_i/R_{Ts} R_{Ti})\,[a/(1-a)^2]$$

$$= (4 \times 5)[(1 \times 1)/(1 \times 1)]$$

$$[1.553/(1-1.553)^2]$$

$$= 101.57$$

Power gain in dB

$$= 10 \log 101.57 = \textbf{20.07 dB}$$

(b) Noise figure

$$F = 1 + 2\,(T_d/T_o)\,[1/\gamma Q + 1/(\gamma Q)^2]$$

$$= 1 + [(2 \times 300)/(300)]\,[1/10 + 1/100]$$

$$= 1.22$$

$$= 10 \log 1.22 = \textbf{0.864 dB}$$

(c) Bandwidth

$$B = (\gamma/2)\sqrt{\left(\frac{f_i}{f_s G}\right)}$$

$$= (0.35/2)\sqrt{5/101.57} = 0.039$$

KEY POINTS

- A parametric amplifier utilizes the variation of a device-parameter for its operation, such as capacitance of a varactor diode.
- Manley-Rowe equation relates the power flowing into and out of an ideal nonlinear reactance and is useful in predicting the power gain in parametric amplifiers.
- The power gain of a parametric amplifier is defined as the ratio of the power delivered by the

capacitor at a frequency $(f_p + f_s)$ to the power absorbed by the capacitor at the frequency f_s. Thus, power gain $= P_{11}/P_{01} = (f_p + f_s)/f_s = f_o/f_s$.

- If the output frequency f_o is the sum of the pump and signal frequencies, such a parametric amplifier is known as up-converter or sum frequency amplifier.

- The important properties of an up-converter are (i) $f_0 = f_s + f_p$, and (ii) no power flows at frequencies other than, f_s, f_p and f_0.

- If the signal frequency is the sum of the pump and the output frequencies, then, power loss occurs. Such a parametric amplifier is known as down-converter.

- The down-converter power loss
$$= (f_s/f_0)[x/(1 + \sqrt{1+x})^2].$$

- When the varactor diode is operated below the threshold of oscillation, the parametric amplifier behaves as a bilateral negative-resistance parametric amplifier.

- The power gain of a bilateral negative-resistance parametric amplifier is $(4f_i/f_s)$ $(R_g R_i/R_{Ts}R_{Ti})$ $[a/(1-a)^2]$

- The optimum noise figure of a negative resistance parametric amplifier is given by $F = 1 + 2(T_d/T_o)$ $[1/\gamma Q + 1/(\gamma Q)^2]$

- The maximum bandwidth of a negative resistance parametric amplifier is given by
$$B = (\gamma/2)\sqrt{f_o/(f_s G)}.$$

- The degenerate parametric amplifier or oscillator is defined as a negative resistance parametric amplifier with $f_s = f_o$. Since the idler frequency $f_i = f_p - f_s$, the signal frequency $f_s = f_p/2$.

- The advantages of up-converters compared to the negative resistance parametric amplifier are (i) The input impedance is positive, (ii) It is absolutely stable, (iii) Power gain is independent of source impedance, (iv) No circulator is required for proper operation and (v) It has a larger bandwidth.

- The parametric amplifiers have the following advantages (i) Noise figure is low (< 2 dB) and (ii) It has wide range of operating frequency (40 to 200 GHz).

- The limitations are (i) The gain is limited to 20 to 80 dB and (ii) The bandwidth is narrow.

- The applications of the parametric amplifiers are (i) as front-end highly sensitive, low noise MW amplifiers in MW receiver and (ii) as MW amplifiers in radar systems.

FURTHER READING

1. Blackwell LA and Kotzebue KL (1961). *Semiconductor Diode Parametric Amplifier*, PH, NJ.
2. Chang KKN (1964). *Parametric and Tunnel Diodes*, PH, NJ.
3. Collins RE (1996). *Foundations of Microwave Engineering*, McGraw Hill, NY.
4. Gandhi OP (1981). *Microwave Engineering and Applications*, Pergamon, NY.

REVIEW QUESTIONS

19.1 What is a parametric amplifier?
19.2 Mention the different types of parametric amplifiers.
19.3 Write down the Manley-Rowe power relation?
19.4 Draw the circuit used to derive Manley-Rowe power relation.
19.5 Give the expression for the power gain of ideal up-converter.
19.6 Draw the circuit of a parametric amplifier.
19.7 What is an idler circuit?
19.8 Give the expression for the noise figure of ideal up-converter.
19.9 Give the expressions for the power gain of ideal down-converter.
19.10 Describe a negative resistance parametric amplifier.
19.11 Give the expressions for the power gain of a negative resistance parametric amplifier.
19.12 Mention the advantages and limitations of parametric amplifiers
19.13 Mention the advantages of up-converter over the negative resistance parametric amplifier.
19.14 Give the applications of parametric amplifiers.

DESCRIPTIVE QUESTIONS

19.1 Explain the principle of operation of a parametric amplifier.
19.2 Derive the Manley-Rowe power relation with necessary circuit diagram.
19.3 Explain the principle of operation of an up-converter.
19.4 Explain the principle of operation of a down converter.

19.5 Explain the principle of operation of a negative resistance parametric amplifier.

PRACTICE PROBLEMS

19.1 An up-converter parametric amplifier has a ratio of the output frequency to the signal frequency of 25, figure of merit γQ of 10 and factor of merit figure γ of 0.4. The diode temperature is $350°K$. Find (a) the power gain in dB, (b) the noise figure in dB and (c) the bandwidth. Assume the room temperature to be $27°C$.

(**Ans:** 9.8 db, 1 dB, 4)

19.2 An up-converter parametric amplifier has a ratio of the output frequency to the signal frequency of 8, figure of merit γQ of 8 and factor of merit figure γ of 0.4. The diode temperature is $300°K$. Find (a) the power gain in dB, (b) the noise figure in dB and (c) the bandwidth. Assume the room temperature to be $27°C$.

(**Ans:** 6.02 dB, 1.072 dB, 2.26)

19.3 A negative resistance parametric amplifier has $f_s = 2GHz$, $f_p = 12$ GHz, $f_i = 10$ GHz, $R_l = 1$ kΩ, $R_s = 1$ kΩ, $R_{Ts} = 1$ kΩ, $R_{Ti} = 1$ kΩ, $\gamma = 0.4$, $\gamma Q = 10$ and $C = 0.01$ pF. The diode temperature is $300°K$. Find (a) the power gain in dB, (b) the noise figure in dB and (c) the bandwidth. Assume the room temperature to be $27°C$.

(**Ans:** 15.85 dB, 0.864 dB, 0.072)

REFERENCE

1. Gentile C (1987). *Microwave Amplifiers and Oscillators*, McGraw Hill, NY.
2. IEEE Trans. Electron Devices (1980). Special Issue on Microwave Solid State Devices, ED-27, No.2.
3. IEEE Trans. Electron Devices (1980). Special Issue on Microwave Solid State Devices, ED-27, No.6.
4. IEEE Trans. Electron Devices (1981). Special Issue on Microwave Solid State Devices, ED-28, No.2.
5. IEEE Trans. Electron Devices (1981). Special Issue on Microwave Solid State Devices, ED-28, No.8.
6. Liao SY (1985). *Microwave Solid State Devices*, PH, NJ.
7. Milnes AG (1980). *Semiconductor Devices and Integrated Electronics*, Van Nostrand, NY.
8. Nanavathi RP (1975). *Semiconductor Devices*, Intext Edn., Scranton , Pa.
9. Pozar DM (1990). *Microwave Engineering*, Addison-Wesley, Mass.
10. Roy SK and Mitra M (2003). *Microwave Semiconductor Devices*, PHI, New Delhi.
11. Sobol W and Sterzer F (1972). Solid State Microwave Power Source, IEEE Spectrum, Vol. 4, No. 32, April.
12. Sze SM (1985). *Semiconductor Devices: Physics and Technology*, John Wiley, NY.
13. Watson A (Ed.) (1969). *Microwave Semiconductor* Devices and their applications, McGraw Hill, NY.

20

Microwave Transistors

Objectives

- Understand the limitations of low frequency transistors.
- Know the constructional features of MW transistors.
- Discuss the principle of operation.
- Explain the applications.
- Analyze the noise considerations.

20.1 INTRODUCTION

Negative resistance diodes such as tunnel diode were the first solid-state devices used for microwave amplification. Parametric amplifiers that use a varactor diode as a variable capacitance and a pump source to vary the junction capacitance were then developed for microwave amplification. An outstanding feature of the parametric amplifiers is the low noise that can be achieved by cooling the diode to liquid-nitrogen temperature. The parametric amplifiers are the most widely used solid-state microwave amplifiers during 1958 to 1970. Improvements in materials preparation and processing technology led to the development of *npn* bipolar transistors for oscillations up to 10 GHz. Then, the design and fabrication of metal semiconductor field effect transistors (MESFET) were established by 1970. These devices are widely used above 5 GHz. The molecular beam epitaxy techniques led to the development of hetero-structures that resulted in the development of high electron mobility transistors (HEMT) that can operate up to 100 GHz.

Microwave amplifiers are usually constructed either as hybrid or monolithic microwave integrated circuits. In hybrid construction, the transmission lines and matching networks are realized as microstrip circuit elements, and then, the discrete components such as chip resistors, capacitors and transistors are connected by using wire-bonding techniques. A monolithic microwave integrated circuit is one in which all active and passive devices are fabricated on a single semiconductor crystal. GaAs is used as substrate material because of its high resistivity in the undoped state and superiority for high-frequency FET construction.

In this chapter, we shall discuss the high frequency limitations of BJP transistors, the physical structures and applications of microwave transistors.

20.2 HIGH-FREQUENCY LIMITATIONS

Microwave transistor is a nonlinear device. Its principle of operation is similar to that of low frequency transistor. However, the requirements of micron dimensions, heat sinking and packaging are more severe at microwave frequencies due to the following limitations.

20.2.1 Junction capacitance

The reactance of the junction capacitance cannot be neglected at microwave frequencies. For example, a capacitance of 0.1 pF at 10 GHz offers a reactance of 159 Ω and is significant as shunt reactance across a 50 Ω transmission line. Because of this, the gain is reduced. The junction capacitance should be as small as possible.

20.2.2 Lead Inductance

The lead inductance also cannot be neglected at microwave frequencies. This results in the loss of signal and hence, gain is reduced. Reduction of the lead length in packaging minimizes this effect

20.2.3 Transit Time

The time taken by majority carriers to cross over from the emitter to the collector is known as *transit time*. This limits the high frequency operation of transistor. The total transit time is emitter-base junction capacitance charging time T_{jeb}, base-region transit time T_b, base-collector region depletion layer transit time T_{bc} and base-collector junction capacitance charging time T_{jbc}. Since the emitter-base junction is forward biased, T_{jeb} may be neglected. The use of narrow p and n regions reduces the transit time.

The cut-off frequency is given by

$$f_T = 1/2\pi T \tag{20.1}$$

$T = T_{jeb} + T_b + T_{bc} + T_{jbc} = T_b + T_{bc}$. T_b is the base region transit time and T_{bc} is the base-collector region transit time.

20.2.4 Power-frequency

As the operating frequency increases, the power capacity of the transistor decreases. The power-frequency limitation is due to:

(a) Maximum velocity v_s of charge carriers in the semiconductors.
(b) Maximum electric field E_m that can be applied to a semiconductor
(c) Base-width that limits the maximum current.

The maximum power P_m available is given by

$$P_m = (E_m v_s/2\pi f_T)^2 X_c \tag{20.2}$$

Here, X_c is the capacitive reactance. Thus, for a given device impedance, the power capacity decreases with increase in cut-off frequency and is inversely proportional to the square of f_T.

20.3 BIPOLAR JUNCTION TRANSISTORS

Microwave bipolar junction transistor is a nonlinear device. Its principle of operation is similar to that of low frequency transistors. However, the higher inter-electrode capacitance, lead inductance and transit time limit its operation in high frequency range. Therefore, the foremost criteria while designing the microwave transistors are:

(i) Proper geometry to reduce the above effects
(ii) Heat sink
(iii) Packaging.

All microwave bipolar transistors are planar in form and is of *npn* type .The *npn* type is preferred because the electron mobility is greater than the hole mobility, they reach the collector faster. This increases the speed of operation and reduces the transit time, thus increasing the operating frequency. The microwave bipolar transistors are capable of generating powers up to 22 GHz. They are fabricated from Si, although GaAs devices offer higher operating frequencies.

The silicon microwave bipolar transistors are predominantly used for low microwave frequency amplification and oscillations because

(i) They are of low cost

(ii) They are more reliable

(iii) They are integrative

(iv) They offer higher gain.

(v) They have low noise figure at microwave frequencies.

20.3.1 Physical Structure

Microwave transistors are fabricated in planar form using Si and *n-p-n* configuration. The geometry of these may be any of the following types:

(i) Inter-digital type

(ii) Overlay type

(iii) Matrix type

Figure 20.1 shows the three types. The inter-digital type is used mostly for small signal and low power applications. The overlay and matrix types are used for power transistors only. These transistors are used in parallel to obtain high output of 2 to 10 W up to 4 GHz.

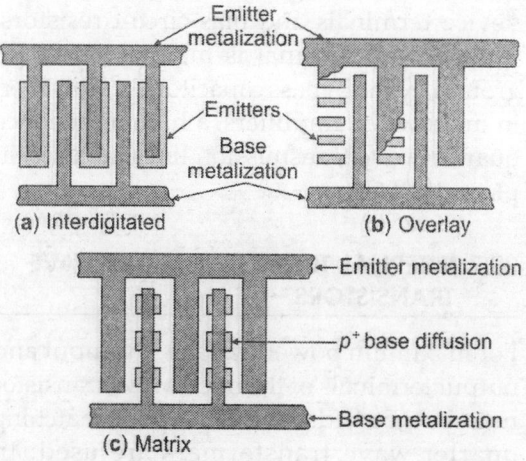

(a) Interdigitated

(b) Overlay

(c) Matrix

Fig. 20.1: Three types of microwave transistor structure

The *n-p-n* structure is used for microwave applications because the electron mobility ($\mu_n = 1500$ cm^2/V·s) is much higher than the hole-mobility ($\mu_p = 450$ cm^2/V·s).

20.4 CE CONFIGURATION

At microwave frequencies, common emitter configuration of transistors is used because it reduces the negative feedback on account of the base-to-collector capacitance. The CE configuration equivalent circuit is shown in Fig. 20.2.

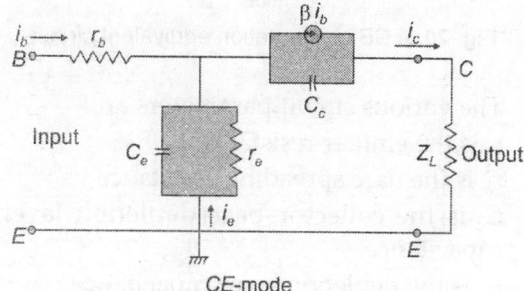

CE-mode

Fig. 20.2: CE configuration equivalent circuit

The various circuit parameters are:

r_b: Base spreading resistance .

C_e: Depletion layer capacitance across the forward biased emitter-base diode.

r_e: A.C. equivalent resistance of the forward biased emitter-base diode.

C_c: Collector–base depletion layer capacitance.

r_c: Resistance of the un-depleted region of the collector.

β: Current gain.

The current gain of the CE transistor is given by

$$\beta(f) = \beta_o / [1 + j(f/f_\beta)] \tag{20.3}$$

Here, $$\beta_o = \alpha_o / (1 - \alpha_o) \tag{20.4}$$

$$f_\beta = (1 - \alpha_o) f_\alpha \tag{20.5}$$

20.5 CB CONFIGURATION

The Common-base configuration is also known as *grounded-base configuration* since the base terminal is grounded. The CB configuration equivalent circuit is shown in Fig. 20.3.

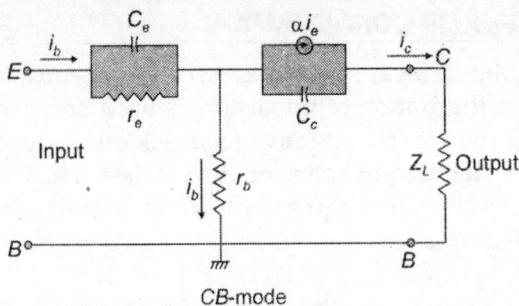

Fig. 20.3: CB configuration equivalent circuit

The various circuit parameters are:

r_e is the emitter resistance

r_b is the base spreading resistance

C_c is the collector–base depletion layer capacitance.

C_e is the depletion layer capacitance

α is the current gain

In *p-n-p* transistors, the largest current components are due to holes and that in *n-p-n* transistors are due to electrons. The holes flow from the emitter to the collector and to the ground through the base.

The maximum allowable power in both configurations is given by

$$P_{max} = (E_m V_s / 2\pi f_T)^2 / \chi_c$$

where E_m is the maximum electric field

v_s is the saturation drift velocity

f_T is the transit time cutoff

20.6 TRANSISTOR BIASING

While designing the transistor biasing circuit, the following main considerations have to be taken into account:

(i) The biasing circuit must provide a stable operating point Q that is independent of variations in device parameters and temperature.

(ii) The biasing circuit must be isolated from high frequency in order to avoid its flow in the biasing circuit.

In order to provide a stable operating point, a dc feedback path is provided in the

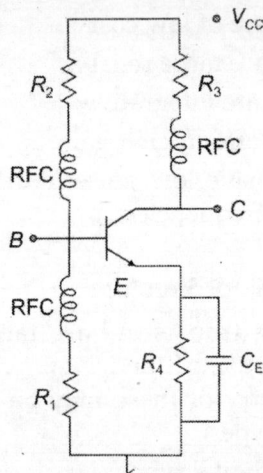

Fig. 20.4: Microwave transistor biasing circuit

biasing circuit. For isolation from the high frequency currents, high impedance RF chokes (RFC) are used in the voltage divider bias and the collector circuit, and a low impedance capacitive bypass circuit across the emitter bias resistance R_E, as shown in Fig. 20.4. This bias circuit provides stable operating point. It is isolated from the transistor by using RF chokes between the device terminals and bias-circuit resistors. The emitter terminal is maintained at RF ground by the bypass capacitor C_E. However, in microwave amplifiers, a high impedance quarter-wave transmission lines are used in place of RFCs.

20.7 INTERNAL TUNING OF MICROWAVE TRANSISTORS

For maximum power transfer, the input and output terminals of the microwave transistor must be matched. For this purpose, matching quarter-wave transformers are used. In recent years, the internal tuning technique is widely used. This technique uses MOS chip capacitors and discrete band wire lengths placed inside the transistor package to increase the input and output impedances to the transmission line impedance (50 Ω). The capacitance and inductance values used are determined from the impedance characteristic of the transistor chips. These devices provide broader bandwidths. The circuit design is also simplified for matching to very low impedances.

20.8 TYPICAL CHARACTERISTICS

The typical characteristics of microwave transistors are given below:

  (i) Frequency of operation: 1 to 8 GHz

  (ii) Output power: 20 W at 1 GHz

                          150 mW at 8 GHz

  (iii) Power gain: 30 to 32 dB

  (iv) Noise figure: 3.3 dB at 4 GHz

                        14 dB at 8 GHz

20.9 COMPARISON BETWEEN Si AND GaAs MICROWAVE TRANSISTORS

GaAs transistors are used for the construction of microwave transistors because of higher frequency of operation and low noise. They can be operated at high temperatures and in the presence of high radiation field. However, its fabrication is complicated and very expensive.

The Si transistors are inexpensive, more reliable, integrative and offer higher gain and durable. They offer 10 dB to 20 dB higher gain than GaAs transistors.

20.10 MICROWAVE FIELD EFFECT TRANSISTORS

The two important characteristics of field-effect transistors that make them superior to bipolar transistors are: (i) low noise and (ii) higher operating frequency. The high operating frequency is due to the higher electron mobility in GaAs that is used in field-effect transistors compared to that in silicon used in bipolar transistors. The higher electron mobility and the absence of shot-noise result in low noise.

The first microwave field-effect transistors were metal-semiconductor field-effect transistors (MESFET). They were realized in 1969 and had a gate length of 1 micron and a maximum frequency of operation of 12 GHz. In 1971, GaAs was used to fabricate the gate length of 1-micron. This increased the frequency of operation to 50 GHz. This is because the GaAs MESFET has higher electron mobility, higher electric field and higher saturation drift velocity than silicon devices. Its operating power was also higher. Because of its higher output power and low noise figure, it is used in microwave integrated circuits for higher power, low noise and broadband amplifier applications. The operation of MESFET is similar to that of JFET. But, the only difference is in MESFET, a metal-semiconductor rectifying contact is used at the gate instead of a *p-n* junction of a JFET. In addition to Si and GaAs, InP is also used as a substrate for MESFET fabrication. The drift velocity is 50% higher in InP than that of GaAs and the frequency of operation is 1.6 times that of GaAs. Thus, *MESFET requires a semi-conductor that has (i) large mobility, (ii) higher maximum drift velocity and (iii) a large avalanche field.* Materials that satisfy these requirements are GaAs and InP.

Two types of field effect transistors are used at microwave frequencies. They are:

  (i) Metal Semiconductor FET (MESFET)

  (ii) High Electron Mobility Transistor (HEMT).

The MESFET is constructed with a metal-semiconductor Schottky-barrier diode. The semiconductor material may be either Si or GaAs. It may be either *n* or *p* channel type. HEMT is a hetero-junction transistor. A *heterojunction* is a junction formed at the interface of an aluminium-gallium-arsenide (AlGaAs) doped alloy and an undoped GaAs layer. The use of hetero-junction enables the channel with very high electron mobility. Hence, it can be operated at higher frequencies with low noise.

20.10.1 Metal-Semiconductor FET

The basic configuration of a typical MESFET is shown in Fig. 20.5. It consists of a moderately doped n-type epitaxial layer on a high resistivity semiinsulating GaAs substrate. Two ohmic contacts, *source* and *drain*, are made on the top surface of the epitaxial layer. Source is the origin of carriers and drain acts as sink. A third contact, a metal-semiconductor-Schottky junction is added between the source and the drain. This is the gate electrode. When the gate is reverse biased, it creates a layer in semiconductor that is completely depleted of carrier electrons. This depletion layer acts as an insulating region and reduces the cross-section available for the flow of current in the n-layer. Thus, the reverse biased gate controls the current flow from the drain to source.

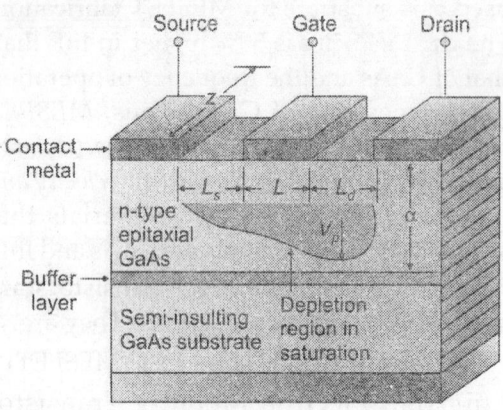

Fig. 20.5: MESFET structure

20.10.2 Principle of Operation

When the gate of a MESFET is reverse biased and the drain is forward biased, the majority carriers (the electrons) flow into the n-type epitaxial layer from the source through the channel beneath the gate and reach the drain. The current flow in the channel cause a voltage drop along its length and the Schottky-barrier gate becomes progressively more and more reverse biased towards the drain. As a result of this, a charge depletion region is set up in the channel and gradually

pinches off the channel against the semi-insulating substrate towards the drain end. As the reverse bias of the gate increases, the height of the depletion region also increases. The channel height of the non-pinched-off region decreases. Hence, the channel resistance is increased. Consequently, the drain current I_{ds} is controlled by the gate voltage V_{gs}. Thus, a set of characteristics of drain current I_{ds} and the source-drain voltage V_{ds} with gate voltage V_{gs} as a variable parameter can be obtained for a GaAs MESFET. This is shown in Fig. 20.6.

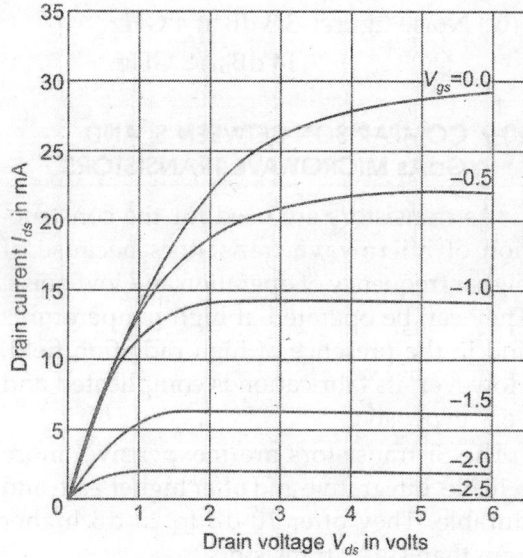

Fig. 20.6: Characteristics of MESFET

20.11 CUT-OFF FREQUENCY AND MAXIMUM OSCILLATION FREQUENCY

The cut-off frequency of GaAs MESFET in a circuit depends on the way the circuit is fabricated. In a wideband lumped circuit, the cut-off frequency is given by

$$f_c = g_m/2\pi C_{gs} = v_s/4\pi L \qquad (20.6)$$

where

g_m is the transconductance of the device

C_{gs} is the gate-source capacitance

v_s is the saturation drift velocity

L is the gate length.

In a distributed circuit, the maximum frequency of oscillation depends on the device transconductance and the drain resistance. It is given by

$$f_{max} = (f_c/2))(g_m R_d)^{1/2}$$
$$= (f_c/2)[R_d/(R_s + R_g + R_i)]^{1/2}$$

(20.7)

where

g_m is the transconductance of the device

R_d is the drain resistance

R_s is the source resistance

R_g is the gate metallization resistance

R_i is the input resistance

20.12 HIGH ELECTRON MOBILITY TRANSISTOR

The basic configuration of an HEMT is shown in Fig. 20.7. It is a selectively doped GaAs-AlGaAs hetero-junction structure. It consists of an undoped GaAs layer and a Si-doped n-type AlGaAs layer successively grown on a higher resistivity semi-insulating GaAs substrate. A *hetero-junction* is a junction formed at the interface of an aluminium-gallium-arsenide (AlGaAs) doped alloy and an un-doped GaAs layer. This provides high electron mobility to the channel. Since mobility is achieved by doping only the large band gap material, AlGaAs, it is also known as *modulation-doped field effect transistor* (MODFET).

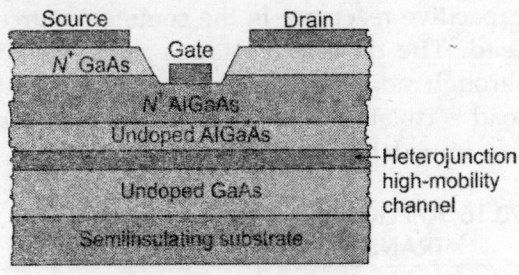

Fig. 20.7: HEMT structure

20.12.1 Typical Characteristics of HEMT

The performance characteristics of HEMT are:

(i) Frequency of operation: up to 100 GHz

(ii) Gain: 4.5 dB at 60 GHz
     4 to 5 dB at 72 GHz

(iii) Noise figure: 6 dB at 57.5 GHz

20.13 FET BIASING

The output drain current I_d versus the drain-source voltage V_{ds} is shown in Fig. 20.8 as a function of the gate voltage V_{gs}. For small signal applications, the operating point is fixed in the vicinity of P_1 and, for maximum dynamic range, in the vicinity of P_2. In both cases, the gate is reverse biased for a depletion mode device. This bias condition is achieved by grounding the gate through a RF choke (RFC) or a high impedance quarter-wave transmission line. Figure 20.9 shows the biasing arrangement. The desired bias voltage is obtained from the voltage drop

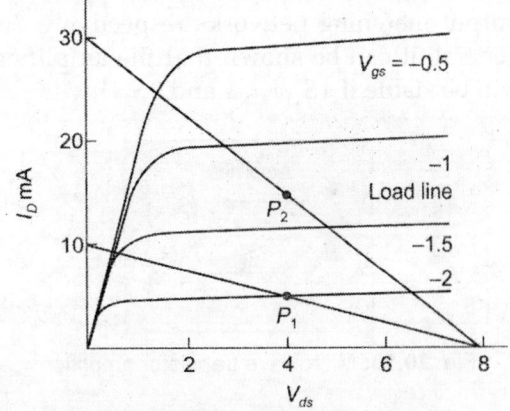

Fig. 20.8: Characteristic of a MESFET

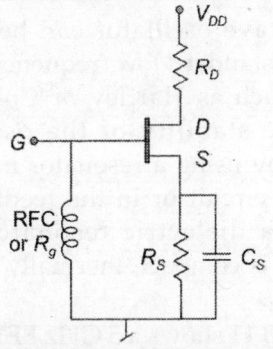

Fig. 20.9: MESFET biasing circuit

across $R_s (= |V_{gs}| / I_d)$. R_s should be bypassed by the capacitor C_s in order to bypass the RF current to the ground.

20.14 MICROWAVE TRANSISTOR AMPLIFIER CIRCUIT

Microwave transistor amplifier consists of the amplifier with input and output matching networks as shown in Fig. 20.10. It is designed using S-parameters. As the transistor is a unilateral device, $S_{12} = 0$. It is matched to the source and the load. Therefore, the maximum gain is obtained. It is given by

$$G_m = |S_{12}|^2/[(1 - |S_{11}|^2)(1 - |S_{22}|^2)]$$
$$= [1/(1 - |S_{11}|^2)] \cdot [|S_{12}|^2] \cdot [(1 - |S_{22}|^2)]$$
$$= G_i G_T G_o \qquad (20.8)$$

Here, G_T is the gain of the transistor and G_i and G_o are determined by the input and output matching networks respectively. In general, it can be shown that the amplifier will be stable if $|S_{11}| < 1$ and $|S_{12}| < 1$.

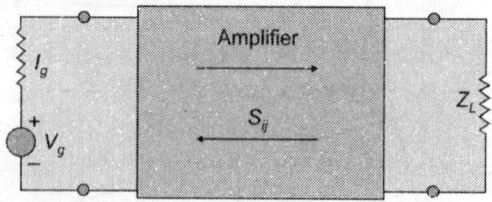

Fig. 20.10: Microwave transistor amplifier

20.15 MICROWAVE TRANSISTOR OSCILLATOR CIRCUIT

A microwave oscillator can be designed using any standard low frequency oscillator circuits such as Hartley or Colpitts. The frequency stability of the oscillator is obtained by using a resonator in the input or output circuit or in the feedback loop. Usually, a dielectric resonator is used because it is compact, thermally stable and has high Q.

Figure 20.11 shows a 5 GHz FET oscillator using strip lines. The input and output are

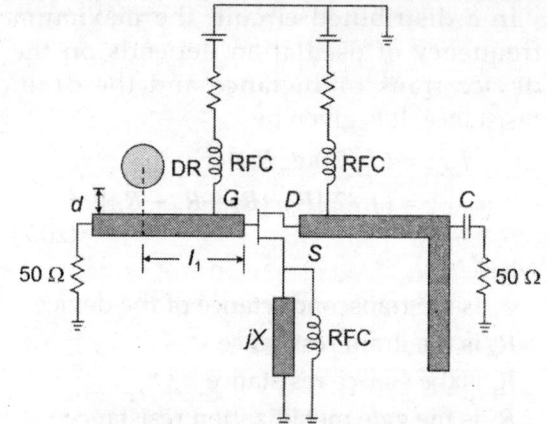

Fig. 20.11: MESFET oscillator

terminated such that both the input and output impedances of the transistor have negative resistance. The oscillations occur at a frequency at which the total reactance in the input and output circuits becomes zero. The frequency is stabilized by using a dielectric resonator (DR) in the input circuit. The magnitude of the source reflection coefficient is adjusted by the coupling to the resonator that can be varied by changing coupling spacing d between the resonator and the micro-strip line. The phase angle of the source reflection coefficient is controlled by the length l_1 of the input line. The output circuit is a standard stub-matched circuit that transforms the 50 ohm load impedance to match the impedance of the oscillator. The circuit is made to oscillate by using a series capacitive reactance in the common source lead. The dc bias voltages are applied through radio-frequency chokes. The output load is isolated from the dc voltages by the low impedance dc blocking capacitor C.

20.16 APPLICATIONS OF MICROWAVE TRANSISTORS

The MW transistors are used as

  (i) Low noise front-end amplifier in radar and microwave communication receivers.
 (ii) Power amplifiers in microwave links.

(iii) Driver amplifiers in high power microwave transmitters.

(iv) Power oscillators.

20.17 TRANSISTOR NOISE FACTOR

Random variations of charge movements within the transistor give rise to noise currents and voltages. These degrade the available signal-to-noise ratio at the input of an amplifier. Usually, the noise factor characterizes the noise performance of an amplifier. Assuming that a source at room temperature is connected to the input of an amplifier, the noise factor F of the combination is defined as

$$F = \frac{\text{Available signal-to-noise power ratio at the input}}{\text{Available signal-to-noise power ratio at the output}}$$

$$= (P_{si}/P_{ni}) \times (P_{no}/P_{so}) \qquad (20.9a)$$

The available power gain G_A is given by

$$G_A = P_{so} / P_{si} \qquad (20.9b)$$

Therefore, the noise factor F may be expressed as

$$F = P_{no} /(G_A P_{ni}) \qquad (20.9c)$$

The available noise power from a source at $T°$ K is

$$P_{ni} = kTB \qquad (20.10)$$

where k is the Boltzman's constant and is equal to 1.38×10^{-23} J/K and B is the bandwidth in Hz over which the noise is spread. At room temperature T_o, the noise factor becomes

$$F = P_{no} /(G_A kT_o B) \qquad (20.11)$$

Hence, the output noise power is given by

$$P_{no} = FG_A kT_o B \qquad (20.12)$$

If the amplifier is noiseless, then the noise output power will be $G_A kTB$, i.e., the input noise power multiplied by the power gain. Because of noise contribution by the amplifier, the output noise is increased by the factor F. Noise factor is a specified parameter for a transistor and it varies with frequency. When it is specified *for one frequency*, it is known as *spot noise factor*. When its value is averaged over a range of frequencies, it is known as *average noise factor*.

Noise factor is a multiplying factor and is a power ratio. The noise figure is the noise factor expressed in decibels. Thus,

$$F_{dB} = 10 \log F \qquad (20.13)$$

20.17.1 Amplifier Input Noise

The total noise at the input of the amplifier may be considered as made up of two components: an amount $kT_o B$ contributed by the source and an amount contributed by the amplifier. The total input noise power is equal to the total output noise power divided by the gain G_A. Hence, we have

$$P_n = FkT_o B \qquad (20.14)$$

The amplifier noise referred to the input is given by

$$P_{ni} = (P_{no}/G_A) - kT_o B$$
$$= FkT_o B - kT_o B$$
$$= (F - 1) kT_o B \qquad (20.15)$$

20.17.2 Amplifiers in Cascade

If two amplifiers are connected in cascade as shown in Fig. 20.12, the noise factor for the combination is given by

$$F = P_{no2} /(G_{A1} G_{A2} kT_o B) \qquad (20.16)$$

This is fed into the second amplifier where already exists a noise input of $(F_2 - 1) kT_o B$. The total input noise to the second amplifier is the sum of these two components. Thus,

$$P_{no2} = G_{A2} (G_{A1} F_1 kT_o B + (F_2 - 1) kT_o B \qquad (20.17)$$

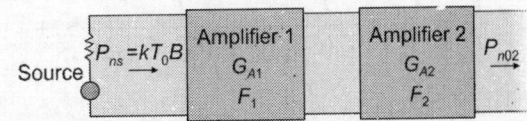

Fig. 20.12: Cascaded amplifier

Substituting Eq. (20.17) in Eq. (20.16) and simplifying, we get

$$F = F_1 + (F_2 - 1)G_{A1} \qquad (20.18)$$

If n amplifiers are connected in cascade, then the noise factor is given by

$$F = F_1 + (F_2 - 1)/G_{A1} + (F_3 - 1)/(G_{A1}G_{A2}] + \ldots + (F_n - 1)/(G_{A1}G_{A2} \cdots G_{A(n-1)}) \qquad (20.19)$$

The above equation is known as *Friis's formula*.

20.18 EQUIVALENT NOISE TEMPERATURE

The total noise at the input of the amplifier is given by $(F - 1)\, kT_oB$. Another way of representing the same is as an available noise power of an amount kT_eB where T_e is an equivalent temperature. Thus,

$$kT_eB = (F - 1)\, kT_oB \qquad (20.20)$$

Hence,

$$T_e = (F - 1)T_o \qquad (20.21)$$

T_e is not a physical temperature that can be measured. It is a mathematical representation of the amplifier noise. Amplifiers and converters used with satellite antennas for home reception usually have noise specified by T_e, a typical value being $100°K$. It is more convenient to use T_e in noise calculations for low-noise amplifiers than noise factor. *Noise temperature is known if noise factor is known and vice versa.*

Friis's formula may be expressed in terms of noise temperature. Subtracting 1 from both sides of Eq. (20.19), we get

$$F - 1 = F_1 - 1 + (F_2 - 1)/G_{A1} + (F_3 - 1)$$
$$(G_{A1}G_{A2}] + \ldots + (F_n - 1)/$$
$$(G_{A1}G_{A2} \cdots G_{A(n-1)}) \qquad (20.22)$$

Substituting for the various $(F_i - 1)$ from Eq. (20.21), we obtain

$$\frac{T_e}{T_o} = \frac{T_{e1}}{T_o} + \frac{T_{e2}}{T_o(G_{A1})} + \frac{T_{e3}}{T_o(G_{A1}G_{A2})} + \ldots +$$
$$\frac{T_{en}}{T_o(G_{A1}G_{A2} \cdots G_{A(n-1)})}$$

or,
$$T_e = T_{e1} + T_{e2}/G_{A1} + T_{e3}/(G_{A1}G_{A2}) + \ldots + T_{en}/(G_{A1}G_{A2} \cdots G_{A(n-1)}) \qquad (20.23)$$

20.19 NUMERICAL EXAMPLES

Example 20.1 A Si microwave transistor has a reactance of 1 ohm, transit time cut-off frequency of 5 GHz, maximum electric field of 2×10^5 V/m and saturation drift velocity of 3×10^5 V/m. Determine the maximum allowable power.

Solution: Given: $X_c = 2\ \Omega$, $f_T = 5$ GHz, $E_m = 2 \times 10^5$ V/m, $v_d = 3 \times 10^5$ V/m

Maximum allowable power
$$P_{max} = (E_m v_s / 2\pi f_T)^2 / X_c$$
$$= [(2 \times 10^5 \times 3 \times 10^5)/$$
$$= (2 \times 3.14 \times 5 \times 10^9)]/2$$
$$= \textbf{3.65 W}$$

Example 20.2 A Si transistor has a reactance of 4 ohm, maximum electric field $E_m = 1.6 \times 10^5$ V/cm, $v_s = 4 \times 10^5$ cm/s and maximum allowable power of 6.48 W Find the transit time cut-off frequency.

Solution: Given:$X_c = 4$, $E_m = 1.6 \times 10^5$ V/cm, $v_s = 4 \times 10^5$ cm/s and P_{max} 6.48 W

The transit time frequency is given by
$$f_c = (1/P_m X_c)^{1/2} (E_m v_s / 2\pi)$$
$$= \left(\frac{1}{1 \times 6.48 \times 4}\right)^{1/2} \left(\frac{1.6 \times 10^5 \times 4 \times 10^5}{6.28}\right)$$
$$= \textbf{2.0 GHz}$$

Example 20.3 A GaAs MESFET has $R_g = 5\Omega$, $R_i = 1\ \Omega$, $g_m = 60 \times 10^{-3}$ mhos, $R_s = 2\ \Omega$, $R_d = 400\ \Omega$, $C_{gs} = 0.5$ pF and $C_{dg} = 0.1$ pF. Calculate (a) f_c and (b) f_{max}.

Solution: Given: $R_g = 5\ \Omega$, $R_i = 1\ \Omega$, $g_m = 60 \times 10^{-3}$ mhos, $R_s = 2\Omega s$, $R_{ds} = 400\Omega$, $C_{gs} = 0.5$ pF, $C_{dg} = 0.1$ pF

(i) The frequency f_c is given by
$$f_c = g_m / 2\pi C_{gs}$$
$$= 60 \times 10^{-3}/(6.28 \times 0.5 \times 10^{-12})$$
$$= \textbf{19.1 GHz}$$

(ii) The frequency f_{max} is given by

$$f_{max} = (f_c/2)[R_d/(R_s + R_g + R_i)]^{1/2}$$

$$= \frac{19.1}{2}\left(\frac{400}{8}\right)^{1/2}$$

$$= \frac{19.1}{2} \times 7.0711$$

$$= 67.53 \text{ GHz}$$

Example 20.4 The available power gain of an amplifier is 20 dB and the bandwidth is 10 MHz. If the noise power output is 8 pW, find the noise factor and the amplifier input noise. Assume a room temperature of 290°K.

Solution: Given: $G_A = 20$ dB $= 100$; $B = 10^7$ Hz; $P_{no} = 8 \times 10^{-12}$ W; $T_o = 290$°K

(a) Noise factor is given by

$$F = P_{no}/G_A k T_o B$$

$$= 8 \times 10^{-12}/(100 \times 1.38 \times 10^{-23} \times 290 \times 10^7)$$

$$= 2.0$$

(b) The amplifier input noise is given by

$$P_{ni} = (F-1)\, kT_o B$$

$$= (2-1) \times 1.38 \times 10^{-23} \times 290 \times 10^7$$

$$= 0.04 \text{ pW}$$

Example 20.5: An amplifier with an available power gain of 30 dB and noise figure of 10 dB is used to feed into a second amplifier of power gain 25 dB and a noise figure of 4dB. Find the overall noise figure of the system.

Solution: Given: $G_{A1} = 30$ dB $= 1000$; $F_1 = 10$ dB $= 10$, $G_{A2} = 25$ dB $= 316.2$; $F_2 = 4$ dB $= 10^{0.4} = 2.5$

The overall noise figure is given by

$$F = F_1 + (F_2 - 1)/G_{A1}$$

$$= 10 + (2.5 - 1)/1000 = 10.0015$$

$$= 10.024 \text{ dB}$$

KEY POINTS

- Microwave amplifiers are usually constructed either as hybrid or monolithic microwave integrated circuits.
- In hybrid construction, the transmission lines and matching networks are realized as microstrip circuit elements, and then, the discrete components are connected by using wire-bonding techniques.
- A monolithic microwave integrated circuit is one in which all active and passive devices are fabricated on a single semiconductor crystal.
- GaAs is used as substrate material because of its high resistivity in the undoped state and superiority for high-frequency FET construction.
- The foremost criteria while designing the microwave transistors are (i) proper geometry, (ii) heat sink and (iii) packaging.
- All microwave bipolar transistors are planar in **form and are of** npn type.
- The npn type is preferred because the electron mobility is greater than the hole mobility. This increases the speed of operation and reduces the transit time, thus increasing the operating frequency.
- Silicon microwave bipolar transistors are of low cost, more reliable, integrative and offer higher gain. They have low noise figure at microwave frequencies.
- The geometry of the npn transistors are (i) interdigital type, (ii) overlay type and (iii) matrix type.
- At microwave frequencies, common emitter configuration of transistors is used because it reduces the negative feedback on account of the base-to-collector capacitance.
- In order to provide a stable operating point, a dc feedback path is provided in the biasing circuit.
- For isolation from the high frequency currents, high impedance radio frequency chokes are used in the voltage divider bias and the collector circuit, and a low impedance capacitive bypass circuit across the emitter bias resistance R_E.
- GaAs transistors offer higher frequency of operation and low noise. They can be operated at high temperatures and in the presence of high radiation field. However, its fabrication is complicated and very expensive.
- The Si transistors are inexpensive, more reliable, integrative and offer higher gain and durable. They offer 10 dB to 20 dB higher gain than GaAs transistors.
- Two types of field effect transistors at microwave frequencies are (i) Metal Semiconductor FET (MESFET) and (ii) High Electron Mobility Transistor (HEMT).
- The MESFET is constructed with a metal-semiconductor Schottky-barrier diode. The semi-

conductor material may be either Si or GaAs. It may be either *n* or *p* channel type.

- MESFET requires a semiconductor that has (i) larger mobility, (ii) higher maximum drift velocity and (iii) a large avalanche field. Materials that satisfy these requirements are GaAs and InP.
- HEMT is a hetero-junction transistor that has very high electron mobility. Hence, it can be operated at higher frequencies with low noise.
- HEMT is a selectively doped GaAs-AlGaAs hetero-junction structure. It consists of an undoped GaAs layer and a Si-doped *n*-type This provides high electron mobility to the channel. Since mobility is achieved by doping only the large band gap material, AlGaAs, it is also known as modulation-doped field effect transistor (MODFET).
- The microwave transistors are used as (i) low noise front-end amplifier in radar and microwave communication receivers, (ii) power amplifiers in microwave links, (iii) driver amplifiers in high power microwave transmitters and (iv) power oscillators.

FURTHER READING

1. Davis WA (1984). *Microwave Semiconductor Circuit Design*, Van Nostrand, NY.
2. Liao SY (1985). *Microwave Solid State Devices*, PH. NJ.
3. Liao SY (1990). *Semiconductor Electron Devices*, PH, NJ.
4. Watson A (Ed.) (1969). *Microwave Semiconductor Devices and Their Applications*, McGraw Hill, NY.

REVIEW QUESTIONS

20.1 What are the limitations of BJT at microwave frequencies?
20.2 Mention the three geometries of microwave transistors.
20.3 Explain the internal tuning of microwave transistors.
20.4 Draw the equivalent circuit of a microwave transistor in CE configuration.
20.5 What are the important considerations while designing a transistor biasing circuit?
20.6 Give the performance characteristics of microwave transistors.
20.7 Compare Si and GaAs microwave transistors.

20.8 Mention the two types of FET used at microwave frequencies.
20.9 Draw the basic structure of a GaAs MESFET.
20.10 Draw the V-I characteristics of GaAs MESFET.
20.11 Describe a HEMT.
20.12 Draw the basic structure of HEMT.
20.13 Why is HEMT is known as MODFET?
20.14 Give the performance characteristics of a HEMT.
20.15 Draw the FET biasing circuit. Give the applications of microwave transistors.
20.16 Define noise factor.
20.17 Differentiate between spot and average noise factor.
20.18 Define noise figure.
20.19 If two amplifiers are in cascade, what is the noise factor?
20.20 If two amplifiers are in cascade, what is the equivalent noise temperatue?

DESCRIPTIVE QUESTIONS

20.1 Discuss, in detail, the limitations of BJT at microwave frequencies.
20.2 With neat sketches, explain the three structures of microwave transistors.
20.3 What are the important considerations while designing a transistor biasing circuit? With a circuit diagram, explain the biasing circuit of a transistor.
20.4 With a circuit diagram, explain the operation of a MW CE transistor amplifier.
20.5 With neat sketch, explain the structure of MESFET.
20.6 With neat sketch, explain the operation of MESFET.
20.7 With neat sketch, explain the structure of HEMT.
20.8 With a circuit diagram, explain the biasing circuit of a field-effect transistor.
20.9 With a circuit diagram, explain the operation of a MW transistor oscillator.
20.10 Define noise factor and noise figure. Derive the expression for noise factor of a transistor.
20.11 Derive the expression for noise factor of two cascaded transistors.
20.12 Derive expression for equivalent noise temperature of two cascaded transistors.

PRACTICE PROBLEMS

20.1 A Si microwave transistor has a reactance of 1 ohm, transit time cut-off frequency of 4 GHz, maximum electric field of 1.6×10^5 V/m and saturation drift velocity of 4×10^5 cm/sec. Determine the maximum allowable power.
[**Ans: 6.48 W**]

20.2 A Si microwave transistor has a reactance of 1 ohm, maximum electric field $E_m = 1.6 \times 10^5$ V/cm, $v_d = 4 \times 10^5$ cm/s and maximum allowable power of 6.48 W Find the transit time cut-off frequency.
[**Ans: 4.0 GHz**]

20.3 A GaAs MESFET has $R_g = 6$ Ω, $R_i = 2$ Ω, $g_m = 60 \times 10^{-3}$ mhos, $R_s = 2$ Ω, $R_{ds} = 400$ Ω, $C_{gs} = 0.5$ pF and $C_{dg} = 0.1$ pF. Calculate (a) f_c and (b) f_{max}.
[**Ans: a) 19.1 GHz, (b) 77.98 GHz**]

20.4 A GaAs MESFET has $R_g = 3$ Ω, $R_i = 2$ Ω, $g_m = 55 \times 10^{-3}$ mhos, $L = 150$ mm, $v_d = 2 \times 10^7$ cm/s, $R_s = 2$ ohms, $R_{ds} = 400$ Ω, $C_{gs} = 0.5$ pF and $C_{dg} = 0.1$ pF. Calculate (a) f_c and (b) f_{max}.
[**Ans: (a) 17.52 GHz, (b) 66.12 GHz**]

20.5 The available power gain of an amplifier is 30 dB and the bandwidth is 10 MHz. If the noise figure is 5 dB, find the noise power output and amplifier input noise. Assume a room temperature of 290°K.
(**Ans: 0.127 nW, 0.04 pW**)

20.6 An amplifier with an available power gain of 25 dB and noise figure of 4 dB is used to feed into a second amplifier of power gain 30 dB and a noise figure of 10 dB, Find the overall noise figure of the system.
(**Ans: 4.1 dB**)

REFERENCE

1. Collins RE (1996). *Foundations of Microwave Engineering*, McGraw Hill, NY.

2. Gentile C (1987). *Microwave Amplifiers and Oscillators*, McGraw Hill, NY.

3. Raymond S and Pengelly RS (1986). *Microwave Field-Effect Transistors; Theory, Design and Applications*, 2nd Ed., Research Studies Press, John Wiley, NY.

4. Gonzalez G (1964). *Microwave Transistor Amplifiers: Analysis and Design*, PH, NJ.

5. Dennis R (1986). *Microwave Technology*, PH, NY.

6. Vendelin GD (1982), *Design of Amplifiers and Oscillators by S-Parameter Method*, John Wiley, NY.

7. Seeger JA (1988). *Microwave Theory, Compo-nents and Devices*, PH, NJ.

8. Bahl IJ and Bhatia P (1988). *Microwave Solid State Circuit Design*, John Wiley, NY.

9. Raymond S and Pengelly RS (1986). *Microwave Field-Effect Transistors; Theory, Design and Applications*, 2nd Ed., Research Studies Press, John Wiley, NY.

Microwave Communication Systems

Objectives

- Understand the MW communication systems.
- Know the details of equipment in earth stations and repeaters.
- Classify the types of fading.
- Examine the methods of reducing fading.
- Design a MW link.

21.1 INTRODUCTION

Microwaves find applications in the field of communications, defense, industries, homes and medicine. They are widely used in communication links for transmission of voice, video, data and other information. These links are known as *microwave links* between two stations linking them directly or via satellite. Microwaves found extensive use during World War II in the development of high-resolution radar systems to detect enemy planes and ships. Nowadays, radars are used in many forms such as *missile tracking radars, fire control radars, air traffic control radars, weather detecting and forecasting radars etc.* In industrial and domestic applications, they are used in microwave ovens, dryers, measurements of moisture-content and thickness. In the field of medicine, they are used for therapeutic, diagnostic and monitoring applications.

In this chapter, we shall discuss the terrestrial microwave communication systems.

21.2 BASIC MICROWAVE COMMUNICATION SYSTEMS

Microwave communication systems are broadly classified as

(i) Terrestrial

(ii) Satellite communication systems.

For both systems, the transmission aspects are common but their parameters differ greatly. Hence, planning methods have to take into account the specifics of the particular system.

Figure 21.1 shows the essential components of terrestrial microwave communication systems. At each end of the microwave link, a transmit-receive terminal unit is required for the purpose of transferring the base band signal to the microwave carrier and receiving the base band signal from the microwave carrier. The base band signal is usually a multiplexed signal carrying a number of voice signals, video signals and data. Direct microwave links are used for distances up to 50 km. For long distance

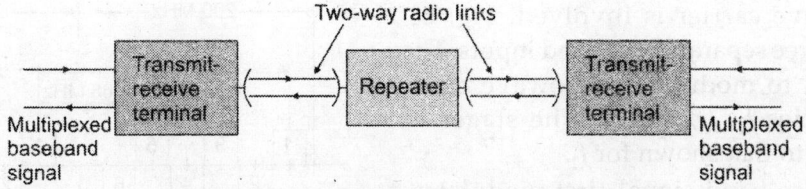

Fig. 21.1: Block diagram of a microwave system

transmission, repeater stations are used at intervals of 50 km. These repeater stations amplify the received signal to compensate for the transmission losses and then transmit to the next hop.

Both analog and digital modulation methods are used in microwave links. In analog systems, the information signal is frequency division multiplexed (FDM) to form multiplexed base band signal and then, the multiplexed base band signal is frequency modulated (FM) onto a microwave carrier. Hence, this is referred as FDM/FM

system. In digital systems, the information signal is time division multiplexed (TDM) to form multiplexed base band signal and then, the multiplexed base band signal is used to phase modulate the microwave carrier. For this, phase shift keying is used. The modern trend is to use digital systems as they provide high efficiency.

21.3 TERMINAL STATIONS

Figure 21.2 shows the details of equipment required at a terminal station. For medium to large capacity systems, more than one

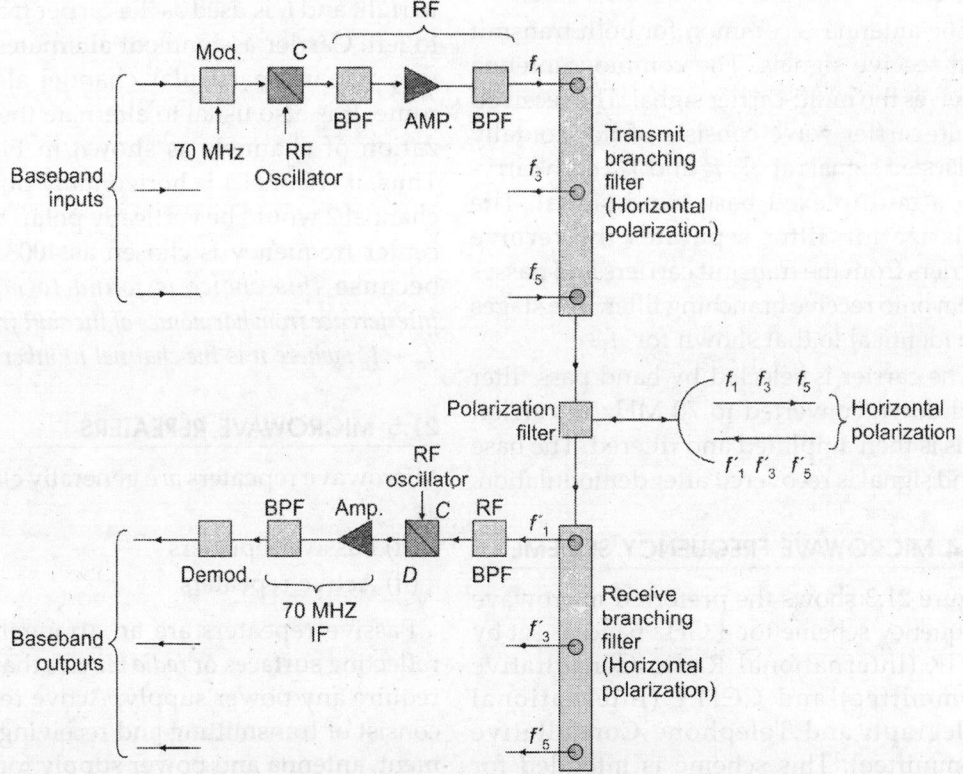

Fig. 21.2: Block diagram of terminal station equipment

microwave carrier is involved. Fig. 21.2 shows three separate base band inputs. They are used to modulate microwave carrier frequencies f_1, f_3, and f_5. The stages are identical to that shown for f_1.

The base band signal first modulates a 70 MHz IF carrier. The modulated signal is then up-converted to the desired microwave carrier frequencies f_1, f_3, and f_5. These microwave carrier frequencies f_1, f_3, and f_5 are then filtered, amplified and passed on to a branch filter to form a FDM signal at the output. Each carrier carries a FDM or TDM base band signal. The output of the branching filter is polarized in the horizontal or vertical direction. The horizontally or vertically polarized multi-carrier signal is passed through a polarization filter to ensure that only the horizontally or vertically polarized wave is passed to the antenna. Figure 21.2 shows horizontally polarized wave.

The antenna is common for both transmit and receive signals. The common antenna receives the multi-carrier signal. The received multi-carrier wave consists of horizontally polarized signals at f_1', f_3' and f_5', each carrying a multiplexed base band signal. The polarization filter separates the receive carriers from the transmit carriers and passes them onto receive branching filter. The stages are identical to that shown for f_1'.

The carrier is selected by band pass filter and down-converted to 70 MHz IF carrier. This is then amplified and filtered. The base band signal is recovered after demodulation.

21.4 MICROWAVE FREQUENCY SCHEME

Figure 21.3 shows the preferred microwave frequency scheme for 4 GHz band as set by CCIR (International Radio Consultative Committee) and CCITT (International Telegraph and Telephone Consultative Committee). This scheme is intended for 600–1800 channel FDM system. To simplify

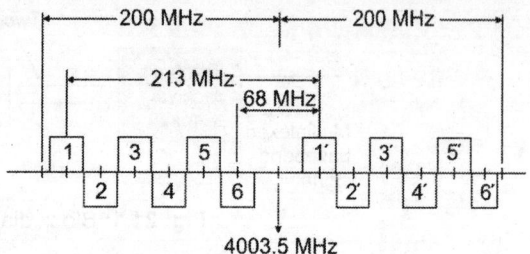

Fig. 21.3: Microwave frequency scheme for 4 GHz band

filtering, all transmit channels are kept in one 200 MHz half of the frequency spectrum,, and all receive channels are kept in the other 200 MHz half, as shown in Fig. 21.3. This keeps the transmit and receive channels widely separated. Two frequencies, f_1 and f_1' are allocated per channel. On any one given section of the route, f_1 is used as the carrier for left to right and f_1' is used as the carrier for right to left. On the following section of the route, f_1' is used as the carrier from left to right and f_1 is used as the carrier from right to left. Carrier assignment alternates in this way for any particular channel along the route. It is also usual to alternate the polarization of channels as shown in Fig. 21.3. Thus, if channel 1 is horizontally polarized, channel 2 would be vertically polarized. The center frequency is chosen as 4003.5 MHz because *this choice is found to minimize interference from harmonics of the shift frequency* $f_n - f_n'$, *where n is the channel number.*

21.5 MICROWAVE REPEATERS

Microwave repeaters are generally classified as

  (i) Passive repeaters

  (ii) Active repeaters

Passive repeaters are an arrangement of reflecting surfaces or *radio mirrors* that do not require any power supply. Active repeaters consist of transmitting and receiving equipment, antenna and power supply for operation.

21.5.1 Passive Repeaters

Passive repeaters are simple reflectors that are used to redirect the microwaves in the same manner as a mirror reflects the light waves. They are used in certain situations. Figure 21.4(a) shows one situation in which parabolic reflector antenna is mounted at the bottom of the microwave tower and an elliptical plane reflector at the top. The plane reflector is mounted at an angle of 45° to the beam so that the beam is bent by 90°. The elliptical perimeter is chosen so that the effective area as seen by the primary antenna is circular. This type of reflector system is known as *periscope system*. It is used with high towers where losses in the long wave-guide feed would be too high. Figure 21.4(b) shows a large, flat *billboard* type reflector used to overcome obstacles.

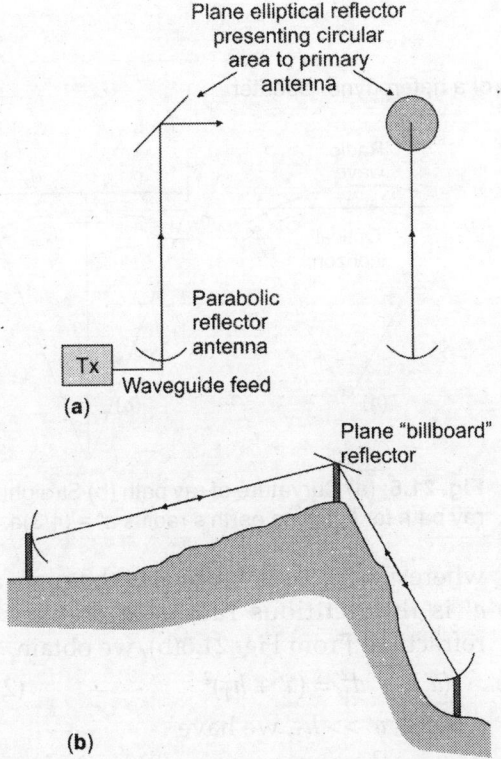

Fig. 21.4: Passive repeater arrangements: (a) Periscope system to replace waveguide feeder (b) Billboard reflector to overcome obstacles

21.5.1.1 Advantages

The advantages of passive repeaters are:
 (a) They do not require any power supply.
 (b) They are easier to install in difficult terrains.

21.5.1.2 Disadvantages

The disadvantage of passive repeaters is that they do not provide gain to compensate for the transmission losses.

21.5.2 Active Repeaters

Figure 21.5 shows the block diagram of a heterodyne repeater. This is commonly used because most of the amplification takes place at heterodyne frequency or 70 MHz IF carrier. The incoming carrier frequencies f_1, f_3 and f_5 from the left side are horizontally polarized. At the repeater, each carrier is converted to 70 MHz IF. It is then up-converted to frequencies f_1', f_3' and f_5'. These are transmitted to the next hop after passing through the branching polarization filters as vertically polarized signals. Similarly, the incoming signals from the right side are vertically polarized at frequencies f_1, f_3 and f_5. They are converted to f_1', f_3' and f_5' horizontally polarized for onward transmission. *The signals are oppositely polarized in order to minimize direct coupling of the transmitted signal on the other side.*

21.6 ATMOSPHERIC REFRACTION

Atmospheric refraction is the bending of the ray path of a radio wave while passing through the earth's atmosphere. The atmosphere is essentially a gaseous dielectric and it has a dielectric constant or relative permittivity that affects the phase velocity of the radio wave. In atmosphere, the phase velocity is given by

$$v_p = c / \sqrt{\varepsilon_r} \qquad (21.1)$$

where c is the free-space velocity of light and ε_r is the relative permittivity and *square root of relative permittivity is the refractive index*. In

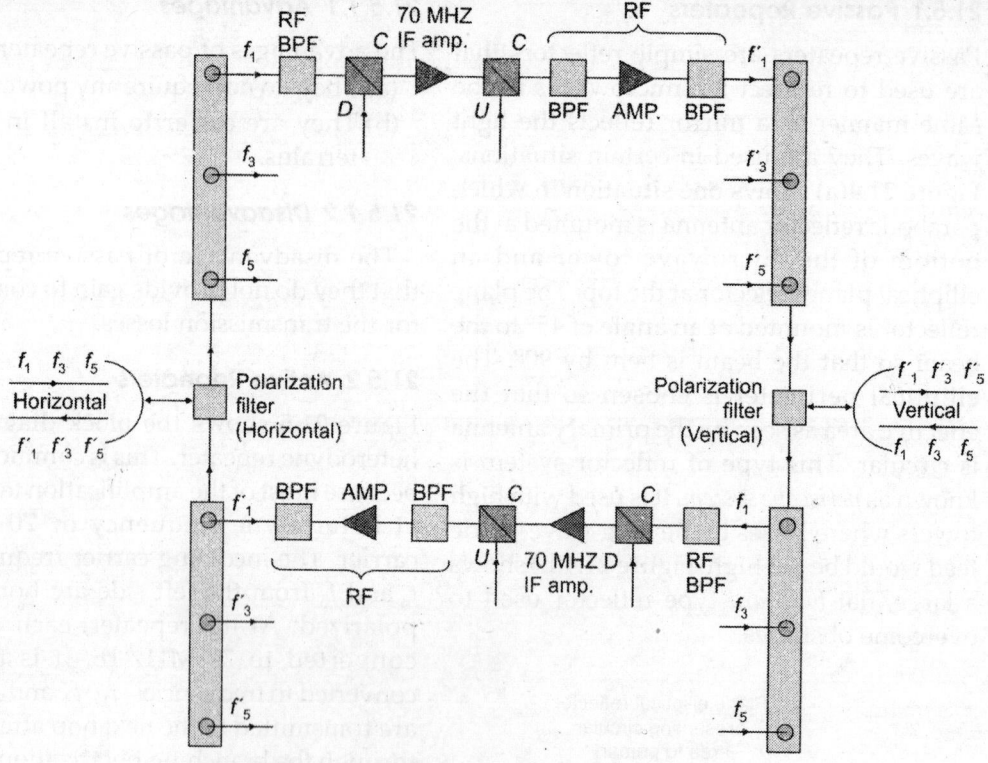

Fig. 21.5: Block diagram of a heterodyne repeater

temperate zones, the refractive index decreases with increase in height above the earth's surface. This causes the wavefront to travel at a greater phase velocity. As the wavefront is always normal to the ray path, the ray path bends towards the earth as illustrated in Fig. 21.6(a). Since the change in refractive index is small, such a curved path is usually modeled by a straight ray path over the spherical earth of radius a' given by $a' = 4/3\,a$ where a is the actual radius of the earth as shown in Fig. 21.6(b). For $a = 6376$ km, $a' = 8501$ km.

21.7 RADIO HORIZON

Assuming straight-line propagation path and smoothly curved earth of radius a', *the radio horizon is the point where the ray path just grazes the earth's surface* as shown in Fig. 21.6(b). Thus,

$$a' = 4/3\,a \qquad (21.2)$$

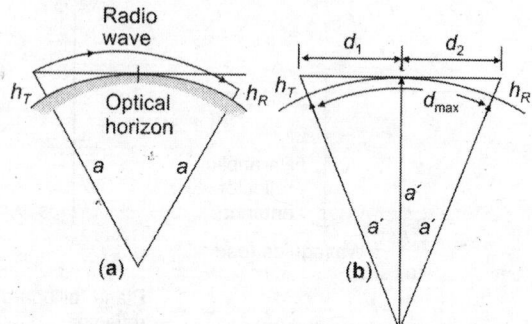

Fig. 21.6: (a) Curvature of ray path (b) Straight-line ray path for fictitious earth's radius $a' = (4/3)a$.

where a is the actual radius of the earth and a' is the fictitious radius to account for refraction. From Fig. 21.6(b), we obtain

$$(a')^2 + d_1^2 = (a' + h_T)^2 \qquad (21.3)$$

Since, $a' \gg h_T$, we have

$$d_1^2 \approx 2a'h_T \qquad (21.4)$$

Similarly,

$$d_2^2 \approx 2a'h_R \qquad (21.5)$$

The maximum radio range d_{max} is given by

$$d_{max} \approx d_1 + d_2 \qquad (21.6)$$

$$= \sqrt{2a'h_T} + \sqrt{2a'h_R}$$

$$= 2a'(\sqrt{h_T} + \sqrt{h_R}) \qquad (21.7)$$

For $a' = (4/3) \times 3960$ miles, the maximum radio range d_{max} is given by

$$d_{max}(\text{miles}) = \sqrt{2}\,[\sqrt{h_T(ft)} + \sqrt{h_R(ft)}] \qquad (21.8)$$

For $a' = 8501$ km, the maximum radio range d_{max} is given by

$$d_{max}(\text{km}) = \sqrt{17}\,[\sqrt{h_T(m)} + \sqrt{h_R(m)}] \qquad (21.9)$$

In practice, *the phenomenon of diffraction extends the range beyond radio horizon.*

21.8 CONTOUR MAPS

The relationship $d = \sqrt{17h}$, a part of Eq. (2.19) is plotted with d in km as abscissa and h in m as ordinates, we obtain a contour as shown in Fig. 21.7(a). An interesting property of this counter is that the distance h' between the tangent at any point P_1 and the curve is related by the equation

$$d'(\text{km}) = \sqrt{17h'(m)} \qquad (21.10)$$

When the curve is inverted, it can be used as a base line. The distance between the tangent point P_1 and the point where the distance between the curve and the tangent is equal to antenna height $h'(m)$, gives the straight line-of-sight distance $d'(km)$ from the antenna to the radio horizon. This is illustrated in Fig. 21.7(b). The profile of the terrain between the transmitter and the receiver is plotted on this graph. This is known as the *contour map*. This map helps to plan obstacle free line-of-sight transmission.

21.9 FRESNEL ZONE

The ray path is usually chosen to avoid obstacles. As the wavefront is spherical, energy from an indirect path from a point such as P will also be received at the receiver in

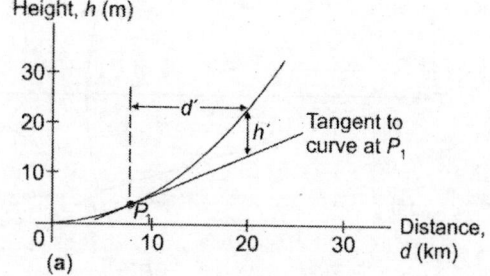

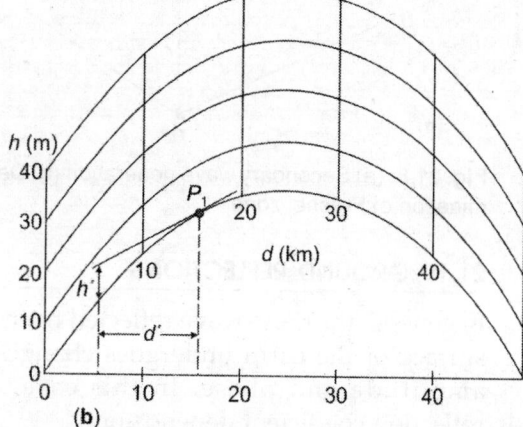

Fig. 21.7: (a) Distance-height graph (b) Contour maps

addition to the direct path as shown in Fig. 21.8(a). This reduces the received energy.

In practice, it is found that the zone defined by the indirect path $TP + PR$ = direct path $TR + \lambda_o/2$ must be cleared for obstructionless transmission. The locus of the point P satisfying the equation $TP + PR = TR + \lambda_o/2$ is an ellipsoid around the direct ray path TR. This ellipsoid of revolution is known as *first Fresnel zone*. From Fig. 21.8, it can be shown that the radius r is given by

$$r = \sqrt{TP' \times P'R\, \lambda_o / TR} \qquad (21.11)$$

The radius r must be cleared for light-of-sight propagation. The maximum clearance distance r_{max} is obtained when $TP' = P'R = TR/2$. It is given by

$$r_{max} = \sqrt{(TR/2) \times (TR/2)\, \lambda_o / TR}$$

$$= \sqrt{(TR \cdot \lambda_o / 4} \qquad (21.12)$$

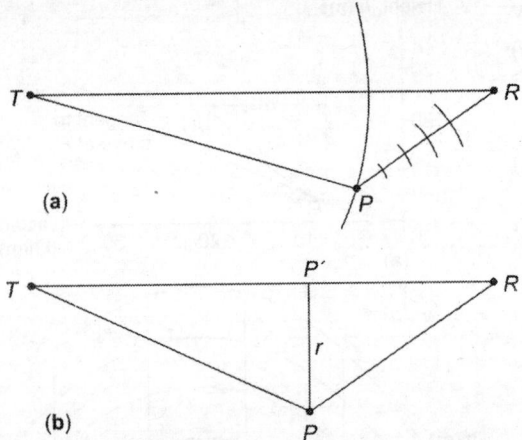

(a)

(b)

Fig. 21.8: (a) Secondary wave generation (b) Determination of Fresnel zone

21.10 GROUND REFLECTIONS

In general, the radio wave reflected from the surface of the earth undergoes changes in amplitude and phase. In this case, the reflection coefficient depends on:

(a) The nature of the reflecting surface such as soil, water etc.

(b) Frequency

(c) Polarization

(d) Angle between the ray path and the reflecting surface.

In most practical situations, the magnitude of reflection coefficient is less than unity but close to it and the phase angle of reflection coefficient is 180° for both horizontally and vertically polarized waves. *The Rayleigh criterion for surface roughness is that the height of surface irregularities should not exceed* 3.6 λ_o/ψ, where ψ is the grazing angle in radians that the ray path makes with the surface. Thus,

$$h \leq 3.6 \, \lambda_o/\psi \qquad (21.13)$$

Calm water acts as a smooth or mirror-like reflector. Vegetation and trees absorb microwave radiation. Hence, in the tree-covered terrain, the ray path should be clear at least by the first Fresnel zone. Reflections from buildings vary widely depending on the shape and the proximity to the antennas in the link. Roofs and walls close to the antenna produce mirror-like reflections. Otherwise, buildings tend to scatter the energy as rough surfaces do.

21.11 SUPER-REFRACTION AND SUBREFRACTION

Irregularities in the earth's atmosphere also affect the tropospheric transmission. When the refractive index of the air decreases with height much more rapidly than normal, the bending of radio wave is much more pronounced than that shown in Fig. 21.6. Then, the radio wave is reflected back from the earth to follow a path as shown in Fig. 21.9(a). This is known as *super-refraction*. This increases the radio range considerably. However, this effect cannot be used for commercial purposes, as it is unreliable.

An increase in temperature with height, known as *temperature inversion*, and an increase in humidity with height give rise to super-refraction. The region in which super-refraction occurs is called *duct*. It can be formed both at earth's surface and in elevated strata as shown in Fig. 21.9(a).

It is quite likely that opposite effect may occur, giving rise to *subrefraction*. This reduces the signal strength by bending the ray path away from the receiver [Fig. 21.9(b)].

Inhomogeneities in the atmosphere give rise to scattering of radio signals as shown

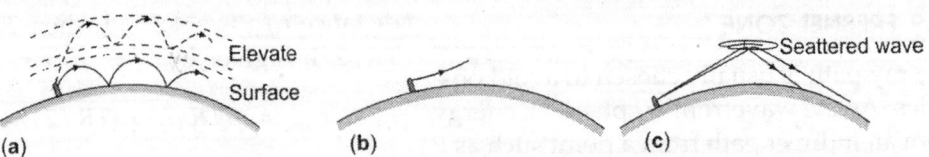

(a)   (b)   (c)

Fig. 21.9: (a) Super-refraction (b) Subrefraction (c) Troposphere scatter propagation

in Fig. 21.9(c). Reliable communication links well beyond the radio horizon can be established by using highly directional high gain antenna. This is referred to *tropospheric scatter* propagation. Ranges up to 650 km have been achieved in the frequency band 40 to 4000 MHz.

21.12 FADING

Fading is the phenomenon in which the strength of received signal is reduced or lost due to atmospheric effects and ground reflections. The types of fading are:

  (a) Absorption fading
  (b) Reflection multipath fading
  (c) Atmospheric multipath fading
  (d) Subrefraction fading

21.12.1 Absorption Fading

Several elements in atmosphere cause attenuation of radio waves due to absorption of energy. These are:

  (i) Rain
  (ii) Cloud
  (iii) Fog
  (iv) Gas molecules in the air.

Heavy rains causes serious attenuation of microwave frequencies above 10 GHz. Moderate rain, cloud and fog seriously attenuate the microwave frequencies above 30 GHz. Hail has effect at frequencies above 100 GHz. Snow has no effect at all frequencies. The gas molecules in the air attenuate the microwaves by absorbing energy due to vibrational resonance. Peak absorption occurs in water vapour molecules at frequencies 22.22 GHz and 176.47 GHz. The oxygen molecule exhibits absorption peaks at 60 GHz and 120 GHz. In microwave communication, these resonance frequencies must be avoided.

21.12.2 Reflection Multipath Fading

The diurnal and seasonal changes in the refractive index cause changes in the relative path lengths between the direct and ground reflected waves as shown in Fig. 21.10(a). The resulting phase change causes reduction in the signal strength or cancellation of the signal. This phenomenon is known as *reflection multipath fading*.

21.12.3 Atmospheric Multipath Fading

Super-refraction can also produce a second atmospheric ray path as shown in Fig. 21.10(a). Hence, phase difference due to path difference between the direct and atmospheric refracted waves can result in signal reduction or cancellation as shown in Fig. 21.10(b). This phenomenon is known as *atmospheric multipath fading. This is the most serious cause of fading at frequencies below 8 GHz.*

21.12.4 Subrefraction Fading

Subrefraction also reduces the signal strength due to bending of ray paths away from the receiver. This phenomenon is known as *subrefraction fading.*

Since fading cannot be eliminated altogether, a fading margin of 30 dB is allowed for in the system design for 99.99% system reliability. The fading is minimized by special techniques known as *diversity schemes*. They are discussed subsequently.

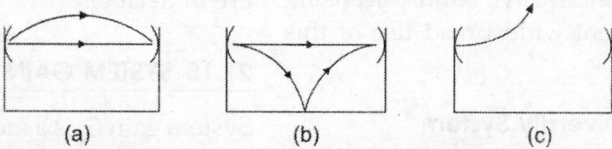

(a)   (b)   (c)

Fig. 21.10: Fading mechanism: (a) Reflection multi-path (super-refraction) fading (b) Atmospheric multi-path fading (c) Subrefraction fading

21.13 DIVERSITY SYSTEMS

Diversity schemes are used to minimize the effect of short-term or rapid fading. The signal is sent over different or diverse paths. The diversity system operates on the statistical principle that separate radio paths are highly unlikely to fade simultaneously for signals that are well separated in space or frequency. Diversity is achieved by setting up different paths in space, known as *space diversity system*, or by using different frequencies, known as *frequency diversity system*. They are shown in Fig. 21.11.

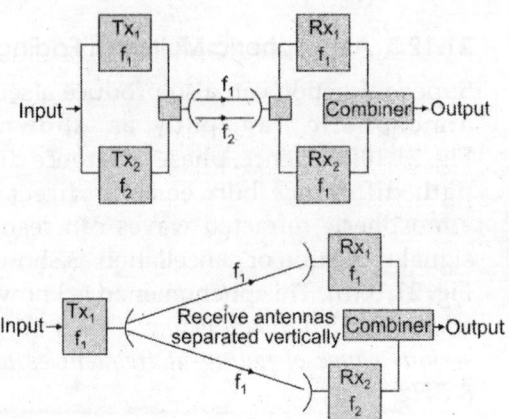

Fig. 21.11: (a) Frequency diversity (b) Space diversity system

21.13.1 Frequency Diversity System

In the frequency diversity system, the signals are sent through *the same path on two different frequencies*. The separation frequency should be equal to or greater than 100 MHz so that the signals do not fade simultaneously. This system requires two transmitters and two receivers. Hence, the system cost is very high. Further, because of very high demand for channels in the microwave bands, licensing restrictions prevent widespread use of this technique.

21.13.2 Space Diversity System

In space diversity system, the vertically polarized signals are transmitted from left

to right through *two different paths in space at the same frequency* f_1 from a single antenna. At the receiving station, two antennas are required. These antennas are spaced vertically at a distance of at least 50 wavelengths. The outputs of the two receivers are combined to give a single desired output. Similarly, right to left transmission is carried out at a different frequency f_2 with horizontal polarization.

21.14 MICROWAVE LINK DESIGN

In microwave communication link design, one has to take into account all the factors that cause signal degradation. The received carrier power must be sufficient enough to be well above the noise level in the receiver. High noise level degrades the signal-to-noise ratio in analog systems and introduces error in digital systems. Hence, the output power of the final transmitter amplifier P_{to} and the minimum detectable receiver carrier power P_{crmin} are important design parameters. In addition, we have to take into account (i) the *transmission path loss* $L_t = 32.5 + 20 \log d + 20 \log f$, where d is the link distance in kilometers and f is the frequency in megahertz, (ii) the *fading margin* f_m, usually 30 dB, (iii) the transmitters and receivers are connected to a single line through filters and circulators. The losses in these are termed as *branching losses* L_b and (iv) the losses in the feeders connecting the transmitter and the receiver to the antennas are known as *feeder loss* L_f. Therefore, we have

$$P_{to} \geq P_{crmin} + f_m + L_t + L_f + L_b - G_T - G_R \tag{21.13}$$

G_T is the transmitter antenna gain and G_R is the receiver antenna gain. All quantities are in decibels.

21.15 SYSTEM GAIN

System gain G_s is a measure of overall system performance. It is defined as

$$G_s = P_{to} - P_{crmin} \tag{21.14}$$

For a well-designed system, the system gain is usually of the order of 100 dB. The higher the system gain, the better. For digital systems operating in the 11 GHz band at a transmission rate of 90 Mb/s, the system gain is about 115 dB.

21.16 ADVANTAGES OF MICROWAVE COMMUNICATION SYSTEMS

The advantages of microwave communication systems are :

(a) They accommodate large number of channels.

(b) They provide high signal-to-noise ratio.

(c) They require small size antennas.

(d) Atmospheric noise and man-made interference such as electric transients, automobile ignition are much less.

21.17 NUMERICAL EXAMPLES

Example 21.1 A terrestrial microwave link of 30 km long is operating at 5000 MHz. Find the free space loss.

Solution: Given: $d = 30$ km, $f = 5000$ MHz.

The free-space loss is given by

$$L_t = 32.5 + 20 \log d + 20 \log f \quad \text{dB}$$
$$= 32.5 + 20 \log 30 + 20 \log 5000$$
$$= 32.5 + 29.54 + 73.98$$
$$= \mathbf{136.02 \ dB}$$

Example 21.2 Find the maximum range for trophospheric transmission for which the antenna heights are 120 ft and 60 ft.

Solution: Given: $h_T = 120$ ft, $h_R = 60$ ft

$$d_{\max}(\text{miles}) = \sqrt{2} \left(\sqrt{h_T \text{ (ft)}} + \sqrt{h_R \text{ (ft)}} \right)$$
$$= 1.414 \times (10.95 + 7.75)$$
$$= \mathbf{26.45 \ miles}$$

Example 21.3 A microwave link of 40 km long is operating at 5 GHz. Find the clearance required at the midpoint.

Solution: Given: $TR = 40, f = 5$ GHz

The maximum clearance is given by

$$r_{\max} = \sqrt{TR\lambda_o / 4}$$
$$\lambda_o = c/f = 3 \times 10^8 / 5 \times 10^9$$
$$= 0.06 \text{ m}$$
$$r_{\max} = \sqrt{TR \cdot \lambda_o / 4}$$
$$= \sqrt{(40 \times 10^3 \times 0.06 / 4}$$
$$= \mathbf{24.5 \ m}$$

Example 21.4 A microwave link is operating at 5 GHz. A ray path makes an angle of 2° with the earth's surface. Find the upper limit for the average wave height for which the surface may be considered as smooth.

Solution: Given: $f = 5$ GHz, $\psi = 2°$.

The average height is given by

$$h = 3.6 \, \lambda_o / \psi$$
$$\lambda_o = c/f = 3 \times 10^8 / 5 \times 10^9$$
$$= 0.06 \text{ m}$$
$$h = 3.6 \times 0.06 \times 57.3/2$$
$$= \mathbf{6.19 \ m}$$

Example 21.5 A microwave link of 40 km long is operating at 5 GHz with a radiated power of 90 W. The transmitting and receiving antennas have 55 dB gain each. Find the received power.

Solution: Given: $d = 40$ km, $f = 5000$ MHz, $G_T = G_R = 55$ dB, $P_{to} = 90$ W, $L_f = L_b = 0$, $f_m = 0$ dB

The received power is given by P_{crmin}.

$$P_{to} = P_{\text{crmin}} + f_m + L_t + L_f + L_b - G_T - G_R$$
$$L_t = 32.5 + 20 \log d + 20 \log f \quad \text{dB}$$
$$= 32.5 + 20 \log 40 + 20 \log 5000$$
$$= 32.5 + 32.04 + 73.98$$
$$= 138.9 \text{ dB}$$
$$P_{\text{crmin}} = P_{to} - L_t + G_T + G_R$$
$$= 10 \log P_{to} \text{(mW)} - 138.9 + 55 + 55$$
$$= 58.73 - 138.9 + 110$$
$$= \mathbf{29.73 \ dBm}$$

Example 21.6 A terrestrial microwave link of 50 km long is operating at 5000 MHz. The gain of each antenna is 50 dB. The fade margin is 40 dB, the branching loss is 2 dB and the feeder loss is 2 dB. Calculate the transmitter power required to meet the minimum received carrier objective of −70 dBm.

Solution: Given: $d = 50$, $f = 5000$, $G_T = G_R = 50$ dB, $f_m = 40$ dB, $L_b = 2$ dB, $L_f = 2$ dB, $P_{crmin} = -75$ dBm

The required transmitter power is given by

$$P_{to} = P_{crmin} + f_m + L_t + L_f + L_b - G_T - G_R$$

$$L_t = 32.5 + 20 \log d + 20 \log f \text{ dB}$$

$$= 32.5 + 20 \log 50 + 20 \log 5000$$

$$= 32.5 + 33.98 + 73.98$$

$$= 140.46 \text{ dB}$$

$$P_{to} = (-75) + 40 + 140.46 + 2 + 2 - 50 - 50$$

$$= \textbf{9.46 dBm}$$

KEY POINTS

- Microwave communication systems are broadly classified as terrestrial and satellite systems.
- MW communication links are widely used for the transmission of voice, video and data to distant places. These links are known as microwave links between two stations linking them directly or via satellite.
- Both analog and digital modulation methods are used in microwave links. In analog systems, FDM/FM is used. In digital systems TDM/PSK is used.
- The radio horizon is the point where the ray path just grazes the earth's surface.
- The contour map is the profile of the terrain between the transmitter and the receiver plotted on the distance-height graph.
- Calm water acts as a smooth or mirror-like reflector. Vegetation and trees absorb microwave radiation.
- Fading is the phenomenon in which the strength of received signal is reduced or lost due to atmospheric effects and ground reflections.

- The types of fading are (a) Absorption fading, (b) Reflection multi-path fading, (c) Atmospheric multi-path fading and (d) Sub-refraction fading
- Rain, cloud, fog and gas molecules in the air absorb the energy in the radio wave. This is known as absorption fading.
- The diurnal and seasonal changes in the refractive index cause changes in the relative path lengths that result in reflection multi-path fading.
- Super-refraction causes signal reduction or cancellation. This phenomenon is known as atmospheric multi-path fading. This is the most serious cause of fading at frequencies below 8 GHz.
- Sub-refraction fading also reduces the signal strength due to bending of ray paths away from the receiver.
- Since fading cannot be eliminated altogether, a fading margin of 30 dB is allowed for in the system design for 99.99% system reliability.
- The fading is minimized by special techniques known as frequency and space diversity systems.
- The frequency diversity system requires two transmitters and two receivers since the signals are sent through the same path over two different frequencies with the separation frequency equal to or greater than 100 MHz.
- In space diversity system, vertically polarized signals are transmitted through two different paths in space at the same frequency from a single antenna. At the receiving station, two antennas spaced vertically at a distance of at least 50 wavelengths receive the signals and combine them to give a single desired output.
- In microwave communication link design, all the factors that cause signal degradation are taken into account.
- The important design parameters are (i) transmitted power, (ii) the minimum detectable receive power, (iii) fading margin, (iv) transmission loss, (v) feeder loss, (vi) branching loss and (vii) gains of transmit and receive antennas.
- Microwaves found extensive use in the development of high-resolution radar systems to detect enemy planes and ships.
- In industrial and domestic applications, they are used in microwave ovens, dryers, measurement of moisture-content and thickness.
- In the field of medicine, they are used for therapeutic, diagnostic and monitoring applications.

FURTHER READING

1. Roddy D and Coolen J (2000). *Electronic Communication*, PHI, New Delhi.
2. Bray WJ (1958). A survey of microwave radio communication, *Electron. Engg.*, Vol. 30.
3. Kennedy G and Davis B (1999). *Electronic Communication Systems*, TMH, New Delhi.
4. Pozar DM (1990). *Microwave Engineering*, Addison-Wesley, Mass.

REVIEW QUESTIONS

21.1 Mention four applications of microwaves.

21.2 What the types of modulation used in microwave links?

21.3 What is meant by FDM/FM and TDM/PSK?

21.4 Draw the block diagram of a microwave terrestrial link.

21.5 What are the important components of terminal stations?

21.6 What is the value of IF carrier?

21.7 Mention the two types of repeaters.

21.8 Which repeater is preferred and why?

21.9 Mention the situations when repeaters are required?

21.10 Define atmospheric refraction.

21.11 What is meant by radio horizon and radio range?

21.12 Give the expression for the radius to be cleared at the midpoint of a microwave link.

21.13 State the Rayleigh criterion.

21.14 What are super and sub refractions?

21.15 What is fading? Mention the types of fading.

21.16 Why fading margin is required while designing a microwave link?

21.17 Give the expression for the transmission path loss.

21.18 Define frequency and space diversity schemes.

21.19 What are the factors to be considered while designing a microwave link?

DESCRIPTIVE QUESTIONS

21.1 Draw the basic microwave terrestrial system and explain briefly.

21.2 Describe the general features of terminal stations used in terrestrial microwave radio links.

21.3 What is the need for repeaters? Explain the passive and active repeaters.

21.4 Briefly explain the atmospheric refraction, radio horizon and contour maps.

21.5 Explain what is meant by (i) Fresnel zone and (ii) Rayleigh criterion and their effects on terrestrial microwave communication.

21.6 Discuss the factors that give rise to fading of microwave signals. How is fading taken care of in the system design?

21.7 Explain the need for diversity systems and explain space and frequency diversity systems.

PRACTICE PROBLEMS

21.1 A terrestrial microwave link of 50 km long is operating at 4000 MHz. Find the free space loss.

(**Ans:** 138.5 dB)

21.2 Find the maximum range for trophospheric transmission for which the antenna heights are 100 ft and 60 ft.

(**Ans:** 25.1 miles)

21.3 A microwave link of 50 km long is operating at 6 GHz. Find the clearance required at the midpoint.

(**Ans:** 25 m)

21.4 A microwave link is operating at 6 GHz. A ray path makes an angle of 2° with the earth's surface. Find the upper limit for the average wave height for which the surface may be considered as smooth.

(**Ans:** 5.16 m)

21.5 A microwave link of 30 km long is operating at 4 GHz with a radiated power of 100 W. The transmitting and receiving antennas have 50 dB gain each. Find the received power.

(**Ans:** 15.9 dBm)

21.6 A terrestrial microwave link of 40 km long is operating at 6000 MHz. The gain of each antenna is 44.8 dB. The fade margin is 39 dB, the branching loss is 2 dB and the feeder loss is 2 dB. Calculate the transmitter power required to meet the minimum received carrier objective of –70 dBm.

(**Ans:** 13.5 dBm)

21.7 A microwave transmission path is to be established over smooth terrain between the transmit and receive antennas mounted on 20 m towers. Find the maximum range possible. (**Ans:** 36.88 km)

REFERENCE

1. Bray WJ (1961). The Standardization of International Microwave Radio Relay Systems.

2. Panther PF. *Communication System Design,* MGH, NY.

3. Wayne Tomasi. *Advanced Electronic Communication Systems*, Pearson Education, 3rd Edition, 2001.

4. Roy Blake. *Electronic Communication Systems,* Thomson Delmar, 2nd Edition, 2002.

5. G Kennedy. *Electronic Communication Systems,* McGraw Hill, 4th Edition, 2002.

6. Miller. *Modern Electronic Communication,* Prentice Hall of India, 2003.

22. Satellite Communication Systems

Objectives

- Understand the communication satellites.
- Know the components of satellite communication systems.
- Discuss the details of equipment in earth stations and transponders.
- Prepare link budget.

22.1 INTRODUCTION

A satellite communication system is a microwave communication system consisting of earth stations and a satellite repeater placed in the sky. The satellite repeater is also known as *transponder*. The transponder receives the signal from the transmitting earth station and retransmits it to the receiving earth station as shown in Fig. 22.1.

The satellite may be passive or active type. A *passive satellite* simply reflects the received signal from transmitting earth station back to the receiving earth station. An active satellite receives the signal from transmitting earth station, shifts the frequency, amplifies and retransmits it towards the receiving earth station.

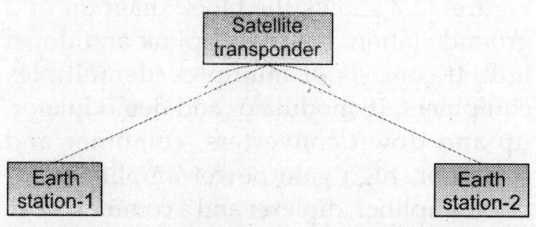

Fig. 22.1: Satellite communication system

22.2 COMMUNICATION SATELLITES

A communication satellite is a spacecraft placed in an orbit around the earth. Most communication satellites are placed in the *geostationary orbit*. The earth's rotational period about its own axis is 23 hours and 56 minutes. A satellite in geo-stationary orbit travels in the same direction as the earth's rotation and completes one revolution about the earth's axis in the same time. Therefore, the satellite appears stationary to an observer on earth. Hence, it is known as the *geostationary satellite*. Three satellites placed 120° apart in geo-stationary orbit can cover the whole world.

A communication satellite carries on board microwave receiving and transmitting equipment capable of relaying signals from one station to other earth stations. As the satellites are at heights well above the ionosphere, microwave frequencies are used because they can penetrate the ionosphere, handle wideband signals and make use of high gain directional antennas required aboard the satellites.

The first communication satellite was launched in 1965. Since then, numerous satellites have been launched for communication purposes. The International Telecommunication Satellite Organization in USA has been launching communication satellites known as INTELSATs (International Satellites). They provide telecommunication services to its member countries throughout the world. Similarly, Indian Space Research Organization (ISRO) in India has been launching communication satellites known as INSATs (Indian Satellites) that provide telecommunication services to the Indian region. The services include telecommunication services such as telephony, telegraphy, telex, digital transmission, wide-area television coverage (known as direct broadcasting by satellite or DBS), videotext, video conferencing and navigational and communication services to aircrafts and ships.

Satellites presently used are active satellites that receive the signals from ground stations, convert the frequency, amplify and transmit them to receiving earth stations. Hence, they have, on board, highly directional transmitting and receiving antennas and complex interconnecting circuits. Accurate positioning and control mechanism are also required for the satellites. The power for on-board equipment is usually obtained from arrays of solar cells with back-up Ni-Cd batteries for periods of solar eclipse.

22.2.1 Advantages of Geo-stationary Satellites

The advantages of using geo-stationary satellites are:
  (a) No tracking of satellite is required
  (b) The satellite is continuously visible from within its service area on earth. Hence, fixed antenna in ground stations establishes the link at all times.
  (c) Doppler shift frequency is negligible as there is no relative movement between the source and the receiver.

22.3 SATELLITE COMMUNICATION SYSTEMS

A satellite communication system consists of earth stations and a satellite repeater placed at a height of 35,786 km above the earth. In this system, the information is transmitted from the ground at microwave frequency, known as *uplink frequency*, using a highly directional antenna to the satellite. The satellite receives the signal through an on-board antenna. The received signal frequency is shifted and amplified by means of a low-nose amplifier (LNA). This is then transmitted towards the earth at a frequency 2 GHz less then the uplink frequency. This frequency is known as *down link frequency*. *This frequency difference is necessary to avoid interference between the uplink and downlink frequencies.*

The satellite frequencies are so chosen that the effect of ionosphere is negligible and atmospheric absorption is also small. The commonly used frequency ranges are 6/4 and 14/12 GHz. The first number in each range gives the uplink frequency to the nearest GHz and the second one the down link frequency. Table 22.1 shows the satellite frequency bands.

Table 22.1: Satellite frequency bands

Frequency band	Frequency range	Direction
6/4 GHz	5.85–6.42 GHz	Up link
	3.7–4.2 GHz	Down link
14/12GHz	14.0–14.5 GHz	Up link
	11.7 – 12.2 GHz	Down link

22.4 GROUND STATION

Figure 22.2 shows the block diagram of a ground station. It has an uplink and down link. It consists of multiplex/demultiplex equipment, IF modulator and demodulator, up and down converters, combiner and separator, high gain power amplifier, low noise amplifier, diplexer and a common large directional antenna.

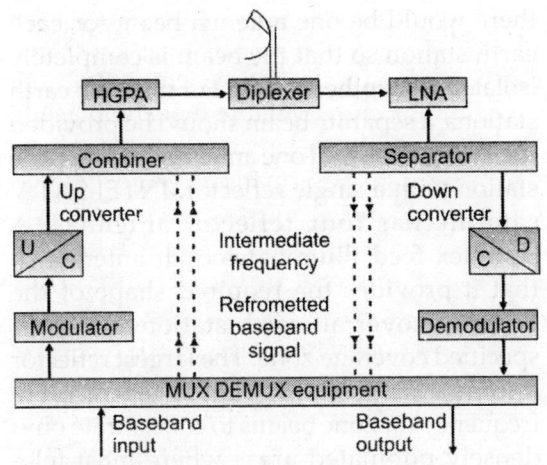

Fig. 22.2: Block diagram of a Ground Station

22.4.1 Uplink

In the uplink, the base band signals are multiplexed. Each channel signal is modulated to IF carrier of 70 MHz and then upconverted. All the channel signals are combined in the combiner and the output power is boosted to the required level by means of a high gain power amplifier. Then, it is transmitted through the common antenna.

22.4.2 Downlink

In the downlink, the signal is received by the common antenna and amplified by the low noise amplifier. Then, the signals are directed into their respective channels by the separator. Each channel signal is down-converted to the IF carrier and then demodulated. The demodulated signal is demultiplexed and the base band is obtained. The diplexer connects

the common antenna to trans/receive position appropriately.

22.4.3 Ground Station Antennas

Each ground station antenna is a large parabolic reflector antenna having high gain and produces narrow pencil-like beam pointing towards the satellite. They may be monopole, dipole, horn, reflector or micro-strip array antennas. The monopole and dipole antennas are primarily used at VHF/UHF for omni-directional coverage in terrestrial communication systems (TCS). Horn antennas are used for global coverage where wide beams are required. The reflector antenna with its feed placed at its focal point produces plane waves with maximum gain and narrow beam to cover a specific zone on earth. The characteristics of earth-station antenna are very important in their design. In a large station like INTELSAT network, a 30 m diameter dish antenna is used. Small stations for reception of direct broadcast by satellite (DBS) use 0.7 m diameter antennas.

As the signal received from the satellite is very weak, the ground station should have low noise temperature. Hence, low noise traveling-wave amplifiers are used.

22.5 SATELLITE TRANSPONDER

The stage between the reception of the uplink signal and the transmission of the down link signal by the satellite is known as a transponder. Figure 22.3 shows the block diagram of a transponder. It consists of receiving and

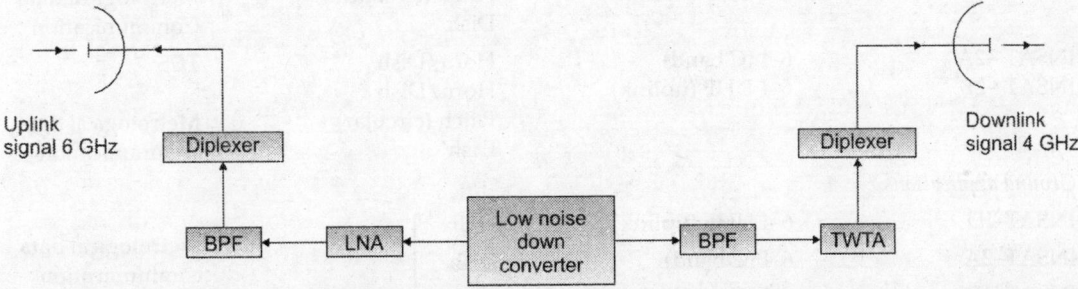

Fig. 22.3: Block diagram of a transponder

transmitting antennas, diplexers, band pass filters and amplifiers. The received uplink signal is passed through the band pass filter in order to reduce the noise temperature. A low noise amplifier then amplifies the signal. Then, a down converter down-converts the frequency. The down converted signal is filtered by a band pass filter, amplified by a TWT amplifier and transmitted to the earth station at the down link frequency.

For television signal transmission, the video signal bandwidth is 4.5 MHz including synchronizing, blanking and equalizing pulses. This signal frequency modulates the microwave carrier. The audio signal is 15 kHz and modulates a 6.8 MHz subcarrier. The audio signal is frequency division multiplexed with the video signal and relayed by a single transponder. The frequency deviation of the video and audio signal is 10.5 MHz and 2 MHz respectively. Hence, the bandwidth required for both sidebands is $2 \times (10.5 + 2 + 6.8) = 38.6$ MHz ≈ 36 MHz for each transponder. Usually, the satellite has 12 transponders. Therefore, including a guard band of 8 MHz, the total bandwidth is accommodated within 500 MHz.

22.5.1 Transponder Antennas

The spacecraft antennas are mounted on the body of the satellite to provide coverage of a specific zone on the earth. In an ideal system, there would be one antenna beam for each earth station so that the beam is completely isolated from other beams. For multiple earth stations, a separate beam should be provided for each station and one antenna feed for each station with a single reflector. INTELSAT V satellite has four reflector antennas. A complex feed illuminates each antenna so that it provides the required shape of the beam to cover all earth stations within a specified coverage zone. The largest reflector antenna is used to transmit at 4 GHz frequency for zone beams to concentrate onto densely populated areas where most telecommunication service traffic is generated. The smaller antennas are used to provide beams to cover hemisphere.

Most domestic satellites do not have complex antenna systems. They use orthogonal polarization frequency reuse system in order to double the effective bandwidth at 6/4 GHz for separate channels, with cross-polarization isolation of 25 dB. Table 22.2 shows the frequency band and antennas used in Indian satellites.

22.6 LINK LOSSES

In a satellite link, the following losses occur.
  (a) Transmission path loss
  (b) Atmospheric absorption and scattering loss

Table 22.2: Indian satellite frequency band and antennas

Satellite	Frequency (GHz)	Antenna type	Use
INSAT–ID	6-4 (C band)	Horn/Dish	TCS
	6-4 UHF (uplink)	Patch (circular)	Metrological data
		Dish	Communication
INSAT –2A	6-4 (C band)	Horn/Dish	TCS
INSAT –2B	6-4 UHF (uplink)	Horn/Dish	
		Patch (circular)	Metrological data
		Dish	communication
Ground applications			
INSAT–ID	6-4 UHF (uplink)	Helix	
INSAT–2A	6-4 (C band)	Dish	Metrological data communication
INSAT–2B	6-4 (C band)	Dish	

22.6.1 Transmission Path Loss

The transmission loss is due to spreading of waves as they propagate outwords from the source. It is given by

$$L_t = 32.5 + 20 \log d + 20 \log f \text{ dB}$$
$$(22.1)$$

where d is the link distance in km and f is the frequency in MHz.

22.6.2 Atmospheric Absorption and Scattering Loss

The absorption and scattering loss is proportional to the length of path in the attenuation medium. This depends on the angle of elevation of the ground antenna and frequency. At 4 GHz for the loss (vertical incidence) is about 0.04 dB whereas at 5° elevation, the loss is about 0.1 dB. Ionospheric absorption is negligible. Heavy rains and clouds also contribute for the loss.

The atmospheric attenuation varies with frequency. In the atmosphere, two absorption peaks are observed: one at a frequency of 22.2 GHz because of absorption due to water vapour molecules that go into vibrational resonance; the other peak occurs at a frequency of 60 GHz due to resonant absorption of oxygen molecules.

In system design, these absorption frequencies should be avoided and a fading margin will be allowed for rainfall and other effects. Its value depends on the geographical location of the ground station.

22.7 LINK BUDGET CALCULATIONS

The power requirement of a satellite link is calculated with the knowledge of the losses and the receiver noise. To reduce the noise temperature, low-noise amplifiers (LNA) are used in the receiving mode. In addition to the amplifier noise, the antenna and various waveguide and branching losses also contribute to the receiver noise. The system noise temperature T_s takes into account all these sources. Then, the noise power density

at the input of the receiver is kT_s watts/Hz or Joules where k is the Boltzmann's constant and is equal to 1.38×10^{-23} j/K.

The received signal power P_R is given by

$$P_R = P_T G_T G_R (0.57 \times 10^{-3})/(df)^2$$
$$(22.2)$$

G_T is the transmitter antenna gain and G_R is the receiver antenna gain.

The received signal-to-noise density ratio C/N_o is given by

$$C/N_o = P_R/kT_s \tag{22.3}$$

22.7.1 Equivalent Isotropic Radiated Power

The important parameter in a satellite receiving system is the ratio of the receiving antenna gain to the system noise temperature G_R/T_s and is given in *decilog* by

$$(G_R/T_s) = 10 \log (G_R/T_s) \text{ dB-K} \tag{22.4}$$

The important parameter in a satellite transmitting system is the *equivalent isotropic radiated power* (EIRP). The EIRP is given by

$$\text{EIRP} = P_T G_T \tag{22.5}$$

Substituting for P_R from Eq. (22.2) we obtain

$$C/N_o = P_T G_T G_R (0.57 \times 10^{-3})/(df)^2 (kT_s)$$
$$= (P_T G_T)(G_R/T_s)[(0.57 \times 10^{-3})/(df)^2](k)$$

$$(C/N_o) = \text{EIRP} + (G_R/T_s) - L_t + 228.6 \text{ dB}$$

Taking into account other losses, we get

$$C/N_o = \text{EIRP} - M - L_t + (G_R/T_s) + 228.6 \text{ dB Hz} \tag{22.6}$$

All quantities are either in decibels or decilogs. The quantity 228.6 is due to the Boltzmann's constant k and is equal to $-10 \log k$. The propagation or transmission loss L_t is given by Eq. (22.1) and M is the total margin in decibels to allow for fading, antenna pointing error and waveguide and branching losses.

In digital systems, the important design parameter is the ratio of energy per bit to noise density E_b/N_o and is usually specified. The received signal-to-noise density ratio C/N_o is given by

$$C/N_o = E_b/N_o + R \qquad (22.7)$$

where R is the transmission rate. All quantities are in decibels or decilogs.

22.6 NUMERICAL EXAMPLES

Example 22.1 In a satellite link, the EIRP is 55 dBW and G_R/T_s is 20 dB-K, $L_t = 200$ dB, fading margin, antenna pointing margin and equipment implementation margin each is 2 dB. Calculate the C/N_o ratio.

Solution: Given: EIRP = 55 dBW, G_R/T_s = 20 dB-K, $L_t = 200$ dB, $M = 6$ dB

$$C/N_o = \text{EIRP} - M - L_t + (G_R/T_s) +$$
$$228.6 \text{ dB-Hz}$$
$$= 55 - 6 - 200 + 20 + 228.6$$
$$= \textbf{97.6 dB-Hz}$$

Example 22.2 The satellite in Example 22.1 is transmitting a digital signal at a rate of 60 Mbps. Calculate the E_b/N_o ratio.

Solution: Given: EIRP = 55 dBW, G_R/T_s = 20 dB-K, $L_t = 200$ dB, $M = 6$ dB, $R = 60$ Mbps.

$$C/N_o = E_b/N_o + R$$
$$E_b/N_o = C/N_o - R$$
$$= 97.6 - 10 \log (60 \times 10^6)$$
$$= 97.6 - 77.8$$
$$= \textbf{19.8 dB}$$

Example 22.3 In a satellite link, the C/N_o ratio is 90 dB-Hz and G_R/T_s is 20 dB-K, $L_t = 200$ dB, fading margin, antenna pointing margin and equipment implementation margin each is 2 dB. Calculate the **EIRP**.

Solution: Given: C/N_o ratio = 90 dB-Hz, G_R/T_s = 20 dB-K, $L_t = 200$ dB, $M = 6$ dB

$$C/N_o = \text{EIRP} - M - L_t + (G_R/T_s) + 228.6$$
$$\text{EIRP} = C/N_o + M + L_t - (G_R/T_s) - 228.6$$
$$= 90 + 6 + 200 - 20 - 228.6$$
$$= \textbf{47.4 dBW}$$

Example 22.4 The satellite in Example 22.3 is transmitting a digital signal at a rate of 6 Mbps. Calculate the E_b/N_o ratio.

Solution: Given: C/N_o ratio = 90 dB-Hz, $R = 10 \log (6 \times 10^6) = 67.8$ dB

The E_b/N_o ratio is given by

$$E_b/N_o = C/N_o - R$$
$$= 90 - 67.8$$
$$= \textbf{22.2 dB}$$

KEY POINTS

- A satellite communication system consists of earth stations and a satellite repeater or transponder placed at a height of 35.86 km from earth. The transponder receives the signal from the transmitting earth station and retransmits it to the receiving earth station.
- A passive satellite simply reflects the received signal from transmitting earth station back to the receiving earth station.
- An active satellite receives the signal from transmitting earth station, shifts the frequency, amplifies and retransmits it towards the receiving earth station.
- A communication satellite is a spacecraft placed in the geo-stationary orbit around the earth.
- A satellite in geo-stationary orbit travels in the same direction as the earth's rotation and completes one revolution about the earth's axis in the same time. Therefore, the satellite appears stationary to an observer on earth. It carries on board microwave receiving and transmitting equipment capable of relaying signals from one station to other earth stations.
- Three satellites placed 120° apart in geo-stationary orbit can cover the whole world.
- The power for on-board equipment is usually obtained from arrays of solar cells, with back-up Ni-Cd batteries for periods of solar eclipse.
- The advantages of using geo-stationary satellites are: (i) no tracking of satellite is required; (ii) the satellite is continuously visible from within its service area on earth. Hence, fixed antenna in ground stations establishes the link at all times and (iii) Doppler shift frequency is negligible as there is no relative movement between the source and the receiver.
- The information is transmitted from the ground at microwave frequency f_1, known as uplink

frequency. The satellite receive, the signal through an on-board antenna, processes and then transmits towards the earth at a frequency 2 GHz less then the uplink frequency. This frequency is known as down link frequency. This frequency difference is necessary to avoid interference between the uplink and down link frequencies.

- The commonly used frequency ranges 6/4 and 14/12 GHz. The first number in each range gives the uplink frequency to the nearest GHz and the second one the down link frequency.
- As the signal received from the satellite is very weak, low noise traveling-wave amplifiers are used for amplification.
- In a satellite link, transmission path loss and atmospheric absorption and scattering loss occur.
- The power requirement of a satellite link is calculated with the knowledge of the losses and the receiver noise.
- The important parameters in a satellite link design are (i) the received signal power P_R, (ii) the received signal-to-noise density ratio C/N_o, (iii) the ratio of the receiving antenna gain to the system noise temperature G_R/T_s, and (iv) the equivalent isotropic radiated power (**EIRP**),
- In digital systems, the important design parameter is the ratio of energy per bit to noise density E_b/N_o and is usually specified. The received signal-to-noise density ratio C/N_o is then $C/N_o = E_b/N_o + R$, where **R** is the transmission rate. All quantities are in decibels or decilogs.

FURTHER READING

1. Roddy D (2001). Satellite Communication, McGraw Hill, New Delhi.
2. Hudson HE (1990). Communication Satellite-Their Development and Impact, Free Press, NY.
3. Pratt T et al. (2003). Satellite Communication, Wiley, NJ.
4. Miller (2003). Modern Electronic Communication, Prentice Hall of India.

REVIEW QUESTIONS

22.1 What is a satellite communication system and what are its important components?
22.2 What is a transponder?
22.3 Draw the block diagram of a satellite communication system.
22.4 Distinguish between the two types of satellites.

22.5 What is a communication satellite and geostationary satellite?
22.6 Mention the advantages of using geo-stationary satellites.
22.7 Why is microwave frequency used for satellite communication system?
22.8 What is an uplink and downlink?
22.9 What are the frequencies used for uplink and downlink?
22.10 Explain why different frequencies are used for uplink and downlink.
22.11 What are the important components of a satellite ground station?
22.12 What are the important components of a satellite transponder?
22.13 Mention the losses in a satellite link.
22.14 What is link budget calculation?

DESCRIPTIVE QUESTIONS

22.1 With a neat block diagram, explain the satellite ground station.
22.2 With a neat block diagram, explain the satellite transponder.
22.3 Explain the major differences between a satellite repeater and terrestrial repeater station.
22.4 Write a brief note on communication satellites.
22.5 Write brief notes on earth station and transponder antennas.
22.6 Explain, in detail, the various link losses.
22.7 Explain, in detail, the satellite link budget calculation.

PRACTICE PROBLEMS

22.1 In a satellite link, the **EIRP** is 54 dBW and G_R/T_s is 17.7 dB-K, $L_t = 210$ dB, fading margin, antenna pointing margin and equipment implementation margin together is 2.95 dB. Calculate the C/N_o ratio.

   (**Ans:** 87.35 dB-Hz)

22.2 The satellite in Problem 22.1 is transmitting a digital signal at a rate of 61 Mbps. Calculate the E_b/N_o ratio.

   (**Ans:** 9.5 dB)

22.3 In a satellite link, the C/N_o ratio is 85.6 dB-Hz and G_R/T_s is 10 dB-K, $L_t = 200$ dB, fading margin, antenna pointing margin and equipment implementation margin together is 3 dB. Calculate the **EIRP**.

(**Ans:** 50 dBW)

22.4 The uplink requirement of a satellite are C/N_o = 71.97 dB, fade margin 0.5 dB, antenna pointing margin 0.5 dB, wave-guide losses 0.2 dB, equipment implementation margin 1 dB, propagation loss 207 dB and G_R/T_s 23.5 dB-K. Calculate the earth station **EIRP** in dBW.

(**Ans:** 29.07 dBW)

22.5 The E_b/N_o ratio required is 9.5 dB at a transmission rate of 1.764 Mbps. The transmission loss is 214 dB, fade margin 2.1 dB, antenna pointing margin 1 dB, wave-guide losses 2 dB and equipment implementation margin 1 dB. The earth station **EIRP** = 50 dBW. Calculate the G_R/T_s ratio in dB-K.

(**Ans:** 13.5 dB-K)

REFERENCE

1. Brown WC (1973). Satellite power stations: a new source of energy, *IEEE Spectrum*, March, p 38–47.

2. Wayne Tomasi. *Electronic Communication Systems,* Pearson Education, 3rd Edition, 2001.

3. Roy Blake. *Electronic Communication Sys-tems,* Thomson Delmar, 2nd Edition, 2002.

4. William Schweber. *Electronic Communication Systems,* Prentice Hall of India, 2002.

5. G. Kennedy. *Electronic Communication Systems,* McGraw Hill, 4th edition, 2002.

6. Indian National Satellite Systems, (1988) ISRO Bulletin, India,

7. Martin J (1978). *Communication Satellite Systems,* PH, N.J.

8. Gagliaredi HM (1987). *Satellite Communication,* Van Nostrand.

9. Lewis GE (1988). *Communication via Satellites,* Blackwell.

10. Elbert VBR (1987). *Introduction to Satellite Communication,* Artech., Mass.

11. Maral G and Bousquet M (1986). *Satellite Communication,* Wiley, N.J.

12. Roddy D (2001). *Satellite Communication,* MGH, NY.

13. Pratt T and Bousquet M (1986). *Satellite Communication,* Wiley, NJ.

23

Radar Systems

Objectives

- Understand the basic principle of radar system.
- Derive radar range equation.
- Classify the types of radars.
- Explain the operation and application of radars.

23.1 INTRODUCTION

Radar is the acronym for *ra*dio *d*etection *a*nd *r*ange. Radar is essentially an echo-sounding system. Radar transmitter sends pulses of high power electromagnetic energy but of very short duration. Objects such as aircrafts, ships, mountains and buildings reflect some of this energy back to the transmitter. The time delay of the returned echo is a measure of the distance from the reflecting objects. For a wave traveling with velocity of light, a delay of one microsecond corresponds to a range of 150 meters. Directional transmitting and receiving antennas are used to obtain the direction of the reflecting object.

However, with development of new radar systems at frequencies well above the microwave band, the radar is defined as "An electromagnetic device for detecting the presence and location of objects. The presence of objects and their distance (range) are determined by the transmission and return of the electromagnetic energy, direction is usually obtained, through use of a movable or rotating directive antenna pattern."

23.2 RADAR CLASSIFICATION

The radar is classified into *primary* and *secondary radar*. In primary radar, a microwave signal is transmitted from the radar station and is reflected by the object to be detected. The reflected signal is picked up at the radar station using the same antenna. Primary radars are used for military applications such as to detect position and flight path of enemy aircrafts, ships and missiles. The flight path of shells can be projected back on the battlefield pinpointing the positions of the enemy guns. It is also used to detect the position and movement of storm centers for weather forecasting.

Secondary radar transmits a signal towards the target and receives a coded signal for identification. In this manner, the identification of commercial airliners in flight and detection of their position and speed are achieved.

22.3 RADAR FREQUENCIES

Microwaves are used for radar because of the following advantages:

(a) Very compact antennas can be designed
(b) High gain and highly directional antennas can be used

Table 23.1 shows the various radar frequency bands used.

Table 23.1: Radar frequency bands		
Frequency band	*Frequency range*	*Wavelength*
HF	3–30 MHz	100–10 m
VHF	30–300 MHz	10–1 m
UHF	300–1000 MHz	1–0.1 m
L	1–2 GHz	30–15 cm
S	2–4 GHz	15–7.5 cm
C	4–8 GHz	7.5–3.75 cm
X	8–12 GHz	3.75–2.5 cm
Ku	12–18 GHz	25–1.67 cm
K	18–27 GHz	1.67–1.11 cm
Ka	27–40 GHz	1.11–0.75 cm
mm	40–300 GHz	7.5 – 1 mm

22.4 BASIC RADAR SYSTEM

Figure 23.1 shows the block diagram of a basic radar system. It consists of a transmitting section, a receiving section, a duplexer and an antenna. The transmitting section consists of a microwave oscillator that is controlled by a modulator or pulser in such a way as to generate periodic pulses of high

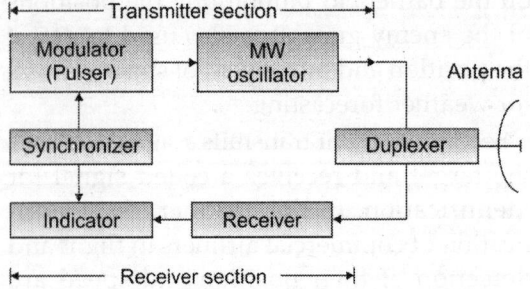

Fig.23.1: Block diagram of a radar system

power but of relatively short duration. The antenna is highly directional and can be rotated so as to direct the beam as desired. A single antenna is commonly used for both transmission and reception. Hence, a switching arrangement known as *duplexer* is used to isolate the receiver while the pulses are transmitted so that the receiver is not damaged due to high power transmitted. It switches the antenna to the receiver in the intervals between pulses during which the reflected energy is received.

The radar receiver is a radio receiver with lowest noise figure, high sensitivity and an appropriate bandwidth. The receiver output is usually displayed on a CRT indicator. The sweep voltage of the CRT display is synchronized with the transmitted pulse so as to indicate the time difference between the outgoing pulses and the returning echoes.

23.5 RADAR RANGE EQUATIONS

The factors that determine the range of a radar are:

(i) R is the range to the target
(ii) σ is the equivalent cross-sectional area of the target
(iii) P_T is the peak transmitted power
(iv) P_{ref} is the peak echo power received by the antenna
(v) G_T is the power gain of the transmitting antenna relative to isotropic radiator
(vi) G_R is the power gain of the receiving antenna relative to isotropic radiator
(vii) λ_o is the wavelength
(viii) A_o is the aperture area of the receiving antenna

23.5.1 Received Power

The radar range equation relates the range of the target R with the characteristics of transmitter, receiver and target. Let P_T and G_T be the transmitted power and gain of the transmitter antenna respectively. The equivalent power in the beam is $P_T G_T$. Let R be the range of the target. The surface area of a sphere of radius R is $4\pi R^2$. Hence

Power density at target

$$P_d = P_T G_T / 4\pi R^2 \qquad (23.1)$$

This energy strikes the target and is scattered in all directions, some being returned to the radar antenna. Let the surface area of the target that intercepts the transmitted signal be σ. This area of the target is known as the *radar cross section of the target*. The echo power P_{ref} received is given by

Echo power received

$$P_{ref} = P_d \sigma \qquad (23.2)$$

The power received by receiving antenna is proportional to the aperture area A_o of the receiving antenna. Hence, the received power is given by

$$P_R = P_d \, \sigma \, A_o \, / 4\pi R^2$$

Using the relationship $A_o = G_R \lambda_o / 4\pi$ and substituting for P_d from Eq. (23.1) and assuming $G_T = G_R = G$, we get

$$P_R = P_T G^2 \lambda_o^2 \sigma / [(4\pi)^3 (R)^4] \qquad (23.3)$$

Thus, the received power is inversely proportional to the fourth power of the range and drops off very rapidly with increase in range.

23.5.2 Receiver Noise and S/N Ratio

The receiver noise is given by

$$N = F k T_o B_n \qquad (23.4)$$

where

F is the receiver noise factor

k is the Boltzmann's constant = 1.38×10^{-23} J/K

T_o is the room temperature in degrees Kelvin

B_n is the noise bandwidth of the receiver

Therefore, the signal-to-noise ratio at the input of the receiver is given by

$$S/N = P_T G^2 \lambda_o^2 \sigma / [(4\pi)^3 (R)^4 \, F k T_o B_n] \qquad (23.5)$$

23.5.3 Losses

The various losses that occur such as atmospheric attenuation and scattering of the microwaves due to heavy rain or precipitation have not been taken into account. Grouping all the losses as L_A, the signal-to-noise ratio is given by

$$S/N = P_T G^2 \lambda_o^2 \sigma / [(4\pi)^3 (R)^4 \, F k T_o B_n L_A] \qquad (23.6a)$$

In decibels, it is expressed as

$$S/N = P_T + 2G + 2\lambda_o + \sigma + 171 \\ - 4R - F - B_n - L_A \qquad (23.6b)$$

All quantities in the above equation are either in *decibels* or in *decilogs*. The constant factor $(4\pi)^3 k T_o$ expressed in decilogs is equal to (-171) dB at 290°K. This equation is the *basic radar equation*. It shows all the parameters of the radar system that affect its performance. Thus, the signal-to-noise ratio is directly proportional to the transmitted power P_T, inversely proportional to the noise factor N and inversely proportional to the fourth power of the range R.

23.5.4 Maximum Range Equation

Let maximum range R_{max} of the target be as that range beyond which the received echo power is negligible. For the minimum received power P_{Rmin}, the maximum range R_{max} is given by

$$R_{max} = [P_T G^2 \lambda_o^2 \sigma / (4\pi)^3 (R)^4 \, F k T_o B_n L_A]^{1/4} \qquad (23.7)$$

This is the basic radar range equation. If λ_o is in meters, σ should be in square meters and R_{max} will be in meters. To double the range, a 16-fold increase in power is required. The range in decibels is given by

$$R_{max} = \tfrac{1}{4}[P_T + 2G + 2\lambda_o + \sigma + 171 - F - B_n - L_A] \qquad (23.8)$$

All quantities in the above equation are either in *decibels* or in *decilogs*. The constant factor $(4\pi)^3 k T_o$ expressed in decilogs is equal to (-171) dB at 290°K. Navigational distances are often expressed in nautical miles. The conversion factor is 1 nautical mile is 1852 meters. This is the international nautical mile.

23.5.5 Radar Cross-section

The radar cross-section s of a target is defined as

$$\sigma = \frac{\text{Power radiated from the target}}{\text{Incident power density on the target}} \quad (23.9)$$

Assuming that all other quantities except σ and R are constant, the received power is proportional to the radar cross-section. Thus,

$$P_R \propto \sigma \quad (23.10)$$

The radar cross-section is a function of the aspect angle θ and so is P_R. The normalized radar cross-section $\sigma(\theta)/\sigma(0)$ of the target can be obtained by measuring the received power for different aspect angles.

23.6 DUPLEXER

When a common antenna is used with a radar system, some arrangements must be used to isolate the transmitter from the receiver. Otherwise, the transmitted high power may burn out the front end of the receiver; or the direct coupling between them may result in inefficient transfer of power to and from the antenna. A unit known as duplexer is used to couple the transmitter or receiver to the antenna and to reduce the coupling between them. A hybrid-T can be used as a duplexer but a 3-dB loss will occur.

A common type of duplexer for use with narrow-band pulsed radar is shown in Fig. 23.2. It makes use of fast acting microwave switches known as TR-ATR switches. Since the operation is controlled by $\lambda/4$ line the arrangement results in a narrow-band system. The two types of duplexers commonly used are *PIN diode switches* and *ferrite circulators*.

23.6.1 PIN Diode Switches

A passive PIN switch is one that switches to its high-conducting state when the incident power is high. An active PIN switch may also be used. In this case, the diode is normally in the reverse-biased condition and hence, in a low-conductance state. Simultaneously with transmission, the diode is forward-biased and becomes a high conductance.

When the transmit power is present on the line, the TR-ATR switches in Fig. 23.2(a) are both closed or shorted. The resulting circuit is shown in Fig. 23.2(b). The branch lines *cd* and *ab* are odd number of quarter-wavelengths long and shorted at the ends *d* and *b* respectively. They have no effect upon the transmitter operation. At the same time, the TR switch approximates a short circuit at *b* and it prevents any little energy reaching *b* from going on to the receiver. Thus, the receiver is isolated. Following the transmitted pulse, the TR-ATR switches rapidly become open circuited. The resulting circuit is shown in Fig. 23.2(c). The open circuit at *d* places very low impedance across the line at *c*. This, in turn, causes the impedance looking

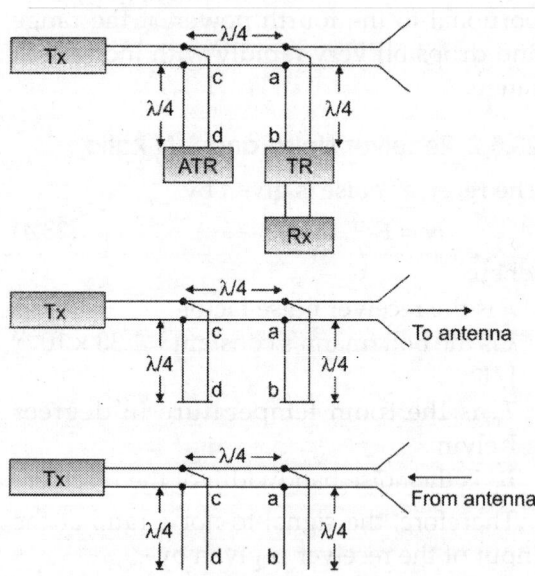

Fig. 23.2: (a) Narrow band duplexer, (b) Transmit mode, (c) Receiver mode

towards the transmitter from a to b very high. As a result, all the received energy reaching a travels towards the receiver and the transmitter is effectively isolated.

23.6.2 Ferrite Circulators

A pair of ferrite circulators can also be used as duplexers. Figure 23.3 shows how TR switching can be achieved using two ferrite circulators. The direction of signal around the circulator depends on the direction of the dc field. The transmit condition is shown in Fig. 23.2(a). The transmitted energy travels from port 1 to port 2 of the first circulator and then, on to the antenna. Most of the energy enters the port 2. Any leakage energy that continues to circulate around enters the second circu-lator through port 3 to port 1' branch. The magnetic field to this circulator is in such a direction as to direct it to port 3' where most of the energy is absorbed by the matched load. Under receive conditions; the magnetic field in the second circulator is reversed as shown in Fig. 23.3(b) The received energy travels around the first circulator from port 2 to port 3 and then enters the second circulator at port 1'. It travels around the second circulator to port 2' where it goes to the receiver. Any leakage energy that continues to circulate in the second circulator is absorbed by the matched load at port 3'. Thus, the received energy is directed to the receiver only.

23.7 PULSED RADAR

In pulsed radar systems, sinusoidal signals cannot be used because of the difficulty in determining the delay time as well as the presence multiple targets. Therefore, pulses of short duration are used. These pulses are obtained by modulating a sinusoidal carrier with a repetitive rectangular pulse wave as shown in Fig. 23.4. The width of the pulse is τ and the pulse repetition frequency is $f_r = 1/T_r$.

23.7.1 Range

For an echo time T_e, the corresponding range R is given by

$$R = c\,T_e/2 \qquad (23.11)$$

where c is the velocity of light. Since T_e is the roundtrip time of the signal, division by 2 occurs in the above equation. Maximum range is obtained when $T_e = T_r$. Hence, the maximum range R_{max} is given by

$$R_{max} = cT_r/2 \qquad (23.12)$$

Minimum range is obtained when $T_e = \tau$. Hence, the minimum range R_{min} is given by

$$R_{min} = c\tau/2 \qquad (23.13)$$

When two targets are present, they can be resolved *only if* the second echo arrives after time τ from that of the first echo. Hence, for proper target resolution, the separation between pulses should be greater than or equal to τ. Thus,

$$T_{e2} - T_{e1} \geq \tau \qquad (23.14)$$

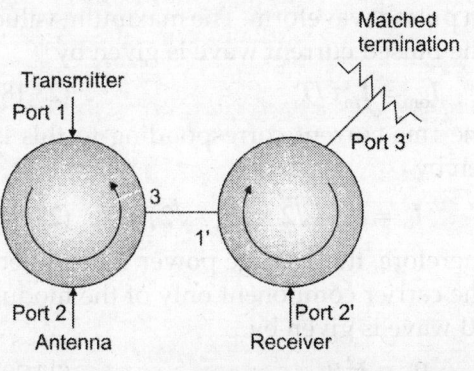
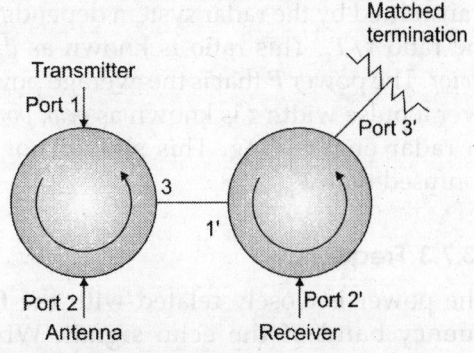

Fig. 23.3: Ferrite duplexer (a) Transmit mode (b) Receive mode

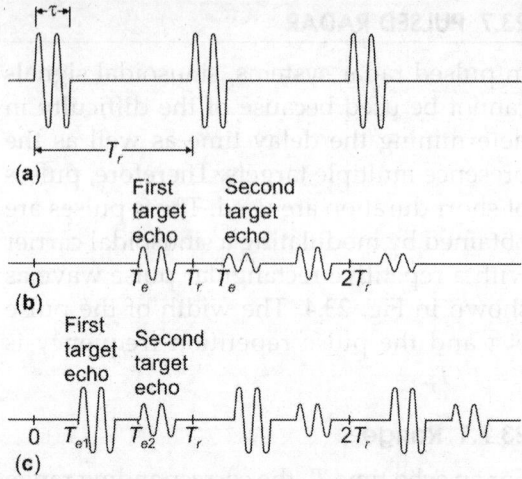

(a)

(b) First target echo / Second target echo

(c) First target echo / Second target echo

Fig. 23.4: (a) Pulsed radar wave (b) Received echo (c) Combination of transmitted and echo signals

23.7.2 Power

Figure 23.5 shows the power wave associated with pulsed radar system. The pulsed current wave has a maximum value I_m. The peak or maximum power P_m is given by

$$P_m = I_m^2 R_{ar} \tag{23.15}$$

where R_{ar} is the antenna radiation resistance. The average power over one pulse width is one half of P_m and is given by

$$P = P_m/2 = I_m^2 R_{ar}/2 \tag{23.16}$$

The average power P_{av} over one complete period T_r is given by

$$P_{av} = P\tau/T_r \tag{23.17}$$

This is the average power the transmitter must deliver to the antenna. Thus, the power transmitted by the radar system depends on the ratio τ/T_r. This ratio is known as *duty factor*. The power P that is the average power over a pulse width τ is known as *peak power* in radar engineering. This should not be confused with P_m.

23.7.3 Frequency

The power is closely related with the frequency band of the echo signal. When sinusoidal carrier of frequency f_0 is modula-

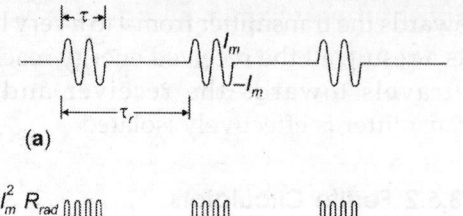

(a)

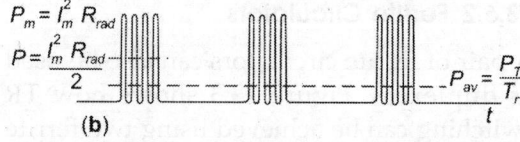

(b)

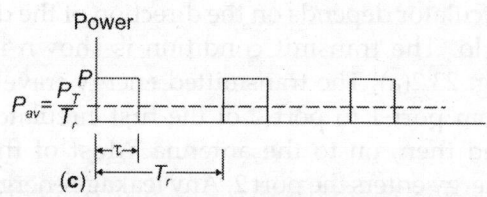

(c)

Fig. 23.5: (a) Pulsed radar waveform (b) Instantaneous power wave (c) Peak average power P and true average P_{av}

ted with a rectangular pulse train of repetition frequency f_r $(= 1/T_r)$, it has an infinite number of side frequencies given by $(f_0 \pm nf_r)$ where $n = 1, 2, 3, \ldots$ If the pulse repetition frequency f_r is low, most of the side frequencies are close to the carrier and hence the complete spectrum will be received. In this case, the power used in Eq. (23.6) is the peak average power P. When the pulse repetition frequency f_r is high, the receiver may have only sufficient bandwidth to receive the carrier component of the spectrum f_0. A Fourier analysis of the pulse waveform in Fig. 23.5 shows the power wave associated with pulsed waveform. The maximum value of the pulsed current wave is given by

$$I_{om} = I_m \tau/T_r \tag{23.18}$$

The rms current corresponding to this is given by

$$I_o = I_{om}/\sqrt{2} = (I_m/\sqrt{2})\tau/T_r \tag{23.19}$$

Therefore, the average power transmitted in the carrier component only of the modulated wave is given by

$$P_o = I_o^2 R_{ar} \tag{23.20}$$

Substituting for I_0 from Eq. (23.19), we obtain

$$P_0 = [(I_m/\sqrt{2})\tau/T_r]^2 R_{at}$$
$$= (I_m^2 R_{ar}/2)(\tau/T_r)^2$$
$$= P(\tau/T_r)^2$$
$$= P_{av}(\tau/T_r) \qquad (23.21)$$

This is the power that must be used in Eq. (23.6) when f_r is high.

23.8 FMCW RADAR

Earlier it was stated that it is necessary to pulse amplitude modulate the carrier to determine the range by measuring the echo time and to allow separation of echo signals from the outgoing signal and from each other. As an alternative to pulse amplitude modulation, frequency modulation is widely used. These radars are known as frequency modulated continuous wave radar.

Let the unmodulated carrier frequency be f_0, the modulation frequency be $f_m(t)$ and the instantaneous FM signal frequency f_i. Then, f_i is given by

$$f_i = f_0 + f_m(t) \qquad (23.22)$$

The received signal frequency f_{ir} is given by

$$f_{ir} = f_0 + f_m(t - T_e) \qquad (23.23)$$

This is due to the fact that the received signal is really the signal that was transmitted T_e earlier. Hence, the frequency difference between the transmitted and received signal is given by

$$f_d = f_i - f_{ir}$$
$$= f_m(t) - f_m(t - T_e) \qquad (23.24)$$

Figure 23.6 shows the commonly used triangular waveform for frequency modulation. Along any straight line section of the modulation waveform, the frequency $f_m(t)$ may be expressed by a straight line equation given by

$$f_m(t) = at + b \qquad (23.25)$$

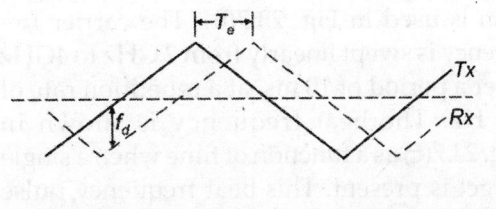

Fig. 23.6: FMCW transmit and receive frequency waveforms

where a is the slope and b is the intercept. Substituting Eq. (23.25) in Eq. (23.24), we get

$$f_d = aT_e \qquad (23.26)$$

The basic range equation is $R = cT_e/2$ and hence the range is given by

$$R = cf_d/2a \qquad (23.27)$$

Thus, the range can be obtained by measuring f_d and a.

Figure 23.7 (a) shows a block diagram of a FMCW radar system. The frequency modula-

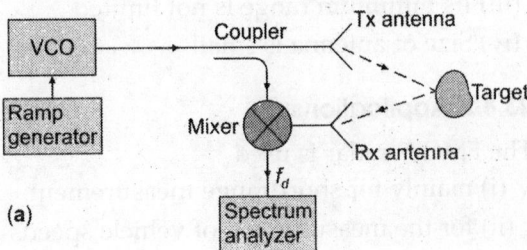

(a)

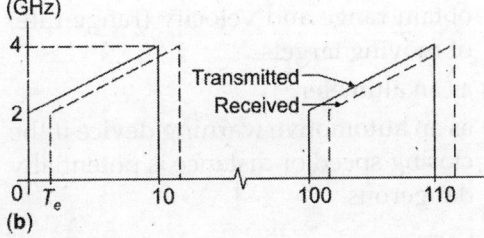

(b)

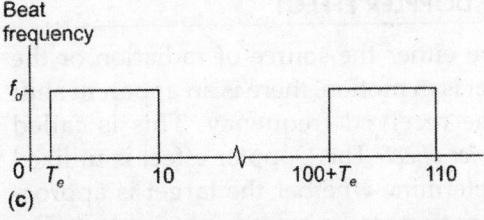

(c)

Fig. 23.7: FWCW radar (a) Configuration (b) Transmit and receive frequency variations (c) Resultant heat frequency

tion is used in Fig. 23.7(b). The carrier frequency is swept linearly from 2 GHz to 4GHz over a period of 10 ms, at a repetition rate of 10 Hz. The beat frequency is shown in Fig. 23.7(c) as a function of time when a single target is present. This beat frequency pulse width is a function of the echo time T_e and this, in turn, is related to target range. Hence, phase velocity of the wave in the medium must be used instead of free space velocity c. With multiple targets, the situation is more complicated and hence, digital signal processing is used to separate out the echo waves.

23.8.1 Advantages

The advantages of FWCW radar are:

(i) It operates with continuous power

(ii) The power level is relatively low

(iii) Its minimum range is not limited

(iv) Size of antenna is small

23.8.2 Applications

The FMCW radar is used

(i) mainly for short-range measurement

(ii) for the measurement of vehicle speeds and closing or separating distances.

(iii) In conjunction with Doppler effect to obtain range and velocity (range rate) of moving targets.

(iv) as an altimeter.

(v) as an automotive warning device if the closing speed or distance is potentially dangerous.

23.9 DOPPLER EFFECT

When either the source of radiation or the target is in motion, there is an apparent shift in the received frequency. This is called *Doppler effect*. The Doppler effect is utilized to determine whether the target is approaching or receding from the radar. The frequency of received echo signal is increased if the target is approaching the radar and is decreased if the target is moving away from the radar.

When the target is moving towards the radar receiver, the increase in frequency is given by

$$f_{dop} = 2 \, (dR \, /dt) \, f_o/c$$
$$= 2 \, (dR \, /dt)/\lambda_o$$
$$= 2v\cos\theta/\lambda_o \qquad (23.28)$$

Here, f_o is the carrier frequency, $(dR \, /dt)$ is the rate at which the range is changing (range rate), c is the free space velocity, λ_o is the wavelength given by c/f_o and θ is the aspect angle of the target as shown in Fig. 23.8. When the target is approaching the radar receiver, the aspect angle lies between 0 and $\pi/2$. The received frequency is increased by the Doppler frequency. When the target is moving away from the radar receiver, the aspect angle lies between $\pi/2$ and π. The received frequency is decreased by the Doppler frequency. When the velocity is perpendicular, $\theta = \pi/2$ and the Doppler shift is zero. By measuring Doppler frequency shift and its polarity with respect to the transmitted frequency, the range rate of the target can be obtained.

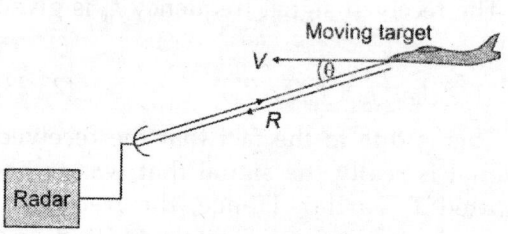

Fig. 23.8: Doppler effect

23.10 FM DOPPLER RADAR

In FMCW radar, for a stationary target, the difference frequency between the transmitted and received signals is positive over the positive slope of the modulating triangular wave and is negative over the negative slope. When the target is moving, this difference frequency will also contain the Doppler shift. This is shown in Fig. 23.9.

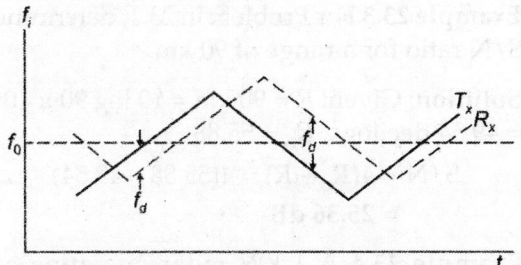

Fig. 23.9: FMCW transmit and receive frequency waveforms with Doppler shift

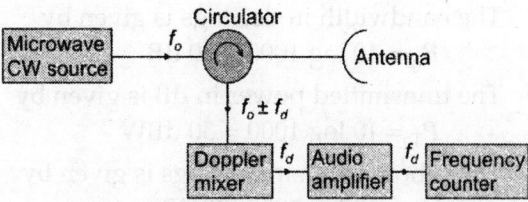

Fig. 23.10: CW Doppler radar system

If the target is moving towards the radar receiver, the frequency difference over the positive slope decreases by an amount f_{dop} and is given by

$$f_+ = f_d - f_{dop} \qquad (23.29)$$

The frequency difference over the negative slope increases by an amount f_{dop} and is given by

$$f_- = f_d + f_{dop} \qquad (23.30)$$

Combining the two equations, we obtain

$$2f_d = f_+ + f_-$$
$$f_d = (f_+ + f_-)/2 \qquad (23.31)$$

Substituting for f_d in Eq. (23.4), we get the range as

$$R = cf_d/2a = c(f_+ + f_-)/4a \qquad (23.32)$$

Subtracting the two Eqs (23.29) and (23.30), we get

$$f_{dop} = (f_+ - f_-)/2 \qquad (23.33)$$

Substituting for f_{dop} in Eq. (23.28) and rearranging, we obtain

$$dR/dt = c(f_+ - f_-)/4f_o \qquad (23.34)$$
$$= \lambda_o(f_+ - f_-)/4 \qquad (23.35)$$

FMCW Doppler radar is used to determine the range and velocity of moving targets.

23.11 CW DOPPLER RADAR

In a CW Doppler radar system, the Doppler shift is utilized to detect the velocity and range of a moving target. When the moving target is detected by a continuous wave radar signal, the received echo signal contains the Doppler frequency shift. Figure 23.10 shows the block diagram of a CW Doppler radar system. It consists of a single antenna for transmission and reception. A circulator is used to separate transmit and receive signals. Sufficient leakage signal is generally present from transmit signal, A Doppler mixer produces the output signal at the Doppler frequency by mixing the received signal with the leaked signal.

23.11.1 Applications of CW Doppler Radar

The Doppler frequency shift is utilized to design low cost CW Doppler radar. This is used as:

(i) Intruder alarms
(ii) Speed detectors
(iii) Traffic signal control

23.12 NUMERICAL EXAMPLES

Example 23.1 A radar system with the common antenna gain of 35 dB operates at 4 GHz. The receiver noise bandwidth is 1 kHz. The noise factor is 5 dB. The transmitted power is 1 kW. The path loss is 10 dB. If the echoing area of the target is 100 sq m., determine the range for unity S/N ratio.

Solution: Given: G = 35 dB, f = 4000 MHz, B_n = 1000 Hz, P_T = 1000 W, F = 5 dB, L_A = 10 dB, σ = 100 sq. m.

Wavelength

$$\lambda_o = c/f = 3 \times 10^8/4 \times 10^9 = 0.075 \text{ m}$$

Expressing it in decilogs, we obtain

$$\lambda_o = 10 \log 0.075 = -11.25 \text{ dB}$$

The bandwidth in decilogs is given by
$$B_n = 10 \log 1000 = 30 \text{ dB}$$

The transmitted power in dB is given by
$$P_T = 10 \log 1000 = 30 \text{ dBW}$$

The echoing area in decilogs is given by
$$\sigma = 10 \log 100 = 20 \text{ dB}.$$

The S/N ratio in dB is given by
$$S/N = 10 \log 1 = 0 \text{ dB}$$

The range R_o for S/N = 0 dB is given by
$$R_o = \frac{1}{4}[P_T + 2G + 2\lambda_o + \sigma + 171 - F - B_n - L_A]$$
$$= \frac{1}{4}[30 + 2 \times 35 + 2 \times (-11.25) + 20 + 171 - 5 - 30 - 10]$$
$$= 55.88 \text{ dB} = 387.3 \text{ km}$$

Example 23.2 A radar system operates at 3 GHz with a common antenna gain of 32 dB. The receiver bandwidth is 1 kHz. The noise factor is 5 dB. The transmitted power is 1 kW. If the echoing area of the target is 100 sq m., determine the range for S/N ratio of 10.

Solution: Given: $G = 32$ dB; $f = 3000$ MHz; $B_n = 1000$ Hz; $P_T = 1000$ W; $F = 5$ dB; $\sigma = 100$ sq.m; $L_A = 0$

Wavelength
$$\lambda_o = c/f = 3 \times 10^8 / 3 \times 10^9 = 0.1 \text{ m}$$

Expressing it in decilogs, we obtain
$$\lambda_o = 10 \log 0.1 = -10 \text{ dB}$$

The bandwidth in decilogs is given by
$$B_n = 10 \log 1000 = 30 \text{ dB}$$

The transmitted power in dB is given by
$$P_T = 10 \log 1000 = 30 \text{ dBW}$$

The echoing area in decilogs is given by
$$\sigma = 10 \log 100 = 20 \text{ dB}.$$

The S/N ratio in dB is given by
$$S/N = 10 \log 10 = 10 \text{dB}$$

The range for S/N ratio of 10 dB is given by
$$R_{max} = \frac{1}{4}[P_T + 2G + 2\lambda_o + \sigma + 171 - F - B_n - L_A - S/N]$$
$$= \frac{1}{4}[30 + 2 \times 32 + 2 \times (-10) + 20 + 171 - 5 - 30 - 0 - 10]$$
$$= 55 \text{dB} = 316.2 \text{ km}$$

Example 23.3 For Problem in 23.1, determine S/N ratio for a range of 90 km.

Solution: Given: $R = 90$ km $= 10 \log 90 \times 10^3$ $= 49.54$ decilogs, $R_o = 55.88$
$$S/N = 4(R_o - R) = 4(55.88 - 49.54)$$
$$= 25.36 \text{ dB}$$

Example 23.4 A 1 kW radar operating at 5 GHZ uses a common antenna with a gain of 35 dB. The receiver bandwidth is 1 kHz. The noise factor is 5 dB. If the echoing area of the target at 10 nautical miles is 10 sq m., determine the minimum S/N ratio.

Solution: Given: $G = 35$ dB, $f = 5000$ MHz, $B_n = 1000$ Hz, $P_T = 1000$ W, $F = 5$ dB, $L_A = 0$, $\sigma = 10$ sq.m, $R = 10$ n-miles

Wavelength
$$\lambda_o = c/f = 3 \times 10^8 / 5 \times 10^9 = 0.06 \text{ m}$$

Expressing λ_o in decilogs, we obtain
$$\lambda_o = 10 \log 0.06 = -12.2 \text{ dB}$$

The bandwidth in decilogs is given by
$$B_n = 10 \log 1000 = 30 \text{ dB}$$

The transmitted power in dB is given by
$$P_T = 10 \log 1000 = 30 \text{ dBW}$$

The echoing area in decilogs is given by
$$\sigma = 10 \log 10 = 2 \text{ dB}.$$
$$R = 10 \text{ n-miles} = 18520 \text{ m}$$
$$= 10 \log 18520 = 42.68$$
$$S/N = P_T + 2G + 2\lambda_o + \sigma + 171 - 4R - F - B_n - L_A$$
$$= 30 + 2 \times 35 + 2 \times (-12.2) + 10 + 171 - 4 \times (42.68) - 5 - 30 - 0$$
$$= 50.88 \text{ dB}$$

Example 23.5 For Example in 23.1, determine the range in nautical miles.

Solution: Given $R_o = 387.3$ km

R_o in nautical miles is given bi
$$R_o = R_o(\text{km}) \times 1000/1852$$
$$= 387.3 \times 1000/1852$$
$$= 209.13 \text{ n-miles}$$

Example 23.6 A 250 kW radar is operating at 10 cm wavelength. The common antenna gain is 2000. The target echoing area is 12.5 sq.m. The receiver noise bandwidth is 1 MHz The noise factor is 14 dB for unity S/N ratio. Find the range.

Solution: Given: G = 2000; l_o = 10 cm; B_n = 1 MHz; P_T = 250 kW; F = 14 dB; L_A = 0 dB; σ = 12.5 sq.m.

The antenna gain in dB is given by
$$G = 10 \log 2000 = 33 \text{ dB}$$

The bandwidth in decilogs is given by
$$B_n = 10 \log 10^6 = 60 \text{ dB}$$

Expressing λ_o in decilogs, we obtain
$$\lambda_o = 10 \log 0.1 = -10 \text{ dB}$$

The transmitted power in dB is given by
$$P_T = 10 \log 250 \times 10^3 = 53.98 \text{ dBW}$$

The echoing area in decilogs is given by
$$\sigma = 10 \log 12.5 = 10.97 \text{ dB}.$$

The S/N ratio in dB is given by
$$S/N = 10 \log 1 = 0 \text{ dB}$$

The range R_o for S/N = 0 dB is given by
$$R_o = \frac{1}{4}[P_T + 2G + 2\lambda_o + \sigma + 171 - F - B_n - L_A]$$
$$= \frac{1}{4}[53.98 + 2 \times 33 + 2 \times (-10) + 10.97 + 171 - 14 - 60 - 0]$$
$$= \textbf{51.99 dB} = \textbf{158.12 km}$$

Example 23.7: A radar system is operating with a pulse repetition frequency (prf) of 1kHz, pulse width of 10 μs and peak power of 1.5 kW. Determine (a) the maximum unambiguous range, (b) the minimum separation between targets that might be resolved, (c) the average power transmitted and (d) the power in the carrier component only.

Solution: Given: prf = 1000 Hz; t = 10 μs; P = 1500 W

(a) $R_{max} = cT_r/2 = 3 \times 10^8 \times 10^{-3}/2$
$$= \textbf{150 km}$$

(b) $R_{min} = ct/2 = 3 \times 10^8 \times 10 \times 10^{-6}/2$
$$= \textbf{1.5 km}$$

(c) The duty factor is given by
$$\tau/T_r = f_r\tau = 10^3 \times 10 \times 10^{-6}$$
$$= 0.01$$
$$P_{av} = P\tau/T_r = 1500 \times 0.01 = \textbf{15 W}$$

(d) The power in the carrier component is given by
$$P_o = P_{av} = P\tau/T_r = 15 \times 0.01$$
$$= \textbf{0.15 W}$$

Example 23.8: In an FMCW radar employing triangular modulation, the rate of change of frequency is 1.5 GHz and the echo produces a beat frequency of 10 kHz. Find the target range.

Solution: Given: a = 1.5 × 10⁹; f_d = 10⁴Hz

The target range R is given by
$$R = cf_d/2a$$
$$= 3 \times 10^8 \times 10^4/2 \times 1.5 \times 10^9$$
$$= \textbf{1.0 km}$$

Example 23.9 An FMCW radar with triangular modulation is operating at a carrier frequency of 6 GHz. The slope is 1 GHz. The beat frequency is 5 kHz over the negative slope and 4.8 kHz over the positive slope. Find (a) the target range, (b) range rate and (c) the direction of the moving target.

Solution: Given: f_o = 6 GHz; f_- = 5000; f_+ = 4800; a = 10⁹

(a) The target range is given by
$$R = c (f_+ + f_-)/4a$$
$$= 3 \times 10^8 \times (4800 + 5000)/4 \times 10^9$$
$$= \textbf{735 m}$$

(b) The range rate is given by
$$dR/dt = c (f_+ - f_-)/4f_o$$
$$= 3 \times 10^8 \times (4800 - 5000)/4 \times 6 \times 10^9$$
$$= \textbf{-2.5 m/s}$$

(c) The beat frequency over the negative slope is greater than that over the positive slope, the target is moving towards the radar.

KEY POINTS

- Radar is the acronym for **ra**dio **d**etection **a**nd **r**ange.
- Radar is essentially an echo-sounding system. Radar transmitter sends pulses of high power electromagnetic energy but of very short duration.
- Objects such as aircrafts, ships, mountains and buildings reflect some of EM energy back to the transmitter.
- The time delay of the returned echo is a measure of the distance from the reflecting objects.
- Directional transmitting and receiving antennas are used to obtain the direction of the reflecting object.
- The radar is classified into primary and secondary radar.
- In primary radar, a microwave signal is transmitted from the radar station and is reflected by the object to be detected. The reflected signal is picked up at the radar station using the same antenna.
- Secondary radar transmits a signal towards the target and receives a coded signal for identification.
- Microwaves are used for radar because very compact antennas can be designed and high gain and highly directional antennas can be used
- A basic radar system consists of a transmitting section, a receiving section, a duplexer and an antenna.
- The radar cross-section σ of a target is defined as the ratio of power radiated from the target to the incident power density on the target
- Assuming that all other quantities except σ and **R** are constant, the received power is proportional to the radar cross-section.
- FMCW radars use continuous waves that are frequency modulated.
- When either the source of radiation or the target is in motion, there is an apparent shift in the received frequency. This is called Doppler effect.
- The Doppler effect is utilized to determine whether the target is approaching or receding from the radar.
- In a CW Doppler radar system, the Doppler shift is utilized to detect the velocity and range of a moving target.
- The pulsed radar is used to determine the range and velocity of targets,

- The advantages of FWCW radar are: (i) It operates with continuous power, (ii) The power level is relatively low, (iii) Its minimum range is not limited and (iv) The size of antenna is small.
- The applications of FMCW radar are: (i)It is mainly used for short-range measurement, (ii) It is used in measurement of vehicle speeds and closing or separating distances, (iii)In conjunction with Doppler effect, it is used to obtain range and velocity (range rate) of moving targets, (iv) It is used as an altimeter and (v) It is used an automotive warning device if the closing speed or distance is potentially dangerous.

FURTHER READING

1. Skolnok MI (1981). *Introduction to Radar Systems*, MGH, NY.
2. Skolnik MI (Ed.) (1978). *Radar Handbook*, MGH, NY.
3. Barton DK (1964). *Radar System Analysis*, Artech., NJ.
4. Kennedy G and Davis B (1999). *Electronic Communication Systems*, TMH, New Delhi.
5. Wheeler GJ (1967). *Radar Fundamentals*, PH, NY.

REVIEW QUESTIONS

23.1 Define the term radar.

23.2 Distinguish between primary and secondary radars.

23.3 Mention the application of primary and secondary radars.

23.4 What are the reasons for using microwave in radar systems?

23.5 Define the range of a radar.

23.6 By what factor, the power should be increased if the range has to be doubled?

23.7 What is the need for a duplexer?

23.8 What are the two types of duplexers used?

23.9 Why unmodulated sinusoidal signal cannot be used in radars?

23.10 Mention the disadvantages of pulsed radar.

23.11 Define the duty factor.

23.12 What is Doppler effect?

23.13 How do you determine whether the target is moving towards or away from the radar transmitter?

23.14 What are the advantages of FMCW radar?

23.15 What are the applications of FMCW radar?

23.16 What are the applications of CW Doppler radar?

23.17 What are the applications of FMCW Doppler radar?

DESCRIPTIVE QUESTIONS

23.1 With a block diagram, explain a basic radar system.

23.2 Derive the radar range equation.

23.3 What is the need for a duplexer? Explain the two types briefly.

23.4 Explain the operation of a pulsed radar with necessary waveforms.

23.5 Explain how the pulse repetition time determines the maximum range of a pulsed radar system.

23.6 Distinguish between maximum power, peak power and the average power in a pulsed radar. Define the duty factor and show how it relates average power to peak power.

23.7 Explain how echo signals may be resolved in a radar using frequency modulation.

23.8 Explain with a block diagram the FMCW radar.

23.9 Explain briefly the Doppler effect and its applications.

23.10 Explain the FMCW Doppler and CW Doppler radars.

23.11 Explain briefly the applications of various types of radars.

PRACTICE PROBLEMS

23.1 A radar system with the common antenna gain of 32 dB operates at 3 GHz. The receiver noise bandwidth is 1 kHz The noise factor is 4.4 dB. The transmitted power is 1 kW. The path loss is 10 dB. If the echoing area of the target is 100 sq m., determine the range for unity S/N ratio.

(**Ans:** 55.15 dB = 327.7 km)

23.2 A radar system operates at 10 GHz with a common antenna gain of 30 dB. The receiver bandwidth is 1 kHz. The noise factor is 5 dB. . The transmitted power is 1 kW. If the echoing area of the target is 10 sq m., determine the range for S/N ratio of 10.

(**Ans:** 77.45 km)

23.3 For Problem in 23.1, determine S/N ratio for a range of 100 km.

(**Ans:** 20.8 dB)

23.4 A 1 kW radar operating at 3 GHZ uses a common antenna with a gain of 30 dB. The receiver bandwidth is 1 kHz. The noise factor is 5 dB. If the echoing area of the target at 10 nautical miles is 10 sq m., determine the minimum S/N ratio.

(**Ans:** 45.3dB)

23.5 For Problem in 23.1, determine the range in nautical miles.

(**Ans:** 176.73)

23.6 A radar system is operating with a pulse repetition frequency (prf) of 1kHz, pulse width of 10 ms and peak power of 1 kW. Determine (a) the maximum unambiguous range, (b) the minimum separation between targets that might be resolved, (c) the average power transmitted and (d) the power in the carrier component only.

(**Ans:** (a) 150 km, (b) 1.5 km, (c) 10 W, (d) 0.1 W)

23.7 In an FMCW radar employing triangular modulation, the rate of change of frequency is 1 GHz and the echo produces a beat frequency of 10 kHz. Find the target range.

(**Ans:** 1.5 km)

23.8 An FMCW radar with triangular modulation is operating at a carrier frequency of 10 GHz. The slope is 1 GHz. The beat frequency is 5 kHz over the negative slope and 4.8 kHz over the positive slope. Find (a) the target range, (b) range rate and (c) the direction of the moving target.

(**Ans:** (a) 735 m, (b) 1.5 m/s, (c) Moving towards the radar)

23.9 A radar transmits an average power of 100 W. The transmit antenna gain is 40 dB. The range is 5 km and the echoing area is 1 sq. m. Determine (a) the power density, (b) the reflected power at the target.

(**Ans:** (a) 3.18 mW/sq.m, (b) 3.18 mW)

23.10 In Problem 23.9, if the same antenna is used to receive the reflected signal and the wavelength is 3 cm, find the received power.

(**Ans:** 7.26 pW)

23.11 The specifications of a radar are: frequency is 2 GHz, transmit power is 10 kW, antenna gain is 35 dB, noise factor is 3 dB and noise bandwidth is 1 kHz path loss is 10 dB and the echoing area is 50 sq.m. Find (a) the range for 0 dB signal-to-noise ratio and (b) the signal-to-noise ratio when the range is one half of the value found in part (a).

(**Ans:** (a) 700 km, (b) 12 dB)

23.12 In a pulsed radar, the peak power is 3 kW and the duty factor is 0.01. Find the average power.

(**Ans:** 0.03 kW)

23.13 An FMCW radar employs triangular modulation. The frequency modulation slope is 3 kHz/μs. The beat frequency is 5 kHz. Find the range of the target.

(**Ans:** 250 m)

23.14 A target is receding from a CW radar transmitter at the rate of 25 m/s. The radar wavelength is 3 cm. Find the Doppler frequency.

(**Ans:** 1666.7 Hz)

REFERENCE

1. Hovanessian SA (1973). *Radar Detection and Tracking Systems*, Artech., Mass.
2. Meyer DF and Meyer HA (1973). *Radar Target Detection*, Acad., NY.
3. Ridenour LN (1978). *Radar System Engineering*, MIT Press, MI.
4. Barton DK (1974). *The Radar Equation*, Artech., Mass.
5. Nahanson FE (1969). *Radar Design Principles*, MGH, N.Y.
6. Terman FE (1955). *Electronic and Radio Engineering*, MGH, Tokyo.

■ Industrial Applications of Microwaves

Objectives

- Understand the heating effect of microwaves.
- Know the principle of operation of MW ovens, dryers and plasma generator.
- Discuss the applications of microwaves in industry and medicine.

24.1 INTRODUCTION

Microwaves are extensively used in industries such as food, chemicals, rubber, textiles, plastics, paper, pharmaceutical, ceramics, leather, cosmetics and others. Most industries utilize the heating effect of microwaves. There are two types of industrial processes. They are:

(i) *Primary industrial processes* such as cooking, baking, drying, puffing, tempering, curing, sterilizing etc.

(ii) *Secondary industrial processes* such as casting, extruding, moulding, sintering etc.

In scientific applications, they are used for moisture content and thickness measurements.

In the field of medicine, they are used for therapeutic, diagnostic and monitoring applications. The microwave frequencies that are presently used for medical applications are 915, 2450, 3300, 5800 and 10,525 MHz.

In this chapter, we shall discuss some of the industrial, scientific and medical applications of microwaves.

24.2 MICROWAVE HEATING

Microwaves are used to heat any lossy dielectric materials since they exhibit conductivity and permittivity. Microwaves penetrate into such materials and the resulting ohmic losses in the equivalent conductance are dissipated as heat. The term *equivalent conductance* is used here because the heating is due to normal conductive losses and rotational and vibrational losses in molecules.

The power density is given by

$$P_D = \sigma |E_i|^2 \quad W/m^2 \qquad (24.1)$$

where

σ is the equivalent conductance in S/m,

E_i is the internal electric field in V/m.

The conductivity is dependent of frequency. Hence, a more useful parameter that is independent of frequency, known as *loss tangent* is used. It is defined as

$$\tan \delta = \sigma / \omega \varepsilon_r' \varepsilon_o \qquad (24.2)$$

where

ω is the angular frequency in rad/s,

ε_r' is the relative permittivity of the dielectric (dielectric constant),

ε_o is free space permittivity and is equal to 8.854 pF/m.

Substituting for σ in Eq. (24.1) we obtain

$$P_D = \omega \varepsilon_r' \varepsilon_o \tan \delta |E_i|^2 \quad W/m^2 \quad (24.3)$$

The internal field E_i need not necessarily be uniform. It may produce *"hot spots"* due to focusing action of high dielectric constant materials and the shape of the cavities formed inside the materials.

The equivalent conductance results in complex permittivity or dielectric constant and is expressed as

$$\varepsilon_r = \varepsilon_r' - j\varepsilon_r'' \quad (24.4)$$

Here ε_r is the relative permittivity and ε_r'' is the loss factor. The loss factor is given by

$$\varepsilon_r'' = \sigma / \omega \varepsilon_o \quad (24.5)$$

The loss tangent can now be expressed as

$$\tan \delta = \varepsilon_r'' / \varepsilon_r' \quad (24.6)$$

The power density is proportional to the frequency if the loss tangent is constant. This is the reason for using microwave frequencies for heating. However, the limitation is that higher frequency microwave sources are not presently available. For domestic micro-

wave ovens, the cavity magnetrons are generally used as microwave source. The standard power ratings for domestic microwave ovens are 600 W and 1000 W.

24.2.1 Depth of Penetration

Microwaves penetrate lossy materials. The depth of penetration or the *skin depth* is defined as the depth at which the internal electric fields reduce by a factor of $1/e$. This depth is given by

$$D = \frac{0.225\lambda}{\sqrt{\varepsilon_r'(\sqrt{1 + \tan^2 \delta} - 1)}} \quad (24.7)$$

The greater penetration depth can be obtained with longer wavelengths or at lower frequencies but this is offset by the reduction in electric field at lower frequencies.

24.3 DOMESTIC MICROWAVE OVENS

Figure 24.1 shows the basic constructional features of a domestic microwave oven. It is a metallic cylinder or cavity that is excited by magnetron oscillator. The microwave frequency chosen for this purpose is 2450 MHz so as to achieve a desired balance between the degree of heat generated within the food and the depth of penetration of

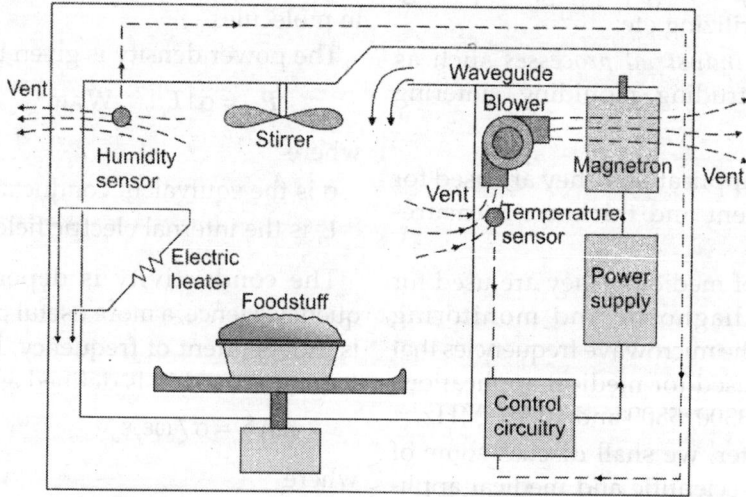

Fig. 24.1: Basic constructional features of a microwave oven

microwave energy. The microwave energy is generated by cavity magnetron oscillator and is launched into the oven cavity through the waveguide aperture as shown in Fig. 24.1. A rotating metallic blade is used as the stirrer and it reflects the microwave energy and produces a multimode field in the oven cavity. This ensures uniform heating throughout the cavity. The stirrer may be driven by convection and the food material be rotated on a turntable to ensure uniform cooking. For environmental protection, a plastic ceiling shield is placed between the stirrer chamber and oven chamber.

Microwaves cook the food material from inside to the outside. This leaves the outside appearing uncooked. Hence, an electric heater is used to brown the food to give the conventional cooked appearance on the outside. Since microwaves penetrate up to a depth of about 3 to 4 cm, large pieces are cooked by the heat conduction up to the center of the food material. The cooking time using microwaves is less and the process is even. Therefore, the food retains its natural flavour and its nutritional value.

Because of short cooking time required using microwaves, it is essential to accurately control the cooking time and temperature. A microprocessor based controller unit is used to control them. The temperature is sensed from the exhaust air from the oven using a thermistor. This, in turn, controls the voltage to a comparator in the control unit. The comparator reference voltage is set proportional to initial exhaust temperature so that the circuit measures the change in temperature. The controller has a built-in compensator for variations in room temperature, differences in food quantity and initial food temperature as well as changes in initial temperature due to quick and repeated use.

24.3.1 Design of MW Ovens

The microwave ovens are designed such that the oven door is a secure seal against leakage

of microwave energy beyond the maximum permissible level as prescribed by international regulations. The direct mechanical contact between the door and oven chamber is not sufficient enough to keep the microwave leakage below the maximum permissible level. Special methods are used for this purpose. A commonly used method is to include a microwave choke in series with the door-to-oven gap as shown in Fig. 24.2. A flange L of quarter-wave length is incorporated in the door so as to form a quarter-wave shorted section. This presents an open circuit at the gap G. The high impedance in series with leakage gap effectively isolates this from the interior of the oven. Further, the choke is filled with special ferrite materials that readily absorbs microwaves and also prevents the entry of foreign matter. The quarter-wave section must be cut accordingly. The oven door is provided with a safety lock that switches off the microwaves automatically once the door is opened.

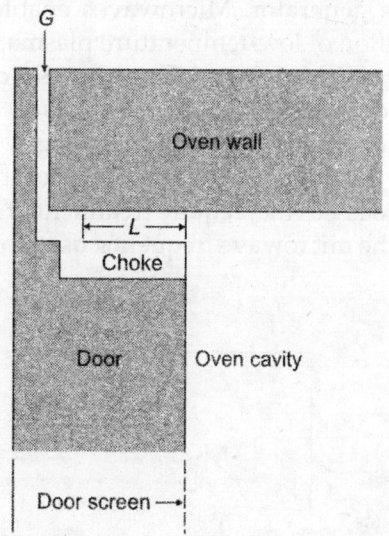

Fig. 24.2: Secure microwave oven door

24.4 INDUSTRIAL MICROWAVE DRYERS

Generally, industrial systems using microwaves must be custom made for specific applications. Microwave drying is gaining acceptance in processing industries. Effective use of microwave energy provides faster drying at lower temperatures. The dryer is operated at atmospheric pressure or under vacuum where evaporation at lower temperatures is required. It consists of a microwave source, wave-guide ducting, microwave traps and a conveyer belt. The material to be dried is fed into the tunnel-oven through the microwave field by conveyor belt. Wave-guide ducting distributes the microwave energy throughout the oven. The microwave traps are plastic pipes with water flowing through them. They prevent the radiation of microwave energy from the end gaps of the conveyer system. The microwave source is a high power magnetron that can deliver up to 30 kW at 915 MHz. It is capable of evaporating 35 kg of water in an hour.

24.5 INDUSTRIAL PLASMA GENERATORS

Another application of microwaves in industries is as a large volume microwave plasma generator. Microwaves enable the generation of low-temperature plasma. This system is used for plasma deposition of polymer coatings on various surfaces. The plasma can be of any desired length. This makes the method very attractive for industrial processes that require treatment of large area. The microwave frequency used for this purpose is 2450 MHz. The power can be varied from zero to 2.5 kW.

24.6 MEASUREMENT OF MOISTURE CONTENT

Measurement of moisture content using microwaves find extensive applications such as determination of moisture content in food, fabrics, paper, grains and seeds. It is also known as *microwave aquametry*. The underlying principle is that the presence of moisture greatly changes the complex permittivity of a material. The complex permittivity controls the attenuation and phase coefficients (propagation coefficient). It also controls the wave impedance and hence, the voltage reflection coefficient at the air-moisture interfaces. The instrumentation system measures the attenuation and phase shift due to passage of the microwaves through the material, known as *transmission-type* measurement, or the complex reflection coefficient, known as *reflection-type* measurements. Figure 24.3 shows the block diagram for transmission-type measurement. In this method, both attenuation A and phase shift ϕ are measured. The relative moisture content m_w is then given by

$$m_w = (Aa_4 - \phi a_2)/[\phi(a_1 - a_2) - A(a_3 - a_4)] \quad (24.8)$$

Here the a's are constants of calibration.

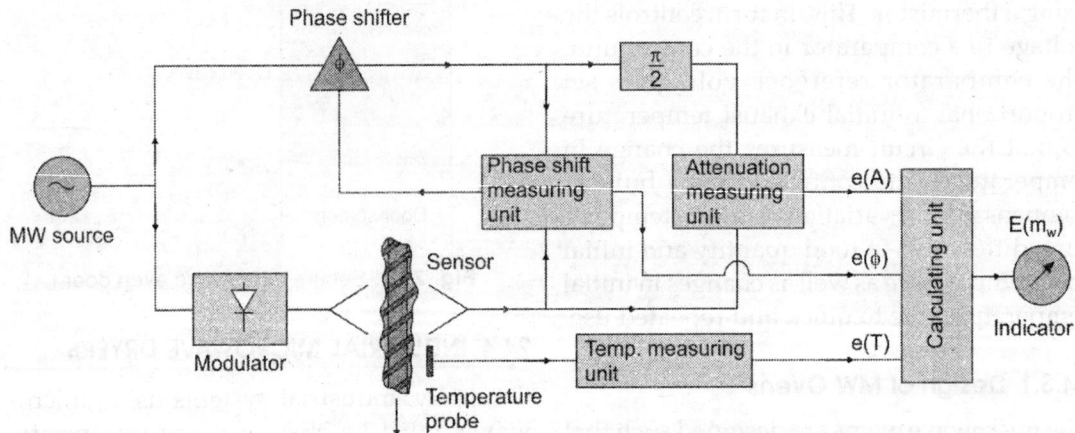

Fig. 24.3: Measurement of moisture content

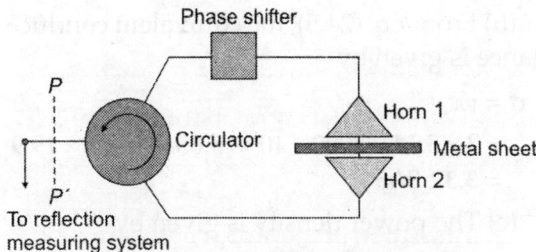

Fig. 24.4: Measurement of thickness

24.7 MEASUREMENT OF THICKNESS

Microwaves are also used to measure the thickness of sheet metals in rolling mills. It is determined by measuring the complex reflection coefficient or the attenuation and phase shift at microwave frequencies. Figure 24.4 shows the thickness measurement system by reflection-type measurements. The sheet metal in the rolling process is passed between two horn antennas placed face to face as shown in figure. The circulator, the connecting wave-guides, phase-shifter and the horn antennas form a resonant cavity. Its resonant frequency is adjusted to that of the microwave source by means of the phase-shifter. For desired thickness of the metal sheet, the reflection coefficient at plane *PP'* is adjusted to be as small as possible. Any change in the thickness of the sheet metal will cause changes in the reflection coefficient. This can be detected and calibrated with known thickness of the metal.

24.8 MICROWAVE APPLICATIONS IN MEDICINE

Applications of microwaves in medicine can be broadly classified as:

(i) Therapeutic applications
(ii) Diagnostic applications
(iii) Monitoring applications

24.8.1 Therapeutic Applications

In the therapeutic applications, the heating effect of microwaves is utilized. Since microwaves can penetrate the fat layers of the body and reach the bones and areas inside the muscles, localized heating can be achieved. The two therapeutic applicators are *diathermy* and *hyperthermia*. In diathermy, the heating effect is used to relieve pain and promote healing of various inflammatory diseases and ailments. In hyperthermia, the heat treatment assists in destroying cancerous cells in conjunction with radioactive and chemotherapy.

24.8.2 Diagnostic Applications

The human body produces radiation over a wide frequency spectrum including microwaves. The radiation intensity is proportional to the temperature of the emitting region. Diseased tissues and malignant tumors have higher temperatures than their surroundings and hence, a sensitive micro-wave receiver can be used to detect the difference in radiation levels for diagnostic purposes.

24.8.3 Monitoring Applications

Movement of heart and arterial valves can be monitored by means of Doppler shift frequency, a highly specialized application of the Doppler radar. Changes in reflection coefficient can be used to monitor the conditions of the lung. The complex permittivity changes due to the accumulation of fluids in the lung, known as *pulmonary edema*. This, in turn, changes the reflection coefficient of the tissue compared to healthy tissue. For the edematous condition, the reflection coefficient amplitude increases and the phase angle decreases compared to normal lung conditions.

24.8.4 Applicators

Microwave energy is launched into a patient using special devices known as *applicators*. All applicators must meet the following operational criteria:

(i) They must be safe for both patient and the operator
(ii) They should not produce discomft to the patient

(iii) They must provide good matching between microwave source and region of application

(iv) They should provide required focusing of microwave energy

24.8.5 Advantages

Microwaves are extensively used for medical applications because of the following advantages:

(i) It is less harmful compared to radioactive or X-ray exposure.

(ii) A better contrast is achieved in the subcutaneous tissues.

(iii) Improved focusing of power is obtained

(iv) It is possible to have selective heating in tissues

(v) The human body radiates microwave energy.

(vi) The radiation intensity is proportional to the temperature of the emitting region.

24.9 NUMERICAL EXAMPLES

Example 24.1 The complex relative permittivity of a dielectric is $25 - j15$. Determine the loss tangent.

Solution: Given: $\varepsilon_r = \varepsilon_r' - j\varepsilon_r'' = 25 - j15$

Loss tangent is given by

$\tan\delta = j\varepsilon_r''/\varepsilon_r' = 15/25 = \mathbf{0.6}$

Example 24.2 The complex relative permittivity of hemoglobin at a frequency of 3000 MHz is $59.9 - j19.9$. Calculate (a) the loss tangent, (b) the equivalent conductivity and (c) the power density for an internal field of 90 mV/m.

Solution: Given: $\varepsilon_r = \varepsilon_r' - j\varepsilon_r'' = 59.9 - j19.9$, $f = 3000$ MHz, $E_e = 90$ mV/m.

(a) The loss tangent is given by

$\tan\delta = j\varepsilon_r''/\varepsilon_r'$

$= 19.9/59.9 = \mathbf{0.3322}$

(b) From Eq. (24.5), the equivalent conductance is given by

$\sigma = \omega\varepsilon_0\varepsilon_r''$

$= 2 \times 3.14 \times 3000 \times 10^6 \times 8.854 \times 10^{-12} \times 19.9$

$= \mathbf{3.32\ S/m}$

(c) The power density is given by

$P_D = \sigma|E_r|^2$ W/m^2

$= 3.32 \times (90 \times 10^{-3})^2$

$= \mathbf{26.9\ mW/m^2}$

Example 24.3 Calculate the depth of penetration for the material in Example 24.2.

Solution: Given: $\varepsilon_r' - j\varepsilon_r'' = 59.9 - j19.9$; $f = 3000$ MHz; $\tan\delta = 0.3322$

The wavelength is given by

$\lambda = c/f$

$= 3 \times 10^8/3 \times 10^9$

$= 10$ cm

The depth of penetration is given by

$$D = \frac{0.225\lambda}{\sqrt{\varepsilon_r'\left(\sqrt{1+\tan^2\delta}-1\right)}}$$

$$= \frac{(0.225 \times 10)}{\sqrt{59.9(\sqrt{1+0.3322^2}-1)}}$$

$= \mathbf{1.25\ cm}$

KEY POINTS

- Microwaves are extensively used in industries such as food, chemicals, rubber, textiles, plastics, paper, pharmaceutical, ceramics, leather, cosmetics and others.

- Most industries utilize the heating effect of microwaves for cooking, baking, drying, puffing, tempering, curing, sterilizing and secondary industrial processes such as casting, extruding, moulding, sintering etc.

- In scientific applications, they are used for moisture content and thickness measurements.

- In the field of medicine, they are used for therapeutic, diagnostic and monitoring applications.

- The microwave frequencies that are presently used are 915, 2450, 3300, 5800 and 10,525 MHz.

- Microwaves can heat any lossy dielectric materials since they exhibit conductivity and permittivity. Microwaves penetrate into such materials and the resulting ohmic losses in the equivalent conductance are dissipated as heat. The term equivalent conductance is used here because the heating is due to normal conductive losses and rotational and vibrational losses in molecules.

- Microwaves penetrate lossy materials. The depth of penetration or the skin depth is defined as the depth at which the internal electric fields reduce by a factor of $1/e$.

- A domestic microwave oven operates at 2450 MHz and the power output is 600 to 900 W.

- The industrial microwave dryers can deliver up to 30 kW at 915 MHz. It is capable of evaporating 35 kg of water in an hour.

- Measurement of moisture content using microwaves find extensive applications such as determination of moisture content in food, fabrics, paper, grains and seeds. The underlying principle is that the presence of moisture greatly changes the complex permittivity of a material.

- Microwaves are also used to measure the thickness of sheet metals in rolling mills.

- Microwaves are used in medicine for therapeutic, diagnostic and monitoring applications.

FURTHER READING

1. Barber H (1981). Microwaves for cooking and heating, *Electronics and Power*, vol. 27, No.5, p 401–402.

2. Special issue on the industrial, scientific and medical applications of microwaves, (1974) Proc. IEEE. Vol. 62, No. 1, Jan.

3. Brown WC (1970). High power microwave generators of the cross field type, *J. Microwave Power*, vol.5, No.4, pp 245–260.

4. Bucksbaun AM (1981). Microwave oven door seal characteristics, *J. Microwave Power*, Vol. 16, No.1.

REVIEW QUESTIONS

24.1 Mention some of the industries using microwaves for industrial processes.

24.2 Mention four primary and four secondary industrial processes.

24.3 Mention two scientific applications and two medical applications.

24.4 What is the principle involved in microwave heating?

24.5 What are the microwave frequencies assigned for industrial applications?

24.6 Define loss tangent and write down the expression.

24.7 Define complex relative permittivity and write down the expression.

24.8 Define skin depth and write down the expression.

24.9 What is the use of microwave oven? What are the frequencies and the power?

24.10 What is a microwave industrial dryer? What are the frequency and the power?

24.11 What is the use of microwave plasma generator?

24.12 What are the applications of microwave aquametry? Mention the principle involved.

24.13 Mention the principle involved in the thickness measurement.

24.14 Mention the MW applications in medicine.

DESCRIPTIVE QUESTIONS

24.1 Describe the main features of a domestic microwave oven.

24.2 Explain the importance of having a tight microwave seal on microwave oven door. Describe one method of seal construction.

24.3 Describe the main features of an industrial microwave dryer.

24.4 Define microwave aquametry. Describe one area of application.

24.5 Explain the applications of microwaves in medicine.

PRACTICE PROBLEMS

24.1 The complex relative permittivity of a dielectric is $50 - j15$. Determine the loss tangent.

(**Ans:** 0.3)

24.2 The complex relative permittivity of hemoglobin at a frequency of 2450 MHz is $33 - j18$. Calculate (a) the loss tangent, (b) the equivalent conductivity and (c) the power density for an internal field of 100 mV/m.

(**Ans:** (a) 0.5·'54, (b) 2.45 S/m, (c) 24.5 mW/m^2)

24.3 Calculate the depth of penetration for the material in Problem 24.2

(**Ans:** 1.5 cm)

REFERENCE

1. Freedman G (1973). The future of microwave heating equipment in the food industries, *J. Microwave Power*, Vol. 7, No. 4.

2. Gupta C (1981). *Microwaves in Medicine, Electronics Power*, Vol. 27, No. 5.

3. Kraszewski A (1980). Microwave Aquametry— A review, *J. Microwave Power*, Vol. 15.

4. Stuchly S et al (1969). Microwaves for continuous control of industrial process, *Microwave Jour.* Vol. 12, No. 9. Aug.

Monolithic Microwave Integrated Circuits

Objectives

- Classify the integrated circuits and scale of integration.
- Know the advantages and disadvantages of ICs.
- Understand the properties of substrate, dielectric and resistive materials.
- Define the different types of MICs.
- Explain the fabrication of MMICs.
- Compare MMICs with HMICs.

25.1 INTRODUCTION

An integrated circuit (IC) is an electronic circuit in which many active and passive devices such as transistors, diodes, resistors and capacitors are fabricated on a single small silicon chip of dimension 50 mils × 50 mils. The fabrication method employed is successive diffusion or ion implantation process. The active devices are silicon planar chips. The passive components are either thin film or thick film elements. In thin film technology, a thin film of conducting (resistor) or non-conducting (capacitor) material is deposited by vacuum deposition on a passive insulated substrate such as glass, ceramic or silicon dioxide. Thick films are of several thousand angstroms thick and are used exclusively to form resistors by silk-screening technique. In this chapter, we shall discuss, in detail, the basic materials and processes necessary for the fabrication of monolithic microwave integrated circuits.

25.2 CLASSIFICATION

Electronic circuits are classified as *discrete circuit, integrated circuit* and *monolithic microwave integrated* circuit.

(i) **Discrete Circuits:** In the discrete circuits, the electronic components are manufactured separately and then connected together by wires.

(ii) **Integrated Circuits:** Integrated circuit consists of both active and passive components and their interconnections fabricated on a single silicon chip of dimension 50 mils × 50 mils. Since a single chip is used, it is known as *monolithic* meaning *single stone*. A monolithic integrated circuit is fabricated on a single crystal. Such circuits are manufactured using the process of *epitaxial growth, masked impurity diffusion, oxidation growth* and *oxide etching*.

(iii) **Monolithic Microwave Integrated Circuits (MMIC):** The monolithic microwave integrated circuits (MMIC) differ from conventional integrated circuits in that the packing density is low. A monolithic microwave integrated circuit with its elements formed on an insulating substrate is known as a *film integrated circuit*. A monolithic microwave integrated circuit that consists of a combination of two or more integrated circuit types such as integrated circuit and discrete components or monolithic and film is known as *hybrid integrated circuit*.

25.3 SCALE OF INTEGRATION

The number of circuits or components that are fabricated on a standard size of silicon chip is known as *scale of integration*. The types of integration are *SSI, MSI, LSI, VLSI* and *ULSI*.

(i) **Small Scale Integration (SSI):** If the number of components contained in a single chip is less than 100, then it is known as *small-scale integration*.

(ii) **Medium Scale Integration (MSI):** If the number of components contained in a single chip is between 100 and 1000, then it is known as *medium scale integration*.

(iii) **Large Scale Integration (LSI):** If the number of circuit components in a single chip is between 1000 and 100,000, then it is known as *large scale integration*.

(iv) **Very Large Scale Integration (VLSI):** If the number of components contained in a single chip is between 10^5 and 10^6, then it is known as *very large scale integration*.

(v) **Ultra Large-Scale Integration (ULSI):** If the number of components contained in a single chip is greater than 1.5×10^6, then it is known as *ultra large-scale integration*.

Advantages

The advantages of monolithic microwave integrated circuits over discrete circuits are:

(a) Extremely small size and light weight
(b) Low cost
(c) Extremely high reliability
(d) Low power consumption
(e) Easy replacement
(f) Fast response.
(g) Ruggedness against shock, vibration
(h) Operability under severe temperature conditions

Disadvantages

The disadvantages of monolithic microwave integrated circuits over discrete circuits are:

(a) It cannot handle high power and withstand excessive heat
(b) It is quite delicate and is liable to be damaged
(c) The whole IC is to be replaced in the case of failure of a component.

25.4 APPLICATIONS

The monolithic microwave integrated circuits are extensively used in space and military applications because of their ruggedness against shock and severe vibrations and temperature conditions.

25.5 MATERIALS FOR MMIC FABRICATION

The basic materials necessary for the fabrication of monolithic microwave integrated circuits are generally grouped into following four categories:

(i) Substrate materials
(ii) Conductor materials
(iii) Dielectric films
(iv) Resistive films

25.5.1 Substrate Materials

The substrate materials used for the fabrication of monolithic microwave integrated circuits are *Alumina, beryllium, ferrite/garnet, GaAs, glass, sapphire* and *rutile*.

25.5.2 Conductor Materials

The conductor materials used for the fabrication of monolithic microwave integrated circuits are *aluminum, copper, gold* and *silver*.

25.5.3 Dielectric Films

The dielectric films used for the fabrication of monolithic microwave integrated circuits are Al_2O_3, SiO, SiO_2, Si_3N_4 and Ta_2O_5.

25.5.4 Resistive Films

The resistive films used for the fabrication of monolithic microwave integrated circuits are Cr, Cr-SiO, NiCr, Ta and Ti.

25.6 PROPERTIES OF SUBSTRATE MATERIALS

A substrate of monolithic microwave integrated circuits is a piece of dielectric substance on which the active and passive elements are fabricated. The ideal properties of substrate materials are:

(i) High dielectric constant as high as 9 or higher

(ii) Dielectric constant should be constant over the desired frequency and temperature range

(iii) High resistivity and dielectric strength

(iv) High thermal conductivity

(v) High purity and constant thickness

(vi) High surface smoothness

(vii) Low dissipation factor or loss tangent

25.7 SELECTION OF SUBSTRATE MATERIALS

The selection of substrate material depends upon the *expected circuit dissipation, the circuit function* and the *type of the circuit*. Table 25.1 shows the important properties of substrate materials used for monolithic microwave integrated circuits.

25.8 PROPERTIES OF CONDUCTIVE MATERIALS

The ideal properties of conductive materials are:

(i) High conductivity

(ii) Low temperature coefficient

(iii) Good adhesion to substrate

(iv) Good etchability and solderability

(v) Easily deposited or electroplated

Table 25.2 lists the properties of conductive materials. These conductive materials have excellent conductivity. They can be deposited by a number of methods. They are capable of photo-etched. They are used to form both conductor pattern and bottom ground plane. To carry 98% of the current density, the thickness of the conductor should be at least four skin depth. From Table 25.2, it is seen that good electrical conductors have poor substrate adhesion and *vice versa*. Aluminium has good conductivity and good adhesion. A good adhesion with high-conductivity can be obtained by using a very thin layer of a

Table 25.1: Substrate materials and their properties

Materials	$\tan \theta (\times 10^4)$ at 10 GHz	Relative dielectric constant ε_r	Thermal conductivity K(W/cm°C)	Applications
Alumina	2	10	0.3	Microstrip, suspended substrate
Beryllia	1	6	2.5	Compound substrate
Ferrite/garnet	2	13–16	0.03	Microstrip, coplanar, compound substrate
GaAs	16	13	0.03	High frequency, microstrip, MMIC
Glass	4	5	0.01	Lumped element
Sapphire	1	9.3–11.7	0.4	Microstrip, lumped element
Rutile	4	100	0.02	Microstrip

Table 25.2: Conductors and their properties

Material	Skin depth δ (μm) at GHz	Surface resistivity (Ω/sq $\times 10^{-7} \sqrt{f}$)	Coefficient of thermal expansion ($\alpha_t/^\circ C \times 10^6$)	Adherence	Deposition method
Ag	1.4	2.5	21	Poor	Evaporation, screening
Cu	1.5	2.6	18	Very poor	Evaporation, plating
Au	1.7	3.0	15	Very poor	Evaporation, plating
Al	1.9	3.3	26	Very poor	Evaporation
W	2.6	4.7	4.6	Good	Evaporation, sputtering, vapour phase, electron beam evaporation
Cr	2.7	4.7	9.0	Good	Evaporation
Mo	2.7	4.7	6.0	Good	Electron beam evaporation, sputtering
Ta	4.0	7.2	6.6	Very good	Electron beam evaporation, sputtering

poor conductor between the substrate and the good conductor. Typical combinations are Cr-Cu, Cr-Au and Ta-Au. An adhesion layer has a surface resistivity from 500–1000 Ω/square. The choice of conductors is determined by compatibility with other materials required in the circuit and the required process. For low losses, the conductors of the order of three to five skin depths in thickness or about 10 μm thickness are used. This can be achieved by evaporation or plating.

25.9 PROPERTIES OF DIELECTRIC MATERIALS

In monolithic microwave circuits, the dielectric materials are used for *blockers, capacitors* and *other coupling structures*. The ideal properties of the dielectric materials are:

(i) Reproducibility

(ii) Capability of withstanding high voltages

(iii) Low RF dielectric loss

(iv) Ability to undergo various processes without developing pin-holes

Table 25.3 shows the dielectrics used in microwave integrated circuits and their properties. The most commonly used dielectric materials are SiO, SiO_2 and Ta_2O_5. Thin-film SiO_2 with high-dielectric Q is obtained by growing the pyrolitic deposition of SiO_2 from silicon and then, densifying it by heat treatment. SiO_2 can also be deposited by sputtering. SiO_2 capacitors in the range of

Table 25.3: Dielectric materials and their properties

Material	Relative dielectric constant (ε_r)	Dielectric Strength (V/cm)	Q at microwave frequencies	Deposition method
SiO	6–8	4×10^3	30	Evaporation
SiO_2	4	10^7	100–1000	Deposition
Si_3N_4	7.6	10^7		Vapour phase, sputtering
	6.5	10^7		
Al_2O_3	7–10	4×10^6		Anodization, evaporation
Ta_2O_3	22–25	6×10^6	100	Anodization sputtering

0.02 to 0.05 pF/sq.mil and with quality factors in excess of 100 have been successfully fabricated with proper processing. Since thin-film SiO_2 is not very stable, it is used only in non-critical applications such as bypass capacitors. Capacitors with break-down voltages in excess of 200 V can be fabricated with film thickness of 0.5 to 1.0 μm with low probability of pin-holes or shorts.

25.10 PROPERTIES OF RESISTIVE MATERIALS

In monolithic microwave circuits, the resistive materials are used for bias circuits, terminations and attenuators. The ideal properties of good microwave resistor materials are:

(i) Good stability

(ii) Good heat dissipation capacity

(iii) Low temperature coefficient

(iv) Sheet resistivity in the range of 10 to 1000 Ω/square

Table 25.4 shows some of the thin-film resistive materials used in monolithic microwave integrated circuits and their properties. The most widely used resistive materials are evaporated nichrome and tantalum nitride. The achievable temperature coefficient depends on the conditions of thin-film formation. Thick-film resistors are utilized in circuits incorporating chip components. The thickness of thick film is of the order of 1 to 500 μm. Here, thick film refers to the process used and not to the film thickness. Thick-film technique involves silk-screening through a mask, such as printing and screening of gold or silver in a glass frit

that is applied on the ceramic and fired at 850°C. Sometimes, microwave thick-film materials are several micrometers thick.

25.11 DEVELOPMENT OF MICROWAVE INTEGRATED CIRCUITS (MMICs)

Microwave integrated circuits are fabricated in the following three forms.

(i) Monolithic form

(ii) Hybrid form

(iii) Quasi-monolithic form

In monolithic microwave integrated circuits (MMIC), active devices are grown on or in the semiconductor substrate. The passive elements are then deposited on the substrate or grown on it.

In the hybrid microwave integrated circuits (HMICs), the active devices are attached to a ceramic, glass or ferrite substrate that contains the passive circuitry.

In the quasi-monolithic microwave integrated circuits (QMMICs), the passive components are realized using integrated technology similar to that of MMICs whereas the active components are mounted individually.

25.12 MONOLITHIC MICROWAVE INTEGRATED CIRCUITS

In monolithic conventional integrated circuits, all required circuit components are simultaneously fabricated. They have been used successfully in analog and digital applications. In most cases, the same device such as BJT or MOSFETs is used for ampli-

Table 25.4: Resistive materials and their properties

Material	Resistivity (ohm/square)	Temp. Coeff. (%/°C)	Stability	Deposition method
Cr	10–1000	−0.100 to +0.100	Poor	Evaporation
CrSiO	600	−0.005 to 0.020	Fair	Evaporation, cermet
Ni–Cr	40–400	+0.002 to +0.100	Good	Evaporation
Ta	5–500	−0.010 to +0.010	Excellent	Sputtering
Ti	5–2000	−0.100 to +0.100	Fair	Evaporation

fiers, diodes, resistors and capacitors without any degradation in performance. Integrated circuits used in computers require large arrays of identical devices and hence they contain very high packing densities. In monolithic microwave integrated circuits, active devices are seldom used for passive components. In addition, very few applications in microwave integrated circuits require identical devices and hence, the packing density in microwave integrated circuits is low.

Because of processing difficulties, low yields and poor performance, monolithic fabrication technology is not suited to microwave integrated circuits. Presently, the microwave integrated circuits are almost exclusively fabricated using hybrid technology in the frequency range of 1 to 15 GHz. HMICs are fabricated on high-quality ceramic, glass or ferrite substrate. The passive components are first deposited on the substrate and then, the active devices are mounted on the substrate and connected to the passive circuit components. The active devices may be in chip form, in chip carriers or in small plastic packages. For good circuit performance, the resistivity of microwave integrated circuits should be much greater than 1000 Ω-cm.

25.13 MMIC FABRICATION METHODS

Monolithic microwave integrated circuits are fabricated using the following techniques:

1. Diffusion and ion implantation
2. Oxidation and film deposition
3. Epitaxial growth
4. Lithography
5. Etching and photo-resist
6. Deposition

25.13.1 Diffusion and Ion Implantation

The two processes used in controlling the quantities of dopants in the fabrication of semiconductor devices are diffusion and ion

implantation. The diffusion process is the process of diffusing impurities into a pure semiconductor material in order to alter its basic electronic characteristics. Ion implantation is used to dope the substrate with high-energy ion impurities. To produce a *p*- or *n*-type layer, both processes are used to dope the semiconductor substrate selectively.

In the ion implantation process, the dopant ions are implanted into the semiconductor by using a high-energy ion beam. The advantages of this method are:

(i) Precise control of the total amount of dopants
(ii) Improved reproducibility
(iii) Reduced processing temperature.

25.13.2 Oxidation and Film Deposition

The four types of thin films used to fabricate discrete and integrated circuits are:

(i) Thermal oxides
(ii) Dielectric layers
(iii) Polycrystalline silicon
(iv) Metal films

Thermal oxidation is used for silicon. It is not used for GaAs because it results in poor electrical insulation. Dielectric layers are then deposited on silicon dioxides and nitrides. They are used for insulation between conducting layers, for diffusion and ion-implantation masks for capping doped films to prevent the loss of dopants and for passivation to protect devices from impurities, moisture and scratches. Polycrystalline silicon is used as gate electrode material for multilevel metallization. Aluminium and silicides are the metal films used to form low-resistance interconnections and ohmic contacts.

25.13.3 Epitaxial Growth

The word *epitaxy* in Greek means an arrangement on. Thus, the epitaxial technology refers to the growth of semiconductor layers on a *single-crystal* semiconductor substrate. The epitaxial process offers a means of controlling precisely the doping profiles so that the device and circuit performances are optimized.

There are three types of epitaxy. They are: (i) Vapour phase epitaxy (ii) Molecular beam epitaxy (iii) Liquid phase epitaxy

(i) **Vapour Phase Epitaxy (VPE):** This is the most important technique for silicon and GaAs devices.

(ii) **Molecular Beam Epitaxy (MBE):** This process involves the reaction of one or more thermal beams of atoms or molecules with a crystalline surface under ultra-high vacuum conditions of approximately 10^{-1} torr. Molecular beam epitaxy can achieve precise control in both chemical composition and doping profiles. Single-crystal multi-layer structures with dimensions of the order of atomic layers are possible with molecular beam epitaxy.

(iii) **Liquid Phase Epitaxy (LPE):** This is the process of growing epitaxial layers by direct deposition from liquid phase on crystalline substrates. This process is particularly useful for growing GaAs and related III–V compounds. Since it has a slow growth rate, it is suited for growing epitaxial layers as thin as 0.2 µm. It is also used to grow multi-layered structures in which precise control of doping and composition are required.

25.13.4 Lithography

Lithography is the process of transferring patterns of geometric shapes on a mask onto a thin layer of radiation-sensitive material, known as *resist*, that covers the surface of a semiconductor wafer. The resist patterns are only replicas of circuit features. The four types of lithography technology are:

(i) Electron beam lithography

(ii) Ion beam lithography

(iii) Optical lithography

(iv) X-ray lithography

25.13.5 Etching and Photo-resist

In the monolithic microwave integrated circuit fabrication, selective removal of SiO_2 is required to form openings through which impurities are diffused. Figure 25.1 shows the photo-etching method used for this removal. During this process, the substrate is coated with a uniform film of a photo-sensitive emulsion such as Kodak Photo Resist (KPR). A negative of the black and white layout of the required pattern is prepared and this is known as *mask*. It is placed over the KPR. It is now exposed to ultraviolet light and the KPR under the transparent region of the mask becomes polymerized. After removing the mask, the substrate is developed in the trichloro-ethylene and the unpolymerized portion of the KPR is dissolved. The substrate is now immersed in an etching solution of hydro-fluoric acid. The acid removes SiO_2 that is not covered by KPR. These are the areas through which impurities are to be diffused. These are known as *windows*. Thick-film technique involves the printing and silk-screening through a mask of gold or silver in a glass frit that is applied on the ceramic and fired at 850°C. After firing, the multi-layer is covered with gold.

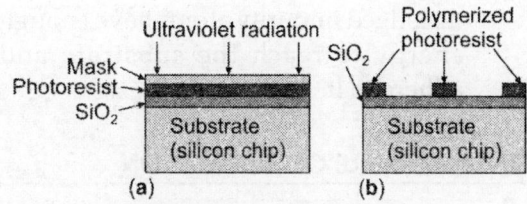

Fig. 25.1: Photo-etching process

25.13.6 Deposition

The commonly used deposition methods for fabricating monolithic microwave integrated circuits are: (i) Vacuum evaporation (ii) Electron beam evaporation (iii) DC or Cathode sputtering.

(i) **Vacuum Evaporation:** In this method, the material to be evaporated is placed in a metallic boat through which a high current is passed. The substrate with mask on it and the heated boat are located in a glass tube. A high vacuum at a pressure of 10^{-6} to 10^{-8} torr is maintained in the glass tube. The substrate is heated slightly while the heated impurities are evaporated. The evaporated impurity vapour deposits itself on the substrate to form a poly-crystalline layer on it.

(ii) **Electron Beam Evaporation:** In this method, a narrow beam of electrons is generated to scan the substrate in the boat to vapourize the impurity.

(iii) **DC or Cathode Sputtering:** The third method of vacuum deposition is the dc or cathode sputtering. A crucible containing the impurity is placed in a vacuum and is used as the cathode and the substrate as the anode of a diode. A slight trace of argon gas is introduced in the vacuum. A glow discharge of argon gas is formed when the applied voltage between the cathode and anode is sufficiently high. The positive argon ions are accelerated towards the cathode. On reaching the cathode, they dislodge the impurity atoms. The dislodged impurity atoms have enough energy to reach the substrate and adhere to it.

25.14 EXAMPLE OF FABRICATION

The photo-resist technique is used to remove the oxide layer in related areas as shown in Fig. 25.2.

The fabrication procedures include the following steps:

(i) *Deposition:* An oxide layer is deposited on the semiconductor material. Then, a photo-resist layer is deposited to cover the oxide layer on the top of the semiconductor chip.

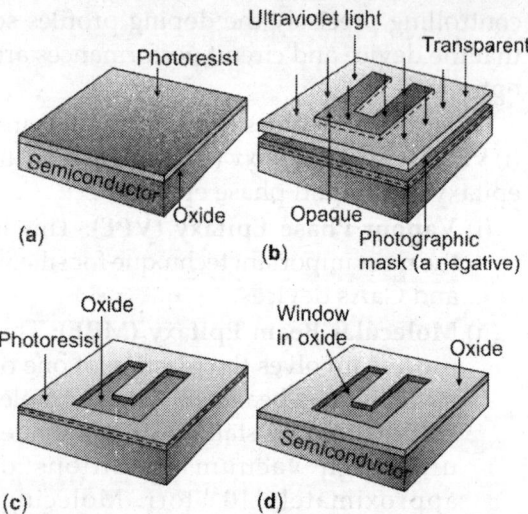

Fig. 25.2: Illustration of etching technique (a) Deposition (b) Mask (c) Chemical etching (d) Etching

(ii) *Mask:* Ultraviolet light is used to illuminate substrate through a precision photographic mask to photo-resist.

(iii) *Chemical Etching:* To remove the selected oxide region, chemical etching with hydrofluoric acid is used

(iv) *Etching:* The photo-resist is finally dissolved with trichloroethylene solvent in the oxide leaving the desired opening.

25.15 DISADVANTAGES OF MMICs

The disadvantages of MMICs are:
1. Unfavourable device-to-chip ratio.
2. Impractical circuit tuning
3. Difficulties in trouble-shooting.
4. Low yield.
5. Performance variation from wafer to wafer.
6. Performance variation within a wafer.

25.16 FABRICATION OF MOSFET

In recent years, the metal-oxide semiconductor field-effect transistors are replacing the bipolar transistors in most electronic applications. This is because of the advantages of MOSFET over the BJT. They are:

(i) Only one diffusion process is involved.

(ii) Fabrication of MOSFET is more efficient

(iii) Structure of MOSFET is simple

(iv) Low-cost

The MOSFET is the most commonly used device in very large-scale integrated circuits such as microprocessors and semiconductor memories. The basic fabrication process is described under three headings: *MOSFET formation, NMOS growth* and CMOS *development*.

25.16.1 MOSFET Formulation

The steps involved in the fabrication of MOSFETs are shown in Fig. 25.3 and discussed below.

(i) **Oxidation**: Select the *p*-type substrate and form a SiO_2 layer on it as shown in Fig. 25.3(a).

(ii) *Diffusion*: Using photo-resist technique, open two windows and diffuse an n^+-layer through them as shown in Fig. 25.3(b).

(iii) *Etching*: By photo-etching technique, remove the center oxide region as shown in Fig. 25.3(c).

(iv) **Oxidation**: Expose the entire surface to dry oxygen so that SiO_2 covers the top surface as shown in Fig. 25.3(d).

(v) *Deposition*: Deposit phosphorous glass over the surface to cover the oxide layer as shown in Fig. 25.3(e).

(vi) *Etching*: Using photo-etching technique, open two windows above the two n^+-type diffused regions as shown in Fig. 25.3(f).

(vii) *Metallization*: Carry out aluminium metallization over the entire surface of the device as shown in Fig. 25.3(g).

(viii) *Etching*: Lastly, etch away the unwanted metal and attach the metal contacts to the diffused gate, drain and source regions as shown in Fig. 25.3(h).

25.16.2 NMOS Growth

The steps involved in the fabrication of NMOS logic gate are shown in Fig. 25.4 and discussed below.

(i) *Deposition* and *Implantation*: The initial *p*-type substrate is lightly doped. Then, a SiO_2 layer is grown on the top of the substrate. On the oxide layer, a Si_3N_4 layer is deposited. An isolation mask is used to define the active areas covered by SiO_2–Si_3N_4 The isolation or field areas are then etched by plasma or reactive ion etching [Fig. 25.4(a)].

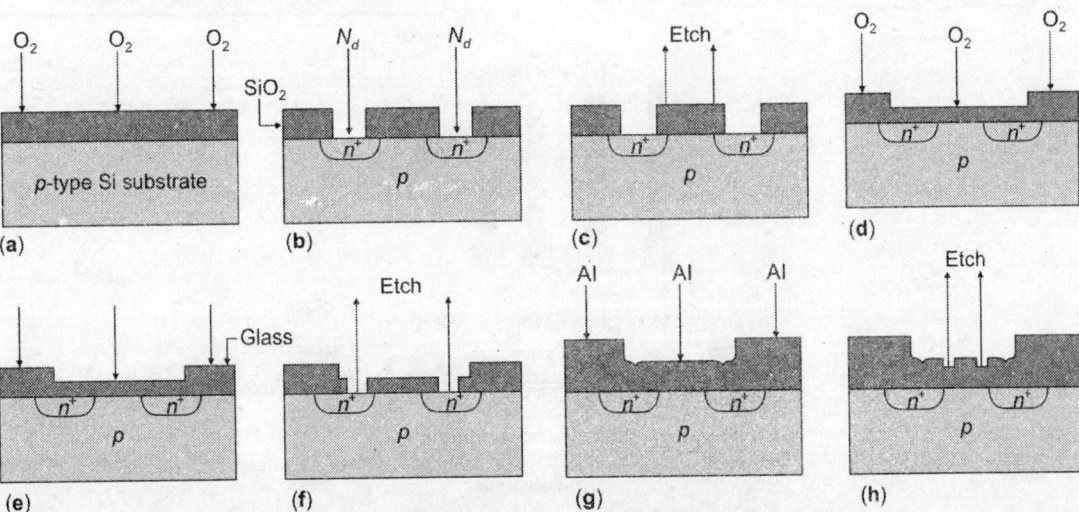

Fig. 25.3: MOSFET fabrication steps (a) Oxidation (b) *n*-type diffusion (c) Masking, etching (d) Oxidation (e) Formation of phosphorous glass (f) Matching, etching (g) Metallization (h) Matching, etching

(ii) *Implantation*: To prevent inversion under the field oxide, boron ions are implanted as the channel stop. Then, the wafer is put in an oxidation furnace to grow a thick layer of field oxide [Fig. 25.4(b)].

(iii) *Implantation (after clearing)*: After clearing the oxide layer, a thin gate oxide of about 20 nm thick is formed. Use photo-resist to mask the enhancement mode device and form the depletion mode device by an *n*-channel implant [Fig. 25.4(c)].

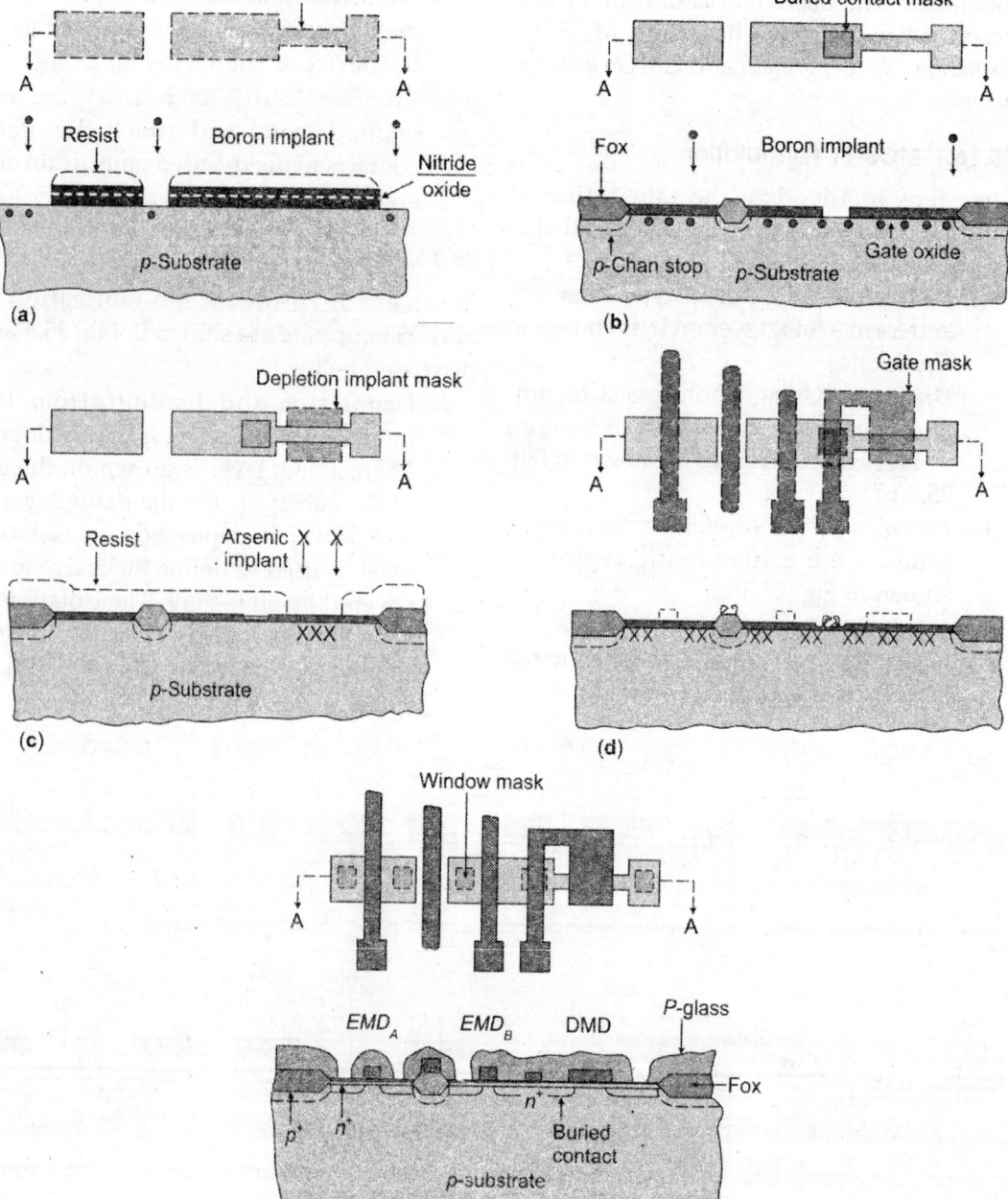

Fig. 25.4: NMOS fabrication process

(iv) **Deposition**: The polysilicon is deposited and patterned as the gates. The gates are also used as the self-aligned mask for source and drain arsenic implantation [Fig. 25.4(d)].

(v) **Metallization**: Metal films are then evaporated and etched to produce the electrode contacts [Fig. 25.4(e)].

25.16.3 CMOS Development

The steps involved in the fabrication of CMOS devices are shown in Fig. 25.5 and discussed below.

(i) **Epitaxy and Deposition**: The initial material is a lightly doped n epitaxy over a heavily doped n^+ substrate. A composite layer of SiO_2 as pad and Si_3N_4 (nitride) is defined. Silicon is exposed over the intended n-tub layer. Phosphorous is implanted at low energy as the n-tub dopant. It enters the exposed silicon region but masked from adjacent region by Si_3N_4 layer [Fig. 25.5(a)].

(ii) **Implantation**: The wafers are selectively oxidized over the n-tub regions. The nitride is stripped and the boron is implanted for the p-tub [Fig. 25.5(b)].

(iii) **Oxidation**: The boron enters the silicon through the thin oxide pad, but masked from the n-tub by the thick oxide layer there. Then, all oxides are stripped and the two tubs are driven in [Fig. 25.5(c)].

(iv) **Deposition**: n^+ poly-silicon is deposited and defined. The source and drain regions are implanted [Fig. 25.5(d)].

(v) **Implantation**: Phosphorous is implanted selectively into the n-channel source and drain regions at a higher dose so that it overcompensates the existing boron [Fig. 25.5(e)].

(vi) **Deposition and Metallization**: A phosphorous glass layer is then deposited. The windows are dry-etched in a phosphorous-glass. Then, aluminium metallization is defined using dry etching [Fig. 25.5(f)].

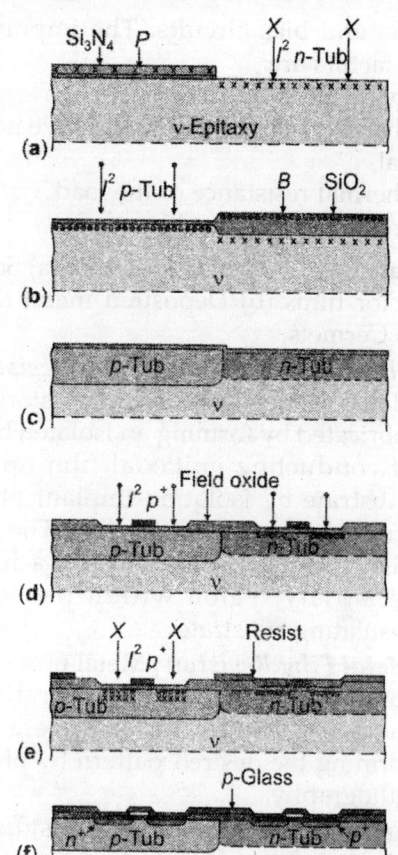

Fig. 25.5: CMOS fabrication process (a) Epitaxy and deposition (b) Implantation (c) Oxidation (d) Deposition (e) Implantation (f) Deposition and metallization

25.17 THICK-FILM FORMATION

In monolithic microwave circuits, planar resistors are utilized in thin-film resistive terminations for couplers, planar inductors for matching purposes and planar capacitors for bias bypass applications. In this section, we shall describe their fabrication methods.

25.17.1 Planar Resistor Film

The planar resistors consist of a thin resistive film deposited on an insulating substrate. The thin-film resistor materials are gold, copper, nichrome, tantalum and titanium. Their resistivity varies from 30 to 1000 Ω^2 square. These planar resistors are used for terminations for couplers, power combiners/

dividers and bias circuits. The important design factors are:

(i) Available sheet resistivity

(ii) Thermal stability of the resistive material

(iii) Thermal resistance of the load

(iv) Frequency bandwidth.

Planar resistors are classified as: (a) Semiconductor films (b) Deposited metal films and (c) Cermets.

(a) *Planar Semiconductor Film Resistors:* Planar semiconductor film resistors are fabricated by forming an isolated band of conducting epitaxial film on the substrate by isolation implant of the surrounding conducting film. They are also formed by implanting a high-resistivity region within the semi-insulating substrate.

(b) *Metal Film Resistors:* Metal film resistors are fabricated by evaporating a metal layer over the substrate and forming the desired pattern by photo-lithography.

(c) *Cermet Resistors:* Cermet resistors are formed from films consisting of a mixture of metal and dielectric. Figure 25.6 shows some configurations of the planar resistors.

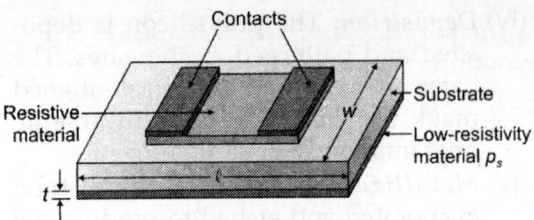

Fig. 25.7: Thin-film resistor

Figure 25.7 shows a thin-film resistor. The resistance of the planar resistor is given by

$$R = \rho_s l/wt \quad \text{ohms} \qquad (25.1)$$

where

ρ_s is the sheet resistivity of the film in ohm-meter,

l is the length of the resistive film in meters

w is the width of the resistive film in meters

t is the thickness of the resistive film in meters.

The units of l and w are chosen to have equal magnitude so that the result is a square. Hence, the unit of resistance R is in ohms per square and is independent of the dimensions of the square.

25.17.2 Planar Inductor Films

Planar inductors for monolithic microwave integrated circuits are realized in a number of configurations. Figure 25.8 shows some configurations.

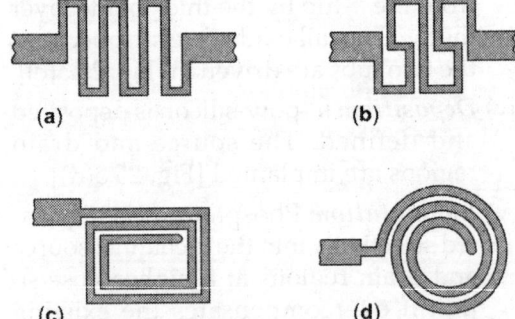

Fig. 25.8: Planar inductor configurations (a) Meander line (b) S line (c) Square spiral (d) Circular spiral

Typical inductance values for monolithic microwave integrated circuits range from 0.5 to 10 nH. We shall describe some configurations here.

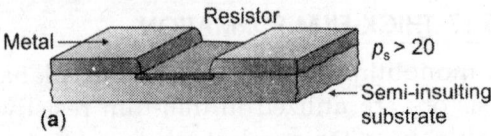

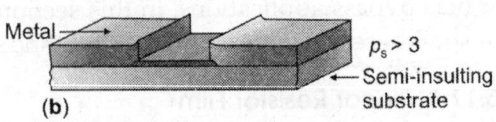

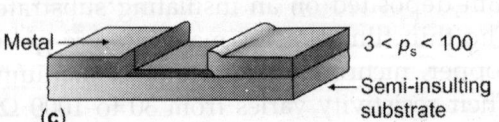

Fig. 25.6: Planar resistor configurations (a) Implanted resistor (b) Mesa resistor (c) Deposited resistor

(i) **Ribbon Inductor:** The inductance of a ribbon inductor is given by

$$L = 5.08 \times 10^{-3} l\{\ln [l/(w + t)] + 1.19 + \\ + 0.022 [(w + t)/l]\ \text{nH/mil} \quad (25.2)$$

where

l is the ribbon length in mils,

w is the ribbon width in mils,

t is the ribbon thickness in mils

(ii) **Round-wire Inductor:** The inductance of a round-wire inductor is given by

$$L = 5.08 \times 10^{-3} l\{\ln [l/d) + 0.386]\ \text{nH/mil} \quad (25.3)$$

where

l is the ribbon length in mils,

d is the wire diameter in mils,

(iii) **Circular Spiral Inductor:** Figure 25.9 shows a circular spiral inductor. The inductance of a circular spiral inductor is given by

$$L = 0.03125\ n^2 d_o\ \text{nH/mil} \quad (25.4)$$

where

$d_o = 5d_i = 2.5\ n(w + s)$ in mils

n is the number of turns

s is the separation in mils

w is the width of the film in mils

(iv) **Circular Loop Inductor:** The inductance of a single-turn flat circular inductor is given by

$$L = 5.08 \times 10^{-3} l\{\ln [t/(w + t)] - 1.76\ \text{nH/mil} \quad (25.5)$$

(v) **Square Spiral Inductor:** The inductance of a square spiral inductor is given by

$$L = 8.5\ A^{1/2}\ n^{5/3}\ \text{nH} \quad (25.6)$$

where

A is the surface area in cm^2,

n is the number of turns.

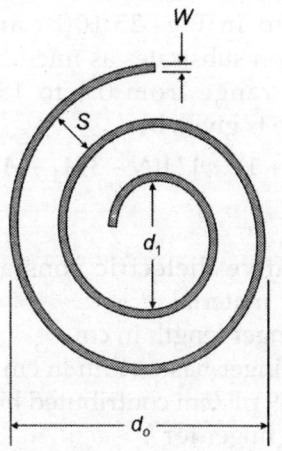

Fig. 25.9: Circular spiral inductor

25.17.3 Planar Capacitors

The commonly used two types of planar capacitors for monolithic microwave integrated circuits are (i) metal-oxide-metal capacitor and (ii) inter-digital capacitor. They are shown in Fig. 25.10.

(i) **Metal-oxide-metal capacitor:** The metal-oxide-metal capacitor has three layers. They are a middle layer sandwiched between a top and bottom electrode layers as shown in Fig. 25.10(a). The capacitance is given by

$$C = \varepsilon_o \varepsilon_r (lw/h)\ \text{farads} \quad (25.7)$$

where $e_o = 8.854 \times 10^{-12}\ \text{F/m}$,

ε_r is relative dielectric constant of the dielectric material,

l is the length of the metal,

w is the width of the metal,

h is the height of the dielectric material.

(ii) **Inter-digital Capacitor:** The inter-digital capacitor is a single-layer structure.

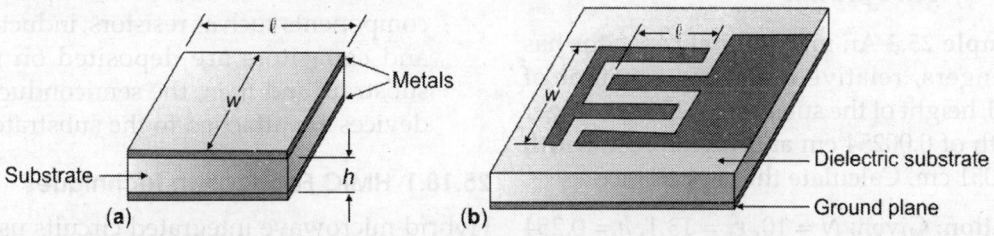

Fig. 25.10: Planar capacitor (a) Metal-oxide-metal capacitor (b) Interdigital capacitor

It is shown in Fig. 25.10(b) and easily fabricated on substrates as microstrip lines. Its values range from 0.1 to 15 pF. The capacitance is given by

$$C = [(\varepsilon_r + 1)/w] \, l \, [(N-3)A_1 + A_2 \text{ pF/cm}^2$$
(25.8)

where

ε_r is relative dielectric constant of the dielectric material

l is the finger length in cm

w is the finger-base width in cm

$A_1 = 0.089$ pF/cm contributed by the interior finger for $h > w$

$A_2 = 0.10$ pF/cm contributed by the two external fingers for $h > w$

Example 25.1 A planar resistor has a resistive film thickness of 1 μm, resistive film length of 10 mm, resistive film width of 10 mm and sheet resistivity of 2.44×10^{-8} Ω m. Calculate the value of the resistor.

Solution: Given: $t = 1$ μm; $l = 10$ mm, $w = 10$ mm; $\rho_s = 2.44 \times 10^{-8}$ Ω m.

$$R = \rho_s l / wt$$
$$= 2.44 \times 10^{-8} \times 10/10 \times 1 \times 10^{-6}$$
$$= \textbf{0.0244 } \Omega\textbf{/square}$$

Example 25.2 A circular spiral inductor has 10 turns, the separation is 100 mils and the film width is 50 mils. Calculate the inductance.

Solution: Given: $n = 10$, $s = 100$ mils, $w = 50$ mils.

$$L = 0.03125 \, n^2 d_o$$
$$= 0.03125 \, n^2 \, [2.5 \, n(w + s)]$$
$$= 0.03125 \times 100 \times [2.5 \times 10 \, (50 + 100)]$$
$$= 3.125 \times 3750$$
$$= \textbf{11.72 } \mu\textbf{H/mil}$$

Example 25.3 An inter-digital capacitor has 10 fingers, relative dielectric constant of 13.10, height of the substrate 0.254 cm, finger length of 0.00254 cm and finger-base width of 0.051 cm. Calculate the capacitance.

Solution: Given: $N = 10$, $\varepsilon_r = 13.1$, $h = 0.254$ cm, $l = 0.00254$ cm, $w = 0.051$ cm

$$C = [(\varepsilon_r + 1)/w] \, l \, [(N-3) \, A_1 + A_2]$$
$$= [(13.1 + 1)/0.051] \times 0.00254 \times$$
$$[(10-3) \times 0.089 + 0.10]$$
$$= 276.5 \times 0.00254 \times 0.723$$
$$= \textbf{0.508 pF/cm}$$

25.18 HYBRID MICROWAVE INTEGRATED CIRCUIT (HMIC) FABRICATION

In the hybrid microwave integrated circuits, active and passive semiconductor circuit elements are fabricated on a dielectric substrate. The passive circuits are lumped or distributed elements or a combination of both. The lumped or distributed elements are formed by using thin or thick film technology. The distributed elements are usually single-layer metallization. The lumped elements are fabricated by multi-level deposition and plating processes or are attached to the substrate in chip form. The hybrid integrated circuits are exclusively used in the frequency range of 1 to 20 GHz. Hybrid microwave integrated circuits are classified into (i) hybrid integrated circuits and (ii) miniature hybrid integrated circuits.

(i) *Hybrid microwave integrated circuits* **(HMIC):** The hybrid microwave integrated circuits use the distributed circuit elements that are fabricated by single-layer metallization process. Then, circuit elements such as semiconductor devices, resistors, inductors and capacitors are attached to the substrate.

(ii) *Miniature hybrid microwave integrated circuits* **(MHMIC):** The miniature hybrid microwave integrated circuits use multi-level elements. All passive components such as resistors, inductors and capacitors are deposited on the substrate and then, the semiconductor devices are attached to the substrate.

25.18.1 HMIC Fabrication Techniques

Hybrid microwave integrated circuits use a single-layer process to form the circuit components on the substrate. The two techniques used for single-layer process are (i) plated-through technique and (ii) etch-back technique.

(i) *Plated-through technique:* In the plated-through technique, the starting material is a substrate coated with a thin layer of evaporated metal. Then, a thick photo-resist is formed on the coated substrate as shown in Fig. 25.11(a). The thickness of the photo-resist is approximately equal to the thickness of the final metal film required. The required pattern is defined on the photo-resist. Then, a second layer is plated up to the desired thickness with precise definition only in the areas where metal is required. Now, the photo-resist layer is removed. Finally, the thin seed metal is etched without any undercut from the undesired areas.

(ii) *Etch-back Technique*: The etch-back technique utilizes either a thick metal layer obtained completely by evapo-ration process or by a combination of a thin evaporated layer and a thick plated layer as shown in Fig. 25.11(b). To define the circuit pattern, a thin photo-resist layer is used as a mask. Then, the unwanted metal areas are etched away. This results in thicker conductors than the plated-through technique.

25.18.2 Advantages of Hybrid Microwave Integrated Circuits

The advantages of the hybrid microwave integrated circuits are:

(i) Higher reliability
(ii) Greater reproducibility
(iii) Better performance
(iv) Smaller size
(v) Lowest cost

25.18.3 Applications

The applications of the hybrid integrated circuits are in:

(i) Satellite communication systems
(ii) Phased-array radar systems

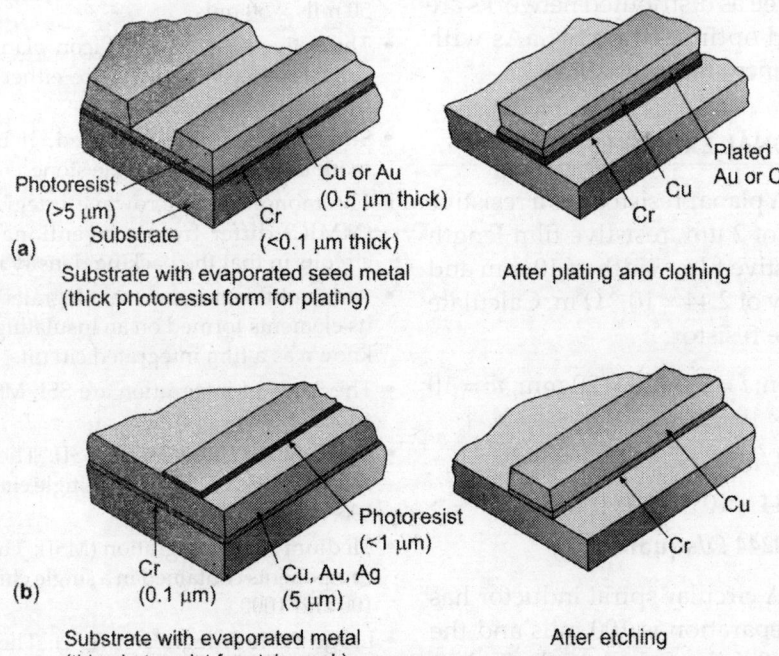

Fig. 25.11: Hybrid MIC fabrication

(iii) Electronic warfare measures

(iv) Commercial and military electronic systems.

25.19 QUASIMONOLITHIC MICROWAVE INTEGRATED CIRCUITS (QMMICs)

Quasimonolithic microwave integrated circuits are also known as *dilithic circuits*. In this, the passive components are realized using integrated technology similar to that of MMICs whereas the active components are mounted individually. This technology overcomes some of the disadvantages of MMIC. QMMICs have the size and batch processing advantages of monolithics as well as superior performance and high yield achievable with discrete-devices. Each circuit component can be tested easily. The active devices can be tested at all process steps. The high-performance active devices are fabricated using Tantalum, Molybdenum and Tungsten for forming Schottky junctions with a thick gold overlay. The lumped circuit components such as resistors, inductors and capacitors as well as distributed networks are developed and optimized on SiGaAs with good performance characteristics.

25.20 ADDITIONAL EXAMPLES

Example 25.4 A planar resistor has a resistive film thickness of 2 μm, resistive film length of 20 mm, resistive film width of 10 mm and sheet resistivity of 2.44×10^{-8} Ω m. Calculate the value of the resistor.

Solution: Given: $t = 2$ μm, $l = 20$ mm, $w = 10$ mm; $\rho_s = 2.44 \times 10^{-8}$ Ω-m.

$$R = \rho_s l / wt$$
$$= 2.44 \times 10^{-8} \times 20/10 \times 2 \times 10^{-6}$$
$$= 0.0244 \ \Omega/\text{square}$$

Example 25.5 A circular spiral inductor has 20 turns, the separation is 100 mils and the film width is 60 mils. Calculate the inductance.

Solution: Given: $n = 20$, $s = 100$ mils, $w = 50$ mils.

$$L = 0.03125 \ n^2 d_o$$
$$= 0.03125 \ n^2 \ [2.5n \ (w + s)]$$
$$= 0.03125 \times 400 \times [2.5 \times 20 (50 + 100)]$$
$$= 93.75 \ \mu\text{H/mil}$$

Example 25.6 An inter-digital capacitor has 20 fingers, relative dielectric constant of 13.10, height of the substrate 0.254 cm, finger length of 0.00254 cm and finger-base width of 0.051 cm. Calculate the capacitance.

Solution: Given: $N = 20$; $\varepsilon_r = 13.1$; $h = 0.254$ cm; $l = 0.00254$ cm; $w = 0.051$ cm

$$C = [(\varepsilon_r + 1)/w] \ l \ [(N - 3)A_1 + A_2]$$
$$= [(13.1 + 1)/0.051] \times 0.00254$$
$$[(20 - 3) \times 0.089 + 0.10]$$
$$= 276.5 \times 0.00254 \times 1.613$$
$$= 1.113 \ \text{pF/cm}$$

KEY POINTS

- Integrated circuit consists of both active and passive components and their interconnections fabricated on a single silicon chip of dimension 50 mils × 50 mils.

- The active devices are silicon planar chips and the passive components are either thin film or thick film elements.

- Since a single chip is used, it is known as monolithic meaning single stone.

- The monolithic microwave integrated circuits (MMIC) differ from conventional integrated circuits in that the packing density is low.

- A monolithic microwave integrated circuit with its elements formed on an insulating substrate is known as a film integrated circuit.

- The types of integration are SSI, MSI, LSI, VLSI and ULSI.

- Small Scale Integration (SSI): The number of components contained in a single chip is less than 100.

- Medium Scale Integration (MSI): The number of components contained in a single chip is between 100 and 1000.

- Large Scale Integration (LSI): The number of components in a single chip is between 1000 and 100,000.

- Very Large Scale Integration (VLSI): The number of components contained in a single chip is between 10^5 and 10^6.
- Ultra Large-Scale Integration (ULSI): The number of components contained in a single chip is greater than 1.5×10^6
- The advantages of monolithic microwave integrated circuits are (i) Extremely small size and light weight, (ii) Low cost, (iii) Extremely high reliability, (iv) Low power consumption, (v) Easy replacement, (vi) Fast response, (vii) Ruggedness against shock, vibration and (viii) Operability under severe temperature conditions
- The disadvantages are (i) It cannot handle high power and withstand excessive heat, (ii) It is quite delicate and is liable to be damaged and (iii) The whole IC is to be replaced in the case of failure of a component.
- The monolithic microwave integrated circuits are extensively used in space and military applications because of their ruggedness against shock and severe vibrations and temperature conditions.
- Monolithic microwave integrated circuits are fabricated in either monolithic or hybrid form.
- In monolithic microwave integrated circuits, active devices are grown on or in the semiconductor substrate. The passive elements are then deposited on the substrate or grown on it.
- In the hybrid circuit, the active devices are attached to a ceramic, glass or ferrite substrate that contains the passive circuitry.
- The hybrid technology is used almost exclusively for microwave integrated circuits in the frequency range of 1 to 15 GHz.
- A hybrid integrated circuit consists of a combination of two or more integrated circuit types such as integrated circuit and discrete components or monolithic and film.
- Hybrid microwave integrated circuits are fabricated on high-quality ceramic, glass or ferrite substrate. The passive components are deposited on the substrate and then, the active devices are mounted on the substrate and connected to the passive circuit components.
- Hybrid microwave integrated circuits are classified into (i) hybrid integrated circuits and (ii) miniature hybrid integrated circuits.
- The hybrid integrated circuits use the distributed circuit elements fabricated by single-layer metallization process. Then, circuit elements such

as semiconductor devices, resistors, inductors and capacitors are attached to the substrate.
- The miniature hybrid integrated circuits are multi-level elements. All passive components such as resistors, inductors and capacitors are deposited on the substrate and then, the semiconductor devices are attached to the substrate.
- Quasimonolithic microwave integrated circuits are also known as dilithic circuits. In this, the passive components are realized using integrated technology similar to that of MMICs whereas the active components are mounted individually.

FURTHER READING

1. Bahl IJ and Bhatia P (ed.) (1988). *Microwave Solid State Circuit Design*, John Wiley, NY.
2. Sze SM (Ed.) (1983). *VLSI Technology*, John Wiley, NY.
3. Nanavathi RP (1975). *Semiconductor Devices*, Intext Edn., Scranton, PA.
4. Liao SY (1990). *Semiconductor Electron Devices*, PH. NJ.

REVIEW QUESTIONS

25.1 List the basic materials for MMICs.
25.2 What are the ideal characteristics of substrate materials?
25.3 What are the ideal characteristics of conductor materials?
25.4 What are the ideal characteristics of dielectric materials?
25.5 What are the ideal characteristics of resistive materials?
25.6 Mention the process involved in MMIC fabrication.
25.7 Mention the four types of thin-films used for MMIC.
25.8 Explain the diffusion and implantation process.
25.9 Explain the oxidation and film deposition process.
25.10 Explain the epitaxial growth process.
25.11 Explain the diffusion and implantation process.
25.12 Explain the lithographic process.
25.13 Mention the steps involved in the MOSFET fabrication.

25.14 Mention the steps involved in the NMOS fabrication.

25.15 Mention the steps involved in the CMOS fabrication.

25.16 What is a planar resistor? What are the types?

25.17 What is a planar inductor? What are the types?

25.18 What is a planar capacitor? What are the types?

25.19 Distinguish between hybrid and monolithic ICs.

25.20 Distinguish between hybrid and miniature hybrid ICs.

25.21 What are the advantages of hybrid ICs?

25.22 What are the applications of hybrid ICs?

DESCRIPTIVE QUESTIONS

25.1 Discuss the discrete, integrated and monolithic microwave ICs.

25.2 What are the ideal properties of dielectric and resistive materials?

25.3 List the steps involved in the fabrication of MMIC.

25.4 Explain the photo-resist process for the fabrication of MMIC.

25.5 Explain in detail the fabrication of MOSFET.

25.6 Explain in detail the fabrication of NMOS logic gate.

25.7 Explain in detail the fabrication of CMOS.

25.8 Explain in detail the fabrication of planar resistors, inductors and capacitors.

25.9 Explain the two techniques used in the fabrication of hybrid IC.

PRACTICE PROBLEMS

25.1 A planar resistor has a resistive film thickness of 0.1 μm, resistive film length of 10 mm, resistive film width of 10 mm and sheet resistivity of 2.44×10^{-8} Ω·m. Calculate the value of the resistor.

(**Ans:** 0.224 Ω/square)

25.2 A circular spiral inductor has 5 turns, the separation is 100 mils and the film width is 50 mils. Calculate the inductance.

(**Ans:** 1.46 μH/mil)

25.3 An inter-digital capacitor has 8 fingers, relative dielectric constant of 13.10, height of the substrate 0.254 cm, finger length of 0.00254 cm and finger-base width of 0.051 cm. Calculate the capacitance.

(**Ans:** 0.383 pF)

REFERENCES

1. Keister FZ (1968). An evaluation of materials and processes for integrated microwave circuits, IEEE. Trans., MTT-19, No. 7.

2. Caulton M and Sobol H (1970). Microwave integrated circuit technology: A survey, *IEEE. J. Solid-State Circuits*, SC-5, No. 6, pp 292–303.

3. Sobol H (1971). Application of integrated circuit technology to microwave frequencies, Proc. IEEE. Vol.59, No. 8, pp 1200–1211.

4. Sobol H (1970). Technology and design of hybrid microwave integrated circuits, *Solid State Technology*, Vol. 13, No. 2, pp 49–59.

5. Nanavati RP (1975). *Semiconductor Devices*, Intext Edu. Pub., PA.

6. Sze SM (Ed) (1983). *VLSI Technology*, Wiley, NY.

7. Liao SY (2000). *Microwave Devices and Circuits*, PHI, New Delhi,

8. Calviello JA et al (1986). Quasimonolithic: An alternative/intermediate approach to fully monolithic, *Microwave J.*, p. 243–256.

9. Capello A et al (1987). A high performance, quasi-monolithic 2 to 18 GHz distributed GaAs FET amplifier, IEEE, MTTs, Intl. Microwave Symp. Did., pp. 833–835.

10. Young Leo (1966). *Advances in Microwaves*, Vol. I, Academic Press, NY.

11. Streetman BG (2000), *Solid State Electronic Devices*, PH, N.J.

Microwave Measurement Devices and Instruments

Objectives

- Know the operating principle of tunable detector and slotted line probe.
- Study the VSWR meter.
- Explain the application of spectrum and network analyzers.
- Understand the principle of power sensors and their applications.

26.1 INTRODUCTION

Microwaves are considerably different from low-frequency waves in respect of transmission structures, resonators, sources and the network representation. Therefore, the measurement techniques and the quantities that are measured are different at microwave frequencies.

At low frequencies, the amplitudes of voltage and current are easily measurable whereas at microwave frequencies they are not easily measurable as they are functions of distance on transmission lines. However, the power transmitted over a loss-less line is independent of location along the line. Therefore, it is more convenient to measure power at microwave frequencies than voltages or currents. Many properties of microwave devices and circuits are obtained from the measurement of power, impedance, frequency, VSWR, S-parameters, phase shift and noise figures.

The microwave measuring devices and instruments such as network analyzer, spectrum analyzer and power meters are expensive. Therefore microwave measurements in the laboratory are often carried out using 1 kHz square-wave modulating signal which amplitude modulates the microwave signal. The transmitted and reflected signals are then demodulated and measured using low-frequency instruments such as oscilloscope and VSWR meters.

In this chapter, we shall discuss some of the important devices and instruments commenly used in microwave measurements such as tunable detector, slotted line and probe, VSWR meter, spectrum analyzer and network analyzer.

26.2 TUNABLE DETECTOR

Detection of microwaves is carried out for relative measurement of microwave power. In order to indicate the relative power levels, it is necessary to detect or rectify the microwave signals and obtain a proportional dc signal. For the purpose of detection, point contact diodes and Schottky diodes are used. These diodes have been described in detail in an earlier chapter. These specially designed diodes are mounted suitably in the microwave transmission line or co-axial line. The diode detector is mounted across one end of the wave-guide or transmission line and the other end is shorted. A tuning plunger is used to vary the distance between the shorted-end and the diode detector. This tuning arrangement is used to tune the detector for a range of signal frequencies. In this way the detector performance is optimized at the desired frequency. The detected output is normally available at a coaxial BNC connector. The tunable detector, coaxial and waveguide types, are shown in Fig. 26.1.

The performance of a microwave detector is expressed in terms of the current sensitivity. This is defined as

$$\beta = \Delta i / P \qquad (26.1)$$

Here Δi is the increase in the short circuit current regulated from the available input power P. Sensitivity β is a function of bias level and is usually in the range of 1 to 15 μA per μW. The highest value for β is usually attained when the bias level is between 10 μA and 100 μA. However, most of the detectors are operated without any bias voltage.

26.3 SLOTTED LINE PROBE

Slotted line is a fundamental tool for microwave measurements. It consists of a section of a waveguide or coaxial line with a longitudinal slot. This slot is approximately 1 mm wide and allows an electric field probe (*E*-probe) to be inserted inside the waveguide or coaxial line for measuring the relative magnitude of the electric field at the location of the probe. The slot is suitably located in the middle of the broad wall of the waveguide such that the disturbance to the wall currents is minimum. The location of the slot and the direction of the wall current in a waveguide and coaxial system are shown in Fig. 26.2(a) and (b) respectively. Slotted line is normally mounted in a carriage as shown in Fig. 26.3. This also supports the probe moving inside the slot.

The *E*-probe is a thin conducting wire, which passes through the slot in the slotted line and couples to the electric field in the waveguide or coaxial line. The amount of insertion of the probe is critical and needs careful adjustment. A small insertion results in a poor sensitivity. Hence, it is difficult to

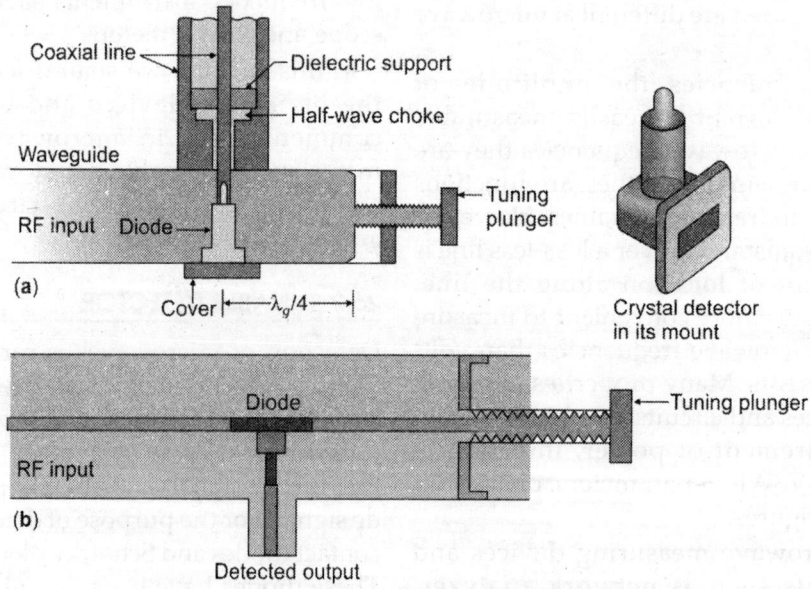

Fig. 26.1: Tunable detector (a) Waveguide (b) Coaxial

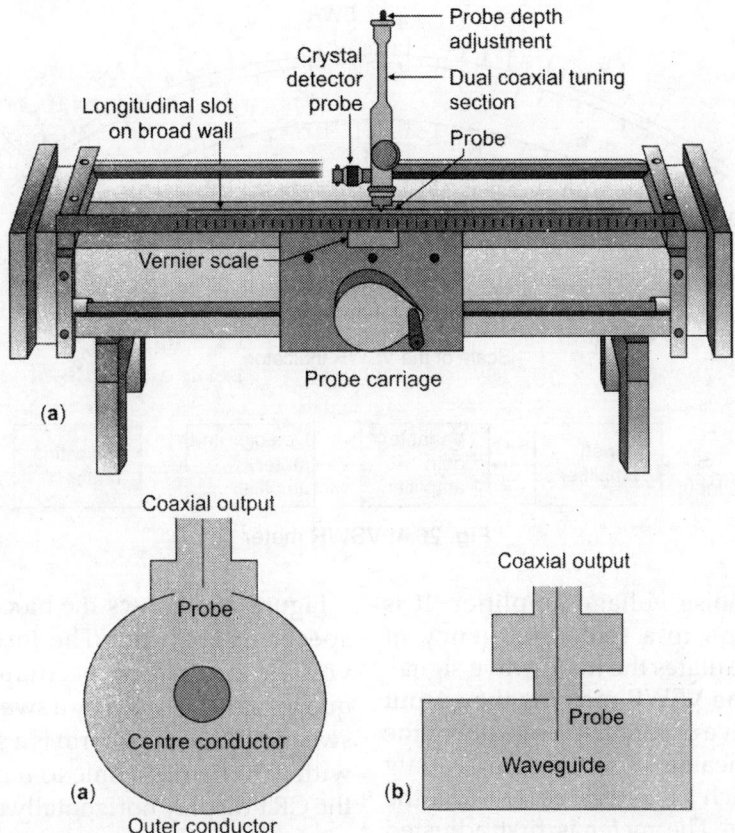

Fig. 26.2: (a) Waveguide system (b) Coaxial system

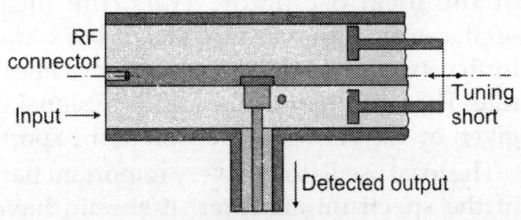

Fig. 26.3: Slotted line

locate the minima of the standing wave pattern. On the other hand, an insertion disturbs the field and may reflect some of the incident input power and thereby lead to inaccurate results. The output of the probe is fed to the detector in a mount. The electric field is proportional to the induced voltage on the probe. The probe carriage contains a stud tunable detector to obtain the 1 kHz modulating signal output to the input oscilloscope or VSWR meter.

This unit is primarily used to determine the location of the voltage standing wave maxima and minima along the line. It is used to measure

1. VSWR and SW pattern
2. Wavelength
3. Impedance
4. Reflection coefficient
5. Return loss

The disadvantage of the slotted line is that amplitude and phase measurements are limited to single frequencies and hence, broadband measurement is expensive and time consuming.

26.4 VSWR METER

The block diagram of a VSWR meter is shown in Fig. 26.4. It is a sensitive, high gain,

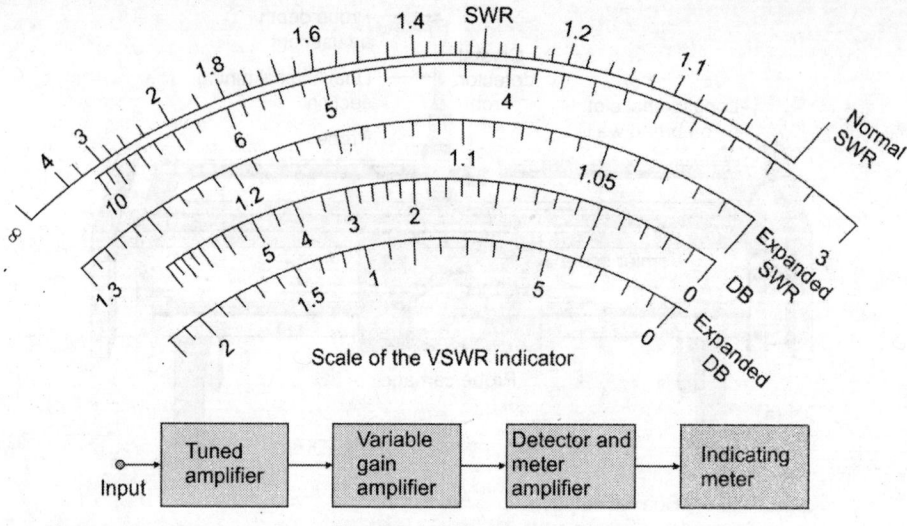

Fig. 26.4: VSWR meter

high Q, low noise voltage amplifier. It is normally tuned to a fixed frequency of 1 kHz that modulates the microwave signal. The input to the VSWR meter is the output of the microwave detector. The output of the amplifier is measured with a square-law voltmeter which is calibrated to read the VSWR directly. The meter is first adjusted for unity VSWR reading for an input corresponding to V_{max}. A gain control is provided to adjust the reading to the desired value. The VSWR meter has an overall gain of 125 dB. This can be varied in steps of 10 dB.

The meter has three scales, *normal VSWR*, *expanded VSWR* and the *dB scale* as shown in Fig. 26.4. The top normal VSWR scale is graduated from 1 to 4, the bottom one from 3.2 to 10. The expanded VSWR scale is used when the reading is less than 1.3 so that more accurate reading can be obtained. The third scale is graduated in dB.

26.5 SPECTRUM ANALYZER

A spectrum analyzer is a broadband superheterodyne receiver which displays the plot of amplitude versus frequency of the received signal or the frequency spectrum of the signal. In other words, a spectrum analyzer displays plot of the amplitude of the Fourier transform of the input signal.

Figure 26.5 shows the block diagram of a spectrum analyzer. The local oscillator is voltage-controlled oscillator whose frequency can be varied by a sweep voltage. The sweep voltage waveform is a saw tooth wave with zero fly back time to move the spot on the CRT display horizontally in synchronism with the frequency sweep so that the horizontal position is a function of frequency of the local oscillator. Thus, the local oscillator is automatically swept back and forth between two frequency limits at a linear rate. The amplitude of the input RF signal is given by the vertical deflection of the spot.

The local oscillator is a very important part of the spectrum analyzer. It should have good stability and spectral purity. The oscillator stability sets the lower limit for the bandwidth resolution achievable in a spectrum analyzer. The important design considerations are:

(i) Frequency sweep rate

(ii) Frequency sweep range

(iii) IF amplifier bandwidth

(iv) IF amplifier center frequency

To obtain highest resolution, the bandwidth should be narrow and hence, the sweep speed should be very low in order to

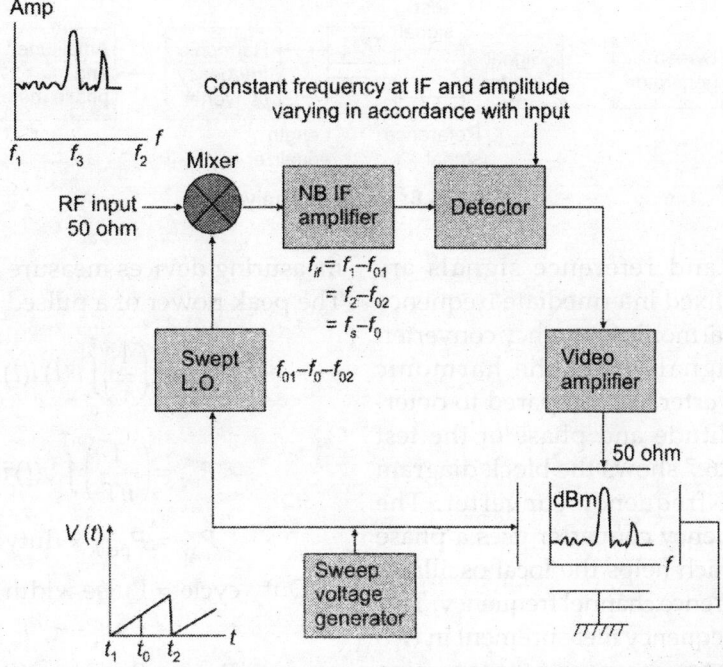

Fig. 26.5: Spectrum analyzer

allow time to build up the voltage in the receiver circuit. The frequency range should also be as small as possible.

The intermediate frequency IF should be so selected that the image frequency is eliminated. Let f_o be the local oscillator frequency, f_s be the signal frequency and f_{if} be the intermediate frequency. Then, f_o and f_i are given by

$$f_o = f_s \pm f_{if}$$

and $\quad f_i = f_o \pm f_{if} = f_s \pm 2 f_{if}$

This image frequency f_i beats with the local oscillator frequency f_o and produce a difference frequency equal to f_{if}. Thus,

$$f_i - f_o = \pm f_{if}$$

For example, when $f_{if} = 460$ KHz and $f_o = 6000$ KHz, the signal with 6460 KHz or 5540 KHz will beat with f_o and produce f_{if}. For $f_{if} = 460$ KHz, the image frequency $f_i = 2 \times 460 = 920$ KHz off the signal frequency which is a bit difficult to tune out. If $f_{if} = 2000$ KHz, the image frequency $f_i = 2 \times 2000 = 4000$ KHz off the signal frequency which can be easily tuned out. The bandwidth and hence the resolution of the spectrum analyzer is determined by the bandwidth of the IF amplifier.

26.6 NETWORK ANALYZER

Network analyzer is another important instrument used for microwave measurements on passive and active microwave components and networks. A network analyzer measures both amplitude and phase of signal over a wide frequency range within a reasonable time. The basic measurement requires an accurate reference signal which must be generated. The amplitude and phase of the test signal are measured with respect to the generated reference signal.

Figure 26.6 shows the block diagram of a network analyzer. The microwave signal from the sweep oscillator is first split by means of a power divider into a test signal and a reference signal. The test signal is transmitted through the Device Under Test (DUT) and the reference signal passes through a phase equalizing length of line.

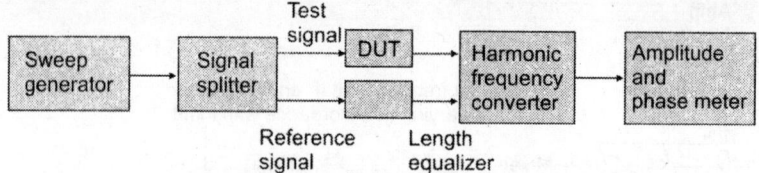

Fig. 26.6: Network analyzer

Both the test and reference signals are converted to a fixed intermediate frequency by means of a harmonic frequency converter. The output signals from the harmonic frequency converter are compared to determine the amplitude and phase of the test signal. Figure 26.7 shows the block diagram of a harmonic frequency converter. The harmonic frequency converter uses a phase locked loop which helps the local oscillator to track the reference channel frequency. This allows swept frequency measurement in two stages. The first mixer converts the incoming RF signal to a fixed IF of 20 MHz and then, after amplification, further converted to another fixed IF of 278 kHz by a second mixer for final amplitude and phase comparison.

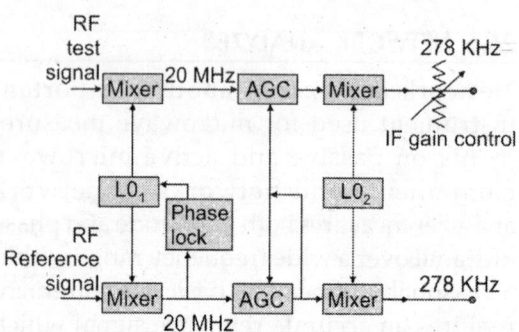

Fig. 26.7: Harmonic frequency converter

26.7 MW REFERENCE POWER SENSORS

At microwave frequencies, transmission lines and wave-guides are employed for transmission of power. Hence voltage and current are no longer measurable. The fundamental quantity that is commonly measured at microwave frequencies is power. Most of the microwave power-measuring devices measure average power. The peak power of a pulsed signal is

$$P_{\text{peak}} = \left(\frac{1}{\tau}\right) \int_0^\tau v(t)\, i(t)\, dt \qquad (26.2a)$$

$$P_{\text{av}} = \left(\frac{1}{nT}\right) \int_0^{nT} v(t)\, i(t)\, dt \qquad (26.2b)$$

$$P_{\text{av}} = P_{\text{peak}} \times \text{duty cycle} \qquad (26.2c)$$

Duty cycle = Pulse width x $p.r.f$

$$= \tau \times f_r = \tau/T \qquad (26.2d)$$

$$P_{\text{peak}} = P_{\text{av}} \cdot T/\tau = (P_{\text{av}}/\tau f_r) \qquad (26.2e)$$

Here τ is the pulse width, T is the period of the pulse and f_r is the pulse repetition frequency. The most convenient unit of power at microwave frequency is dBm. In this case, the reference power is assumed to be 1 milliwatt. Thus

$$P_{\text{dBm}} = 10 \log\left[P/1\ \text{mW}\right] \qquad (26.3)$$

A power of 30 dBm is 1 W and –30 dBm is 1 µW.

26.8 MW POWER SENSORS

The microwave power meter consists of a power sensor. The sensors used for power measurements are Schottky barrier diode, bolometer and thermocouple.

26.8.1 Schottky Barrier Diode Sensor

The constructional details of this diode have been discussed in Chapter 14. A zero-biased Schottky barrier diode is used as a square-law detector for measuring microwave signal as shown in Fig. 26.8. The output of the circuit is proportional to the input RF power. This is used to measure low power.

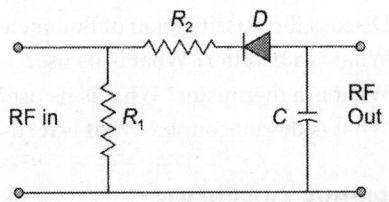

Fig. 26.8: Schottky diode MW power sensor

26.8.2 Bolometer Sensor

Bolometer is a power sensor whose resistance varies with temperature as it absorbs microwave power. There are two most common types of Bolometer. They are (i) baretters (ii) thermistors.

26.8.2.1 Baretters

Baretters consist of a short length of very fine platinum wire suitably encapsulated. They have a positive temperature coefficient. Baretters are very delicate and are easily burnt out at high power.

26.8.2.2 Thermistors

Thermistors consist of small beads of semiconductor material placed on two wires as shown in Fig. 26.9. The lead material may be a mixture of manganese and nickel oxides combined with finely divided copper particles to control the resistivity. The lead is coated with a thin film of glass to make the assembly strong, heat resistant and stable. They have negative temperature coefficient.

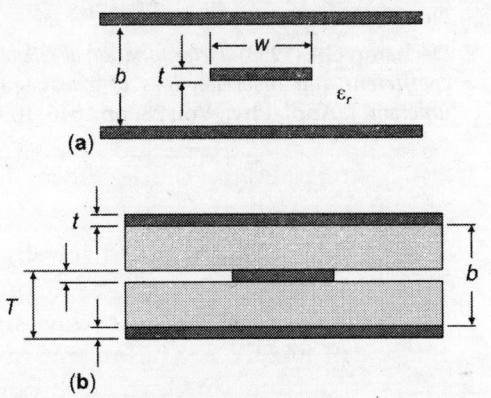

Fig. 26.9: Thermistor

They can be easily mounted on microwave lines. Thermistors are more sensitive than baretters but require higher bias current. Thermistor-mounts provide good isolation from thermal and physical shock and good shielding against energy leakage.

26.8.3 Thermocouples

Thermocouples consist of thin films of antimony and bismuth deposited on thin resistive strips. When the two ends of thermocouples are at different temperatures, a thermo-emf is generated. The microwave power incident on the resistive strip causes the difference in temperature of the two ends of the thermocouples. These devices are used to measure very low power.

KEY POINTS

- It is more convenient to measure power at microwave frequencies than voltages or currents.
- Many properties of microwave devices and circuits are obtained from the measurement of power, impedance, frequency, VSWR, S-parameters, phase shift and noise figures.
- The microwave measuring instruments such as network analyzer, spectrum analyzer and power meters are expensive. Therefore microwave measurements in the laboratory are often carried out using 1 kHz square-wave modulating signal which amplitude modulates the microwave signal. The transmitted and reflected signals are then demodulated and measured using low-frequency instruments such as oscilloscope and VSWR meters.
- The slotted line probe is used to measure (i) VSWR and SW patterns, (ii) Wavelength, (iii) Impedance, (iv) Reflection coefficient and (v) Return loss.
- VSWR meter is a sensitive, high gain, high Q, low noise voltage amplifier. It is normally tuned to a fixed frequency of 1 kHz that modulates the microwave signal.
- The important design considerations of the spectrum analyzer are (i) Frequency sweep rate, (ii) Frequency sweep range, (iii) IF amplifier bandwidth and (iv) IF amplifier center frequency.

- A network analyzer measures both amplitude and phase of signal over a wide frequency range within a reasonable time.
- The sensors used for power measurements are Schottky barrier diode, bolometer and thermo-couple.

FURTHER READING

1. Lebedev I (1973). *Microwave Engineering*, MIR Publications, Moscow.
2. Collins RE (1996). *Foundations of Microwave Engineering*, McGraw Hill, NY.
3. Reich HJ (1978). *Microwave Principles*, East-West, New Delhi.
4. Ginzton EL (1957). *Microwave Measurements*, McGraw Hill, NY.

REVIEW QUESTIONS

26.1 How does the microwave differ from low frequency waves?
26.2 Mention three instruments used in microwave measurements.
26.3 What is a tunable detector? What is its use?
26.4 What is a probe?
26.5 What is a slotted line?
26.6 Mention the use of a slotted line with probe.
26.7 For what measurements would you use a slotted line carriage? What should be the minimum length of the slot in it?
26.8 What is a VSWR meter?
26.9 Mention the use of the spectrum analyzer.
26.10 What are the important design considerations in spectrum analyzer?
26.11 Mention the use of the network analyzer.
26.12 What are the measurements that can be performed using (a) spectrum analyzer and (b) network analyzer?
26.13 What is the value of reference power for dBm?
26.14 Mention the sensors used for microwave power measurements.

26.15 Discuss the classification of Bolometers.
26.16 What is a baretter? What is its use?
26.17 What is a thermistor? What is its use?
26.18 What is thermocouple? What is its use?

DESCRIPTIVE QUESTIONS

26.1 Describe, with a neat sketch, the tunable detector.
26.2 Describe, with a neat sketch, the slotted line and probe.
26.3 Describe, with a neat sketch, the VSWR meter.
26.4 Describe, with a neat block diagram, the spectrum analyzer.
26.5 Describe, with a neat block diagram, the network analyzer.
26.6 Describe, with a neat block diagram, the microwave sensors.

REFERENCE

1. Montgomery CG (1947). *Technique of Microwave Measurements*, McGraw Hill, NY.
2. Lebedev I (1973). *Microwave Engineering*, MIR Publications, Moscow.
3. Collins RE (1996). *Foundations of Microwave Engineering*, McGraw Hill, NY.
4. Reich HJ (1978). Microwave Principles, East-West, New Delhi.
5. Barrington AE and Rees JR (1958). A Simple 3-cm Q-meter, Proc. IRE, vol.105, pp 511–512, November.
6. Surber WH Jr and Crouch GE Jr (1948). Dielectric measurement methods for solid at microwave frequencies, J. Appl. Phy., Vol. 19, No. 12, December.
7. Dechamp GA (1953). *Determination of reflection coefficient and insertion loss of a waveguide junction*, J. Appl. Phy., Vol. 28, pp 1046–1050.

Microwave Measurement Techniques

Objectives

- Know the method of measuring.
- Microwave power.
- Insertion loss
- VSWR.
- Impedance.
- Frequency.
- Q of the resonant cavity.
- Dielectric constant.
- Antenna parameters.
- Noise factor.

27.1 INTRODUCTION

In the previous chapter, we have studied the devices and instruments required for the measurement of various quantities at microwave frequency. In this chapter, we shall discuss, in detail, the various microwave measurement techniques. The measurement of microwave power, VSWR, insertion loss, attenuation, impedance, scattering parameters, Q of a cavity, dielectric constant, antenna radiation pattern and noise factor are described in detail.

27.2 MICROWAVE POWER MEASUREMENTS

The measurement of power at microwave frequencies is classified into four types:
  (a) Very low power ($P < 1$ mW)
  (b) Low power (1 mW $< P <$ 10 mW)
  (c) Medium power (10 mW $< P <$ 10 W)
  (d) High power ($P >$10 W)

27.2.1 Very Low Power Measurement

A microwave thermocouple instrument to measure very low power is shown in Fig. 27.1. The coupling loop couples the microwave power to the instrument and also provides a dc return path for the meter current. If the coupler is a probe, then a quarter-wavelength stub may be used to provide the dc path. The thermocouple indicator circuit is simple. But the sensitivity is low.

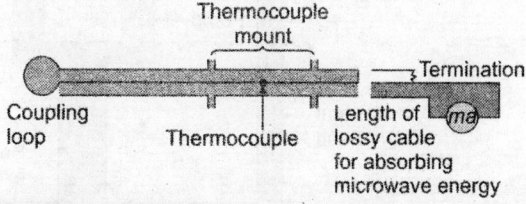

Fig. 27.1: Measurement of very low microwave power

27.2.2 Low Power Measurement

Bolometers are used to measure low microwave power. The basic measuring device is a simple Wheatstone bridge (Fig. 27.2). The Bolometer forms one of the arms of the bridge. The bridge is initially balanced with an audio frequency power. When the R.F. power is applied to the Bolometer, the balance is disturbed. The audio frequency power is removed after the bridge is again balanced. The amount of audio frequency power removed is amplified and displayed on the indicating meter and the reading is equal to true power substitution.

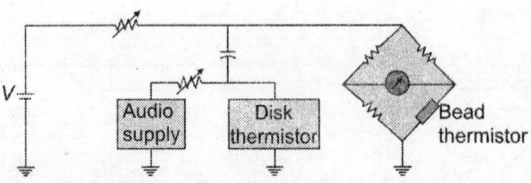

Fig. 27.2: Measurement of low microwave power

In such simple arrangement, the bridge can become unbalanced due to ambient temperature. To compensate this, another bolometer is placed close to the Bolometer in one of the other arms of the Wheatstone bridge so that both are affected equally by changes in ambient temperature.

27.2.3 Medium and High Power Measurement

Calorimeter techniques are used to measure medium and high power. It measures the temperature rise of a known quantity of liquid used with the load. The flow-calorimeter consists of a self-balancing bridge with identical temperature compensating resisters or gauges in two arms of the Wheatstone bridge, an indicating meter and two load resisters, one for input power and the other for comparison power as shown in Fig. 27.3

The bridge consists of two halves of secondary of a transformer and the two gauges. The primary of the transformer is excited by a 1200 Hz sine wave. The audio power across one half of the secondary of the transformer is fed to the comparison load. The heat exchanger maintains the temperature of the

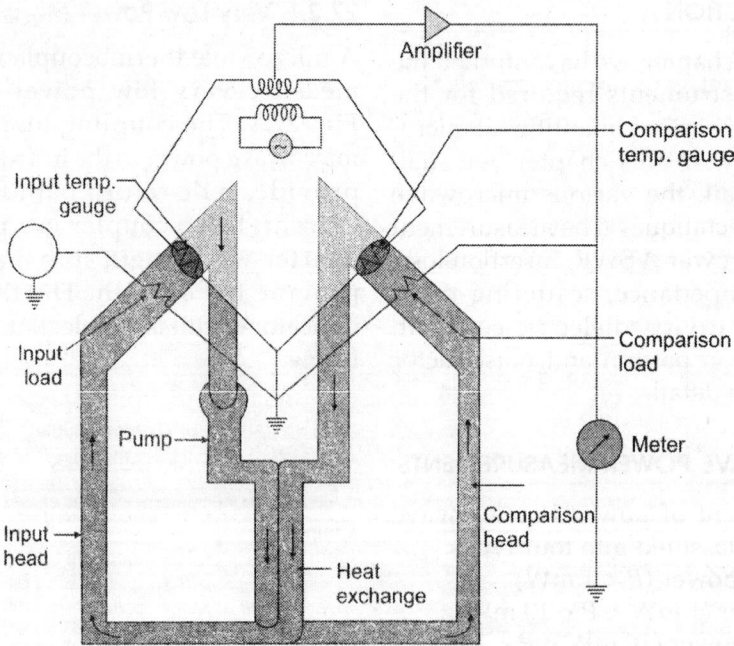

Fig. 27.3: Measurement of medium and high microwave power

oil entering the two arms to be same. When the R.F. power is applied to the input load, this raises the temperature of the liquid. The input gauge senses this unbalance in temperature and the bridge becomes unbalanced. The regulating voltage is amplified by a high gain amplifier and is applied to the comparison load.

The comparison gauge senses the resulting rise in temperature and the bridge is once again balanced. The indicating meter is calibrated in terms of power required to bring the bridge into balance. Accuracies better than 5% can be achieved by minimizing frequency and impedance mismatch effects.

27.2.4 Error in Power Measurement

The common errors in power measurements are:

   (i) Instrumental error

   (ii) Substitution error

   (iii) Mount inefficiency error.

The instrumental error is minimized by maintaining the stability of bias sources and by the degree of ambient temperature compensation.

The substitution error arises from the difference in heating effects of radio frequency and audio frequency power.

The mount inefficiency error is due to mismatch of impedances, resistive losses in the walls of the mount, poor contacts and loose nature of the dielectric.

27.2.5 Disadvantages

The disadvantages of calorimetric method are:

   (i) Thermal material causes time lag between the application of microwave power and the final reading.

   (ii) It cannot be adapted to measure low power.

   (iii) The accuracy is low, about 5%

27.3 INSERTION LOSS AND ATTENUATION MEASUREMENTS

When a device or network is inserted in transmission lines, a small part P_r of the input signal power P_i is reflected or returned from the input terminals of the device or network. This is known as return loss and is given by

Return Loss

$$= 10 \log P_r/P_i$$
$$= 20 \log |\Gamma| \ \text{dB} \qquad (27.1)$$

where Γ is the reflection coefficient.

The power that actually enters the network is $P_i - P_r$. Because of the loss or attenuation of the network, the output power P_o is therefore less than P_i. The attenuation is defined as the ratio of output power to the input power of the network. Thus

Attenuation

$$= 10 \log P_o/(P_i - P_r) \ \text{dB} \qquad (27.2)$$

The total loss due to the insertion of the network is the insertion loss. It defined as the ratio of the input power P_i to the output power P_o. Thus.

Insertion Loss

$$= 10 \log P_o/P_i \ \text{dB} \qquad (27.3)$$
$$= 10 \log [P_o/(P_i - P_r)] [(P_i - P_r)/P_i]$$
$$= 10 \log [P_o/(P_i - P_r)] +$$
$$\quad 10 \log [(P_i - P_r)/P_i] \qquad (27.4)$$
$$= \text{Attenuation} + \text{Reflection loss}$$

Thus reflection loss is given by

Reflection loss

$$= 10 \log (P_i - P_r)/P_i \ \text{dB} \qquad (27.5)$$

27.4 VSWR MEASUREMENTS

In a microwave system, when the waveguide or coaxial line is not matched, there exists a reflected wave which combines with the incident wave to create standing wave along the length of the transmission path. The voltage standing wave ratio (VSWR) is defined as the ratio of the maximum voltage to the minimum voltage. It may vary from unity to infinity. It is one of the most important parameter to be measured at microwave frequencies. Its measurement is also required in determining the unknown impedance in microwave systems. The accuracy of the unknown impedance depends on the accurate measurement of VSWR.

The measurement of VSWR is divided into the following two categories:

(i) Low VSWR (S < 10)
(ii) High VSWR (S > 10)

27.4.1 Low VSWR Measurement (S < 10)

VSWR meter, slotted line and travelling tunable probe detector are used to measure low VSWR. The experimental setup is shown in Fig. 27.4. The variable attenuator is adjusted to 10 dB. The microwave source is set to the required frequency. The 1 kHz modulation is adjusted for maximum reading on the VSWR meter in 30 dB scale. The probe carriage stub is tuned for maximum detected signal in VSWR meter. The probe carriage is slided along the slot from the load end towards the generator end until a peak reading is obtained in the VSWR meter. The meter gain control is adjusted to get the meter reading of 1, corresponding to the position of voltage maximum. The probe is now moved towards the generator end to an adjacent voltage minimum. The corresponding reading in the VSWR meter directly gives the VSWR.

27.4.1.1 Limitations

The possible sources of error in this method are:

(i) Presence of harmonics and spurious signals in the source may cause error in measurement.

(ii) The measurement of V_{max} and V_{min} may not be in the square-law region of the detector.

(iii) The probe thickness and depth of penetration may introduce errors.

(iv) If the 1 kHz modulating signal is not a perfect square wave, it would be difficult to locate the V_{min} sharply. This introduces error in reading the voltage minimum position.

(v) The VSWR connector produces significant error in low (<1.05) VSWR measurement.

27.4.2 High VSWR Measurement (S > 10)

For high VSWR, it would be difficult to remain in the square-law region of the detector. Therefore, *double minimum method* is used. In this case, measurements are carried out at two positions around the voltage minimum point as shown in Fig. 27.5. The probe is moved to a voltage minimum point. The probe depth and gain control are adjusted to read 3 dB in the VSWR meter. The probe is first moved to one side of the minimum point to read 0 dB in the meter. Let this position be x_1. The probe is then moved to the other side of the minimum point to read 0 dB. Let this position be x_2. Then the wave-guide length λ_g is found by moving the probe between two successive minima, a distance equal to $\lambda_g/2$. Now the VSWR is given by

$$\text{VSWR} = \lambda_g / [\pi(x_1 \sim x_2)] \qquad (27.6)$$

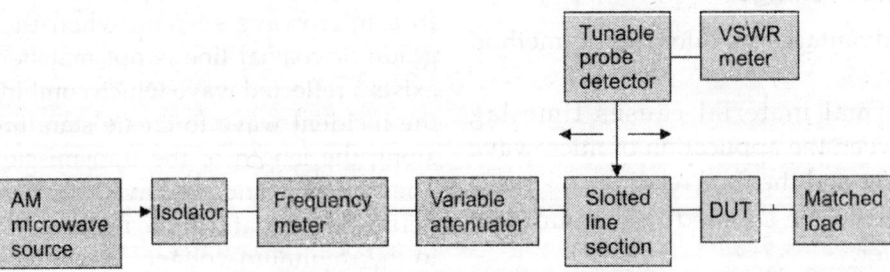

Fig. 27.4: Measurement of low VSWR

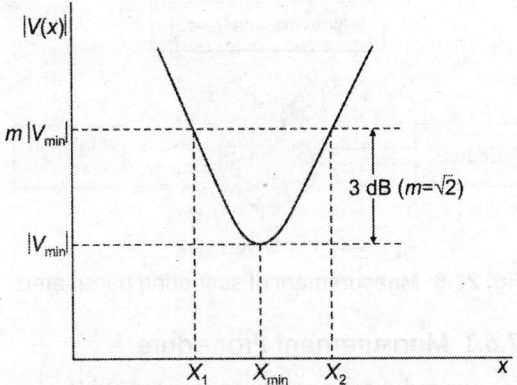

Fig. 27.5: Measurement of high VSWR

27.5 IMPEDANCE MEASUREMENTS

The unknown impedance at microwave frequencies are determined by using

  (i) Slotted line and a probe

  (ii) Network analyzer.

27.5.1 Slotted Line Method

This is the simplest method of measuring unknown impedances at microwave frequencies. The measurement setup is shown in Fig. 27.6. The unknown impedance Z_L is connected at the end of the slotted line. Microwave power is fed from the other end. The unknown impedance reflects a part of this power. The reflection coefficient Γ_L is measured by probing the standing wave fields in the slotted line by suitable arrangement.

The unknown impedance Z_L is given by

$$Z_L = Z_o(1 + \Gamma_L)/(1 - \Gamma_L) \qquad (27.7)$$
$$\Gamma_L = \rho_L \angle \phi_L \qquad (27.8)$$

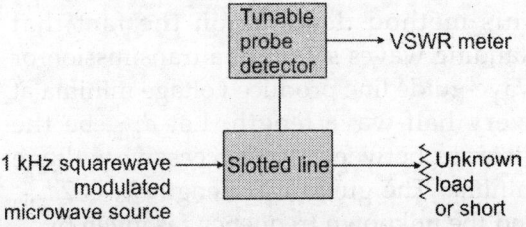

Fig. 27.6: Measurement of impedance by slotted line method

Here Z_o is the characteristic impedance of the transmission line. ρ_L is found from VSWR measurement. Thus

$$\rho_L = (\text{VSWR} - 1)/(\text{VSWR} + 1) \quad (27.9)$$

27.5.1.1 Measurement Procedure

The procedure for measurement of microwave power using slotted line is enumerated below.

1. Determine the unknown load VSWR to find ρ_L from Eq. (27.9).
2. Determine the distance d between two successive voltage minima to find $\lambda_g = 2d$ and $\beta = 2\pi/\lambda_g$.
3. Determine the distance d_{min} of the first voltage minimum from the load end towards the generator end.
4. The phase angle $\phi_L = 2\beta d_{min} - \pi$.
5. The unknown impedance is given by $Z_L = Z_o(1 + \Gamma_L)/(1 - \Gamma_L)$.

27.5.2 Network Analyzer Method

The slotted line method of measuring unknown impedance is time-consuming and does not lend itself for automation. When rapid measurement of impedance over a broad frequency range or variation of impedance with respect to some circuit parameter is to be measured, the network analyzer is more suitable and convenient.

Measurement Procedure

The method is based on the direct measurement of the complex reflection coefficient Γ. Reflection coefficient is defined as the ratio of the reflected wave to the incident wave amplitudes. If the incident wave and the reflected wave are separated and a mechanism is designed to evaluate their complex ratio, the complex impedance can be measured directly. A network analyzer performs these functions. A measurement setup is shown in Fig. 27.7. Two directional couplers are used to sample the incident and reflected

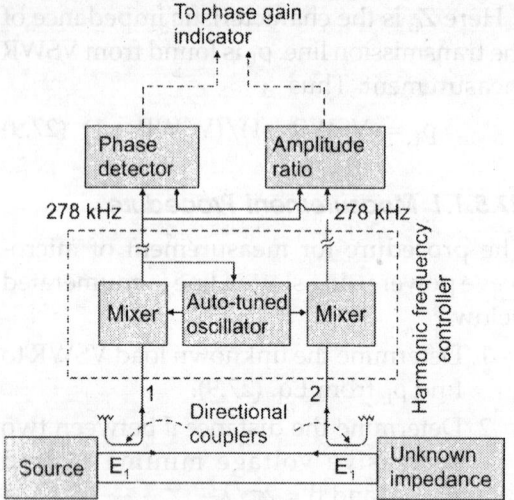

Fig. 27.7: Impedance measurement using network analyzer

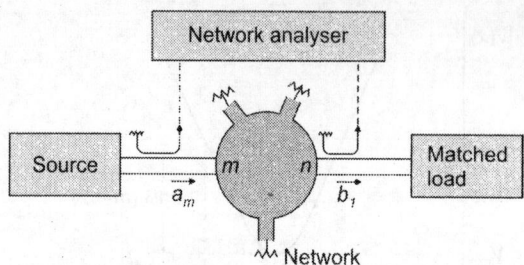

Fig. 27.8: Measurement of scattering parameters

waves. The directional coupler 1 couples a fraction of the incident power to branch 1; and directional coupler 2 feeds a fraction of the reflected power to branch 2. The outputs of these two directional couplers are fed into a harmonic frequency converter. This translates the microwave frequency to a fixed 278 kHz frequency. An auto-tuning local oscillator and two identical mixers are used for this purpose. The frequency conversion is usually carried out in two stages. The two outputs at 278 kHz preserve the relative amplitude and the phase relationship of the incident and the reflected waves at microwave frequency. The amplitude and the phase comparison are carried out at 278 kHz by suitably designed low frequency circuit. The phase and amplitude information are given to the CRO for direct display of the impedance on a Smith chart overlay placed over the CRO screen.

27.6 MEASUREMENT OF SCATTERING PARAMETERS

Scattering parameters are defined as the ratio of the outgoing waves to the incident waves. Thus the scattering parameter S_{nm} is the ratio of b_n to a_m. The setup for measurement of S_{nm} is shown in Fig. 27.8.

27.6.1 Measurement Procedure

The procedure for measurement of scattering parameters is enumerated below.

1. Connect a source to port m and a matched load to port n of the network. These two ports are connected to a network analyzer.

2. Terminate all other ports of the network with matched loads so that all other a's are zeros.

3. The network analyzer indicates the complex value of S_{nm} in terms of amplitude and phase.

27.7 MEASUREMENT OF FREQUENCY

A number of mechanical and electronic techniques are used for the measurement of microwave frequency. The mechanical devices are slotted lines and resonant cavities or wave meters. Both these devices depend on a precise measurement or calibration of physical dimensions for their operation and accuracy. The electronic devices are high frequency heterodyne systems. These devices are very accurate.

27.7.1 Slotted Line Method

This method depends on the fact that standing waves set up in a transmission or wave-guide line produce voltage minima at every half-wave length. Let d_{min} be the distance between two successive voltage minima. The guide wavelength λ_g is $2d_{min}$ and the unknown frequency f is given by

$$f = 30/\lambda_o \qquad (27.10)$$

Here f is in GHz and λ_o is in cm. The wavelength λ_o is given by

$$\lambda_o = \lambda_g \left[1 + \left(\frac{\lambda_g^2}{4a^2} \right) \right]^{-1/2} \quad \text{for waveguide}$$

(27.11)

$$= \lambda_g \sqrt{\varepsilon_r} \quad \text{for coaxial line}$$

(27.12)

The accuracy of measurement is about 1% because the wavelength depends upon the wave-guide dimensions. However, frequency measurement in coaxial system is independent of physical dimensions of the slotted line.

27.7.2 Wave Meter Method

This is the most commonly used method for measuring microwave frequencies. The key element in the wave meter is a cylindrical or coaxial resonant cavity. Fig. 27.9 shows a commonly used frequency meter. An adjustable plunger can be used to vary the cylindrical cavity and can be moved by a calibrated dial knob assembly. The range of the meter depends on the tuning range of the cavity. The cavity is so designed that, for a given position of the plunger, the cavity is resonant

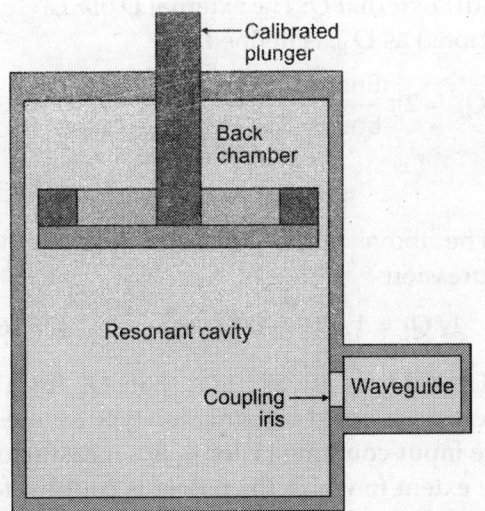

Fig. 27.9: Wave meter method of measuring frequency

at only one frequency in the specified range. The Q-factor of the cavity is made high, as high as 5000.

(i) Measurement Procedure

The cavity is coupled to the waveguide through an iris in the narrow wall of the waveguide. If the unknown frequency of the wave passing through the waveguide is different from the resonant frequency of the wave-guide, the transmission through the wave-guide is not affected. However, if these two frequencies coincide, a resonant field is set up inside the cavity. Because of power loss associated with the cavity, the wave passing through the wave-guide is attenuated by 1 to 3 dB approximately. If an indicating meter such as a VSWR or power meter is connected such that the frequency meter is between the source and the indicating meter, the indicating instrument will show a dip in the reading. The unknown frequency can be read from the calibrated wave meter. Accuracy greater than 0.1% can be obtained in this method.

(ii) Limitations

The limitation of this method is that the frequency meters are usually affected by temperature and humidity. The effects are minimized by using hermitically sealed cavity and special temperature compensating elements.

27.7.3 Heterodyne or Down Conversion Method

The microwave frequency can be measured accurately by this method. Figure 27.10 shows the setup. A heterodyne converter down-converts the unknown microwave frequency f_x by mixing it with an accurately known frequency f_a. The difference frequency $f_{if} = f_x - f_a$ is amplified and measured by the meter. The frequency $f_a = nf_1$ where f_1 is the accurately known input frequency to the harmonic generator that generates a series of harmonics of f_1. The frequency f_1 is

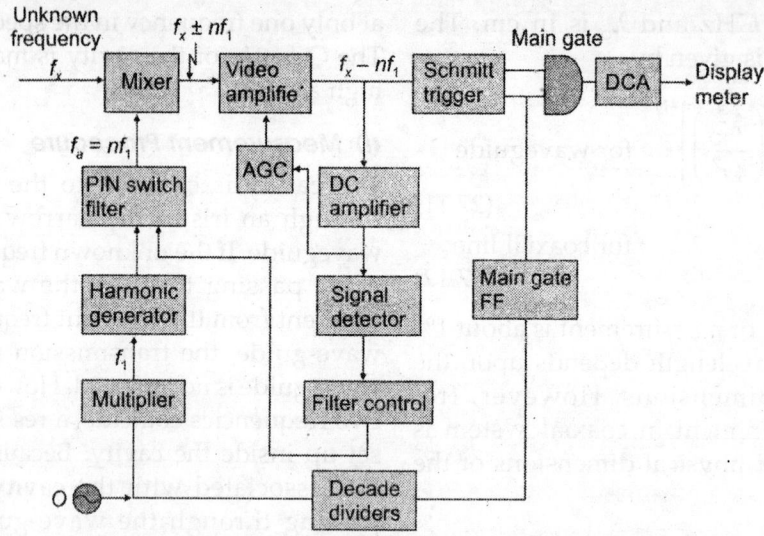

Fig. 27.10: Down conversion method of measuring frequency

a multiple of the local oscillator frequency. The frequency f_a is selected by the tuning cavity such that f_a is added with the meter reading to obtain the unknown frequency f_x. For the range of f_x up to 20 GHz, the frequency f_1 may be from 100 MHz to 500 MHz. For better accuracy, low noise oscillator and noise-less multiplier are employed.

27.8 MEASUREMENT OF CAVITY Q

The accurate measurement of Q at microwave frequencies for cavities having very high Q is very difficult. This is due to the fact that the 3 dB bandwidth of the high Q cavity response curve is a very small fraction of the resonance frequency. Moreover, the cavity gets loaded during measurement and the Q becomes lower.

27.8.1 Definitions of different Qs

There are three different definitions of Q depending on the associated circuits.

(i) **Unloaded** Q: The unloaded Q of a cavity, denoted as Q_o, is defined as

$$Q_o = 2\pi \frac{\text{Energy stored in the cavity}}{\text{Energy lost per cycle in cavity}}$$

(25.13)

Q_o is the selectivity factor of the cavity and depends on the geometrical portion of the cavity.

(ii) **Loaded** Q: The loaded Q of a cavity, denoted as Q_L, is defined as

$$Q_L = 2\pi \frac{\text{Energy stored in the cavity}}{\begin{array}{c}\text{Energy lost per cycle in cavity}\\\text{and external system}\end{array}}$$

(25.14)

(iii) **External** Q: The external Q of a cavity, denoted as Q_E, is defined as

$$Q_E = 2\pi \frac{\text{Energy stored in the cavity}}{\begin{array}{c}\text{Energy lost per cycle in the}\\\text{external system}\end{array}}$$

(25.15)

The above three Q's are related by the expression

$$1/Q_L = 1/Q_o + 1/Q_E$$

(27.16)

Thus, Q_L is always less than Q_o for all aperture-coupled transmission type cavities. The input-coupling factor β_1 is a measure of the extent to which the power is coupled to the cavity and the output-coupling factor β_2 is a measure of the extent to which the power is coupled from the cavity to the output. The two coupling factors are given by

$$\beta_1 = 4/[4S_o - (S_o + 1)^2 T(f_o)] \quad (27.17)$$

$$= 1 \text{ for critical coupling} \quad (27.18)$$

$$< 1 \text{ for under-coupling} \quad (27.19)$$

$$> 1 \text{ for over-coupling} \quad (27.20)$$

$$\beta_2 = \beta_1 S_o - 1 \quad (27.21)$$

Here S_o is the VSWR at resonance frequency f_o.

$$T(f_o) = P_{out}/P_{in} \quad (27.22)$$

Here $T(f_o)$ is the transmission loss at f_o. The relationship between loaded and unloaded Q of the cavity is given by

$$Q_o = Q_L (1 + \beta_1 + \beta_2) \quad (27.23)$$

Measurement of both $T(f_o)$ and at S_o resonance are necessary for calculating β_1 and β_2 and determining Q_o. We shall describe below a few methods of determining Q of a cavity resonator.

27.8.2 Slotted Line Method

Figure 27.11 shows the setup for measurement of the Q of a reflection type cavity. This type of cavity is commonly used in a microwave tube. In this method, the VSWR of the cavity is measured at the resonant frequency f_o and the two half-power frequencies f_1 and f_2. The VSWR of terminating

impedance Z_{in} in a lossless line of Z_o is given by

$$S = [\,|Z_{in} + Z_o| + |Z_{in} - Z_o|\,]/$$
$$[\,|Z_{in} + Z_o| - |Z_{in} - Z_o|\,] \quad (27.24)$$

Figure 27.12 shows the equivalent circuit of a cavity in the vicinity of the resonant frequency. Therefore, we assume that the line is terminated with $Z_{in} = R + jX$. Since $X = 0$ at f_o, Eq.(27.24) becomes

$$S_o = R/Z_o \quad \text{if } R > Z_o \quad (27.25)$$

$$= Z_o/R \quad \text{if } R < Z_o \quad (27.26)$$

At half power frequencies, f_1 and f_2 of the unloaded cavity, $X = R$. Hence

$$S_1 = (a + b)/(a - b) \quad (27.27)$$

Here $\quad a = \sqrt{(R + Z_o)^2 + R^2}$

and $\quad b = \sqrt{(R - Z_o)^2 + R^2}$

Since the factor inside the radical is small, we can show that

$$S_1 = S_o + \frac{1}{2S_o} + \sqrt{S_o^2 + \left(\frac{1}{4S_o^2}\right)} ; R > Z_o \quad (27.28)$$

$$= \frac{1}{S_o} + \left(\frac{S_o}{2}\right) + \sqrt{\frac{1}{S_o^2} + \left(\frac{S_o^2}{4}\right)} ; R < Z_o \quad (27.29)$$

From the above measurement, the unloaded Q can be determined as

$$Q_o = f_o/(f_2 - f_1) \quad (27.30)$$

For the loaded cavity, the resistance R in Eq. (27.27) should be taken as the sum of

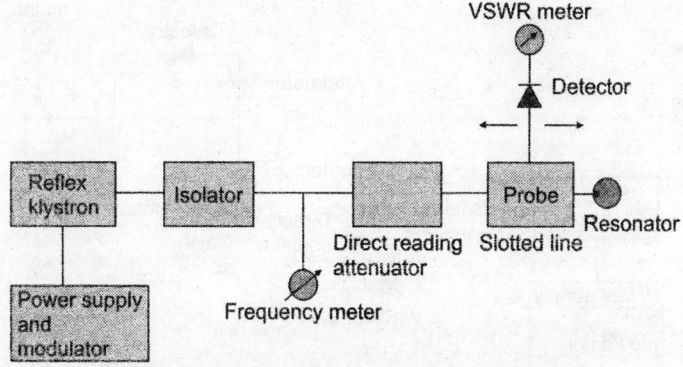

Fig. 27.11: Slotted line method of measuring Q

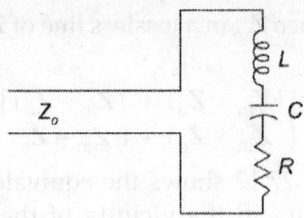

Fig. 27.12: Equivalent circuit of a cavity

equivalent resonator resistance and equivalent load resistance. Thus, Eq. (27.27) equally applies for loaded or unloaded resonators. However, the value of S_o and $(f_2 - f_1)$ increase resulting in lower value of Q.

27.8.3 Transmitted Power Method

This method can be used for both transmission and reflection type cavities for determining loaded Q. In this method, the power transmitted through the cavity as a function of frequency is measured. Figure 27.13 shows the setup for determining loaded Q. The RF signal is square-wave modulated and a VSWR is used at the output of the square-law detector to indicate the transmitted power at the resonance frequency f_0 and half-power frequencies $f_o \pm (\Delta f/2)$. Then, Q is given by $f_0/\Delta f$. In order to avoid error due to non-square-law response of the crystal detector at different power levels, a calibrated attenuator is used to keep the input power level low and the same in all measurements.

27.8.4 Errors in Measurement

In this method of measurement, the common errors are:

1. Departure from square-law behaviour of the probe.
2. Frequency instability of the probe.
3. Microwave generator mismatch.
4. Probe and generator interaction at high VSWR.

27.9 MEASUREMENT OF DIELECTRIC CONSTANT

The dielectric constant ε_r of a material is defined as the ratio of the permittivity of the material ε to that of the air or free space ε_o. Thus,

$$\varepsilon_r = \varepsilon/\varepsilon_o \qquad (27.31)$$

Here $\varepsilon_o = (10^{-9}/36\pi)$ farad per meter. The dielectric constant is a complex quantity because of the dielectric loss due to non-zero conductivity. Therefore, it may be represented as

$$\varepsilon_r = \varepsilon_r' + j\varepsilon_r'' \qquad (27.32)$$

The loss tangent tan δ is given by

$$\tan \delta = \varepsilon_r''/\varepsilon_r' \qquad (27.33)$$

The measurement of the dielectric constant is important not only in scientific applications but also for industrial applications such as microwave ovens and to study the biological effect of microwaves.

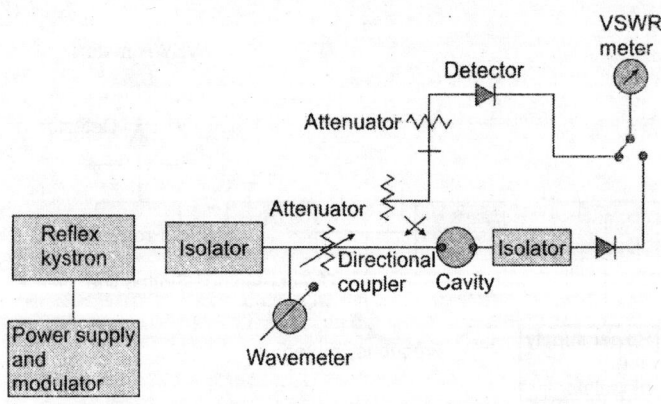

Fig. 27.13: Transmitted power method of measuring Q

The dielectric constant ε_r is frequency dependent. However, it may be considered to be constant over a wide frequency band for most microwave applications. On the other hand, the percent variation in ε_r'' is always greater than ε_r'. Hence ε_r'' should be measured at or near the frequency of interest.

There are several methods available for measurement of dielectric constant. The waveguide method alone is described below.

27.9.1 Waveguide Method

In the waveguide method, the dielectric material is assumed to be lossless. Figure 27.14 shows the waveguide method of the mea-suring dielectric constant. The length *AB* of the waveguide is completely filled with the dielectric sample. The end is terminated with a short as shown. Let a voltage standing wave minimum be observed in the slotted line at *C*. Let

$l_e = AB$

= length of the dielectric sample

$l_o = BC$

= the voltage minimum distance from *B*

Then, $AC = AB + BC = l_e + l_o$ (27.34)

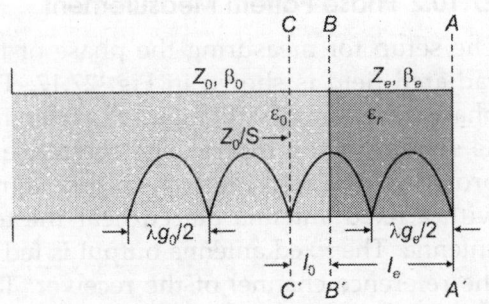

Fig. 27.14: Waveguide method of of measuring dielectric constant

Looking from the plane at *C* towards the right and left, the impedance equation is given by

$Z_o \tan \beta_o l_o = -Z_e \tan \beta_e l_e$ (27.35)

Here Z_o and Z_e are the characteristic impedances, and β_o and β_e are the propagation constants of the empty and filled waveguide respectively.

Assuming that the dielectric is non-magnetic, we have

$Z_o / Z_e = \beta_e / \beta_o$ (27.36)

or $Z_o = Z_e \beta_e / \beta_o$ (27.37)

Substituting Eq. (27.37) in Eq. (27.35), we get

$$\frac{Z_e \beta_e \tan \beta_o l_o}{\beta_o} = -Z_e \tan \beta_e l_e$$ (27.38)

The above equation may be written as

$$\frac{l_o \tan \beta_o l_o}{(\beta_o l_o)} = -\frac{l_e \tan \beta_e l_e}{(\beta_e l_e)}$$ (27.39)

or, $\left(\dfrac{l_o}{l_e}\right)\left[\dfrac{(\tan Y)}{Y}\right] = -\left(\dfrac{\tan X}{X}\right)$ (27.40)

Here $X = b_e l_e$

and $Y = b_o l_o$.

For the dominant mode,

$\beta_o = 2\pi / \lambda_{go}$ (27.41)

$\lambda_{go} = 2 d_{min}$ (27.42)

Here d_{min} is the distance between successive voltage minimum points. d_{min} can be measured by a slotted line. l_o and l_e are read from the slotted line. Hence the left hand side Eq.(27.40) is known and let its value be α. Then

$(\tan X)/X = -\alpha$ (27.43)

The above equation is solved to obtain $X = \beta_e l_e$.

The propagation constant β_e is given by

$$\beta_e = 2\pi / \lambda_{ge}$$

$$= (2\pi / \lambda_o)\sqrt{\varepsilon_r - (l_o / \lambda_c)^2}$$ (27.44)

Here $\lambda_c = 2a$ is the cut-off wavelength and a is the dimension of the wave-guide broad wall. Since β_e is known, ε_r can be determined from the above equation. This equation has an infinite number of solutions for ε_r. Hence

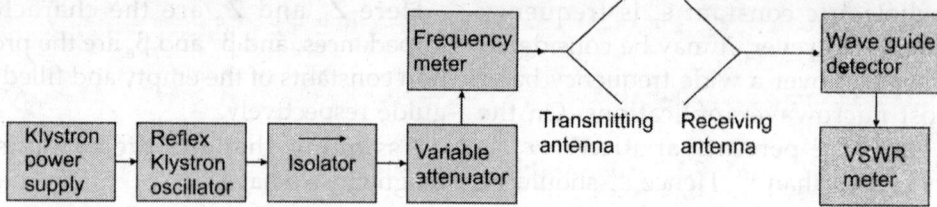

Fig. 27.15: Radiation pattern measurement

measurements are taken for two different lengths of the sample. Let the two lengths be l_e and l'_e. Then, we get two equations of the form of Eq. (27.44). The two equations are solved and the desired value of ε_r is the solution that is common for both the sample length.

27.10 MEASUREMENT OF ANTENNA PARAMETERS

The most important parameters of the microwave antenna are radiation amplitude pattern, phase pattern, gain, directivity and bandwidth.

27.10.1 Radiation Amplitude Pattern Measurement

A short dipole antenna radiates equal power in all directions and is known as *isotropic radiator*. But a practical antenna like horn does not radiate equal power in all directions. The field strength or the power intensity as a function of the elevation angle θ and the azimuth angle φ at a constant distance from the radiating antenna is known as *the radiation pattern of the transmitting antenna*. Due to the reciprocal properties of antennas, the test antenna is placed in the receiving mode and the measurements are carried out. Figure 27.15 shows the setup for determining the radiation pattern. Initially, the two antennas are aligned in line of their maximum radiation direction by adjusting the angle and height. The distance between the antennas should be greater than $2D^2/\lambda_o$ where D is the maximum size of the aperture. The microwave source is switched on and

suitable power level is obtained in the meter. The received power is recorded. The transmitting antenna is rotated in step of 5° on both the sides and the received power is recorded. The polar plot of the received power gives the radiation pattern. A typical radiation pattern is shown in Fig. 27.16.

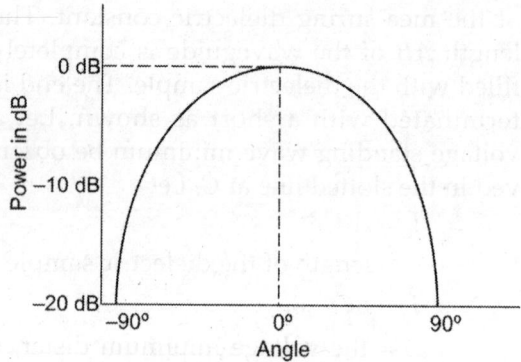

Fig. 27.16: Typical radiation pattern

27.10.2 Phase Pattern Measurement

The setup for measuring the phase of the radiated field is shown in Fig. 27.17. The phase is measured with respect to a reference as shown in the figure. The reference is provided by receiving transmitted signal with a fixed antenna placed near the test antenna. The fixed antenna output is fed to the reference channel of the receiver. The phase pattern is recorded as the antenna under test is rotated in step of 5° in the horizontal plane.

27.10.3 Beamwidth Measurement

The radiation pattern of the test antenna is determined and plotted as shown in

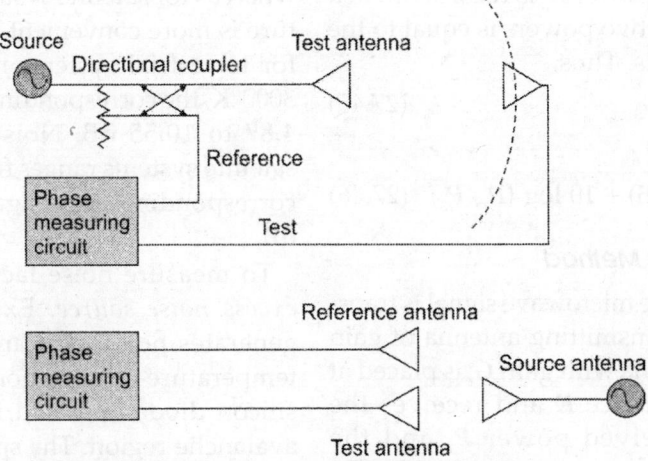

Fig. 27.17: Measurement of phase pattern

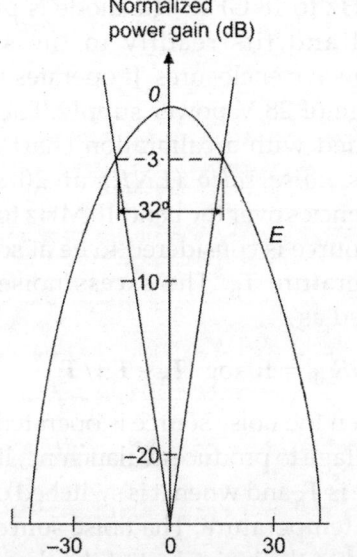

Fig. 27.18: Measurement of beam width

Fig. 27.18. The beam width of the antenna is the angle θ subtended by the 3 dB points on both sides of the maximum radiation in the main beam.

27.10.4 Gain Measurement

The gain of an antenna is the most important parameter because it is used directly in the microwave link calculations. To determine the gain of the antenna, two methods are described below.

(i) Standard Antenna Method

Figure 27.19 shows the setup for the gain measurement. This method uses two set of measurements; one with the test antenna and the other with a standard antenna. The test antenna with gain G_r is used in the receiving mode and the received power P_r is recorded. Without changing the transmitted power and geometrical configuration, the test antenna is replaced by a standard antenna of gain G_s

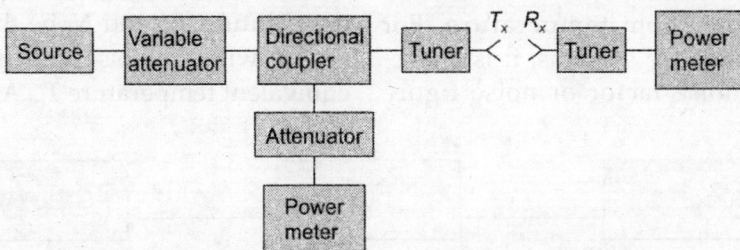

Fig. 27.19: Measurement of gain by standard antenna method

and the received power P_s is recorded. Then the ratio of these two powers is equal to the ratio of their gains. Thus,

$$P_r/P_s = G_r/G_s \qquad (27.45)$$

Hence,

$$G_r(dB) = G_s(dB) + 10 \log (P_r/P_s) \quad (27.46)$$

(ii) Two Antenna Method

In this method, the microwave signal is transmitted from a transmitting antenna of gain G_t. The test antenna with gain G_r is placed at the far-field distance R and receives the signal. The received power P_r and the transmitted power P_t are measured. The received power P_r is given by

$$P_r = P_t G_t G_r \lambda^2/(4\pi R)^2 \qquad (27.47)$$

Hence,

$$G_r(dB) + G_t(dB) = 20 \log (4\pi R/\lambda) + 10 \log (P_r/P_t) \qquad (27.48)$$

If the two identical antennas are used, the $G_t = G_r$. Hence,

$$G(dB) = G_r(dB) = G_t(dB)$$
$$= 10 \log (4\pi R/\lambda) + 5 \log(P_r/P_t) \qquad (27.49)$$

By measuring R, λ, G_t and P_r, the gain G is obtained.

27.11 MEASUREMENT OF NOISE FACTOR

In an earlier chapter, we have studied that the noise factor F and noise temperature T_e are used to specify the noise performance of an amplifier or any two port network. They are related as

$$T_e = (F - 1) T_o \qquad (27.50)$$

where T_o is the room temperature. For terrestrial microwave systems, it is convenient to use noise factor or noise figure whereas for satellite systems, noise temperature is more convenient. Noise temperature for terrestrial systems ranges from 800 to 3000°K, the corresponding noise figure being 4.87 to 10.55 dB. Noise temperature for satellite systems ranges from 35 to 120°K, the corresponding noise figure being 0.5 to 1.5 dB.

To measure noise factor, we require an *excess noise source*. Excess noise source generates noise over and above the room temperature thermal noise. This source is a silicon diode operated in the reverse bias avalanche region. The spontaneous generation of charge results in wideband noise covering the frequency spectrum from 10 MHz to 18 GHz. The diode is physically small and fits readily in the standard microwave enclosures. It operates from low voltage of 28 V power supply. Each source supplied with a calibration chart showing *excess noise ratio (ENR)* at 20 selected frequencies over the band 10 MHz to 18 GHz. The source is considered to be at some high temperature T_h. The excess noise ratio is defined as

$$ENR_{dB} = 10 \log (T_h - T_o)/T_o \qquad (27.51)$$

When the noise source is operated at rated dc voltage to produce avalanching, its temperature is T_h and when it is switched off, it is at room temperature. The noise source is connected to the input port of the device under test *(DUT)* and a power meter is connected at the output as shown in Fig. 27.20.

Let N_2 be the noise power output with the noise source on and at the equivalent temperature T_h, and N_1 be the noise power output with the noise source off and at the equivalent temperature T_o. Assume T_e is the

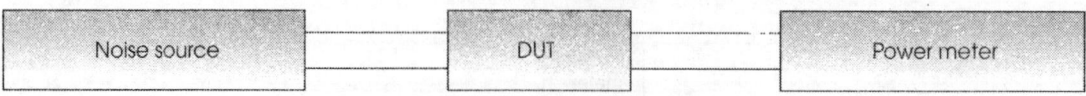

Fig. 27.20: Noise factor measurement

noise temperature of the device under test. Then,

$$N_2 = k (T_h + T_e) B \qquad (27.52)$$

$$N_1 = k (T_o + T_e) B \qquad (27.53)$$

Then, Y is defined as

$$Y = N_2/N_1 = (T_h + T_e)/(T_o + T_e) \qquad (27.54)$$

Solving for T_e in terms of Y, we obtain

$$T_e = (T_h - YT_o)/(Y-1) \qquad (27.55)$$

Using the calibration chart supplied with the noise generator, T_h is determined from Eq. (27.51). With this T_h and measured value of Y, T_e is calculated from Eq. (27.55). Then, F is obtained from Eq. (27.50).

27.12 NUMERICAL EXAMPLES

Example 27.1 The signal power at the input device is 20 mW and the output is 0.40 mW. Calculate the insertion loss in dB.

Solution: P_i =20 mW, P_o = 0.4 mW

The insertion loss is given by

$$IL = 10 \log P_o/P_i$$

$$= 10 \log (0.4/20)$$

$$= -16.99 \text{ dB}$$

Example 27.2 A crystal detector generates a signal of 10 mV when the incident power is – 20 dBm. Find the detector sensitivity in mV/mW.

Solution: Given:

$$V_s = 10 \text{ mV},$$

$$10 \log P_{mw}/1 \text{mW} = -20;$$

$$P_{mW} = 10^{-2} \text{ mW}$$

Detector sensitivity

$$V_s/P_{mW} = 10/10^{-2} = 10^3 \text{ mV/mW}.$$

Example 27.3 A rectangular pulse of width 1 ms modulates a microwave signal. If the average power is 100 mW and the pulse repetition frequency is 400 pps, compute the peak power.

Solution: Given: Pulse width = 1 μs, P_{av} = 100 mW, prf = 400

$$P_{peak} = P_{av}/\text{Duty cycle};$$

Duty cycle = Pulse width × prf

$$= 1 \times 10^{-6} \times 400$$

$$= 4 \times 10^{-4}$$

$$P_{peak} = 100/4 \times 10^{-4}$$

$$= 25 \times 10^4$$

$$= 250 \text{ W}.$$

Example 27.4 Measurement of noise figure using excess noise source resulted in $Y = 4.91$ dB with an ENR of 5.83 dB. Assuming T_o to be 300°K, find (a) the noise figure in dB and (ii) the equivalent noise temperature.

Solution: Given: $Y = 4.91$ dB $= 10^{4.91/10} = 3.1$, ENR = 5.83 dB, $T_o = 300°K$

(a) Noise factor is given by

$$F = 10^{ENR/10}/(Y-1)$$

$$= 10^{5.83/10}/(3.1 - 1)$$

$$= 3.83/2.1 = 1.826$$

$$\therefore \quad F_{dB} = 10 \log F = 10 \log 1.826$$

$$= 2.61 \text{ dB}$$

(b) The equivalent noise temperature

$$T_e = (F-1)T_o = (1.826 - 1) \times 300$$

$$= 247.8°K$$

Example 27.5: The noise temperature of an amplifier is known to lie in the range 60 to 120°K. Find the range expected for Y in dB when an excess noise source with an ENR of 6.02 dB is used to measure the noise temperature. Assume $T_o = 290°K$.

Solution: Given: $T_e = 60$ to 120°K, ENR = 6.02 dB, $T_o = 290°K$

$$Y = (T_h + T_e)/(T_e + T_o)$$

$$ENR = 6.02 \text{ dB}$$

$$\therefore (T_h - T_o)/T_o = 10^{6.02/10}$$

$$= 4.17$$

$$T_h = 4.17 \times T_o + T_o$$

$$= 1209.3 + 290$$

$$= 1499.3°K$$

(a) For $T_e = 60$:

$$Y = (1499.3 + 60)/(60 + 290)$$

$$= 1559.3/350 = 4.46$$

$$= \textbf{6.49 dB}$$

(b) For $T_e = 120$:

$$Y = (1499.3 + 120)/(120 + 290)$$

$$= 1619.3/410 = 3.95$$

$$= \textbf{5.97 dB}$$

The range of Y is 5.97 to 6.49 dB.

KEY POINTS

- The measurement of power at microwave frequencies is classified into (i) very low power ($P < 1$ mW), (ii) low power (1 mW $< P < 10$ mW), (iii) medium high power (10 mW $< P < 10$ W) and (iv) high power ($P > 10$ W).

- A microwave thermocouple instrument is used to measure very low power. Bolometers are used to measure low microwave power. Calorimeter techniques are used to measure medium and high power.

- The common errors in power measurement are: (i) instrumental error, (ii) Substitution error and (iii) Mount inefficiency error.

- The instrumental error is minimized by maintaining the stability of bias sources and by the degree of ambient temperature compensation.

- The measurement of VSWR is divided into the following two categories: (i) Low VSWR (S < 10) and (ii) High VSWR (S > 10)

- The unknown impedance at microwave frequencies determined by using (i) slotted line and a probe and (ii) Network analyzer.

- Scattering parameters are measured using network analyzer.

- The unknown impedance at microwave frequencies can be determined by using (i) slotted line and a probe and (ii) Network analyzer.

- Frequency is measured using (i) slotted line, (ii) wave meter and (iii) Heterodyne or Down Conversion Method.

- Q of the cavity is measured by (i) slotted line method and (ii) transmitted power method.

- Dielectric constant is measured by wave-guide method.

- Noise factor is measured using an excess noise source.

FURTHER READING

1. Montgomery CG (1947). *Technique of Micro-wave Measurements*, McGraw Hill, NY.
2. Ginzton EL (1957). *Microwave Measurements*, McGraw Hill, NY.
3. Sucher M and Fox J (1963). *Handbook of Microwave Measurements*, Vol. I, John Wiely, NY.

REVIEW QUESTIONS

27.1 Mention the categories of microwave power measurements.

27.2 Mention the sensor used for very low microwave power measurements.

27.3 Mention the sensor used for low microwave power measurements.

27.4 Mention the sensor for high microwave power measurements.

27.5 Mention the errors in microwave power measurements.

27.6 What are the limitations of power measurements using Wheatstone bridge?

27.7 Define the return loss.

27.8 Define the insertion loss.

27.9 Define the reflection loss.

27.10 Define the transmission loss or attenuation.

27.11 Mention the two classifications of VSWR measurement.

27.12 What are the limitations in low VSWR measurement?

27.13 Mention the methods used for impedance measurement.

27.14 Compare the impedance measurement using slotted line and spectrum analyzer.

27.15 Mention the errors in impedance measurement.

27.16 Mention the methods used for frequency measurement.

27.17 Define unloaded, loaded and external Q of a cavity resonator. Give the relationship among them.

27.18 What are the errors in cavity Q measurement?

27.19 Mention the important antenna parameters to be measured.

27.20 Define the radiation pattern of an antenna.

27.21 Define the phase pattern of an antenna.

27.22 Define the gain of an antenna.

27.23 Define the beam width of an antenna.

27.24 Mention the two methods used for antenna gain measurement.

27.25 Why is the microwave signal amplitude modulated before applying to the detector?

DESCRIPTIVE QUESTIONS

27.1 Describe with a neat block diagram, the measurement of very low microwave power.

27.2 Describe with a neat block diagram, the measurement of low microwave power.

27.3 Describe, with a neat block diagram, the measurement of microwave medium and high power.

27.4 Explain in detail, the measurement of losses in microwave networks.

27.5 Explain, with a neat block diagram, the measurement of low VSWR.

27.6 Explain, with a neat block diagram, the measurement of high VSWR.

27.7 Explain the double minima method of measuring VSWR.

27.8 Explain, with a neat block diagram, the measurement of impedance by slotted line method.

27.9 Explain, with a neat block diagram, the measurement of impedance by network analyzer.

27.10 Explain, with a neat block diagram, the measurement of scattering parameters.

27.11 Explain, with a neat block diagram, the measurement of frequency by slotted line method.

27.12 Explain, with a neat block diagram, the measurement of frequency by wave meter method.

27.13 Explain, with a neat block diagram, the measurement of frequency by heterodyne method.

27.14 Explain, with a neat block diagram, the measurement of cavity Q by slotted line method.

27.15 Explain, with a neat block diagram, the measurement of cavity Q by transmitted power method.

27.16 Explain, with a neat block diagram, the measurement of dielectric constant of a dielectric sample by wave-guide method.

27.17 Explain, with a neat block diagram, the measurement of radiation pattern.

27.18 Explain, with a neat block diagram, the measurement of phase pattern.

27.19 Explain, with a neat block diagram, the measurement of gain of an antenna.

27.20 Explain, with a neat block diagram, the measurement of beam width of an antenna.

27.21 Explain the method of measuring noise factor of a transistor.

PRACTICE PROBLEMS

27.1 The signal power at the input device is 10 mW and the output is 0.30 mW. Calculate the insertion loss in dB.
[**Ans:** –15.23 dB]

27.2 A crystal detector generates a signal of 10 mV when the incident power is –25 dBm. Find the detector sensitivity in mV/mW.
[**Ans:** 3.162×10^3 mV/mW]

27.3 A rectangular pulse of width 1 µs modulates a microwave signal. If the average power is 200 mW and the pulse repetition frequency is 500 pps, compute the peak power.
[**Ans:** 400 W]

27.4 Measurement of noise figure using excess noise source resulted in Y = 4.91 dB with an ENR of 5.83 dB. Assuming T_0 to be 290°K, find (a) the noise figure in dB and (ii) the equivalent noise temperature.
(**Ans:** 2.61 dB, 239.5°K)

27.5 The noise temperature of an amplifier is known to lie in the range 100 to 200°K. Find the range expected for Y in dB when an excess noise source with an ENR of 6.02 dB is used to measure the noise temperature. Assume T_0 = 300°K.
(**Ans:** 5 to 6.15 dB)

REFERENCE

1. Lebedev I (1973). *Microwave Engineering*, MIR Publications, Moscow.

2. Collins RE (1996). *Foundations of Microwave Engineering*, McGraw Hill, NY.

3. Reich HJ (1978). *Microwave Principles*, East-West, New Delhi.

4. Barrington AE and Rees JR (1958). A Simple 3-cm Q-meter, Proc. IRE, vol.105, pp 511–512. November.

5. Surber WH Jr and Crouch GE Jr (1948). Dielectric measurement methods for solid at microwave frequencies, *J. Appl. Phy.*, Vol. 19, No. 12, December.

6. Dechamp GA (1953). Determination of reflection coefficient and insertion loss of a wave-guide junction, *J. Appl. Phy.*, vol. 28, pp 1046–1050.

7. Lebedev I (1973). *Microwave Engineering*, MIR Publications, Moscow.

8. Ginzton EL (1957). *Microwave Measurements*, McGraw Hill, NY.

Microwave Radiation Hazards

- Understand the features of MW radiation.
- Know the biological effects of radiation.
- Explain the MW hazard levels and protection.

28.1 INTRODUCTION

Microwaves are used for domestic cooking, industrial heating and drying as well as scientific and defense applications. Hence, the personnel are exposed to microwave radiation. It may cause damage to biological systems. Though researchers have carried out extensive studies on microwave bio-effects, no conclusive cause has been so far established for causing biological damage.

Any dielectric material, with some conductivity and relative permittivity greater than unity, absorbs microwave radiation and dissipates this as heat. Biological substances such as blood, bone, brain matter, muscle and fat are affected by excessive microwave radiation.

In this chapter, we shall discuss some of these effects and the preventive measures against excessive radiation exposure.

28.2 FEATURES OF MICROWAVE RADIATION

The important features of microwave radiation are described below.

(i) Microwave radiation must be distingui-

shed carefully from the ionizing radiation or radioactivity. Ionizing radiation causes cellular damage whereas microwave radiation produces molecular vibrations.

(ii) Wavelengths at microwave frequencies are of the same order of magnitude as the dimensions of the human body. In many cases, a close coupling exists between the microwave field and the body. Hence, the body absorbs large amount of microwave energy and the heat generated may cause severe damage.

(iii) Biological damage is directly related to the microwave electric field.

(iv) Microwave effects are not cumulative unless permanent damage has already been caused by previous exposures.

(v) Generally, microwave effects are reversible. When the microwave radiation is removed, the system returns to normal.

28.3 MICROWAVE RADIATION LEVELS

Microwave radiation generates heat under the skin without any tanning effect whereas the sunshine generates heat on the surface of the skin with tanning effect. The most widely used parameter to measure microwave radiation is the *average power density*. Table 28.1 shows some typical average power density levels.

Table 28.1: Typical average power density levels

Sunshine on warm days	100 mW/cm²
At 12 GHz satellite antenna trailer unit	32 mW/cm²
Microwave oven	1 mW/cm²
Warmth sensation threshold (1 sec. Exposure at 3 GHz)	58.6 mW/cm²
Threshold of pain (20 sec. exposure at 3 GHz)	3.1 mW/cm²

The average power density for a plane, sinusoidal TEM wave in free space is given by

$$P_D = EH \qquad (28.1)$$

where

E is the rms electric field strength in V/m,
H is the rms magnetic field strength in A/m.

The electric and magnetic fields are related by the expression

$$E = Z_o H = 377\, H \qquad (28.2)$$

where Z_o is the free space wave impedance and is equal to 377 ohms. Hence, average power density is given by

$$P_D = EH = E^2/377 \qquad (28.3)$$
$$= 377\, H^2 \qquad (28.4)$$

In practice, the electric field is measured and P_D is calculated. Unfortunately, most hazardous fields are more complicated than the simple plane sinusoidal wave. Some of the factors that give rise to complicated fields are:

(i) Standing waves
(ii) Near fields
(iii) Polarization
(iv) Modulation

28.3.1 Standing Waves

Incident waves are reflected by nearby objects, surfaces, field-personnel and measuring probes. The reflected waves in combination with the incident wave produce standing waves. In the presence of standing waves, the electric field strength can be high at the maxima while, in the same region, the average power density can be low or even zero.

28.3.2 Near Fields

Near fields exist which alternately store and return the energy to the source similar to the electric field of a capacitor and the magnetic field of an inductor. The electric field strength may be high even with low radiated power density.

28.3.3 Polarization

In many cases, the total electric field is a combination of waves with different polarization. As an example, leakage from vertical and horizontal cracks in a microwave oven can combine and produce complex polarization.

28.3.4 Modulation

Amplitude modulation may occur in many ways. Very high peak fields of short duration can occur in pulsed radars. Rotating antennas will also cause effective amplitude modulation at a fixed location. The stirrers in microwave ovens may cause amplitude modulation.

28.4 BIOLOGICAL INTERACTIONS

Because of the above complications, maximum permissible exposure levels in protection standards are more involved. Table 28.2 shows the exposure standards in force in various countries. In case of the complicated nature of the electric fields, the parameters used in connection with this are:

(i) Penetration depth
(ii) Specific absorption rate

Table 28.2: USSR, US, Canada, and Sweden Exposure Standards [5]

Standard	Type	Frequency	Exposure limit	Duration	CW/Pulsed
USSR Govt. 1977	Occupational	10–30 MHz	20 V/m	Working day	Both
		30–50 MHz	10 V/m	Working day	Both
			0.3 A/m	Working day	Both
		50–300 MHz	5 V/m	Working day	Both
		0.3–300 GHz	10 μW/cm²	Working day	Both
			100 μW/cm²	Working day	Both
			100 μW/cm²	2 hours	Both
			1 mW/cm²	2 hours	Both
			1 mW/cm²	20 mins	Both
USSR Govt. 1970	General public	0.3–300 GHz	1 μW/cm²	24 hours	Both
US ANSI 1974	Occupational	10 MHz–100 GHz	10 mW/cm²	No limit	CW
			20 V/m	8 hours	CW
			0.5 A/m	8 hours	CW
			1 m W/cm²	0.1 hour	Pulsed
US Army and Air Force 1965	Occupational	10 MHz–300 GHz	10 mW/cm²	No limit	Both
US Industrial Hygientist 1971	Occupational	100 MHz–100 GHz	10 mW/cm²	8 hours	Both
			25 mW/cm²	10 min.	Both
Canada Can. Std. Asso. 1966	Occupational	10 MHz–100 GHz	10 mW/cm²	No limit	CW
			1 mW/cm²	0.1 hour	Pulsed
Sweden Worker Protection Authority	Occupational	0.3–300 GHz	1 mW/cm²	8 hours	Both
		10–300 MHz	5 mW/cm²	8 hours	Both
		100 MHz–300 GHz	25 mW/cm²	Any	CW, pulsed averaged over 1 sec

28.4.1 Penetration Depth

Penetration or skin depth is defined as the depth at which the electric field has dropped to e^{-1} of its maximum value. The electric field decays exponentially with distance and is given by

$$E_x = E_0 e^{-x/D} \qquad (28.5)$$

Here, E_x is the field strength at position x within the medium, E_0 is the maximum field strength and D is the penetration or skin depth. Penetration depth is a function of frequency. The dielectric constant and conductivity of the fat are less than those of blood or muscle. Hence, the penetration depth for fat is much greater than that in blood or muscle. The power dissipated in fat is much greater and the wave is rapidly attenuated with increased penetration depth.

28.4.2 Specific Absorption Rate (SAR)

Specific absorption rate is defined as the power absorbed per unit mass of substance and is given by

$$\text{SAR} = \sigma E^2 / m_d \ \text{W/kg} \qquad (28.6)$$

where σ is the conductivity of the material in S/m, E is the rms electric field strength within the material in V/m and m_d is the mass density of the material in kg/m³. While computing SAR, two important effects occur. They are (a) hot spots and (b) body size and orientation.

(a) *Hot Spots:* When the dielectric constant within the body is higher, microwave penetration generates *hot spots* due to the focusing action of the high dielectric constant and the shape of body cavities formed by the bones. Computer simulation studies have shown that the hot spots occur inside the human skull in the frequency range of 918 to 2450 MHz and for within the eyeball they occur at about 1500 MHz.

(b) **Body Size and Orientation:** In determining the SAR, the variations in body size and orientation in relation to frequency are important. The average SAR peaks at 0.8 W/kg for rats at 700 MHz, while for human beings it is 0.03 W/kg for an incident power density of 1 mW/cm^2. At 70 MHz, the average SAR peaks at 0.25 W/kg for human beings; at this frequency the average height of a person is approximated to half wavelength.

28.5 INTERACTIVE MECHANISMS

The interactive mechanisms are grouped as
  (i) Thermal effects
  (ii) Micro-thermal effects

28.5.1 Thermal Effects

The biological materials absorb microwave energy and heat is generated. The rate at which the temperature changes is given by

$$dT/dt = Q/s_h \ °C/s \qquad (28.7)$$

where T is the temperature in °C. The heat Q produced per unit mass is given by

$$Q = SAR + W_M - W_L \qquad (28.8)$$

where

W_M is the metabolic rate of heat production per unit mass in W/kg

W_L is the rate of heat loss per unit mass in W/kg

s_h is the specific heat of the material in kcal/kg·°C

When the rise in temperature is known, then, the SAR can be calculated from

$$SAR = 4185 \ s_h \ dT/dt \ \ W/kg \qquad (28.9)$$

When SAR is high, the temperature initially increases rapidly over a period of a few minutes. Then, the thermoregulatory system of the body functions to stabilize the temperature and to reduce it through vasodilation. However, if the thermoregulatory system is not able to remove the excess heat at the rate it is produced, the temperature of the body again increases. This may lead to collapse due to *hypothermia*. Figure 28.1 shows the temperature variations in a dog subjected to a steady microwave radiation.

When SAR is low, the metabolic rate of heat generation automatically reduces to compensate for the additional SAR component. As a result, the subject appears to suffer from general lethargy and loss of appetite.

28.5.2 Microthermal Mechanism

In this case, the body temperature rise is very small, of the order of a few microdegrees in very short duration of a few microseconds. This causes microwave heating. The microthermal mechanism occurs in the brain matter and sets up a pressure wave. This reaches the cochlea through bone conduction and generates audible clicks and buzzes.

28.6 BIOLOGICAL EFFECTS

The biological effects are extremely temperature sensitive and it is difficult to separate the thermal effects from other effects. Table 28.3 shows the range of effects studied due to exposure to microwaves. When small animals are exposed to low-level microwave radiation, certain changes occur in the blood and the blood does not return to normal even after several months. This effect of microwaves on blood is known as *hematopoiesis*. Blood changes also occur in groups of workers occupationally exposed to low and medium level radiation.

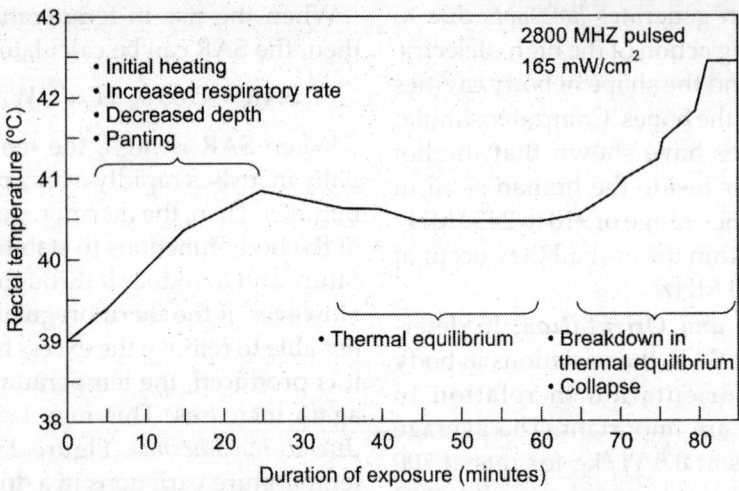

Fig. 28.1: Temperature variations with exposure time

Table 28.3: Microwave exposure effects

Auditory response
Cardiovascular effects
Cataract
Cellular effects
Effects on nervous system
Hematopoiesis
Implanted cardiac pace maker interference
Neuro-endocrine responses

28.7 HAZARD LEVELS AND PROTECTION

The radiation hazard levels are specified after taking into account the skin depth and specific absorption rate. The hazard levels may be classified as

  (i) Hazards to occupational personnel
 (ii) Hazards to ordnance
(iii) Hazards to electro-explosive devices
(iv) Hazards to vapourizing fuel

28.7.1 Hazards to Occupational Personnel

This refers to personnel who are working in the vicinity of radiation field for 8 hours a day. These personnel should not be exposed to an average power density above 10 mW/cm², averaged over any 6 minute period in the frequency range of 10 MHz to 100 GHz. If the exposure to radiation is not continuous, the upper limit is 100 mW/cm².

The protection measures are:
  (i) They should not enter the beam area of the transmit antenna.
 (ii) They should not go close to any radiation generators or propagating medium.
(iii) The personnel in areas where high power radars are used, must wear radiation absorptive suits made of stainless steel woven into fire-resistant synthetic fibers. The suit is usually light, easy to wear and comfortable. The attenuation produced by such suits is about 20 dB at 2450 MHz, 20 to 35 dB from 650 to 1150 MHz and 35 to 40 dB from 1 to 11 GHz.

28.7.2 Hazards to Ordnance

Microwave radiation is also dangerous to ordnance such as weapon systems and electronic warfare systems. It may cause accidental triggering to these systems. Ordnance is more susceptible to radiation than personnel because of the fact that they do not have heat dissipation system. Therefore, the limit for ordnance is lower than that for humans. Ordnance reacts to peak power density whereas the human beings react to average power density. They should be kept at a safe distance from the radiation field.

28.7.3 Hazards to Electro-explosive Devices

The electro-explosive devices are very sensitive to radiation. They can be easily triggered unintentionally by the radiation. They are usually protected from the radiation effects by enclosing them with metallic enclosures.

28.7.4 Hazards to Vapourizing Fuel

This hazard occurs due to handling and loading of inflammable fuels in the proximity of high radiation field. Arcs produced by high-radiation field may accidentally ignite the inflammable fuel. The handling and loading of the fuel should be carried out as far away as possible from the high-radiation field.

28.8 NUMERICAL EXAMPLES

Example 28.1 The radiation limit for the frequency range 50 to 300 MHz is 5 V/m. Find the incident power density.

Solution: Given: $E = 5$ V/m

Incident power density is given by

$$P_D = E^2/377 \text{ W/m}^2$$
$$= 5 \times 5/377$$
$$= 0.0663 \text{ W/m}^2$$

Example 28.2 If a biological material has a conductivity of 150 S/m and a mass density of 1.3×10^3 kg/m^3, find the specific absorption rate for an electric field of 5 V/m.

Solution: Given: $\sigma = 150$ S/m; $m_d = 1.3 \times 10^3$ kg/m^3, $E = 5$ V/m

The specific absorption rate is given by

$$\text{SAR} = \sigma E^2/m_d \text{ W/kg}$$
$$= 150 \times 25/1.3 \times 10^3$$
$$= 2.88 \text{ W/kg}$$

Example 28.3 If the specific absorption rate of a biological material is 2.88 W/kg and a specific heat of 1.2 kcal °C/kg, find the rate of temperature rise.

Solution: Given:
SAR = 2.88, $s_h = 1.2$ kcal °C/kg

From Eq. (28.9), the rate of change in temperature is given by

$$dT/dt = \text{SAR}/4185\, s_h \text{ °C/s}$$
$$= 2.88/(4185 \times 1.2)$$
$$= 5.73 \times 10^{-4} \text{ °C/s}$$

Example 28.4 Calculate the rate of change in temperature if the rate of metabolic heat production is 0.2 W/kg, the rate of heat loss is 0.18 W/kg, the SAR is 0.08 W/kg and the specific heat of the material is 0.8 kcal °C/kg.

Solution: Given: $W_M = 0.2$, $W_L = 0.18$, SAR = 0.08, $s_h = 0.8$.

The rate of change in temperature is given by

$$dT/dt = Q/s_h$$
$$= (\text{SAR} + W_M - W_L)/s_h$$
$$= (0.08 + 0.2 - 0.18)/0.8$$
$$= 0.125 \text{ °C/s}$$

KEY POINTS

- Exposure to microwave radiation may cause biological damage.
- Biological substances such as blood, bone, brain matter, muscle and fat are affected by excessive microwave radiation.
- Wavelengths at microwave frequencies are of the same order of magnitude as the dimensions of the human body. Hence, the body absorbs large amount of microwave energy and the heat generated may cause severe damage.
- Factors that give rise to complicated fields are (i) standing waves , (ii) near fields, (iii) polarization and (iv) modulation
- In many cases, the total electric field is a combination of waves with different polarization.
- Very high peak fields of short duration can occur in pulsed radars. Rotating antennas will also cause effective amplitude modulation at a fixed location. The stirrers in microwave ovens may cause amplitude modulation.
- When the dielectric constant within the body is higher, microwave penetration generates hot

spots due to the focusing action of the high dielectric constant and the shape of body cavities formed by the bones. The hot spots occur inside the human skull in the frequency range of 918 to 2450 MHz and at about 1500 MHz within the eyeball.

- When exposed to low-level microwave radiation, certain changes occur in the blood and the blood does not return to normal even after several months. This effect is known as hematopoiesis.

- The hazard levels may be classified as (i) hazards to occupational personnel, (ii) hazards to ordnance, (iii) hazards to electro-explosive devices and (iv) hazards to vapourizing fuel.

- The personnel protection measures are that (i) they should not enter the beam area of the transmit antenna, (ii) they should not go close to any radiation generators or propagating medium and (iii) the personnel in areas where high power radars are used, must wear radiation absorptive suits made of stainless steel woven into fire-resistant synthetic fibers.

- Microwave radiation may cause accidental triggering to ordnance such as weapon systems and electronic warfare systems.

- Ordnance is more susceptible to radiation than personnel because of the fact that they do not have heat dissipation system.

- The electro-explosive devices can be easily triggered unintentionally by the radiation. They are usually protected from the radiation effects by enclosing them with metallic enclosures.

- Arcs produced by high-radiation field may accidentally ignite the inflammable fuel. The handling and loading of the fuel should be carried out as far away as possible from the high-radiation field.

FURTHER READING

1. Preclusion of Ordnance Hazards in Electromagnetic Fields" (1986). General requirement for, MIL-STD 1385 B, Aug.

2. Standards for Safety Levels with respect to Human Exposure to Radio Frequency Electromagnetic Fields – 3 KHz to 300 KHz", (1991) IEEE. C 95.1-1982/ANSI C 95.1

3. Michaelson SM (1978). *Biological and pathophysiologic effects of exposure to microwaves*, Trans. Intl. Microwave Power Inst., Vol.8.

REVIEW QUESTIONS

28.1 Distinguish between ionizing and non-ionizing radiation. Which category is the microwave radiation?

28.2 Which field, electric or magnetic, of microwave radiation interacts with biological materials?

28.3 Mention the biological substances that absorb microwave radiation.

28.4 What are the important features of microwave radiation?

28.5 Give expression for the average power density in terms of electric field alone, magnetic field and electric and magnetic fields.

28.6 What is complicated electric field?

28.7 What are the factors that give rise to complicated field?

28.8 Mention the two parameters used in the case of complicated field.

28.9 Define penetration depth and express the field strength at any position.

28.10 Define specific absorption rate and give its expression.

28.11 What are the factors that affect the determination of SAR?

28.12 What are hot spots?

28.13 Express SAR in terms of temperature rise.

28.14 Mention the classification of interactive mechanism.

28.15 Mention the radiation hazard levels for personnel and their protective measures.

28.16 Mention the radiation hazard to ordnance and the protective measures.

28.17 Mention the radiation hazard to EED and the protective measures.

28.18 Mention the radiation hazard to fuel and the protective measures.

DESCRIPTIVE QUESTIONS

28.1 Discuss the features of microwave radiation.

28.2 Discuss the factors that give rise to complicated field.

28.3 Explain skin depth and specific absorption rate.

28.4 Discuss thermal and micro-thermal mechanism.

28.5 Explain the classification of radiation hazards and the protective measures.

PRACTICE PROBLEMS

28.1 The radiation limit for the frequency range 50 to 300 MHz is 10 V/m. Find the incident power density.
(**Ans:** 0.265 W/m^2)

28.2 If a biological material has a conductivity of 150 S/m and a mass density of 1.3×10^3 kg/m^3, find the specific absorption rate for an electric field of 10 V/m.
(**Ans:** 11.5 W/kg)

28.3 If the specific absorption rate of a biological material is 2.4 W/kg and a specific heat of 1.2 kcal °C/kg, find the rate of temperature rise.
(**Ans:** 4.78×10^{-4})

28.4 Calculate the rate of change in temperature if the rate of metabolic heat production is 0.2 W/kg, the rate of heat loss is 0.2 W/kg, the SAR is 0.08 W/kg and the specific heat of the material is 0.8 kcal/kg °C.
(**Ans:** 0.1 °C/s)

REFERENCE

1. Stuchly MA and Repacholi MH (1978). *Microwave and radio frequency protection standards*, Trans. Intl. Microwave Power Inst., Vol. 8.

2. Bowman RR (1978). *Quantifying hazardous microwave fields*, Trans. Intl. Microwave Power Inst., Vol.8.

3. Michael K (1986). *Radiation Protection in Small to Extra-Large, Microwaves and RF*, p 41–42, July.

4. Michaelson SM et al (1967). Biological Effects of Microwave Exposure, RADC-TR-67-461, Vol. 138.

5. Health Aspects of Radio Frequency and Microwave Exposure, (1978) Healh and Welfare, Canada.

6. IRPA guidelines on limits of exposure to RF electromagnetic fields in the range from 100 MHz to 300 GHz (1988).

29

■Microwave Antennas

Objectives

- Study the characteristics of the microwave antennas.
- Classify the microwave antennas.
- Study the various antenna structures and the radiation patterns.

29.1 INTRODUCTION

The use of microwave energy generally requires transfer of energy by means of radiation. In a communication link, the microwave signal is radiated into space by an antenna at the transmitting end and picked up from space by another antenna at the receiving end. The radiating antenna is known as transmitting antenna and the antenna that picks up the radiated microwave energy is known as receiving antenna. The same antenna can be used for both transmission and reception.

Antennas are constructed from an assemblage of conducting wires or rods. A familiar example is the household TV antenna. However, at microwave frequencies, even small discontinuities in the feeder lines and mountings give rise to reflections and phase changes which alter the antenna characteristics significantly. Because of short wavelengths involved, microwave antennas are more efficiently designed and constructed from apertures, lenses and mirror type reflectors.

29.2 ANTENNA CHARACTERISTICS

The typical antenna characteristics are:
- (i) Antenna efficiency
- (ii) Antenna gain
- (iii) Antenna directivity
- (iv) Effective area of aperture
- (v) Radiation patterns and side lobes
- (vi) Beam width
- (vii) Polarization.

These are discussed in detail in subsequent sections.

29.3 ANTENNA EFFICIENCY

An antenna transfers energy to and from space. In this process, certain amount of energy is dissipated in the antenna structure as heat This is because of conduction losses in the metallic parts of the antenna and losses in the dielectric supports. The efficiency of an antenna is defined as the ratio of useful power to total power. Thus, the efficiency of an antenna his given by

η_a = Useful power/total power

= Useful power/useful power + losses

(29.1)

In case of transmitting antennas, the useful power is the power radiated into the space with the antenna matched with the feeder line. In case of receiving antennas, the useful power is the power delivered to the matched load from a lossless antenna. With MW antennas, it is difficult to identify the individual source of power loss. Therefore, the determination of antenna efficiency depends upon the ability to measure the total power input and the power radiated. According to the reciprocity theorem, for a given antenna, the antenna efficiency is same for transmit and receive modes of operation.

Mismatch between antenna and feeder line is another source of power loss. Any mismatch between the two is measured in terms of the reflection coefficients. The matching efficiency is given by

$$\eta_r = 1 - \rho_L^2 \qquad (29.2)$$

where ρ_L is the magnitude of the reflection coefficient. This applies for both transmit and receive modes of operation. In the transmit mode, it is assumed that the feeder line is perfectly matched with the transmitter. In the receive mode, it is perfectly matched to the receiver. Thus, the mismatch occurs only between the feeder line and antenna. Stub is inserted between the feeder line and the antenna to reduce the mismatch. Ideally, the reflection coefficient should be zero.

29.4 ANTENNA GAIN

Most of the antennas have well-defined maximum in their radiation pattern. The gain Gm of the antenna is defined for this maximum. For comparison purpose, a reference antenna is required. This hypothetical antenna is known as *isotropic* radiator. *Isotropic* simply means *equally in all directions*. Since it is a hypothetical radiator, it can be safely assumed as lossless. Then, the gain of the antenna is defined for the direction of maximum radiation. Thus, the ratio of the power per unit solid angle radiated by the actual antenna to the power per unit solid angle radiated by the loss-less isotropic radiator. Therefore, the antenna gain G_m is given by

$$G_m = \frac{\text{Power/unit solid angle}}{\text{Power per unit solid angle}} \qquad (29.3)$$
$$\frac{\text{radiated by the antenna}}{\text{of isotropic radiator}}$$

A receiving antenna is a collector of electromagnetic (EM) energy from the space. As the EM wave sweeps over the antenna, the power density of the EM wave in W/m^2 gives rise to a power flow in watts in the load connected to the receiving antenna. The receiving antenna may be considered as having an effective area that relates the power density to the power by a relation of the form

$$P_R = P_D A_{eff} \qquad (29.4)$$

where P_R is the received power in watts delivered to a matched load, P_D is the power density in W/m^2 of the wave and A_{eff} is the effective area in m^2. Equation (29.4) applies when the receiving antenna is pointing in the direction of maximum reception. In any other direction, the power will be reduced by the factor $g(\theta, \phi)$, the radiation pattern where θ and ϕ are the angular spherical coordinates of direction. Thus, the effective aperture area is analogous to maximum gain. The effective area in any other direction is given by

$$A(\theta, \phi) = A_{eff}\, g(\theta, \phi) \qquad (29.5)$$

The effective area of an aperture antenna is proportional to the power gain. For any antenna, the effective area to gain ratio is given by

$$A_{eff}/G = \lambda^2/4\pi \qquad (29.6)$$

The effective area of an aperture antenna is not equal to the physical area of the aperture because the antenna itself produces reflections that modify the way by which the aperture is illuminated. The pyramidal horn antenna in Fig. 29.1 has an effective area given by

$$A_{eff} = 0.8\, ab \qquad (29.7)$$

where a and b are the length and width of the physical aperture.

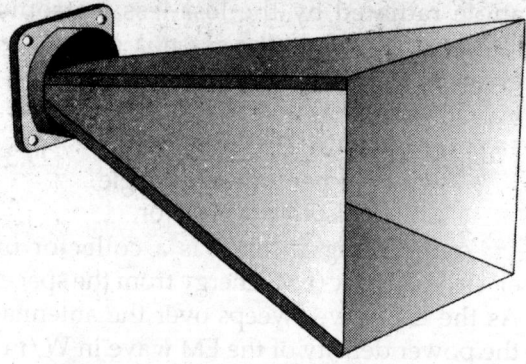

Fig. 29.1: Pyramidal horn antenna

29.5 RADIATION PATTERN AND SIDE LOBES

The function $g(\theta, \phi)$ is the radiation pattern and gives the three-dimensional plot of the power density in the far-field zone. In the far-field zone, only one component of the total radiation is significant. This is a plane transverse EM wave that is proportional to λ/d^2. Radio communication links make use of the far-field radiation. An empirical formula that gives the distance from the antenna to the far-field zone is

$$d = 2D^2/\lambda \qquad (29.8)$$

where d is the distance, D is the largest antenna dimension and λ is the wavelength, Eq. (29.8) applies for $D \gg \lambda$.

The radiation pattern of most MW antennas has a main lobe and a number of side lobes as shown in Fig. 29.2. The main lobe is

usually very narrow and hence referred as pencil beam. Cartesian plots are used to show the details of the radiation pattern. Two Cartesian planes are normally used for this purpose. One plane contains the electric field or *E*-vector and the other the magnetic field or *H*-vector. Both the planes contain the line of maximum radiation. The *E*-plane and the *H*-plane radiation pattern for the pyramidal horn antenna are shown in Fig. 29.3. The radiation pattern is usually plotted in decibels. This eliminates the confusion whether a power gain ratio or field strength ratio is plotted. The field strength is proportional to the square of the power density. Hence, the field strength radiation pattern is proportional to the square-root of the power gain radiation pattern. The *E*-plane graph of Fig. 29.3 re-plotted using decibels is shown in Fig. 29.4. It may be noted that nulls in Fig. 29.3 is not shown in Fig. 29.4 since $\log 0 = -\infty$.

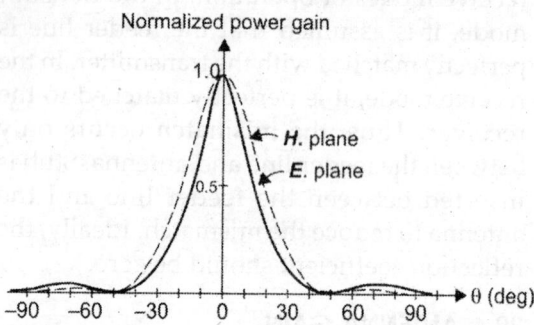

Fig. 29.3: Normalized power gain for pyramidal horn

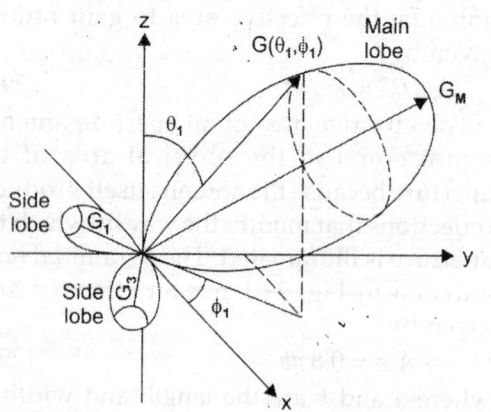

Fig. 29.2: Radiation pattern of a typical antenna

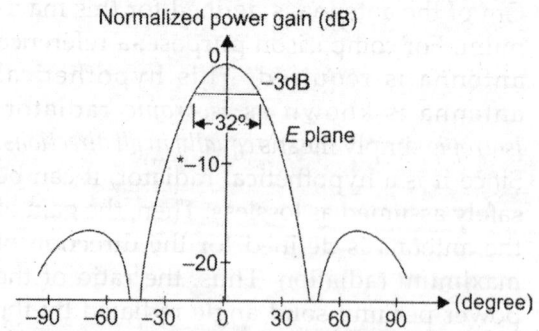

Fig. 29.4: Normalized power gain in decibels

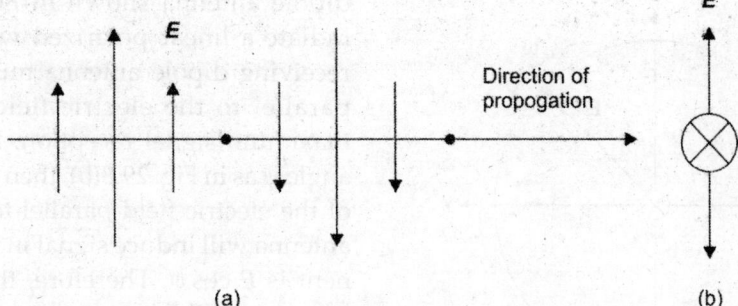

(a)   (b)

Fig. 29.5: Linear polarization as viewed on (a) Axis of propagation (b) Along the direction of propagation

29.6 BEAM WIDTH

The beam width of an antenna is the total angle subtended at the origin of the radiation pattern by the –3 dB points and is usually expressed in degrees. This is shown in Fig. 29.4.

29.7 POLARIZATION

In the far-field zone, the polarization of the EM wave is defined by the direction of the electric field in relation to the direction of propagation. When both are in the same plane, it is *linear polarization*. It is shown in Fig. 29.5.

A linear polarized EM wave that is propagated across the earth's surface is said to be *vertically polarized* when the electric field vector is vertical and *horizontally polarized*

when the electric field vector is parallel to earth's surface.

In certain situations, the electric field vector may rotate about the line of propagation. This is caused by the interaction by the wave with the earth's magnetic field in the F_2 layer of the ionosphere or by the type of antenna used. The path traced out by the tip of the electric field vector may be an ellipse as shown in Fig. 29.6(a). This is known as *elliptical polarization*. If the rotation is in the clockwise direction while looking along the direction of polarization it is known as *right-handed polarization*. If it is anticlockwise, then it is known as *left-handed polarization*. In Fig. 29.7, the direction of propagation is into the paper, so the polarization is right-handed. As shown in Fig. 29.6, the elliptical polarization can be resolved into two linear

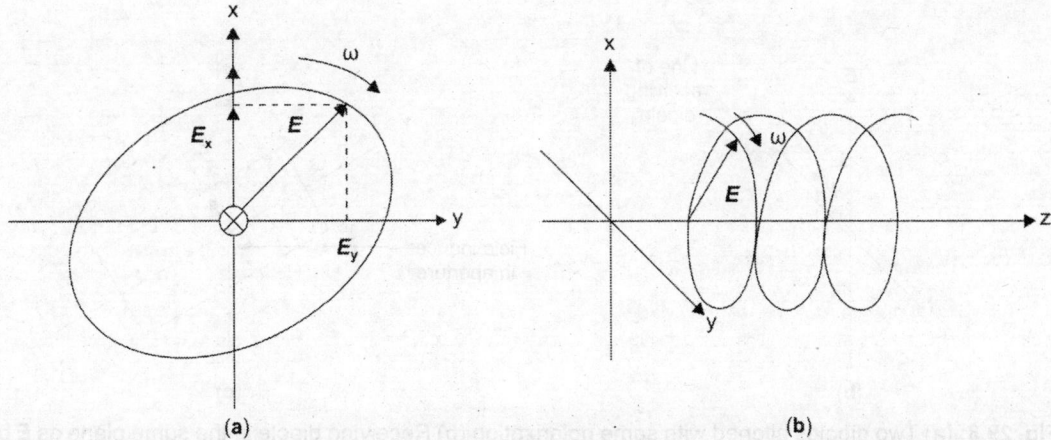

(a)   (b)

Fig. 29.6: Elliptical polarization as viewed (a) Along the direction of propagation (b) On axis of propagation

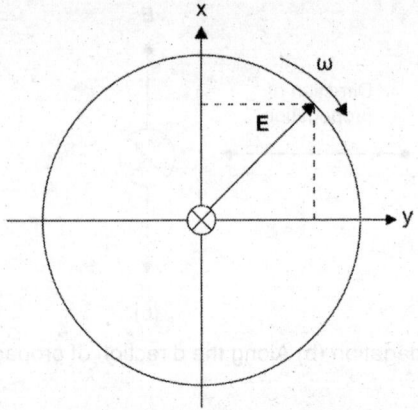

Fig. 29.7: Circular polarization

vectors, E_x and E_y. Linear polarization results when one of these is zero.

In order to receive maximum signal, the polarization of the receiving and transmitting antennas should be the same. A wire

dipole antenna shown in Fig. 29.8(a) will radiate a linear polarized wave. A similar receiving dipole antenna must be oriented parallel to the electric field vector E for maximum signal reception. If it is at some angle ψ as in Fig. 29.8(b), then the component of the electric field parallel to the receiving antenna will induce signal in it. This component is $E \cos \psi$. Therefore, the polarization loss factor, PLF is

$$PLF = \cos \psi \qquad (29.12)$$

A similar situation can exist with an aperture antenna as in Fig. 29.8(c). The angle ψ is the angle between the induced field in the aperture and the incoming electric field. In this case also, PLF = $\cos \psi$. In both cases, the direction of propagation is normal to the plane of the antenna.

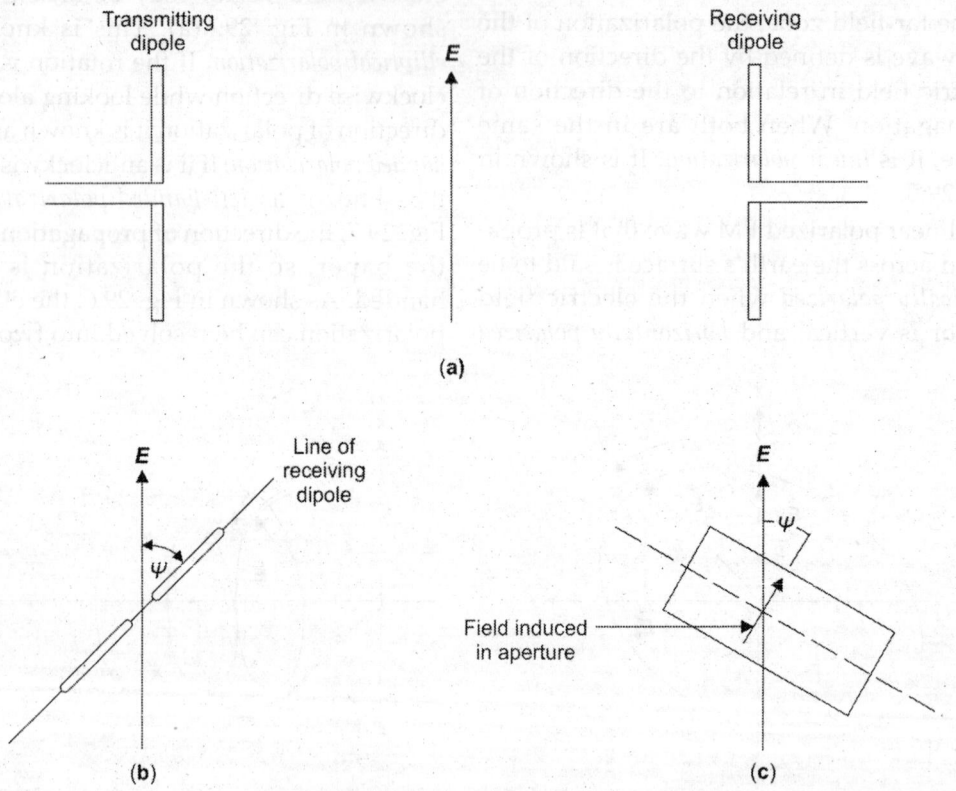

Fig. 29.8: (a) Two dipoles aligned with same polarization (b) Receiving dipole in the same plane as E but polarization misaligned (c) Incoming wave E in the same plane as aperture misaligned

29.8 CLASSIFICATION OF ANTENNAS

The antennas are classified based on their structure as

   (i) Half-wave dipole antennas

  (ii) Horn antennas

 (iii) Reflector antennas

 (iv) Lens antennas

  (v) Slot antennas

 (vi) Micro-strip antennas

(vii) Semiconductor dipole antennas

   They are discussed in detail in the following sections.

29.9 HALF-WAVE DIPOLE ANTENNA

The half-wave dipole antenna consists of two conductors lying in a straight line. It is shown in Fig. 29.9. The overall length from tip to tip is approximately one-half wavelength. The spacing between the conductors should be negligible compared to the overall length. This is difficult to achieve at microwave frequencies. The wave velocity along the antenna wire is slightly less than that of the free space. Hence, the antenna wavelength is slightly less than 95% of the free space value. The antenna must be at this shorter length for resonance as shown in Fig. 29.9(b). The impedance of the antenna under these conditions is 73 ohms resistive.

   The dipole antenna is a balanced antenna. Therefore, it should be fed from a balanced feeder. If a coaxial feeder is used, a balanced-to-unbalanced feed is required. Fig. 29.10(a) shows one form of slot feed to dipole antenna. A narrow slot is cut along the outer conductor of the coaxial feed as in Fig. 29.10(a). The dipole antenna is connected at the ends of the slotted section. The inner conductor is connected to the end of one half of the slotted section, the connecting post usually being in line with the dipole as shown in Fig. 29.10(b). If it is assumed that the slot width is very much smaller than one wavelength, the **TEM** wave on the coaxial line will extend into the slotted section as shown in Fig. 29.10(b). If it is assumed that the connecting post is a perfect conductor, the electric field along this must be zero. This condition is met by the post giving rise to a reflected wave in the TE_{11} mode. The TE_{11} electric field is shown in Fig. 29.10(c). The combined **TEM** and TE_{11} fields is shown in Fig. 29.10(d). It can be seen that zero field exists along the connecting post as required by the boundary conditions. A maximum field exists between inner and outer conductors diametrically opposite to the post. Since the top element of the dipole is connected via the post to the inner conductor and the lower element is connected to the outer conductor, E_{max} also appears across the dipole. It is shown in Fig. 29.10(e). In MW systems, the half-wave dipole is seldom used by itself as the main antenna.

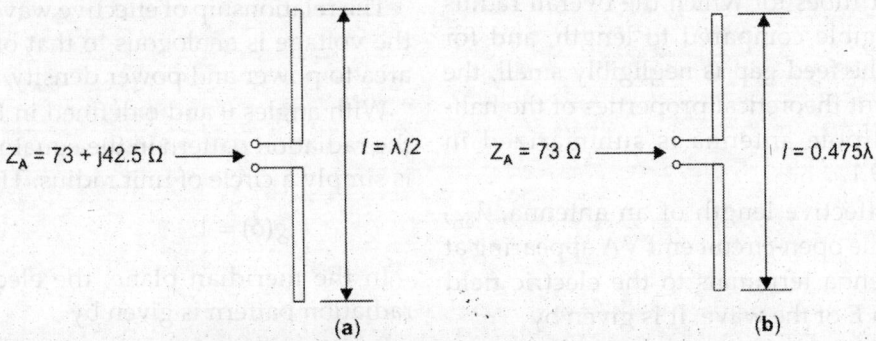

$$Z_A = 73 + j42.5\ \Omega \longrightarrow \qquad l = \lambda/2$$

$$Z_A = 73\ \Omega \longrightarrow \qquad l = 0.475\lambda$$

(a)   **(b)**

Fig. 29.9: Impedance of (a) l/2 dipole (b) 0.475 l

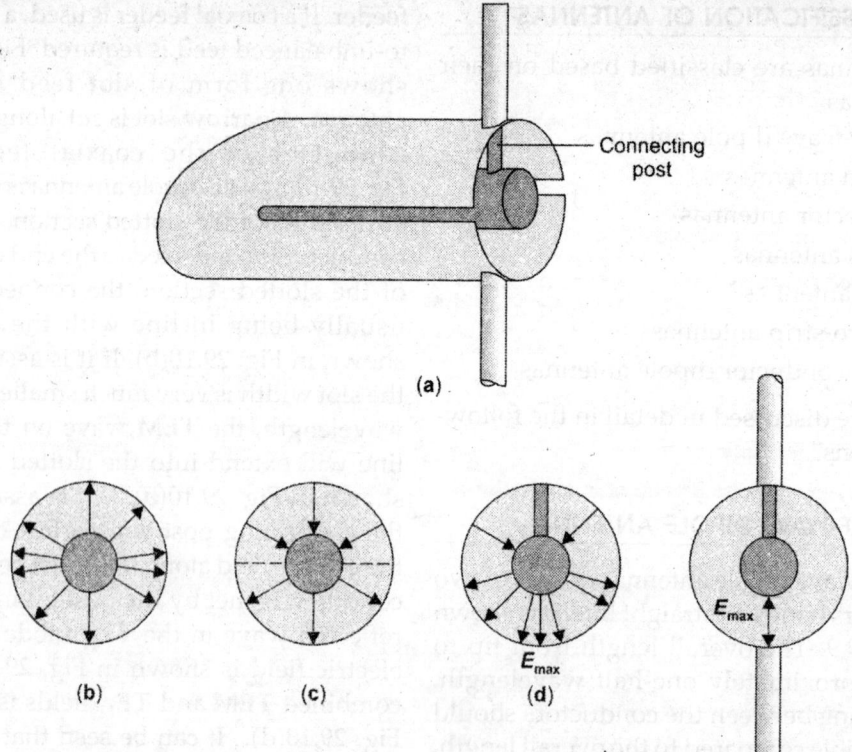

Fig. 29.10: (a) Dipole slot fed (b) Coaxial TEM wave (c) Reflected TE$_{11}$ wave (d) Combined wave (e) Excitation of dipole through E_{max}

Usually, it is used as a feeder antenna for a reflector system, or it may form the basic element in a microstrip array. The feed to the dipole forms a significant part of the antenna. The theoretical results for the half-wave dipole antenna provides only as a guide to antenna performance at microwave frequencies. For a half-wave dipole made of thin wires or tubes for which the overall radius is negligible compared to length, and for which the feed gap is negligibly small, the important theoretical properties of the half-wave dipole antenna is summarized in Table 29.1.

The effective length of an antenna, λ_{eff}, relates the open-circuit emf VA appearing at the antenna terminals to the electric field strength E of the wave. It is given by

$$VA = E\lambda_{eff} \tag{29.10}$$

Table 29.1: properties of the half-wave dipole antenna

1.	Resonance impedance	73 ohms
2.	Isotropic power gain	2.16 dB
3.	–3 dB beam width	78°
4.	Effective area	0.13λ^2
5.	Effective length	λ/π

The relationship of effective wavelength to the voltage is analogous to that of effective area to power and power density.

With angles θ and ϕ defined in Fig. 29.11, the radiation pattern in the equatorial plane is simply a circle of unit radius. Therefore,

$$g(\phi) = 1 \tag{29.11}$$

In the meridian plane, the electric field radiation pattern is given by

$$F(\theta) = \cos\left[\,(\pi/2 \cos\theta)\right]/\sin(\theta) \tag{29.12}$$

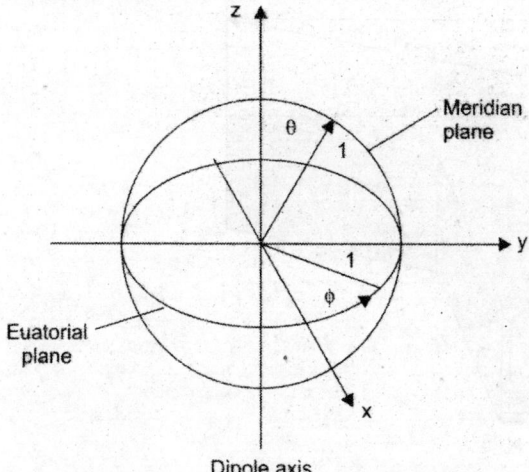

Fig. 29.11: Planes for the dipole radiation patterns g(ϕ) and g(θ)

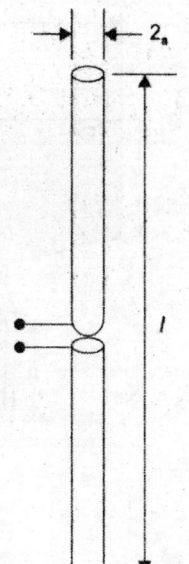

Fig. 29.12: Cylindrical antenna

The power radiation pattern is this function squared. Thus

$$g(\theta) = F^2(\theta) \qquad (29.13)$$

The half-wave dipole antenna is an omni-directional antenna with bidirectional radiation pattern. The current distribution is sinusoidal. It is used as feed element for reflector antennas.

29.9.1 Cylindrical Dipole Antenna

Figure 29.12 shows a cylindrical dipole antenna. It consists of two cylindrical tubes of negligible thickness and radius. The tubes are perfectly conducting ones and the feed gap is negligibly small. The terminal impedance of such a cylindrical dipole antenna is given by

$$R_d = 122.65 - 641.2\,(l/\lambda) + 1085.66\,(l/\lambda)^2 \qquad (29.14)$$

$$X_d = 162.5 - 120\,[ln\,(l/a) - 1]\cos\,(\pi l/\lambda) \\ - 439.82\,(l/\lambda) + 394.78\,(l/\lambda)^2 \qquad (29.15)$$

Therefore,

$$Z_d = R_d + jX_d \qquad (29.16)$$

The above three equations are valid for values of $0.001588 \leq a/\lambda \leq 0.009525$ and $0.4138 \leq (l/\lambda) \leq 0.5411$, where a is the radius of the cylindrical tube.

29.10 HORN ANTENNAS

Electromagnetic energy can be transmitted and received through the open end of a waveguide. But, this is not an efficient way of coupling a waveguide to space because the sudden change in the cross-section area gives rise to reflections. More efficient coupling is achieved by flaring the wave-guide at one end. The resulting structure is known as waveguide horn antenna. Fig. 29.13(a) shows an *H*-plane sectorial horn antenna since the flare is in the same direction as the magnetic field vector *H* at the center of the aperture. The waveguide dimension a' is expanded to a while b remains constant. The slant length l_H is shown in Fig. 29.13(a). Fig. 29.13(b) shows an *E*-plane sectorial horn antenna. The flare in this case is in the same direction as the electric field vector *E*. The waveguide dimension b' is expanded to b while a remains constant. The slant length l_E is shown in Fig. 29.13(b). When both dimensions are flared, it is known as pyramidal horn antenna shown in Fig. 29.1.

The gain of the horn antenna depends on wavelength, aperture dimensions (a and b)

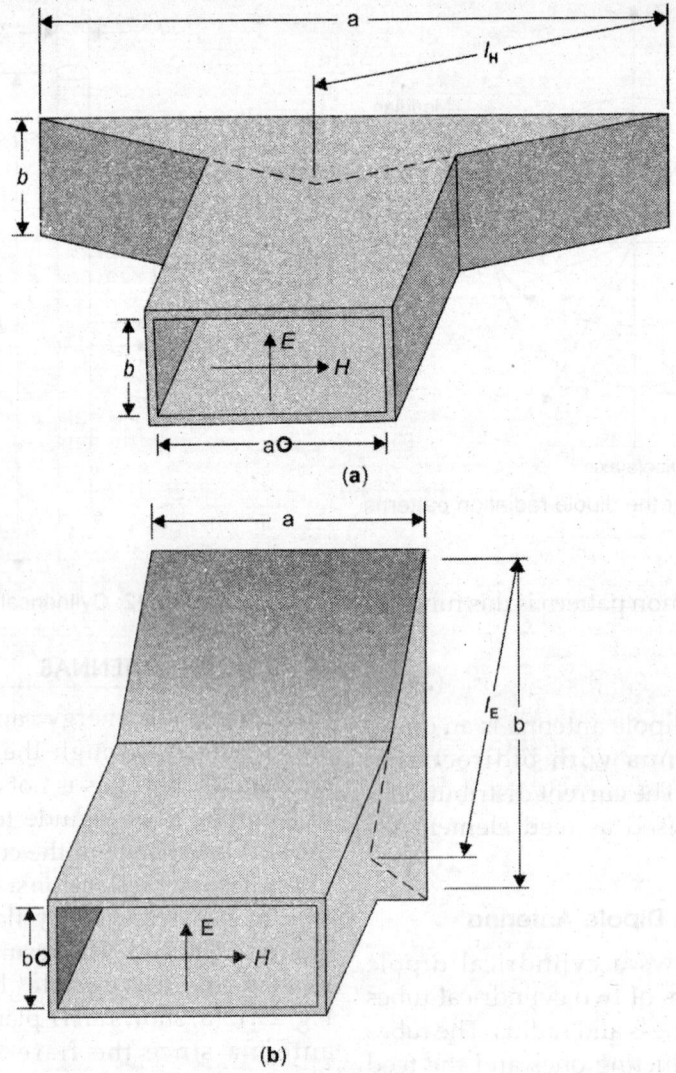

Fig. 29.13: (a) *H*-plane (b) *E*-plane horn antenna

and slant length. The isotropic power gain for a rectangular horn antenna is given by

$$G = G_o R_E R_H \qquad (29.17)$$

where R_E and R_H are gain reduction factors taking into account the *E*-plane and *H*-plane flares of the horn antenna and the effect of finite radiation distance. The variation in R_E and R_H are shown in Fig. 29.14. The x-axis is a generalized coordinate. When R_E curve is used, a is substituted for d and l'_E for l. When RH curve is used, b is substituted for d and l'_H for l. The parameters l'_E and l'_H take into

account the range r and the slant heights. They are given by

$$l'_E = r l'_E / (r + l_E) \qquad (29.18)$$

$$= r l'_H / (r + l_H) \qquad (29.19)$$

G_o is the far-field gain of the rectangular aperture and is given by

$$G_o = 32 ab / \pi \lambda^2 \qquad (29.20)$$

The gain G_o in decibels is

$$G_o \text{ (dB)} = 10 \log (32 ab / \pi \lambda^2) \qquad (29.21)$$

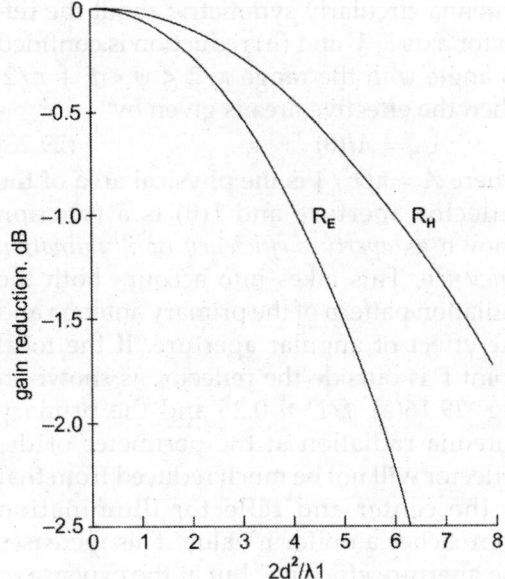

Fig. 29.14: Gain reduction factors R_E and R_H

The gain of the pyramidal horn antenna in dB is given by

$$G_{dB} = G_{odB} + R_{EdB} + R_{HdB} \quad (29.22a)$$

The gain of the *E*-plane sectorial horn is

$$G_{EdB} = G_{odB} + R_{EdB} \quad (23.22b)$$

The gain of the *H*-plane sectorial horn is

$$G_{HdB} = G_{odB} + R_{HdB} \quad (23.22c)$$

Gain can be accurately calculated for horn antennas. As a result, they are used extensively as standard gain antennas for comparing the gains of other antennas. The pyramid antenna shown in Fig. 29.1 is such a standard antenna.

29.11 REFLECTOR ANTENNA

The most widely used microwave antenna is the paraboloidal reflector antenna. It consists of a primary radiator antenna at the focal point of the paraboloidal reflector. The primary radiator antenna may be a dipole antenna or horn antenna. The physical structure of the reflector is circular. The reflector contour, projected into any plane containing focal point F and the vertex V forms a parabola as shown in Fig. 20.15(a). The path lengths FAB and FA'B' in Fig. 29.15(b) are equal for this curve. The reflector focuses parallel rays onto the focal point. Conversely, it can produce a parallel beam from a radiator situated at focal point. Fig. 29.15(c) illustrates this. In addition to the desired beam, some of the rays are not captured by the reflector. Such rays constitute *spill over*. In the receiver antenna, spill over increases the noise pick up. Some radiation from the primary radiator also occurs in the forward direction. This is known as *back lobe radiation* since it is from

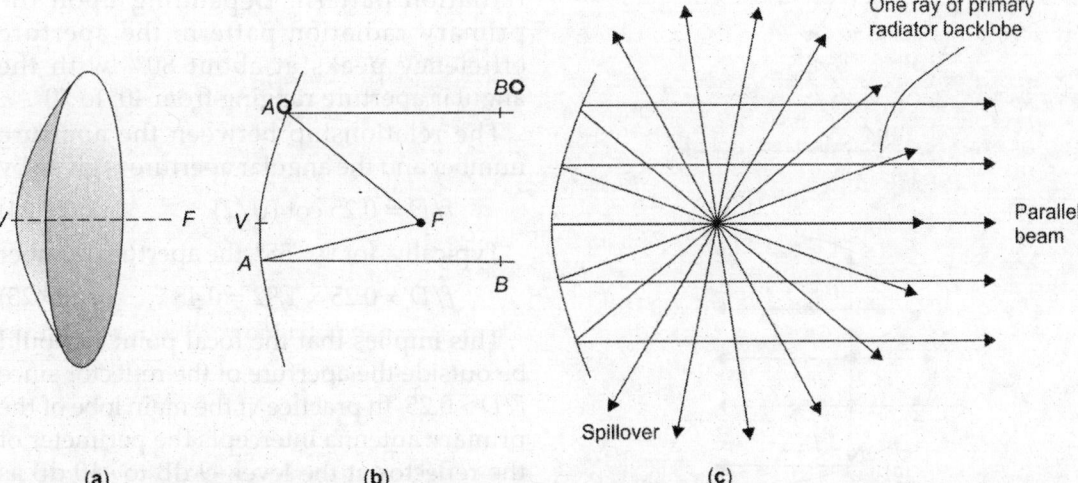

Fig. 29.15: (a) Paraboloidal reflector antenna (b) Parabola (c) Radiation from paraboloidal reflector antenna and primary radiator antenna

the back-lobe of the primary radiator. Back-lobe radiation is undesirable because it interferes destructively with the reflected beam. Practical radiators are designed to eliminate or minimize this. The isotropic radiator at the focal point will radiate spherical waves and the parabolic reflector converts them into plane waves. Thus, over the aperture of an ideal reflector, the wave-front is of constant amplitude and constant phase.

The directivity of the paraboloidal reflector is a function of the primary antenna directivity and the ratio of focal length to reflector diameter f/D. This is known as *aperture number*. This determines the angular aperture of a reflector 2ψ shown in Fig. 29.16(a). This, in turn, determines the quality of the primary radiation intercepted by the reflector. Assume that (i) radiation from the primary

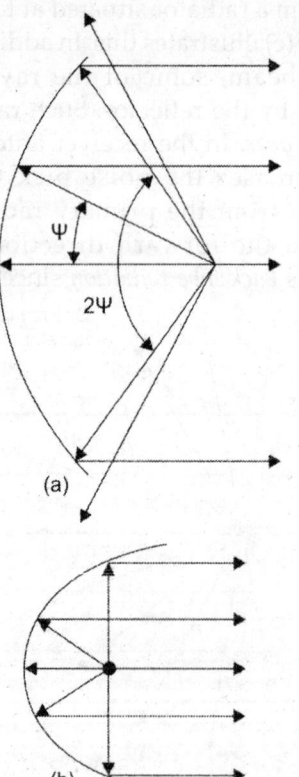

(a)

(b)

Fig. 29.16: Focal point (a) outside and (b) inside the reflector

antenna circularly symmetric about the reflector axis $F–V$ and (ii) reduction is confined to angle ψ in the range $\pi/2 < \psi < E + \pi/2$. Then the effective area is given by

$$A_{eff} = AI(\theta) \qquad (29.23)$$

where $A = \pi D^2/4$ is the physical area of the reflector aperture and $I(\theta)$ is a function known as *aperture efficiency* or *illumination efficiency*. This takes into account both the radiation pattern of the primary antenna and the effect of angular aperture. If the focal point F is outside the reflector as shown in Fig. 29.16(a), $f/D > 0.25$ and the primary antenna radiation at the perimeter of the reflector will not be much reduced from that at the center and reflector illumination approaches a uniform value. This increases the aperture efficiency but at the expense of spill over occurring. Too large f/D increases spill over to the extent that aperture efficiency decreases. If f/D is < 0.25, the focal point is placed inside the reflector as shown in Fig. 29.16(b) and no spill over occurs. But, the illumination of reflector tapers from maximum at the center to zero within the reflector region. This non-uniform illumination tends to reduce aperture efficiency. If the primary antenna is placed close to the reflector, it results in the reflector affecting the primary antenna impedance and the radiation pattern. Depending upon the primary radiation pattern, the aperture efficiency peaks at about 80% with the angular aperture ranging from 40° to 70°.

The relationship between the aperture number and the angular aperture is given by

$$f/D = 0.25 \cot (\psi/2) \qquad (29.24)$$

Typically, for $\psi = 55°$, the aperture number

$$f/D = 0.25 \times 1.92 = 0.48 \qquad (29.25)$$

This implies that the focal point F should be outside the aperture of the reflector since $f/D > 0.25$. In practice, if the main lobe of the primary antenna intercepts the perimeter of the reflector at the level –9 dB to –10 dB as shown in Fig. 29.17, satisfactory results are obtained.

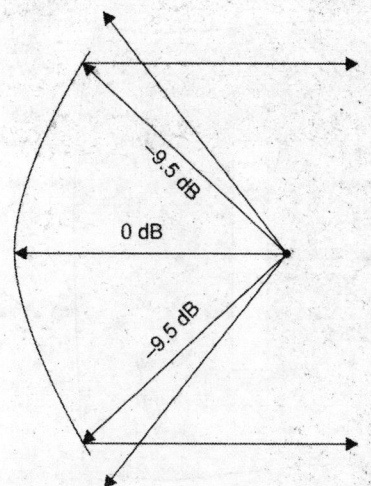

Fig. 29.17: Edge illumination from the primary antenna is 9 dB to 10 dB below that at vertex

Substituting $A = \pi D^2/4$ in Eq. (29.23) and from Eq. (29.9), we obtain the gain G is as

$$G = I(\theta)\,(\pi D^2/4) \qquad (29.26)$$

The reflector antennas are simple and easy to construct. It is used in home TV antennas. It is used as a passive target for radar and communication applications.

Beam Width

The beam width also depends on the primary radiator and its position. In practice, for most types of feed line, the –3 dB beam width is given by

$$BW_{(-3\,dB)} = 70\lambda/D \text{ degrees} \qquad (29.27)$$

The beam width between nulls is given by

$$BW_{(nulls)} = 2\,BW_{(-3\,dB)}$$
$$= 140\lambda/D \text{ degrees} \qquad (29.28)$$

29.12 LENS ANTENNAS

The directivity of parabolic and horn antennas results from a field distribution corresponding to a plane wave across an aperture. The same result is obtained by employing a point source of radiation in conjunction with a lens. Such an arrangement is known as *lens antenna*.

Electromagnetic radiation is refracted when it passes from a lower dielectric constant medium to a higher dielectric constant medium. The relationship between the angles of incident ϕ_i and refraction ϕ_r is given by Snell's law [(Fig. 29.18(a)].

$$\sin\phi_r/\sin\phi_i = (\varepsilon_{ri}/\varepsilon_{rr})^{\frac{1}{2}} = 1/n \qquad (29.29)$$

for waves entering the region of high dielectric constant where n is the refractive index of the material. The refractive property is reciprocal. Therefore, the same relationship holds good when the radiation passes from a higher dielectric constant medium to a lower dielectric constant medium except that the subscript are interchanged. Thus,

$$\sin\phi_i/\sin\phi_r = (\varepsilon_{ri}/\varepsilon_{rr})^{\frac{1}{2}} = 1/n \qquad (29.30)$$

The material used for the lens is usually a high dielectric plastics such as polystyrene or teflon.

Figure 29.18 illustrates the principle of collimating lens. It is used to transform a diverging beam of radiation into a parallel beam traveling in one direction only with a

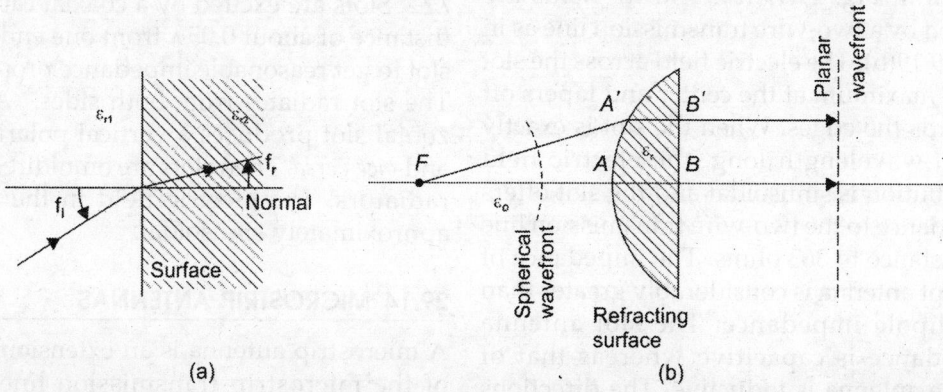

Fig. 29.18: Dielectric lens antenna (a) Snell' law of refraction (b) Principle of collimating lens

planer wavefront. The lens in this case is a convex one. Radiation along the axis of the lens passes through both the surfaces at right angles and hence, no refraction takes place.

Radiation at an angle from the axis is incident at the curved interface at an angle other than normal and hence, refracted towards the normal as it passes into the lens at *A'*. The curvature of the lens is such that, after refraction, the rays are all parallel to the axis.

Radiation at angle along *FA'* takes a little longer path to reach the refractive surface *A'* and arrives with a little time lag compared to that along the lens axis *FA*. Since the velocity of propagation within the dielectric is slower than that in the air, a compensating delay occurs in the radiation along the axis *AB* compared to that along *A'B'*. Hence, all the radiation arrives at the flat surface *BB'* in phase. The result is a planar waveform leaving the lens.

The functions of lens antenna are to generate plane wavefront from spherical wavefront, to converge the incoming wavefront at its focus, collimate the EM waves and control the aperture illumination.

29.13 SLOT ANTENNAS

The slot antenna makes use of the fact that the electromagnetic energy is radiated when a RF field exists across a narrow slot in a metallic sheet. A typical slot antenna is shown in Fig. 29.19.(a). The RF fields are excited by a two-wire transmission line as in Fig. 29.19(b). The electric field across the slot is the maximum at the center and tapers off towards the edges. When the slot is exactly a half-wavelength long, the electric field distribution is sinusoidal and the slot offers impedance to the two-wire transmission line a resistance to 363 ohms. The impedance of the slot antenna is considerably greater than the dipole impedance. The slot antenna impedance is capacitive whereas that of dipole antenna is inductive. The directions of the electric field *E* and the magnetic field

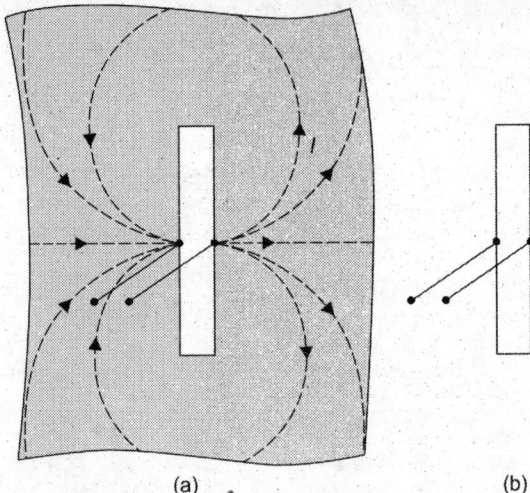

(a) (b)

Fig. 29.19: (a) Narrow slot antenna (b) Narrow rectangular loop

H are shown in Fig. 29.20(a). The slot antenna is center fed. The complementary half-wave dipole antenna is shown in Fig. 29.20(b). The electric field *E* is horizontally polarized for slot antenna. The radiation pattern of the slot antenna is given by Eq. (29.13).

Impedance data for a slot dipole antenna are usually presented in terms of an equivalent cylindrical dipole antenna. A good approximation to a slot dipole antenna of width *w* and thickness *t* is a cylindrical dipole antenna of radius *a*, where

$$a = (w + t)/4 \qquad (29.31)$$

A slot antenna can be rectangular, circular or of any shape. The resonant slot has a length of $\lambda/2$ and its width is much less than $\lambda/2$. Slots are excited by a coaxial cable at a distance of about 0.05λ from one end of the slot to get reasonable impedance properties. The slot radiates from both sides. A horizontal slot produces a vertical polarization and *vice versa*. Then slots are omnidirectional radiators. The electric field in the slot is approximately sinusoidal.

29.14 MICROSTRIP ANTENNAS

A microstrip antenna is an extension of the of the microstrip transmission lines. The simplest antenna elements is a patch antenna

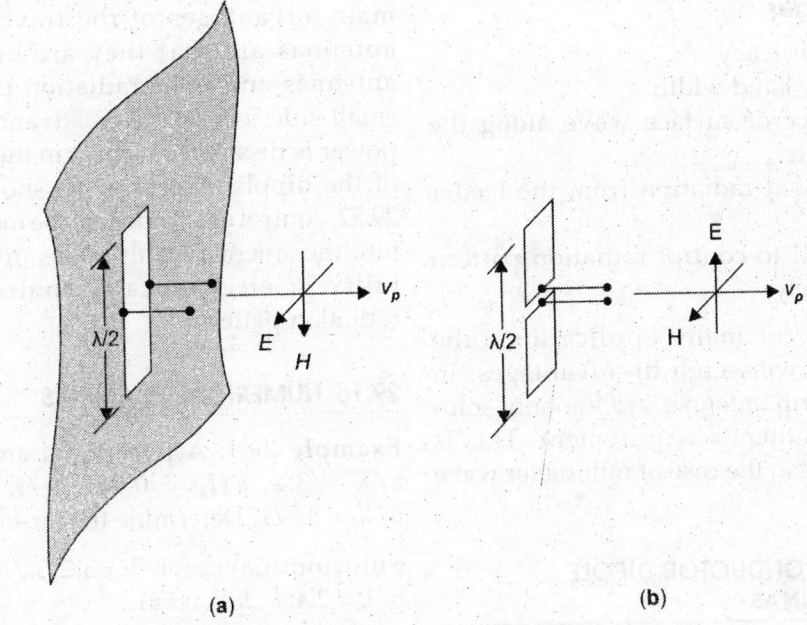

Fig. 29.20: (a) Slot antenna with E and H field directions

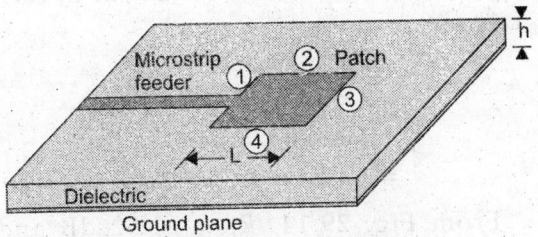

Microstrip feeder ① ② Patch ③ ④ L Dielectric Ground plane

Fig. 29.21: Patch antenna

shown in Fig. 29.21.The EM wave traveling along the microstrip feed line spreads out under the patch. At the perimeter, the wave meets an open circuit. Hence reflections take place. These set up a standing wave pattern under the patch. The patch is resonant if $L = \lambda/2$, where $\lambda = l_o\sqrt{\varepsilon_r}$. ε_r is the effective relative permeability of the microstrip. The far-field radiation from ends 1 and 3 is in phase whereas that from ends 2 and 4 is in opposite phase. Hence, they tend to cancel. Since the height h of the substrate is very much less than the line wavelength, the patch antenna may be considered as a resonant slot antenna. The radiating slot is the total perimeter of the patch and most of the radiation occurs from the far end and the feed end.

Microstrip antennas are easily fabricated. These are arrays of basic elements that are configured to give the desired radiation pattern and polarization.

Applications of Microstrip Antennas

Microstrip antennas are particularly suited for those applications where flat profile antennas are required. Microstrip antennas are used in:

(i) Missile guidance systems

(ii) Portable radar systems

These antennas are easily fabricated to the required shapes.

Advantages

The advantages of microstrip antennas are:

(i) Simple

(ii) Light weight

(iii) Easy to fabricated to the required shapes

(iv) Inexpensive

(v) Easily integrated with circuits

Disadvantages

(i) Low efficiency

(ii) Narrow band width

(iii) Presence of surface wave along the substrate

(iv) Unwanted radiation from the feeder line

(v) Difficult to control radiation pattern accurately

However, for many applications, the advantages overweigh disadvantages. In fact, microstrip antennas are the only solutions to an antenna requirement. This is specially true in the case of millimeter wave systems.

29.15 SEMICONDUCTOR DIPOLE ANTENNAS

Semiconductor dipole antennas are recent developments in the millimeter wave antennas. The basic form of the semiconductor dipole antenna is shown in Fig. 29.22. In this, the dipole elements are semiconductor layers deposited on an insulating substrate. The current along the dipole is controlled by the doping density. Therefore, the current can be varied along the length in such a way that the current becomes negligible at the ends. This eliminates the occurrence of the reflected current wave The radiation pattern is determined by the forward traveling wave along the dipole. The main advantages of the traveling wave antennas are that they are broad band antennas and their radiation pattern has small side lobes. The disadvantage is that power is dissipated as heat in the resistance of the dipole structure. As shown in Fig. 29.22, control electrodes can be incorporated into the antennas. This opens up the possibility of electronically controlling the radiation pattern.

29.16 NUMERICAL EXAMPLES

Example 29.1: A pyramidal antenna has $a/\lambda = 3.2$, $a/l_E = 0.782$, $b/\lambda = 2.4$ and $b/l_H = 0.521$. Determine the far-field gain.

Solution: Given: $a/\lambda = 3.2$, $a/l_E = 0.782$, $b/\lambda = 2.4$, $b/l_H = 0.521$.

For calculation of far-field gain, $l_E = l'_E$ and l'_H. The abscissa values $s = 2d^2/\lambda l$ in each case are:

$$s_a = 2(a/\lambda)(a/l_E)$$
$$= 2 \times 3.2 \times 0.782 = 5$$
$$s_b = 2(b/\lambda)(b/l_H)$$
$$= 2 \times 2.4 \times 0.521 = 2.5$$

From Fig. 29.14, $R_E = -1.52$ dB and $R_H = -0.18$ dB.

The gain G_o is calculated from Eq. (29.23) as

$$G_o = 32 \times 3.2 \times 2.4/\pi = 78.23$$

or, $G_o(dB) = 18.93$ dB.

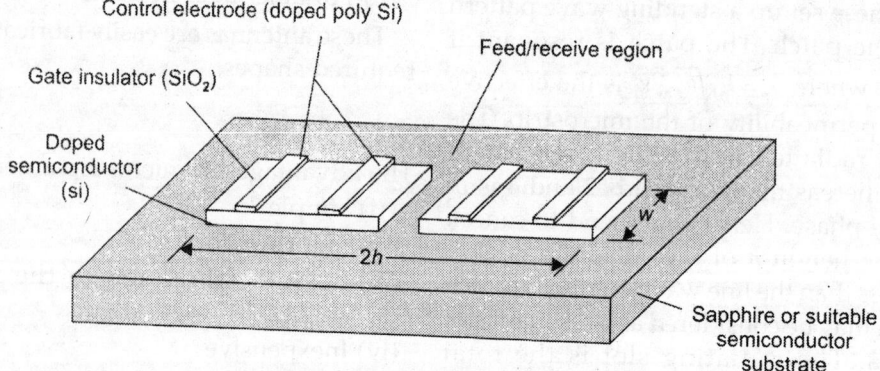

Fig. 29.22: Semiconductor dipole antenna

Hence, using Eq. (29.22a), we get

$$G(dB) = 18.93 - 1.52 - 0.18$$
$$= \textbf{17.23 dB}$$

Example 29.2: Determine the gain, bandwidth and the effective area for a paraboloidal reflector antenna for which the reflector diameter is 6 m and the illumination efficiency is 0.65. The operating frequency is 9 GHz.

Solution: Given: $D = 6$, $\eta = 0.65$, $f = 9 \times 10^9$ Hz.

$$\lambda = c/f = 3 \times 10^8/9 \times 10^9$$
$$= 0.033 \text{ m} = 3.3 \text{ cm}$$
$$A = \pi D^2/4 = 3.14 \times 6 \times 6/4$$
$$= 28.26 \text{ m}^2$$
$$A_{eff} = \eta A = 0.65 \times 28.26$$
$$= 18.4 \text{ m}^2$$
$$G_o = 4\pi A_{eff}/\lambda^2$$
$$= 4 \times 3.14 \times 18.4/3.3 \times 3.3$$
$$= 212217.$$
$$G_o(dB) = \textbf{53.27 dB}$$
$$BW_{(-3dB)} = 70\lambda/D = 70 \times 3.3/600$$
$$= \textbf{0.385}°$$
$$BW_{(null)} = 2 \times BW_{(-3dB)} = 2 \times 0.385$$
$$= \textbf{0.77}°$$

Example 29.3: A slot of 1 mm wide is cut in a highly conducting sheet of thickness 0.27 mm to operate at 6 GHz. Calculate the slot impedance (a) when the length is exactly half-wave length and (b) when it is $0.95\lambda/2$. The dipole impedance $Z_d = 73.46 + j\,41.28$.

Solution: Given: $t = 0.27$ mm, $f = 6 \times 10^9$ Hz, $Z_d = 73.46 + j\,41.28$.

(a) Slot antenna impedance Z_s is given by

$$Z_s = (60\pi)^2/Z_d = \textbf{367.6} - \textbf{j\,206.6 ohms}$$

(b) From Eq. (29.34),

$$a = (1 + 0.27)/4 = 0.3175 \text{ mm}$$
$$\lambda = c/f = 3 \times 10^8/6 \times 10^9 = 0.05 \text{ m}$$
$$= 5.0 \text{ cm}$$
$$\therefore \quad a/\lambda = 0.3175/50 = 0.00635$$
$$l/a = 0.475/0.00635 = \textbf{74.8}$$

For $l = 0.95\,\lambda/2$:

$$l/\lambda = 0.95/2 = 0.475$$
$$R_d = 122.65 - 641.2 \times l/\lambda + 1085.66\,(l/\lambda)^2$$
$$= 122.65 - 641.2 \times 0.475 + 1085.66 \times 0.475^2$$
$$= 122.65 - 304.57 + 244.95$$
$$= \textbf{63.03 ohms}$$
$$X_d = 162.5 - 120\,[\ln(l/a) - 1]\cot(\pi l/\lambda)$$
$$\quad - 439.82\,(l/\lambda) + 394.78(l/\lambda)^2$$
$$= 162.5 - 31.3 - 208.91 + 89.07$$
$$= 11.35$$
$$\therefore Z_d = (60\pi)^2/Z_d = (60\pi)^2/(63.03 + j\,1.35)$$
$$= \textbf{546} - \textbf{j\,98.3 ohms}$$

KEY POINTS

- Typical characteristics of antennas are efficiency, gain, directivity, aperture area, radiation pattern, beam width and polarization.
- Antenna efficiency is the ratio of useful power to the total power.
- Gain of an antenna is the ratio of the power per unit solid angle radiated by the antenna to the power per unit solid angle radiated by the lossless isotropic antenna.
- Directivity is the ratio of the maximum to average power per unit solid angle.
- Aperture area is the ratio of the received power in watts delivered to a matched load to the power density in W/m².
- Radiation pattern is a 3-dimensional plot of the power density in the far-field zone.
- Beam width of an antenna is the total angle subtended at the origin by the –3 dB points.
- Polarization of an EM wave is the direction of the electric field in relation to the direction of propagation.
- Antennas are classified as half-wave dipole antennas, horn antennas, reflector antennas, lens antennas, slot antennas, microstrip antennas and semiconductor dipole antennas.
- Half-wave dipole antenna consists of two conductors lying in a straight line.
- Cylindrical dipole antenna consists of two cylindrical tubes, lying in a straight line, of negligible thickness and radius.

- Horn antenna is wave guide flared at one end.
- Reflector antenna consists of a primary antenna at the focal point of a paraboloidal reflector.
- The primary antenna is a dipole or horn antenna.
- Lens antenna consists of a point source of radiation in conjunction with a lens.
- Slot antenna is a slot cut in a metallic sheet which, when excited by microwaves, radiates EM waves.
- Microstrip antenna is a patch antenna which, when fed with EM energy, radiates the energy through the perimeter of the patch.
- Microstrip antennas are used in missile guidance and portable radar systems because they provide many advantages.
- Semiconductor dipole antenna consists of the d pole elements as the semiconductor layers deposited on an insulation substrate.

FURTHER READING

1. Kraus John D (1950). Antennas, MGH, NY.
2. Elliot Robert S (1981). Antenna Theory and Design, PH, NJ.
3. Jain FC and R Bansai (1984). Monolithic mm-wave antenna, Microwave J, July issue.
4. James AR et al (1981). Microstrip Antennas, Peter peregrinus, England.

REVIEW QUESTIONS

29.1 Mention the antenna characteristics.
29.2 Define the efficiency of an antenna.
29.3 Define the gain of an antenna.
29.4 Define the directivity of an antenna.
29.5 Define the aperture area of an antenna.
29.6 Define the radiation pattern of antenna.
29.7 Define the beam width of an antenna.
29.8 Define the polarization of an antenna.
29.9 Describe the structure of a half-wave antenna.
29.11 Describe the structure of a horn antenna.
29.12 Describe the structure of a reflector antenna.
29.13 Describe the structure of a lens antenna.
29.14 Describe the structure of a slot antenna.
29.15 Describe the structure of a microstrip antenna.
29.16 Describe the structure of a semiconductor antenna.

DESCRIPTIVE QUESTIONS

29.1 What are the characteristics of an antenna? Discuss any two characteristics.
29.2 Explain the antenna efficiency and gain.
29.3 Discuss the antenna directivity and radiation pattern.
29.4 Explain the effective aperture area, polarization of EM waves and beam width.
29.5 Describe the various types of polarization and polarization loss factor.
29.6 How are the antennas classified? Explain any two types.
29.7 Explain in detail the half-wave dipole antenna and derive an expression for its radiation pattern.
29.8 Discuss in detail the pyramidal horn antenna and derive an expression for the gain.
29.9 Describe in detail a reflector antenna.
29.10 Explain the lens and slot antennas.
29.11 What is microstrip antenna? Mention the advantages, disadvantages and applications.
29.12 Write short notes on (i) semiconductor antenna, (ii) lens antenna and (iii) slot antenna.

PRACTICE PROBLMS

29.1 Calculate the impedance of a cylindrical half-wave dipole antenna with $a/\lambda = 0.002$.
(**Ans:** $73.46 + j\,41.28$)
29.2 A 50 ohms feeder line is connected to a 73 ohms antenna. The input power to the line is 5 kW. The total power radiated is 4.2 kW. Determine (i) the antenna efficiency and (ii) power loss in the antenna.
(**Ans:** 0.87, 0.625 W)
29.3 What is the effective area of an isotropic radiator in terms of wavelength and a pyramidal horn antenna of aperture dimensions 2 cm × 3 cm?
(**Ans:** $\lambda^2/4\pi$, $4.8\ cm^2$)
29.4 Find the gain, beam width and effective area of a paraboloidal reflector antenna with reflector diameter 6 m and illumination efficiency 0.65. The operation frequency is 10 GHz
(**Ans:** 54.1 dB, 0.35°, 0.70°)
29.5 An antenna has a gain of 45 dB at a frequency of 4 GHz. Calculate the effective area.
(**Ans:** $12.6\ m^2$)

29.6 In a resonant slot antenna, $l/\lambda = 0.475$ and $l/a = 248.8$. determine the slot antenna impedance and slot dimensions.

(**Ans:** 563.7 ohms, $w = 0.00764\,\lambda$, $l = 0.475\,\lambda$)

29.7 A dipole receiving antenna is aligned so that its plane is normal to the direction of propagation of the wave. Determine the polarization loss factor if the line of the dipole makes an angle of 25° with the electric vector of the wave.

(**Ans:** 0.9063 b).

29.8 Repeat Prob. 29.7 with 10° angle.

(**Ans:** 0.9848)

29.9 A half-wave dipole antenna is operated at a frequency of 500 MHz. Find the effective area and the effective length.

(**Ans:** 468 cm², 19.1 cm)

29.10 A cylindrical dipole antenna of radius 0.3 cm and length 30 cm is operated at the resonant frequency of 500 MHz. Calculate the impedance at 500 MHz and 500 ± 5%.

(**Ans:** $73.46 + j41.28$ ohms, $85.26 + j74.45$ ohms, $63.03 + j8.61$ ohms)

29.11 Calculate the effective area of a rectangular aperture 2 cm × 3 cm.

(**Ans:** 4.86 cm²)

29.12 Calculate the gain in dB for a 3m diameter parabolic dish antenna with an aperture efficiency of 0.55 and an operating frequency of 4 GHz.

(**Ans:** 39.4 dB).

REFERNECE

1. Jull EV, (1970) Finite range gain of sectorial and pyramidal horns, *Electron. Lett.*, vol.6, pp 680-681.

2. Love AW (Ed.), (1976). Electromagnetic Horn Antenna, IEEE Press, USA.

3. Roddy D (1986). *Microwave Technology*, PH, NJ.

4. Rudge AW et al (1982). *The Handbook of Antenna Design*, Peter peregrinus, England.

5. Silver Samuel (Ed.) (1949). *Microwave Antenna Theory and Design*, MGH, NY.

Glossary

Radio waves: Radio waves consist of mutually perpendicular electric and magnetic fields.

Modulation: Modulation is the process of varying the amplitude, frequency or phase of the R.F. carrier wave.

Amplitude modulation: Amplitude modulation is the process of varying the amplitude of the R.F. wave in accordance with the instantaneous value of the message wave.

Frequency modulation: Frequency modulation is the process of varying the frequency of the R.F. wave in accordance with the instantaneous value of the message wave.

Bandwidth: Bandwidth is the range of frequency assigned to a transmitting station. It is usually 5 kHz on either side of the carrier frequency.

Antennas: Antennas are used to transmit and receive the radiated space waves.

Detection: Detection is the process of recovering the message signal from the RF waves.

Microwaves: Microwaves are electromagnetic (EM) waves with wavelengths ranging from 30 cm to 3 mm. The microwave (MW) frequency range is from 1 GHz (= 10^9 Hz) to 100 GHz (= 10^{11} Hz).

Lossy line: It is a transmission line with high values of resistance R.

Loss-less line: It is a transmission line with R = 0.

Attenuation constant: An electromagnetic wave travelling in the z-direction gets reduced or attenuated by a factor of e^{-az}, where a is known as attenuation constant.

Characteristic impedance: It is the ratio of the voltage to the current in an individual wave and is equal to the impedance of a finite length of a line when $Z_L = Z_o$.

Phase velocity: It is the product of wavelength λ and the corresponding frequency f.

Open-circuited: A transmission line is said to be open-circuited if the load at the load or receiving end is infinity.

Short-circuited: A transmission line is said to be short-circuited if the load at the load or receiving end is zero.

Travelling wave: It is the result of incident and reflected wave.

Transmission coefficients: R, L, G and C per unit length of the line.

Smith chart: It is a plot of normalized impedance or admittance or reflection coefficient in a unity circle. The magnitudes are directly read in the radial directions and phase in the angular directions. It is useful for the analysis.

Standing wave: These are due to the simultaneous presence of the incident and reflected waves travelling in opposite directions in a transmission line.

Standing wave ratio: It is the ratio of the maximum voltage or current to the minimum voltage or current on a standing wave pattern.

Matching: Cancellation of reactive component and transformation of real part of the impedance to R_o.

Narrow-band matching: Impedance matching over a narrow band of frequencies.

Broad-band matching: Impedance matching over a broad band of frequencies.

Stub matching: Matching the impedance with a short transmission line.

Tuning screws: Variable capacitance device used to tune or resonate with line impedance.

Waveguide: Metallic hallow tube in rectangular or cylindrical form to guide EM waves.

WG windows/irises/diaphragms: Thin metallic barriers placed perpendicular to the axis of the WG to neutralize the reactance.

Posts: Thin cylindrical posts extending fully across the narrow width of the WG.

Tapered line: A transmission line in which Z_o varies gradually and continuously.

Matched terminations: WG terminations that absorb incident power without any reflection

E-stub: WG short plunger placed across the wide dimensions of a rectangular WG. Offers series reactance.

H-stub: WG short plunger placed across the narrow dimensions of a rectangular WG. Offers shunt reactance.

E-H tuner: Combination of E and H stubs. Used to match wide range of impedances.

k_c: Cut-off wave number.

a_g: WG attenuation constant; defined as power loss over unit length/twice power transmitted through the WG.

Degenerative modes: Two or more modes having the same cut-off frequency.

Dominant mode: Mode with lowest cut-off frequency. Dominant mode in rectangular wave guide is TE_{10} mode. Dominant mode in circular wave guide is TE_{11} mode.

Z-parameters: Z-parameters are the impedances of two port networks measured with ports open-circuited.

Y-parameters: Y-parameters are the admittances of two port networks measured with ports short-circuited.

h-parameters: h-parameters are hybrid or mixed parameters of a two port network and correspond to voltage gain, current gain, impedance and admittance.

ABCD-parameters: ABCD-parameters are transmission line parameters.

Reciprocal network: A reciprocal network has symmetrical impedance and admittance matrices.

Scattering matrix: Scattering matrix represents the linear relationships between incident and reflected waves.

Γ_1: The reflection coefficient at port 1.

Γ_2: The reflection coefficient at port 2.

Coaxial cables: Coaxial cables are shielded two core cables used as MW transmission lines.

Connectors: Connectors are used to connect the coaxial lines and wave guides.

Adapters: Adapters are passive devices with different connectors at their ends.

WG flanges: WG flanges are used to connect two wave guides.

WG corners and bends: They are used to change the direction of propagation of EM waves.

WG twist: WG twist is used to change the polarization by $90°$.

Coupling loops and apertures: Coupling loops and apertures are used to couple EM waves in wave guides.

Attenuators: Attenuators absorb MW power and are used to control the power flow.

Phase shifter: Phase shifters are used to vary the phase of the travelling waves.

WG tees: WG tees are waveguides with three independent ports.

E-plane T: *E*-plane *T* is a three port device whose side arm axis is parallel *E*-field.

H-plane T: *H*-plane *T* is a three port device whose side arm axis is parallel *H*-field.

Magic T: Combination of E and *H* plane tees.

Duplexer: Duplexer couples the circuit to the same load.

E-H tuner: *E-H* tuner is a wide range impedance matching device in WG systems.

Impedance bridge: Impedance bridge is used to determine unknown impedance.

Balanced mixer: Balanced mixer is used to balance the local oscillator noise.

Balanced phase detector: Balanced phase detector is used to determine phase difference between two MW signals.

Coaxial line: Two-conductor MW transmission line, one inner and the other outer conductor. Dominant modes are **TEM** modes.

J_n: n^{th} order Bessel function.

Isolator: Isolates one MW component loading the other MW component.

Circulator: Multi-port device; power flows from *i*-th port to $(i + 1)$-th port.

Directional coupler: A 4-port WG junction; couples the MW power to a port in a secondary WG.

Directivity: Discriminating power of a directional coupler.

Center-hole coupler: A WG coupler with a hole at the central point of two rectangular wave-guides placed one over the other at an optimum angle θ.

Offset-hole coupler: A WG coupler with an offset aperture that couples MW power from one rectangular WG to the other placed one over the other with θ = 0.

Two-hole coupler: A WG coupler with two central apertures spaced λ/4 apart.

Binomial coupler: A WG coupler with flat response characteristic.

Tchebyshev coupler: A WG coupler with equi-ripple response characteristic.

Multi-section coupler: A coupler with wide bandwidth and directional characteristics.

Branch line coupler: A coupler with direct-coupled transmission line in which the main line directly couples the MW power to the secondary line by two shunt branches.

Hybrid ring coupler: When a wave is incident at port 1, half of it appears at port 2 and the other half at port 4. Port 1 and 3 are decoupled. Similarly, when a wave is incident at port 2, half of it appears at port 3 and the other half at port 1. Port 2 and 4 are decoupled.

Schwinger coupler: A coupler with the directivity is less dependent on the frequency

Long slot coupler: A coupler with a single long slot for MW power coupling.

Lange coupler: A coupler with several coupled lines; provides large coupling.

Capacitance loop coupler: A coupler with short loop.

Power divider: A device that splits the power into a number of smaller amounts.

Power combiner: A device that combines the power from a number of smaller amounts.

Cavity: Space enclosed by conducting walls.

Resonator: MW tuned circuit.

Re-entrant cavity: A resonant cavity with opposite sides brought closer together to form a re-entrant structure.

Cavity Q: A measure of selectivity of a cavity.

Loaded Q: Q of a cavity with external load.

Unloaded Q: Q of a cavity when not connected to any external load.

Critical coupling: Matching of resonator with the external load; $\beta_{el} = 1$; $Q_L = Q_o/2$.

Overcoupling: $\beta_{el} > 1$; $Q_L = Q_o/(1 + \beta_{el}) > Q_o$.

Undercoupling: $\beta_{el} < 1$; $Q_L = Q_o/(1 + \beta_{el}) < Q_o$.

Filter: A frequency selective circuit.

Low-pass filter (LPF): Transmits frequencies below the cut-off frequency w_c and highly attenuates the frequency above cut-off frequency.

High-pass filter (HPF): Transmits frequencies above the cut-off frequency w_c and highly attenuates the frequencies below cut-off frequency.

Band-pass filter (BPF): Transmits frequencies between low cut-off frequency w_1 and high cut-off frequency w_2 and highly attenuates the frequencies below the low cut-off frequency and above the high cut-off frequency.

Band-stop filter (BPF): Transmits frequencies below the low cut-off frequency w_1 and above the high cut-off frequency w_2 and highly attenuates the frequencies between low and high cut-off frequencies.

Insertion loss: Loss due to mismatch of impedances.

Frequency scaling: Achieved by multiplying inductances and capacitances of prototype low-pass filter elements by the cut-off frequency. Resistance value is not altered.

Impedance scaling: Achieved by multiplying inductances and resistances of prototype low-pass filter elements by the cut-off frequency and by dividing capacitances by the cut-off frequency.

Transit time: Time duration for an electron to reach anode from cathode.

Skin effect: H.F. current flows through the surface of the conductor with higher losses.

Velocity modulation: Variation in electron velocity.

Current modulation: Bunching of electrons causes variation in current density.

Drift space transit time: Time duration for an electron to travel the drift space.

Beam loading: Loading of the electron beam with excess energy.

Electronic efficiency: Ratio of MW output power to the input dc power.

Mutual conductance: Ratio of induced current to the input voltage.

Plasma frequency: Frequency at which the electrons oscillate in the beam.

Applegate diagram: Distance-time plot of the electron trajectories in the drift space..

TWT: Traveling wave tube, MW amplifier tube.

Slow wave structure: Non-resonant periodic structure to provide high *gain-bandwidth product*.

Helix: A slow wave structure in the form of helical coil.

Brillouin diagram: A graphical representation of variation of angular frequency with β in a helical slow wave structure

Electronic equation: Equation that determines the convection current induced by the axial electric field.

Circuit equation: Equation that gives the variation of axial electric field with spatial electron beam current.

Harmonic distortion: Distortion caused by the presence of harmonic frequencies due to non-linearity of TWT amplifier characteristics.

Phase delay distortion: Distortion caused by the phase delay between the input and output of a TWT amplifier.

Reflex klystron: Reflex klystron is a single cavity klystron that generates MW power.

Mode number: Mode number is the number at which energy transfer takes place and is given by $N = (n + 3/4)$ cycles.

Beam coupling coefficient: Beam coupling coefficient is the coupling coefficient between the electron beam and the resonator cavity.

Mode curves: Mode curves are the variations of output power with frequency.

Round trip transit time: Round trip transit time is the time taken by an electron to traverse the resonator cavity gap twice.

Electronic admittance: Electronic admittance is the admittance of the reflex Klystron equivalent circuit. It varies along a spiral with respect to variation in the repeller voltage.

Magnetron: Magnetron is a cross-field MW oscillator and generates power up to 40 kW.

Amplitron: Amplitron is a cross-field MW amplifier.

Carcinotron: Carcinotron is a cross-field MW oscillator.

Hull cut-off magnetic field: Hull cut-off magnetic field is the magnetic field that is just able to return the electrons back to the cathode.

π-mode: π-mode is the oscillator mode at which the phase difference between adjacent anode poles is π radians.

Strapping: Strapping is the method of separating the π-mode from other modes using two rings.

C-ring: C-ring is used to tune or vary the resonant frequency.

Hull cut-off voltage: For a given axial magnetic field B_o, the critical anode voltage that returns the electrons to the cathode.

Cyclotron frequency: Cyclotron frequency is the angular frequency of the circular motion of electrons.

Coaxial magnetron: Coaxial magnetron is the magnetron with an inner single high-Q cavity operating in TE_{011} mode.

Voltage tunable magnetron: Voltage tunable magnetron is a broad band magnetron oscillator whose frequency can be varied by varying the voltage between anode and sole.

Rieke diagram: Rieke diagram is the performance chart of a magnetron as a function of anode voltage or magnetic field.

Crystal diode: Crystal diode consists of a tungsten wire spring pressing on the surface of a suitably doped silicon wafer.

Schottky diode: Schottky diode is a barrier diode used for detection of MW signals.

PIN diode: PIN diode is a heavily doped p and n region separated by an undoped intrinsic region.

Digital phase shifter: Digital phase shifter shifts the phase of a MW by a finite phase angle.

PIN diode attenuator: PIN diode attenuator is an electronically controlled attenuator.

PIN diode modulator: PIN diode modulator is a 3-port device used to modulate microwaves.

PIN diode limiter: PIN diode limiter protects the MW subsystem when the voltage is excessive.

Gunn diode: Gunn diode is a transferred electron device that generates microwaves.

Gunn effect: Gunn effect is the periodic fluctuations of current in an n-type GaAs specimen above a critical voltage.

Transferred electron effect: Transferred electron effect is the negative resistance property exhibited by an n-type GaAs when all electrons are transferred to upper valley.

Transferred electron device: Transferred electron device is the device that use the transferred electron effect.

High-field domain: High-field domain is the domain near the cathode of an n-type GaAs where high electric field is formed when the applied voltage exceeds the threshold value.

Dipole domain: Dipole domain is the domain that separates the positive and negative charges by a small distance.

Transit time mode: Transit time mode is the mode in which the period of oscillation in a Gunn oscillator is equal to the transit time.

LSA mode: LSA mode is the mode in which the Gunn diode is incorporated as a part of the resonant circuit.

Bias circuit oscillation mode: Bias circuit oscillation mode is the mode in which oscillation occurs when the bulk diode is biased to threshold voltage.

Stable amplification mode: Stable amplification mode is the mode in which the amplification is stable.

InP diode: InP diode is a three level diode.

CdTe diode: CdTe diode is a Gunn diode using CdTe diode.

Avalanche multiplication: Avalanche multiplication is the rapid rate at which electron-hole pair are generated.

Avalanche region: Avalanche region is the thin p-region at which avalanche multiplication occurs.

Drift region: Drift region is the intrinsic region through which the generated holes drift or move to the p^+ region.

Read diode: Read diode is the first avalanche transit time diode invented by Read.

IMPATT diode: IMPATT diode is an impact avalanche transit time diode that exhibits differential negative resistance by impact ionization.

TRAPATT diode: TRAPATT diode is a trapped plasma avalanche triggered transit diode.

BARITT diode: BARITT diode is a barrier injection transit time diode .

Esaki diode: Esaki diode is the tunnel diode exhibiting a negative resistance characteristic named after the inventor Esaki.

Varactor diode: Varactor diode is an electronically variable reactance diode.

Parametric amplifier: Parametric amplifier is an amplifier that utilizes the variation of a device parameter for its operation.

Idler frequency: Idler frequency is the sum and difference frequency of the input signal frequency and the pump frequency.

Idler circuit: Idler circuit is the output circuit that does not require any excitation.

Up-converter: Up-converter is the parametric amplifier with the output frequency greater than signal frequency.

Down-converter: Down-converter is the parametric amplifier with the output frequency less than signal frequency.

Negative resistance parametric amplifier: Negative resistance parametric amplifier is a parametric amplifier that uses the varactor diode that provides the required negative resistance for proper operation.

Degenerative parametric amplifier: Degenerative parametric amplifier is a negative resistance parametric amplifier with output frequency equal to the signal frequency.

MW transistor: MW transistor is the transistor fabricated in the planar form using Si and *npn* configuration for operation at MW frequencies.

Internal tuning: Internal tuning is the matching of input and output impedances of MW transistor circuits to the transmission line impedance of 50 Ω.

MESFET: MESFET is the metal semiconductor field effect MW transistor.

HEMT: HEMT is high mobility electron MW transistor.

Hetrojunction: Hetro-junction is the junction formed at the interface of an AlGaAs doped alloy and an undoped GaAs layer.

MODFET: MODFET is also HEMT.

Noise factor: Noise factor is defined as the ratio of S/N power at the input to the S/N power at the output.

Noise figure: Noise figure is the noise factor expressed in dB.

Equivalent noise temperature: Equivalent noise temperature is the fictitious temperature that represents amplifier noise.

Terrestrial communication system: Terrestrial communication system is the line-of-sight MW communication system on earth.

Satellite communication system: Satellite communication system is the MW communication system that uses satellite as repeaters.

Passive repeaters: Passive repeaters are MW repeaters requiring no power supply.

Active repeaters: Active repeaters are MW repeaters that receive the MW signals, amplify them and transmit to the earth station at a different frequency.

Radio horizon: Radio horizon is the point

where the line-of-sight ray path grazes the earth's surface.

Contour map: Contour map is the profile of the terrain between the transmitter and receiver.

Super-refraction: Super-refraction is the bending of radio waves and reflecting them back to earth.

Subrefraction: Subrefraction is the bending of radio wave path away from the receiver.

Tropospheric propagation: Tropospheric propagation is the propagation of radio waves using highly directional high gain antenna.

Absorption fading: Absorption fading is the fading of signals due to absorption of energy by rain, cloud and fog.

Multipath fading: Multipath fading is the fading due to receipt of signals along multiple paths that may reduce or cancel the signal.

Frequency diversity system: Frequency diversity system is the transmission and reception of radio signals over the same path on two different frequencies.

Space diversity system: Space diversity system is that in which two antennas spaced vertically at a distance of 50λ are used to receive the transmitted signal and combine them to give the net signal.

Communication satellite: Communication satellite is a space craft placed in an orbit around the earth for communication purpose.

Geo-stationary satellite: Geo-stationary satellite is the satellite in geo-stationary orbit travelling in the same direction and completing one revolution in the same time as that of earth and appears to be stationary with respect to earth.

Uplink frequency: Up link frequency is the MW frequency used to transmit signals from earth station to the satellite.

Downlink frequency: Down link frequency is the MW frequency used to transmit signals from the satellite to earth station.

Transponder: Transponder is the stage between the reception of the up link signal and the transmission of the down link signal by the satellite.

Link losses: Link losses are the losses due to transmission path and attenuation and absorption loss.

EIRP: EIRP is the equivalent isotropic radiated power and is the product of transmitted power and the transmitter antenna gain.

Radar: Radar is radio detection and range. It is an echo sounding system to detect objects.

Primary radar: Primary radar is the radar that receives a part of the transmitted signal reflected back by the object.

Secondary radar: Secondary radar is the radar that transmits a signal towards the target and receives a coded signal for identification.

Radar range equation: Radar range equation gives the maximum range upto which the objects can be detected with the given set up.

Radar cross section: Radar cross section is the ratio of radiated power from the target to the incident power density on the target.

Duplexer: Duplexer is the unit used to couple transmitter or receiver to the radar antenna and to reduce the coupling between them.

Pulsed radar: Pulsed radar is a radar system that transmits pulses of short duration.

FMCW radar: FMCW radar is the radar system that transmits frequency modulated continuous signals.

Doppler effect: Doppler effect is the apparent shift in the received frequency when either the radiation source or the target is in motion.

Primary industrial processes: Primary industrial processes are cooking, baking, drying, tempering, curing etc.

Secondary industrial processes: Secondary industrial processes are casting, extruding, moulding etc.

Skin depth: Skin depth is the depth of penetration of microwaves at which the internal electric field reduces by a factor of $1/e$.

Diathermy: Diathermy is the use of MW heating effect to relieve pain and promote healing.

Hyperthermia: Hyperthermia is the MW heat treatment which assists to destroy cancerous cells.

Pulmonary edema: Pulmonary edema is the accumulation of fluid in the lung.

Applicator: Applicator is a special device used to launch MW energy into a patient.

Strip line: Strip line has a central thin conducting strip whose width is much greater than its thickness.

Launcher: Launcher is a thin flat small center conductor used to excite the strip lines.

Microstrip line: Microstrip line is a thin strip conductor in a dielectric substance above the ground plane.

Parallel strip lines: Parallel strip lines are two perfectly parallel strip lines separated by a perfect dielectric slab of uniform thickness.

Slot line: Slot line is a two conductor line separated in a single plane on the dielectric substrate.

Coplanar line: Coplanar line is a parallel thin three conductor line consisting of thin center strip and two thin ground strips on a dielectric substrate.

Shielded strip line: Shielded strip line has its conductors embedded in a dielectric medium with its top and bottom ground planes having no connection.

Discrete circuit: Discrete Electronic components are connected together by wires to form a discrete circuit.

Integrated circuit: Active and passive components and their interconnections are fabricated on a single silicon chip.

Monolithic microwave integrated circuit: A monolithic integrated circuit of MW components with low packaging density.

Small scale integration (SSI): An integrated circuit with less than 100 components on a single chip.

Medium scale integration (MSI): An integrated circuit with components between 100 and 1000 on a single chip.

Large scale integration (LSI): An integrated circuit with components between 1000 and 10000 on a single chip.

Very large scale integration (VLSI): An integrated circuit with components between 10^5 and 10^6 on a single chip.

Ultra large scale integration (ULSI): An integrated circuit with components greater than 1.5×10^6 on a single chip.

Diffusion: The process of diffusing impurities into a pure semiconductor material.

Ion implantation: The process of doping the semiconductor substrate with high-energy impurities.

Epitaxial growth: The process of growing a semiconductor layer on a single-crystal semiconductor substrate.

Lithography: The process of transforming patterns of masks onto a thin layer of photo-resist.

MMIC: Monolithic microwave integrated circuit.

HMIC: Hybrid microwave integrated circuit.

QMMIC: Quasi-monolithic microwave integrated circuit.

Tunable detector: Tunable detector is a diode detector arrangement with a tuning plunger to tune the detector for a range of frequencies.

Slotted line probe: Slotted line probe is a section of a WG or coaxial line with a longitudinal slot through which an electric field probe can be inserted.

E-probe: E-probe is a thin conducting wire that passes through a slot in the slotted line and couples to the electric field in the WG or coaxial line.

Spectrum analyzer: Spectrum analyzer is a broadband superheterodyne receiver that displays the plot of amplitude versus frequency of the applied signal or the frequency spectrum of the signal.

Network analyzer: Network analyzer is the instrument used for measurement of both amplitude and phase of a signal over a wide range of frequency within a reasonable time.

Bolometer sensor: Bolometer sensor is a power sensor used to measure MW power.

Baretters: Baretters are a short length fine platinum wire suitably encapsuled and are used to measure MW power.

Thermistors: Thermistors are small semiconductor beads placed on two wires and are used to measure MW power.

Thermocouples: Thermocouples are temperature sensitive devices that generate thermo-emf when their two ends are at different temperatures.

Standing wave: Standing wave is the result of reflected waves interacting with the incident waves.

Specific absorption rate: Specific absorption rate is defined as the power absorbed per unit mass of substance.

Hot spots: Hot spots are generated within the body due to microwave penetration.

Occupational hazards: Occupational hazards are hazards to personnel working in the vicinity of radiation field.

Ordnance hazard: Ordnance hazard is the hazard due to microwave radiation dangerous to ordnance such as weapon system and electronic warfare systems.

Electro-explosive hazard: Electro-explosive hazard is the hazard to electro-explosive devices.

Vaporizing fuel hazard: Vaporizing fuel hazard is the hazard to handling and loading of inflammable fuels.

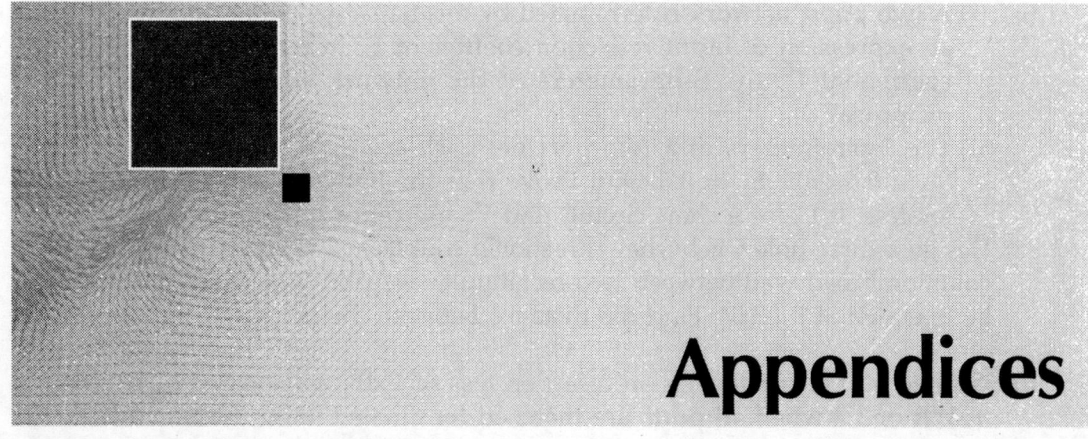

Appendices

APPENDIX I: UNIVERSITY QUESTION PAPERS

MICROWAVE ENGINEERING

Paper 1

Part A (10 × 2 = 20 marks)

1. State the properties of S-matrix of a two port lossless, reciprocal, perfectly matched network.
2. Find S-matrix of a length l of a lossless transmission line terminated by matched impedance.
3. How choke flange is designed?
4. What impedances are offered by a tuning screw on the broad wall of rectangular, waveguide when depth of penetration varies?
5. Explain why optimum rf power output from reflex klystron is more at higher magnitude of repeller voltage and lower mode.
6. Explain why TWTA has a broader bandwidth than two cavity klystron amplifier.
7. What are the differences between Transferred Electron Devices and Avalanche Transit-time Devices?
8. What are the advantages and disadvantages of parametric amplifiers?
9. Why reflex klystron is square wave 1 kHz pulse amplitude modulated while microwave measurements are done using VSWR meter?
10. What are the sources of error in return loss measurement using a w/g reflectometer and reflex klystron source?

Part B (5 × 16 = 80 marks)

11. (a) (i) Explain why Z or Y or $ABCD$ parameters are not preferred in microwave circuit analysis but S-parameters are used.
    (ii) With the help of a 3 port network, establish relationship between S and Z matrices.

Or

(b) (i) A two poprt network is terminated by mismatch generator and load. Derive an expression of input reflection coefficient Γ_1 in terms of load reflection coefficient Γ_2 and S-parameters of the network when it is lossless and reciprocal.

(ii) The S-parameters of a two-port network are $S_{11} = 0.2\angle0°$, $S_{22} = 0.1\angle0°$, $S_{12} = 0.6\angle90°$, $S_{21} = 0.6\angle90°$. Prove that the network is reciprocal but not lossless. If Γ_2 for a short circuit, find Γ_1 and return loss in dB.

12. (a) Design a three-hole Chebyshev directional coupler using centre apertures in the common broad wall between two rectangular w/g of dimensions 0.9″ × 0.4″ to be operated at 9 GHZ. Find the distance between the holes.

Or

(b) A three port circulator has an insertion loss of 1 dB, an isolation of 20 dB, and VSWR of 1.2 when all ports are matched terminated. Find the S matrix of the junction and the output power at ports 2 and 3 for an input power of 100 mW at port 1.

13. (a) A reflex klystron is operated at 5 GHz with dc beam voltage 1000 V, beam current 20 mA, repeller space L cm for $1^3/_4$ mode, cavity gap 2 mm, repeller voltage 500 V. Calculate optimum repeller space, rf power output, efficiency and the bandwidth over $\Delta V_R = 1$ V.

Or

(b) A cylinderical magnetron is operated at 5 GHz with cathode radius 3 cm, anode radius 5 cm, 16 resonant cavities, anode voltage 20 kV, dc magnetic flux density 0.05 T. Calculate cut-off voltage, cut-off magnetic flux density, Hartee voltage.

14. (a) (i) Explain using multivalley energy diagram, the I–V characteristics of Gunn diodes. Draw and explain electrical equivalent circuit. Explain LSA mode of operation.

(ii) A GaAs Gunn diode oscillator operates at 10 GHz with drift velocity of electrons 10^5 m/s. Determine the effective length of the active region. What is the required dc voltage for oscillation? Critical field is 3 µv/cm.

Or

(b) Explain the I–V characteristics of Tunnel diode and its electrical equivalent circuit. Obtain an expression of resonant frequency. With the help of a diagram explain operation and obtain power gain expression for a reflection amplifier. What are the advantages of tunnel diode?

15. (a) (i) Describe the operation of tunable probe detector used in slotted line with the help of a neat diagram. What are the possible sources of error in low VSWR measurements using slotted line?

(ii) A crystal detector generates a signal of 10 mV for an incident microwave power of –25 dBm. What is the detector sensitivity in mV/mW?

Or

(b) (i) Describe with neat diagram and mathematical formulation how dielectric constant of a solid material is determined/measured using rectangular waveguide as sample holder.

(ii) Explain how gain of an antenna is measured using three antenna method. What care should be taken for accuracy in measurements?

MICROWAVE ENGINEERING

Paper 2

Part A (10 × 2 = 20 marks)

1. Write down the scattering matrix of an ideal lossless transmission line of length l units.

2. Write down the transmission parameters of an ideal lossless transmission line of length l units.

3. Find the magnitudes of the scattering parameters for a reciprocal two-port microwave component having the VSWR as 1.4 and the insertion loss as 1 dB.

4. A waveguide load is used to absorb 2 W of average power. The reflected power is 3 mW. Find the magnitude of VSWR.

5. State any two differences between TWT and Klystron amplifier.

6. Draw the electrical equivalent of a cavity type magnetron.

7. Give any two differences between microwave transistors and transferred electron devices.

8. Draw the equivalent circuit of a PIN diode under reverse bias.

9. Compare a Barretter with a thermistor.

10. What are the minimum and maximum values of VSWR? Give the corresponding values of Reflection coefficients.

Part B (5 × 16 = 80 marks)

11. State and prove the properties of scattering matrix. (4 × 4 = 16)

12. (a) (i) In a 'two hole' directional coupler, prove that the power coming out in the coupled port is finite and that in the fourth port is zero. (6)

    (ii) Find the attenuation in decibels for an ideal rotary vane attenuator for vane rotation of $\theta = 0°$ and $60°$. (4)

    (iii) Deduce the formula used in the above subdivision (ii). (6)

Or

(b) Find the scattering matrix of an ideal, symmetrical, lossless magic T junction. (16)

13. (a) (i) Draw the schematic diagram of a two cavity klystron amplifier. (4)

    (ii) From the first principle, derive the expression for the power output and efficiency of the two cavity klystron amplifier. (12)

Or

(b) (i) Draw four types of slow wave structures used in TWT.

    (ii) For a travelling wave tube, $I_0 = 300$ mA, $V_0 = 5$ kV, and the impedance of the helix is 30 ohms. Find the length l of the helix that will give a gain of 60 dB at 9 GHz.

14. (a) (i) Using Ridley-Watkins-Hilsum theory, explain two valley model of GaAs. (8)

    (ii) Hence or otherwise show how negative resistance characteristics is obtained in a Gunn diode. (8)

Or

(b) Show how a PIN diode is used as
  (i) a switch (5)
  (ii) an attenuator (5)
  (iii) a phase shifter (6)

15. (a) (i) What are the three quantities to be measured to determine the impedance of a load at microwave frequencies. (6)

(ii) Draw the experimental set up to find the frequency of a microwave generator (without using the frequency meter) and mention the procedure. (10)

Or

(b) (i) Prove the relationship among guide wavelength, cutoff wavelength and free space wavelength of a rectangular waveguide. (6)

(ii) Draw the experimental set up to find the High VSWR and mention the procedure. (10)

MICROWAVE ENGINEERING

Paper 3

Part A (10 × 2 = 20 marks)

1. State the properties of Scattering Matrix.
2. Define a Reciprocal Network.
3. What should be the minimum radius of curvature for E plane bend and H plane bend? Validate your answer.
4. When can you say that a termination is matched to a system? Give the structure of any such termination and state the significance of that structure.
5. What are slow wave structures? Why and where are they used?
6. Can a Two Cavity Klystron Amplifier be used as an oscillator? If yes, how?
7. Define Gunn Effect.
8. What is the necessary condition for an IMPATT diode to produce oscillations?
9. For what measurements would you use a slotted line carriage? What should be the minimum length of the slot in it?
10. What are the measurements that can be performed using (a) Spectrum Analyser (b) Network Analyser?

Part B (5 × 16 = 80 marks)

11. Prove that it is not possible to construct a perfectly matched, lossless, reciprocal 3 port junction. (16)

12. (a) (i) Explain the working of a Faraday rotation isolator. (6)

(ii) Explain how power splitting occurs in (1) E plane tee (2) H plane tee (3) Magic tee.

Or

(b) (i) Define coupling factor and directivity of a directional coupler. Give the significance of these terms. (4)

(ii) Explain the coupling mechanism in a Bethe-hole directional coupler and two hole directional coupler. (12)

13. (a) (i) Describe the π mode of oscillations in a Magnetron. (6)

(ii) Derive the Hull cutoff voltage equation for a Magnetron. (10)

Or

(b) Derive the Manley-Rowe power relation. (16)

14. (a) With the help of energy band diagrams explain the working of a Tunnel diode.
(16)

Or

(b) With Mathematical substantiation explain the velocity modulation and bunching process in a reflex klystron. (16)

15. (a) (i) Discuss the classification of Bolometers. (4)

(ii) Explain the frequency measurement technique using (1) slotted line (2) resonant cavities. (6)

(iii) Explain the double minima method of VSWR measurement. (6)

Or

(b) Explain the waveguide method for measuring the dielectric constant of a dielectric sample. (16)

APPENDIX II

Classification of Microwave Solid State Devices

Category	Devices	Applications
MW diodes	Crystal and Schottsky diodes	Mixers and detectors
	PIN diodes	Switches, phase shifters, attenuators, modulators and limiters
	Varactor diodes	Frequency multipliers and parametric amplifiers
	Tunnel diodes	Amplifiers, oscillators and tuners
Avalanche transit time devices (ATTD)	READ diodes	Oscillators
	IMPATT diodes	Amplifiers and oscillators
	TRAPATT diodes	Oscillators
	BARITT diodes	Oscillators
Transferred electron devices (TED)	Gunn diode	Amplifiers and oscillators
	LSA diode	Oscillators
	InP diode	Oscillators
	CdTe diode	Oscillators
MW transistors	BJT, HEMT, MESFET	Amplifiers and oscillators

APPENDIX III

Applications of MW Solid State Devices

Device	Applications	Advantages
Transistors	Communications, Telemetry and Radar Systems	Low cost, low power supply, light weight, high CW power output, reliable
TED	Wideband amplifiers and Radar Systems	Low cost, low power supply, light weight, reliable, low noise, high gain
IMPATT	Millimeter wave communication system	Low cost, low power supply, light weight, reliable, high CW power output
TRAPATT	Radar Systems	Low cost, low power supply, reliable, high peak and average power
BARITT	Communications and Radar Systems.	Low cost, low power supply, reliable, low noise

APPENDIX IV

Standard Multiples and Submultiples

Prefix	Symbol	Factor
Exa	E	10^{18}
Peta	P	10^{15}
Tera	T	10^{12}
Giga	G	10^{9}
Mega	M	10^{6}
kilo	K, k	10^{3}
hecto	h	10^{2}
deka	da	10
deci	d	10^{-1}
centi	c	10^{-2}
milli	m	10^{-3}
micro	μ	10^{-6}
nano	n	10^{-9}
pico	p	10^{-12}
femto	f	10^{-15}
atto	a	10^{-18}

APPENDIX V

Greek Letters

A α	B β	G γ	D δ	E ϵ	Z ζ	H η	Θ θ	I ι	K κ	Λ λ	M μ
Alpha	Beta	Gamma	Delta	Epsilon	Zeta	Eta	Theta	Iota	Kappa	Lambda	Mu
N ν	Ξ ξ	O o	Π π	P ρ	Σ σ	T τ	U υ	Φ ϕ	X χ	Ψ ψ	Ω ω
Nu	Xi	Omicron	pi	Rho	Sigma	Tau	Upsilon	Phi	Chi	Psi	Omega

APPENDIX VI

Physical Constants

Charge of an electron $e = 1.602 \times 10^{-19}$ C

Mass of an electron $m = 9.107 \times 10^{-31}$ kg

Charge to mass ratio $e/m = 1.759 \times 10^{-11}$ C/kg

Electron Volt eV $= 1.60 \times 10^{-19}$ J

Boltzmann constant $k = 1.380 \times 10^{-23}$ J/°K

Plank's constant $h = 6.547 \times 10^{-34}$ J-s

1 Ångström = Å $= 10^{-10}$ m

1 micron = 1 μm $= 10^{-6}$ m

APPENDIX VII

Properties of Free Space

Velocity of light
$c = 2.998 \times 10^{8}$ m/s $\approx 3 \times 10^{8}$ m/s

Permittivity of vacuum
$\epsilon_o = 10^{-9}/36\pi = 8.854 \times 10^{-12}$ F/m

Conductivity of free space
$\sigma_o = 10^{-14}$ mho/m

Permeability of free space
$\mu_o = 4\pi \times 10^{-7}$ H/m

Impedance of free space
$Z_o = 120\pi = 376.7$ ohms

APPENDIX VIII

Pascal's Triangle

n	Binomial coefficients	Sum of coef. $= 2^n$
2	1 2 1	4
3	1 3 3 1	8
4	1 4 6 4 1	16
5	1 5 10 10 5 1	32
6	1 6 15 20 15 6 1	64
7	1 7 21 35 35 21 7 1	128
8	1 8 28 56 70 56 28 8 1	256
9	1 9 36 84 126 126 84 36 9 1	512
10	1 10 45 120 210 252 210 120 45 10 1	1024
11	1 11 55 165 330 462 462 330 165 55 11 1	2048
12	1 12 66 220 495 792 924 792 495 220 66 12 1	4056

APPENDIX IX

Characteristics of Single Stage Solid State MW Amplifiers

Device	Gain (dB)	Center Frequency (GHz)	Noise Figure dB
BJT	4–10	1–10	2–6
FET	3–30	10–28	2–5
Tunnel diode	5–15	4–15	5
TED	7–10	5–35	15
IMPATT diode	5–10	6–10	20

APPENDIX X

Electromagnetic Frequency Spectrum

Class	Frequency Range	Wave length
Sonic or audio	20 Hz–20 KHz	15×10^6 m–15×10^3 m
Voice	300 Hz–3500 Hz	1×10^6 m–8.57×10^3 m
Ultrasonic	Above 40 KHz	$< 7.5 \times 10^3$ m
RADIO WAVES		
AM Bands;		
Medium Wave	550 KHz–1650 KHz	5.46×10^2 m–1.88×10^2 m
Short wave-1	2 MHz–8 MHz	150 m–37.5 m
Short wave-2	8 MHz–30 MHz	37.5 m–10 m
FM Band	88 MHz–110 MHz	3.41 m–2.73 m
Infra-red	75 GHz–300 GHz	400 μm–1 μm
Optical (visible)	300 THz–750 THz	1 μm–0.4 μm
Ultra-violet	750 THz–2500 THz	4000 Å–1 Å
X-rays	2500 THz–3×10^6 THz	120 Å–1 Å
Gamma rays	3×10^6–3×10^8 THz	1 Å–0.01 Å
	3×10^8–3×10^{-12} THz	10^{-2}–10^{-6} Å

APPENDIX XI

Visible Spectrum

Colour	Wave length	Frequency
Red	0.71 microns	423 THz
Orange	0.62 microns	483 THz
Yellow	0.57 microns	525 THz
Green	0.52 microns	576 THz
Blue	0.47 microns	639 THz
Indigo	0.44 microns	682 THz
Violet	0.41 microns	732 THz

APPENDIX XII

Television Channels

Band	Frequency range (MHz)	No. of channels (7 MHz width)
I	41–68	1 to 4 (VHF)
II	88–108	FM Radio (VHF)
III	174–230	5 to 12 (VHF)
IV	470–582	13 to 28 (VHF)
V	609–790	Not used in India

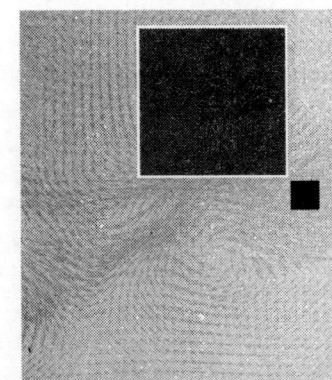

Index

READER'S NOTES

READER'S NOTES